User's guide to the book

This book features the following didactical elements for easy reference and quick access to structures looked for.

– Each chapter has its own **color-code**.

– The **menu bar** located at the top of each double-page spread shows the user's present position. The sub-chapter is shown in boldface type.

– The **subject of each page** is shown in italics.

– Many figures feature a **compass rose**, whose numbers correspond to the figures of adjacent regions, so that the sequence of a structure can easily be followed over several pages.

– Small **supplement drawings** located next to complex views show visual angles and intersecting planes.

– **The colored dots placed** at the end of leader lines on topographic illustrations assist in quickly locating arteries, veins, muscles and nerves.

– Many figures are **cross-referenced**.

– Enclosed is a **separate booklet with tables** pertaining to muscles, joints and nerves, which can easily be taken along or used for quick reference. The relevant table can be placed next to a selected illustration for direct comparison.

– **Cross-references between figures and tables** enable swift correlation of illustrations and table texts.

– **A list of abbreviations, terms for anatomical directions and positions, as well as explanatory notes on information in parentheses** can be found at the end of the book.

Perfect orientation – the new Navigation System

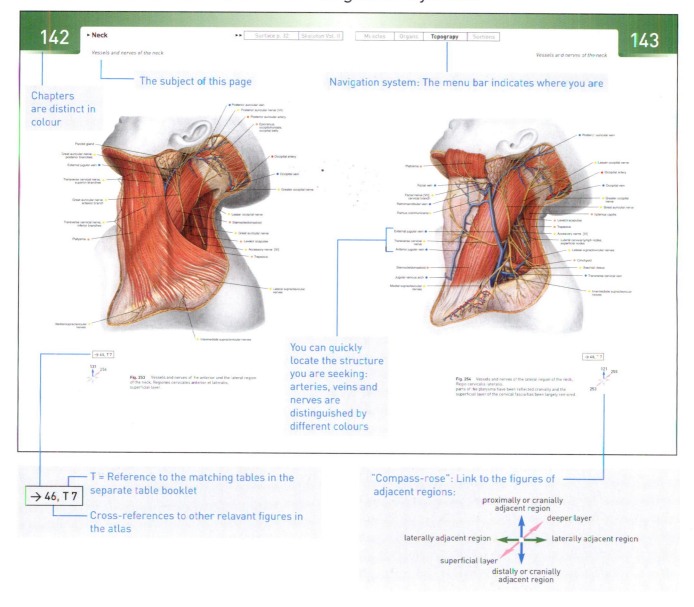

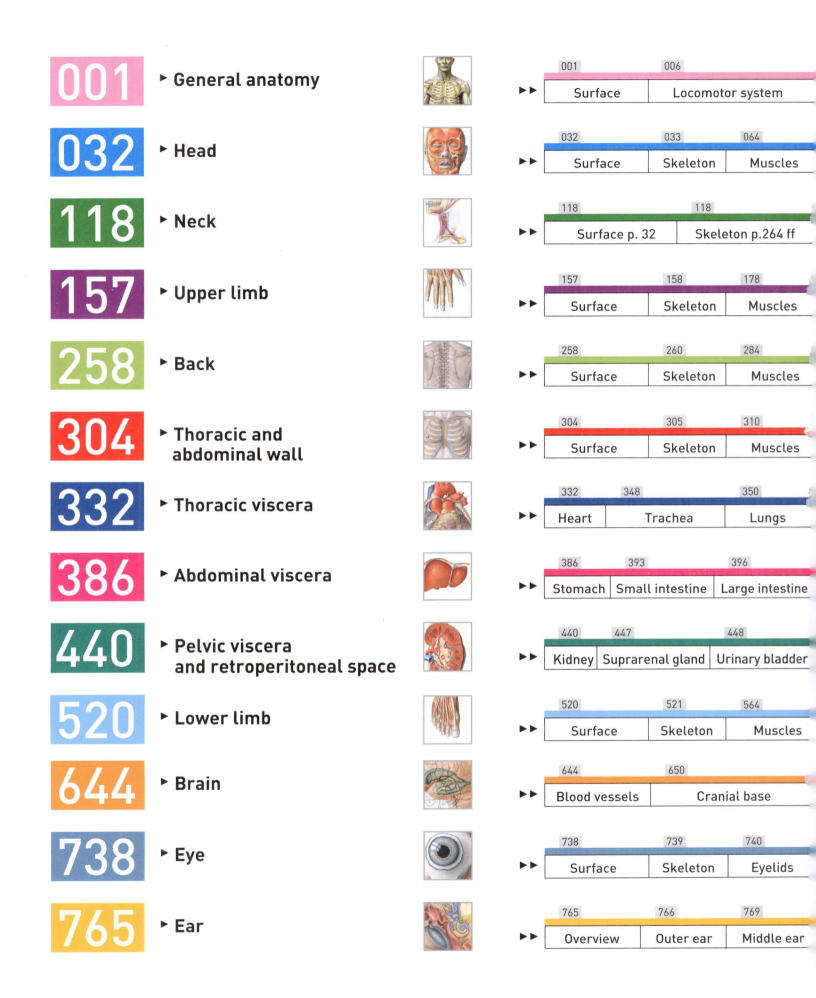

Overview

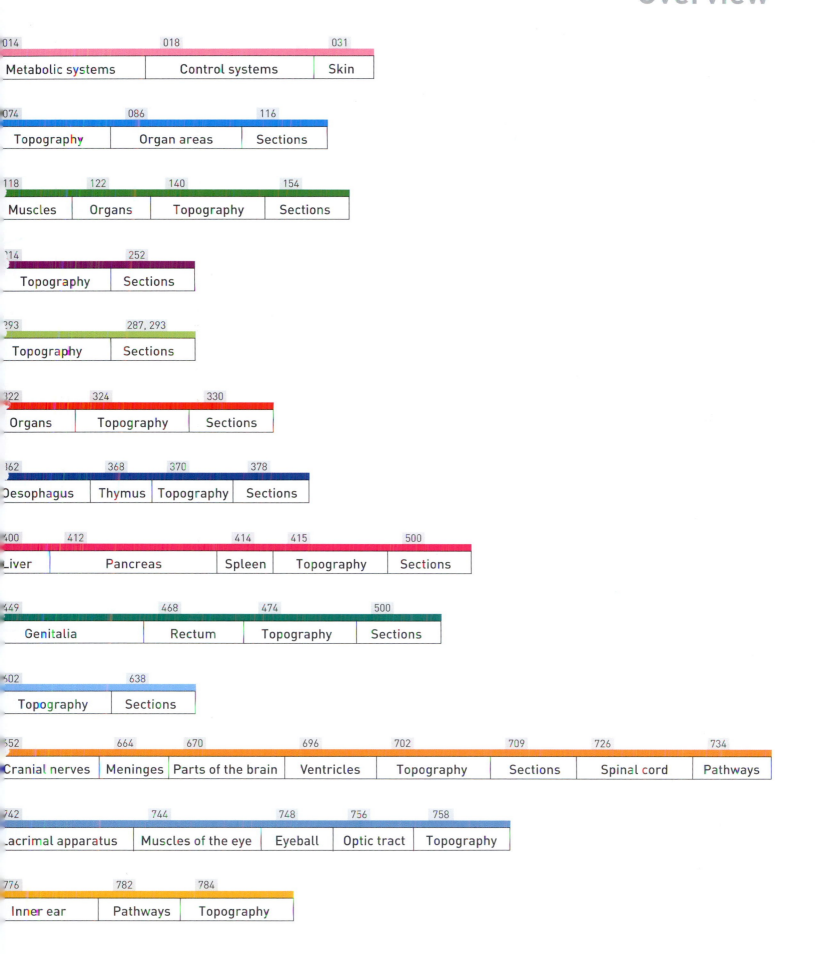

014	018	031
Metabolic systems	Control systems	Skin

074	086	116
Topography	Organ areas	Sections

118	122	140	154
Muscles	Organs	Topography	Sections

214	252
Topography	Sections

293	287, 293
Topography	Sections

322	324	330
Organs	Topography	Sections

362	368	370	378
Oesophagus	Thymus	Topography	Sections

400	412	414	415	500
Liver	Pancreas	Spleen	Topography	Sections

449	468	474	500
Genitalia	Rectum	Topography	Sections

602	638
Topography	Sections

652	664	670	696	702	709	726	734
Cranial nerves	Meninges	Parts of the brain	Ventricles	Topography	Sections	Spinal cord	Pathways

742	744	748	756	758
Lacrimal apparatus	Muscles of the eye	Eyeball	Optic tract	Topography

776	782	784
Inner ear	Pathways	Topography

Sobotta

Atlas of Human Anatomy
One Volume Edition

Edited by R. Putz and R. Pabst
In collaboration with Renate Putz

Head, Neck, Upper Limb, Thorax, Abdomen, Pelvis, Lower Limb

14th edition, newly edited
1431 colour plates with 1984 figures
Booklet (tables of muscles, joints and nerves)

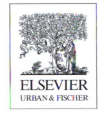

ELSEVIER
URBAN & FISCHER

URBAN & FISCHER
München · Jena

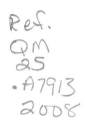
Correspondence and feedback should be addressed to:
Elsevier GmbH, Urban & Fischer Verlag, Department for Medical Student Information, Dr. Helmar Weiß, Karlstraße 45, 80333 Munich, Germany
e-mail: medizinstudium@elsevier.de

Addresses of the editors:

Professor Dr. med. Reinhard Putz
Vizepräsident der
Ludwig Maximilians-Universität
Geschwister-Scholl-Platz 1
80539 München
Germany
e-mail: putz@lmu.de

Professor Dr. med. Reinhard Pabst
Leiter der Abteilung
Funktionelle und Angewandte Anatomie
Medizinische Hochschule Hannover
Carl-Neuberg-Straße 1
30625 Hannover
Germany
e-mail: pabst.reinhard@mh-hannover.de

Bibliographic information published by Die Deutsche Bibliothek

Die Deutsche Bibliothek lists this publication in the Deutsche National-bibliografie; detailed bibliographic data is available in the Internet at http://dnb.ddb.de.

The contents of this edition are identical with the 22nd in two volumes. The order of the chapters has been changed.

Editorial staff at Elsevier: Dr. med. Dorothea Hennessen
                                Alexander Gattnarzik
                                Dr. Andrea Beilmann
                                Alexandra Frntic
Editorial staff and translation: Ulrike Kriegel, buchundmehr, Munich
Illustrators: Ulrike Brugger, Munich; Rüdiger Himmelhan, Heidelberg; Horst Ruß, Munich; Henriette Rintelen, Velbert
Book production: Renate Hausdorf, buchundmehr, Munich
Composed by: Mitterweger&Partner, Plankstadt
Printed and bound by: MKT Print Ljubljana
Cover design: Carsten Tschirner, Munich
Printed on Nopacoat 115 g

Printed in Slovenija
ISBN-13: 978-0-7020-3323-0

This atlas was founded by Johannes Sobotta†, former Professor of Anatomy and Director of the Anatomical Institute of the University of Bonn, Germany.

German Editions:
1st Edition: 1904–1907 J. F. Lehmanns Verlag, Munich
2nd–11th Edition: 1913–1944 J. F. Lehmanns Verlag, Munich
12th–20th Edition: 1948–1993 Urban & Schwarzenberg, Munich
13th Edition: 1953, editor H. Becher
14th Edition: 1956, editor H. Becher
15th Edition: 1957, editor H. Becher
16th Edition: 1967, editor H. Becher
17th Edition: 1972, editors H. Ferner and J. Staubesand
18th Edition: 1982, editors H. Ferner and J. Staubesand
19th Edition: 1988, editor J. Staubesand
20th Edition: 1993, editors R. Putz and R. Pabst
21st Edition: 2000, editors R. Putz and R. Pabst, Urban & Fischer Verlag, Munich
22nd Edition: 2006, editors R. Putz and R. Pabst, Elsevier GmbH, Munich

Foreign Editions:
Arabic Edition
Modern Technical Center, Damascus
Chinese Edition (complex characters)
Ho-Chi Book Publishing Co, Taiwan
Chinese Edition (simplified Chinese edition)
Elsevier, Health Sciences Asia, Singapore
Croatian Edition
Naklada Slap, Jastrebarsko
Dutch Edition
Bohn Stafleu van Loghum, Houten
English Edition (with nomenclature in English)
Atlas of Human Anatomy
Lippincott Williams & Wilkins
English Edition (with nomenclature in Latin)
Atlas of Human Anatomy
Elsevier GmbH, Urban & Fischer
French Edition
Atlas d'Anatomie Humaine
Tec & Doc Lavoisier, Paris
Greek Edition (with nomenclature in Greek)
Maria G. Parissianos, Athens
Greek Edition (with nomenclature in Latin)
Maria G. Parissianos, Athens
Hungarian Edition
az ember anatómiájának atlasza
Alliter Kiadái, Budapest
Indonesian Edition
Atlas Anatomi Manusia
Penerbit Buku Kedokteran EGC, Jakarta
Italian Edition
Atlante di Anatomia Umana
UTET, Torino
Japanese Edition
Igaku Shoin Ltd., Tokyo
Korean Edition
ShingHeung MedScience, Seoul
Polish Edition
Atlas anatomii cztowieka
Urban & Partner, Wroclaw
Portuguese Edition (with nomenclature in English)
Atlas de Anatomia Humana
Editora Guanabara Koogan, Rio de Janeiro
Portuguese Edition (with nomenclature in Latin)
Atlas de Anatomia Humana
Editora Guanabara Koogan, Rio de Janeiro
Spanish Edition
Atlas de Anatomia Humana
Editorial Medica Panamericana, Buenos Aires/Madrid
Turkish Edition
Insan Anatomisi Atlasi
Beta Basim Yayim Dagitim, Istanbul

Current information by www.elsevier.com and www.elsevier.de

Contents

Preface

It was just over a hundred years ago that Johannes Sobotta set out to publish the first edition of his Atlas of Human Anatomy. Since then, this piece of work has evolved step by step as a result of the constant interaction between students, lecturers and editors. It has not only been the most modern basis for the complex subject of macroscopic anatomy throughout many generations of doctors, but has also developed into a lasting work of reference for both clinical training and advanced medical education. All in all, it has become a book for a medical doctor's life. Once again, in this new edition the additional figures have been drawn strictly on the basis of original specimens.

The 14th edition has been particularly designed to meet the demands of a reformed medical curriculum, emphasizing the integration of clinical medicine into the preclinical curriculum. For this purpose, the new edition has been extended to include the following features:
- Surface anatomy including projection of internal organs (45 colour photos)
- Anatomical diagrams next to imaging figures
- Integration of imaging techniques to a greater extent (ultrasound, X-ray, CT, MRI; 119 figures)
- Endoscopic, intraoperative colour images and figures exemplifying techniques of puncture and examination (54 figures)
- Images of patients presenting with typical palsies
- Diagrams of the most important arterial variations (93 figures)
- Frequent variations in the location of internal organs (24 figures)
- Integration of histology at low magnification of important internal organs (intestine, liver, kidney, etc.)

In order to improve the presentation of the knowledge, the following features have been introduced:
- Clear-cut arrangement of the chapters according to the different regions of the body
- Thematically corresponding figures presented on double pages
- A concise, separate booklet contains tables of muscles, joints and nerves, enabling the reader to place it next to any figure in the atlas

One particular aim of the new edition is to facilitate finding of specific structures. The SOBOTTA depicts anatomical structures precisely without the reader loosing the greater picture. Therefore, specific didactic tools have been improved and new aspects included:
- Each chapter has been allocated to a particular colour
- A "menu bar" on each double page ensures precise orientation within a given chapter
- The number of outlines depicting spatial orientation has been significantly increased (270 figures)
- Overviews of total body regions ensure general orientation

- New diagrams of particular muscles clarify their location and course (24 figures)
- Confusion is kept to a minimum by only depicting limbs of the right side of the body
- "Compass roses" point to adjacent figures, thus facilitating following a given structure over several pages
- Continuous leader lines facilitate finding of structures
- Coloured dots at the end of leader lines in topographic diagrams mark arteries, veins, nerves, and muscles
- The figures in the booklet relate directly to the figures in the atlas
- The larger dimensions of the book improve clarity

With the exception of discussions about the general concept of the atlas and mutual correction, the editors have worked separately on individual chapters, with the work divided as follows:
R. Putz: General anatomy, upper limb, brain, eye, ear, back, lower limb;
R. Pabst: Head, neck, thoracic and abdominal walls, thoracic, abdominal and pelvic viscera.

The inclusion of a large number of new figures is the result of the extraordinary capability of the following medical illustrators: Ulrike Brugger, Rüdiger Himmelhan and Horst Ruß. It is to their credit that the classic "SOBOTTA style" has been retained. Several of the diagrams have been generated on the computer by Henriette Rintelen. We also gratefully acknowledge our clinical colleagues for making clinical illustrations available to us (see picture credits). We owe a debt of gratitude to our colleagues from the institutes for their understanding and helpful suggestions. Dr. N. Sokolov and A. Buchhorn have put meticulous efforts into generating the specimen preparations. S. Fryk and G. Hoppmann have supported us in text processing.

The staff of the editorial office of Elsevier publishers, in particular Dr. D. Hennessen and A. Gattnarzik, has our sincere thanks. Some of the creative development of the work is a result of very fruitful discussions. We would also like to thank R. Hausdorf for tremendous efforts in the production of the atlas. R. Putz together with G. Meier were responsible for the proofreading and simplification of page design and legends. Our special thanks go to Dr. U. Osterkamp-Baust for generating the index, and all others involved in the corrections. With our joint efforts, the SOBOTTA has been once more modernized both in contents and design.

We have included many of the helpful suggestions made over the years by students and colleagues, and would therefore ask all readers of this edition to pass on to us any criticism or suggestions on the new format of this atlas.

Munich and Hannover, September 2005
R. Putz and R. Pabst

Univ.-Prof. Dr. med. Reinhard Putz

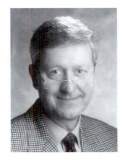

Born in Innsbruck/Austria

1962–1968	Studied medicine at the Leopold-Franzens-University of Innsbruck
1968	Received a doctorate
1968–1982	University assistant at the Institute of Anatomy at the University of Innsbruck
1978	Lecturer in anatomy
1979	Consultant for anatomy
1982–1989	Chair of the Anatomical Institute at the Albert-Ludwigs-University of Freiburg
since 1989	Chair of the Anatomical Institute at the Ludwig-Maximilians-University of Munich
1992–1994	President of the European Association of Clinical Anatomists
1993	Registration to practise medicine
1998–1999	Chairman of the Anatomical Society
1999	Member of the Akademie der Naturforscher und Ärzte (Leopoldina)
2002	Dr. h.c. of the University of Constanta, Romania
2003	Prorector I of the Ludwig-Maximilians-University of Munich

Research and fields of interest

- Functional anatomy of the passive locomotor system
- Evolution and functional anatomy of the vertebral column
- Form-function-relations of joints
- Applied anatomy (anatomical basics of orthopaedics, surgery, radiology)
- Questions about the contents and organisation of the medical curriculum
- Development of didactic training programmes at universities

Univ.-Prof. Dr. med. Reinhard Pabst

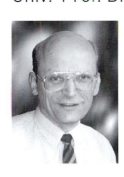

Born in Posen, grown up in Lüneburg

1965–1970	Studied medicine at the Hannover Medical School, and in Glasgow/Scotland
1970	University degree and doctorate
1971	Registration to practise medicine
1971–76	Scientific associate in the Department of Clinical Physiology, University of Ulm
1976	Lecturer for Clinical Physiology, University of Ulm, and new lectureship at the Hannover Medical School
1976–80	Senior assistant in the Department of Functional and Applied Anatomy, Hannover Medical School
1978	Extension of the Venia legendi to include anatomy
1980–1992	Head of the Department of Topographic Anatomy and Biomechanics
since 1992	Head of the Department of Functional and Applied Anatomy, Hannover Medical School
1986–1990	Prorector for studies and education, Hannover Medical School
1993–1997	Dean of the Hannover Medical School
1997–1998	Chairman of the Anatomical Society
1999–2003	Prorector of Research of the Hannover Medical School
2001	Member of the Akademie der Naturforscher und Ärzte (Leopoldina)

Research and fields of interest

- Functional anatomy of lymphatic organs
- Proliferation and migration of lymphocytes
- Development of the intestinal immune system
- Function of the pulmonary immune system
- Questions of a clinically orientated anatomy in the medical curriculum
- Evaluation of teaching

Picture credits

The editors sincerely thank all clinical colleagues that made ultrasound, computed tomographic and magnetic resonance images as well as endoscopic and intraoperative pictures available:

Prof. Altaras, Centre for Radiology, University of Gießen (Fig. 741, 763, 764)

Dr. Baumeister, Department of Radiology, University of Freiburg (Fig. 889)

PD Dr. Burgkardt, Orthopaedic Clinic, Technical University of Munich (Fig. 1163)

Prof. Brückmann & Dr. Linn, Neuroradiology, Institute for Diagnostic Radiology, University of Munich (Fig. 1367, 1431 a, b, 1432 a, b)

Prof. Daniel, Department of Cardiology, University of Erlangen (Fig. 631, 632, 633, 705)

Prof. Degenhardt, Bielefeld (Fig. 865, 867)

Prof. Galanski & Dr. Kirchhoff, Department of Diagnostic Radiology, Hannover Medical School (Fig. 944, 945, 994, 996)

Prof. Galanski & Dr. Schäfer, Department of Diagnostic Radiology, Hannover Medical School (Fig. 603 a, b, 659, 703, 723, 926, 936, 939, 941)

Prof. Gebel, Department of Gastroenterology, Hepatology and Endocrinology, Hannover Medical School (Fig. 242, 749, 758, 759, 770, 771, 806, 824)

Dr. Goei, Radiology, Heerlen, The Netherlands (Fig. 882, 883) (with permission from Radiology 173; 137–141: 1989)

Dr. Greeven, St.-Elizabeth-Hospital, Neuwied (Fig. 150, 970)

Prof. Hoffmann & PD Dr. Bektas, Clinic for Abdominal and Transplantation Surgery, Hannover Medical School (Fig. 772, 960)

Prof. Hohlfeld, Clinic for Pneumology, Hannover Medical School (Fig. 661, 662)

Prof. Jonas, Urology, Hannover Medical School (Fig. 834 a, b, 835)

Prof. Kampik & Prof. Müller, Ophthalmology, University of Munich (Fig. 1362)

Dr. Kirchhoff & Dr. Weidemann, Department of Diagnostic Radiology, Hannover Medical School (Fig. 773, 825, 834, 928, 930, 932, 934, 937)

Prof. Kremers, Department for Restorative Dentistry and Periodontology, University of Munich (Fig. 169)

Prof. Kunze, von Haunersches Children's Hospital, University of Munich (Fig. 327–330)

Dr. Meyer, Department of Gastroenterology, Hepatology and Endocrinology, Hannover Medical School (Fig. 676, 719 a, b, 724, 877, 878)

Prof. Müller-Vahl, Neurology, Hannover Medical School (Fig. 128 a, b)

Prof. Pfeifer, Radiology, Institute for Diagnostic Radiology, University of Munich (Fig. 293, 294, 310, 312, 449, 451, 501–504, 539–542, 987, 1018, 1019, 1049, 1050)

PD Dr. Rau, Department of Radiology, University of Freiburg (Fig. 644, 657, 658)

Prof. Ravelli †, formerly Institute of Anatomy, University of Innsbruck (Fig. 499)

PD Dr. Rieger, Radiology, Institute for Diagnostic Radiology, University of Munich (Fig. 1127)

Prof. Reich, Orofacial Surgery, University of Bonn (Fig. 113 a, b)

Prof. Reiser & Dr. Wagner, Institute for Diagnostic Radiology, University of Munich (Fig. 436, 449, 451, 453, 524, 1276, 1277, 1278, 1281, 1282)

Prof. Rudzki-Janson, Department of Orthodontics, University of Munich (Fig. 72, 73)

Dr. Scheibe, Department of Surgery, Rosman Hospital, Breisach (Fig. 1011 a–c)

Prof. Scheumann, Clinic for Abdominal and Transplantation Surgery, Hannover Medical School (Fig. 243, 244, 245)

Prof. Schillinger, Department of Gynaecology, University of Freiburg (Fig. 866)

Prof. Schliephake, Orofacial Surgery, Göttingen (Fig. 152, 196, 197)

Prof. Schlösser, Centre for Gynaecology, Hannover Medical School (Fig. 864 a, b, 872, 873, 910)

Prof. Schumacher, Neuroradiology, Department of Radiology, University of Freiburg (Fig. 1166 a, b)

Dr. Sommer & PD Dr. Bauer, Radiologists, Munich (Fig. 1022–1024, 1367)

Prof. Stotz, Paediatrics, University of Munich (Fig. 971, 972)

PD Dr. Vogl, Radiology, University of Munich (Fig. 436, 453, 1349, 1350)

Prof. Vollrath, Ear-Nose-Throat Department, Mönchengladbach (Fig. 229, 230, 231)

Prof. Wagner †, Diagnostic Radiology II, Hannover Medical School (Fig. 684, 796, 797, 801, 804, 884)

Prof. Wenz, formerly Department of Radiology, University of Freiburg (Fig. 500)

Prof. Witt, Department of Neurosurgery, University of Munich (Fig. 405)

Dr. Willführ, formerly Clinic for Abdominal and Transplantation Surgery, Hannover Medical School (Fig. 783)

PD Dr. Wimmer, Department of Radiology, University of Freiburg (Fig. 531)

Additional illustrations were obtained from the following textbooks:

Benninghoff-Drenckhahn: Anatomie, Band 1 (Drenckhahn D., Hrsg.), 16. Aufl., Urban & Fischer, München 2003 (Fig. 555, 556, 580, 581, 582)

Welsch, U.: Lehrbuch Histologie, Urban & Fischer, München 2003 (Fig. 654, 752, 829, 854, 855)

Welsch, U. (Hrsg.): Sobotta, Atlas Histologie, 6. Aufl., Urban & Fischer, München 2002 (Fig. 857 a, b, 869, 917)

Wicke, L.: Atlas der Röntgenanatomie, 3. Aufl., Urban & Schwarzenberg, München–Wien–Baltimore 1985 (Fig. 675 a, b)

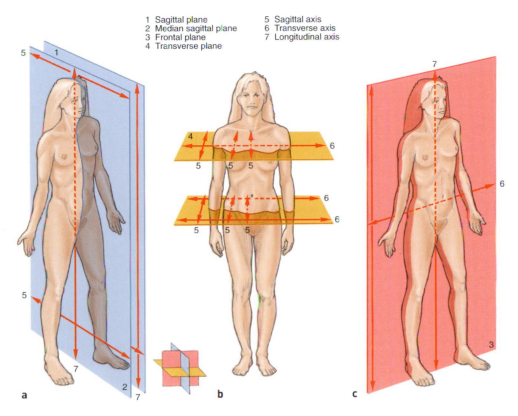

1 Sagittal plane
2 Median sagittal plane
3 Frontal plane
4 Transverse plane
5 Sagittal axis
6 Transverse axis
7 Longitudinal axis

Fig. 1 a–c Planes and axes.
a Sagittal plane, sagittal and longitudinal axes
b Transverse plane (= horizontal plane), transverse and sagittal axes
c Frontal plane (= coronal plane), longitudinal and transverse axes

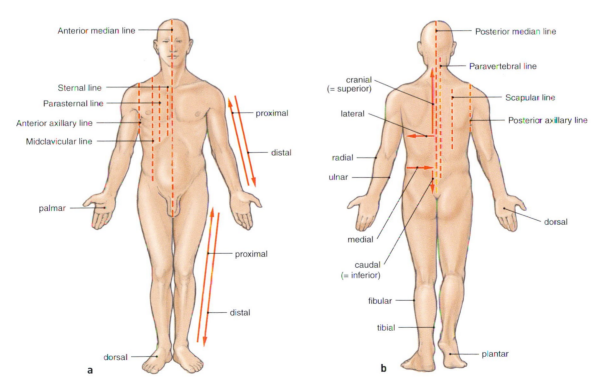

Fig. 2 a, b Orientation lines of the human body and terms of direction and position.
a Ventral view (ventralis, anterior)
b Dorsal view (dorsalis, posterior)

Parts of the human body

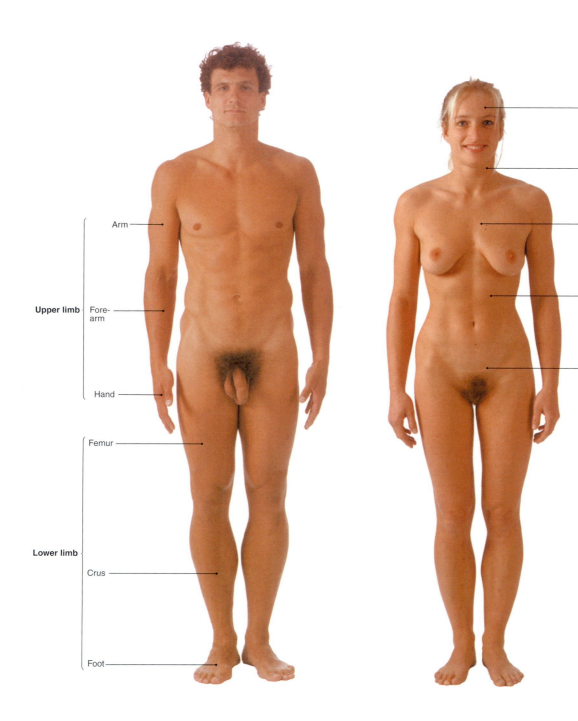

Head	
Neck	
Arm	Thorax
Upper limb	Fore-arm
Hand	Abdomen **Body**
Femur	Pelvis
Lower limb	
Crus	
Foot	

Fig. 3 Surface anatomy of the male.   **Fig. 4** Surface anatomy of the female.

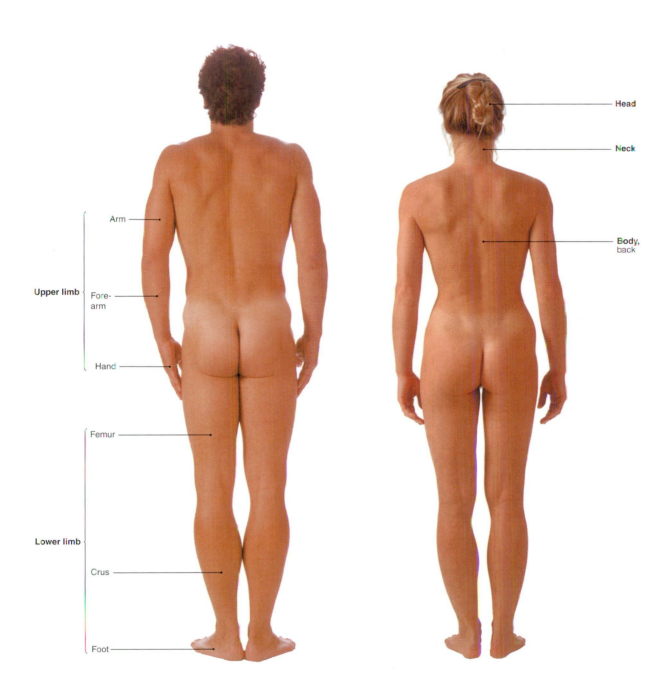

Fig. 5 Surface anatomy of the male. **Fig. 6** Surface anatomy of the female.

Regions of the human body

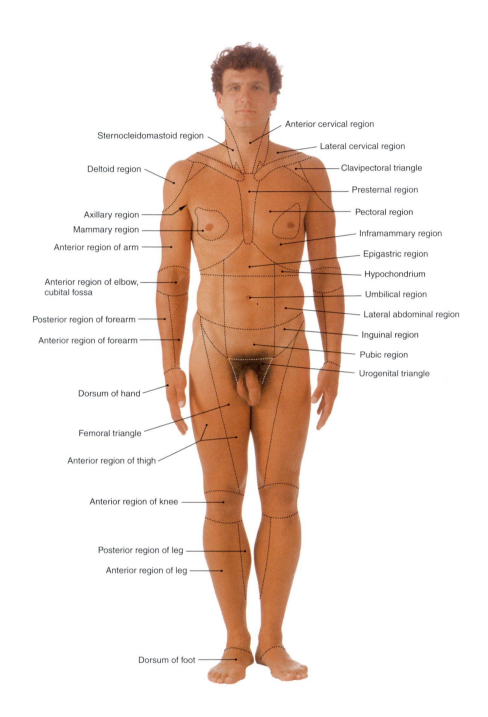

Sternocleidomastoid region

Anterior cervical region

Lateral cervical region

Deltoid region

Clavipectoral triangle

Presternal region

Axillary region

Pectoral region

Mammary region

Inframammary region

Anterior region of arm

Epigastric region

Hypochondrium

Anterior region of elbow,
cubital fossa

Umbilical region

Lateral abdominal region

Posterior region of forearm

Inguinal region

Anterior region of forearm

Pubic region

Urogenital triangle

Dorsum of hand

Femoral triangle

Anterior region of thigh

Anterior region of knee

Posterior region of leg

Anterior region of leg

Dorsum of foot

Fig. 7   Regions of the human body.

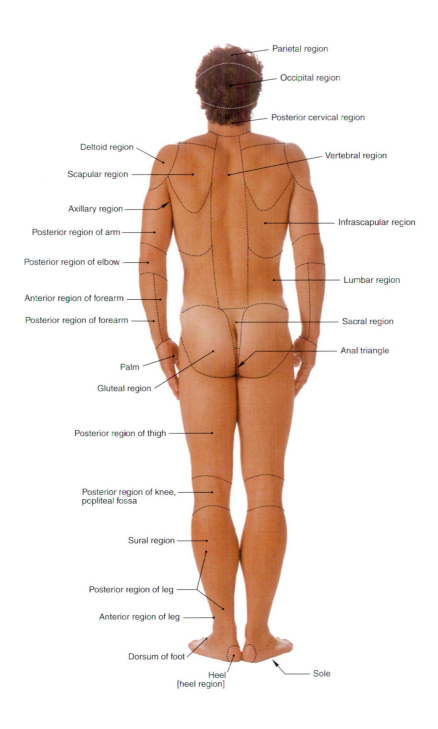

Fig. 8 Regions of the human body.

Skeleton

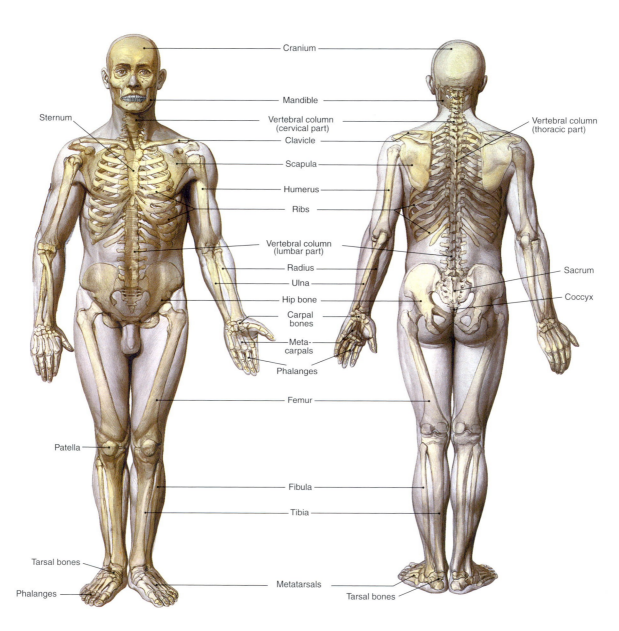

Fig. 9 Overview of the skeleton.

Fig. 10 Overview of the skeleton.

Parts of the human body

Head

Neck

Trunk
Thorax
Abdomen
Pelvis

Upper limb
Shoulder girdle
Arm

Lower limb
Pelvic girdle
Leg

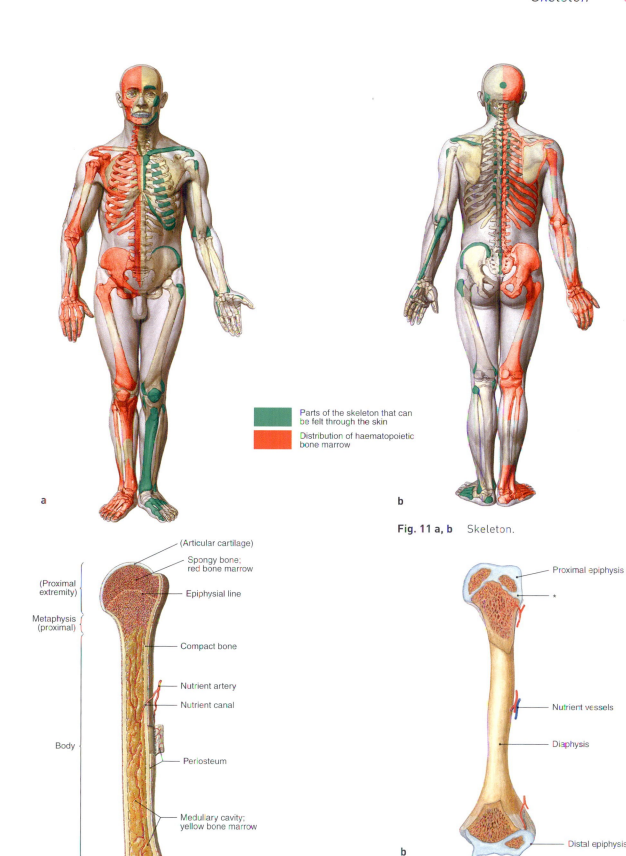

Parts of the skeleton that can be felt through the skin

Distribution of haematopoietic bone marrow

a

b

Fig. 11 a, b   Skeleton.

(Articular cartilage)

Spongy bone; red bone marrow

(Proximal extremity)

Epiphysial line

Metaphysis (proximal)

Compact bone

Nutrient artery

Nutrient canal

Body

Periosteum

Medullary cavity; yellow bone marrow

Metaphysis (distal)

Olecranon fossa

(Distal extremity)

Spongy bone; red bone marrow

Articular cartilage

a

Proximal epiphysis

*

Nutrient vessels

Diaphysis

Distal epiphysis

b

Fig. 12 a, b   Structure of tubular bones; longitudinal sections.
a   Humerus of an adult
    Ossified epiphyses (epiphyseal lines) are only poorly visible.
b   Humerus of a child
    The epiphyses consist of hyaline cartilage.

* Epiphysis, epiphyseal plate

Bone development

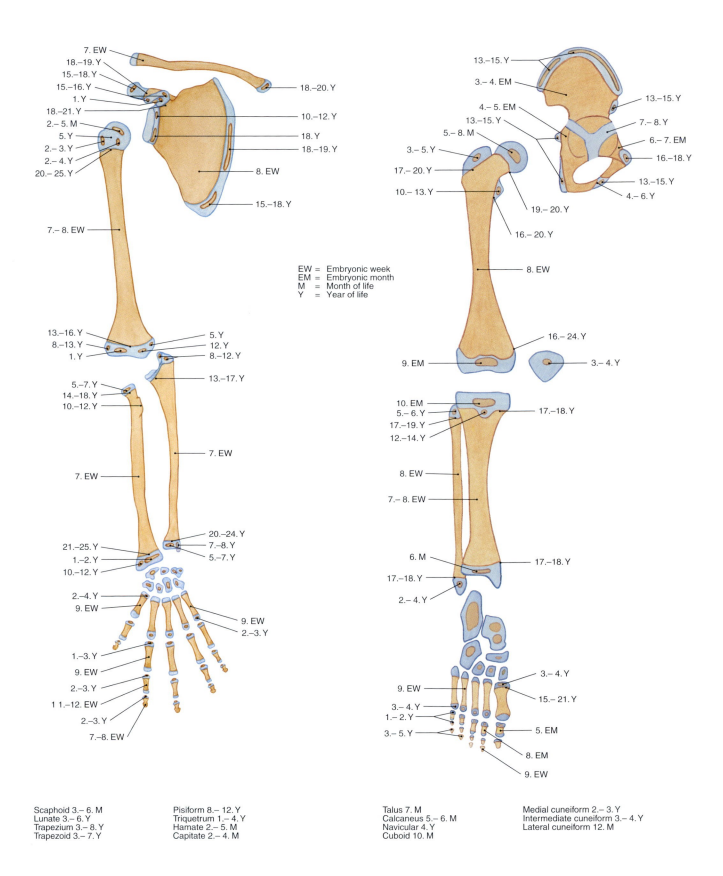

EW = Embryonic week
EM = Embryonic month
M = Month of life
Y = Year of life

Scaphoid 3.– 6. M
Lunate 3.– 6. Y
Trapezium 3.– 8. Y
Trapezoid 3.– 7. Y

Pisiform 8.– 12. Y
Triquetrum 1.– 4. Y
Hamate 2.– 5. M
Capitate 2.– 4. M

Talus 7. M
Calcaneus 5.– 6. M
Navicular 4. Y
Cuboid 10. M

Medial cuneiform 2.– 3. Y
Intermediate cuneiform 3.– 4. Y
Lateral cuneiform 12. M

Fig. 13 Appearance of ossification centres and synossification at the epiphyses of the upper limb (means according to v. LANZ, 1956; EXNER, 1990; HEUCK and BAST, 1994).

Fig. 14 Appearance of ossification centres and synossification at the epiphyses of the lower limb (means according to v. LANZ, 1956; EXNER, 1990; HEUCK and BAST, 1994).

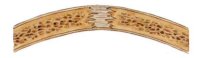

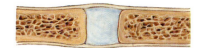

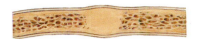

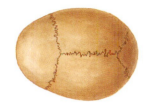

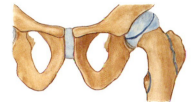

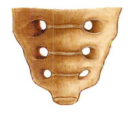

Fig. 15 Fibrous joint, exemplified by the sutures of the skull.

Fig. 16 Cartilaginous joint, exemplified by the pubic bone symphysis.

Fig. 17 Osseous joint, exemplified by the sacrum.

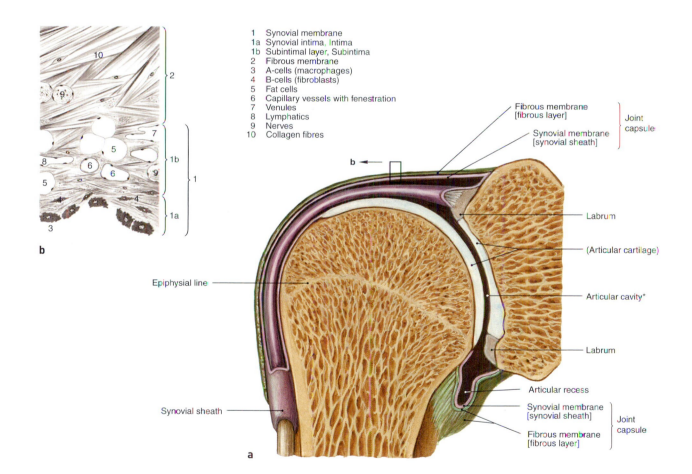

1   Synovial membrane
1a Synovial intima, Intima
1b Subintimal layer, Subintima
2   Fibrous membrane
3   A-cells (macrophages)
4   B-cells (fibroblasts)
5   Fat cells
6   Capillary vessels with fenestration
7   Venules
8   Lymphatics
9   Nerves
10 Collagen fibres

Fibrous membrane
[fibrous layer]   Joint
                                   capsule
Synovial membrane
[synovial sheath]

Labrum

(Articular cartilage)

Epiphysial line

Articular cavity*

Labrum

Articular recess

Synovial membrane
[synovial sheath]   Joint
                               capsule
Synovial sheath

Fibrous membrane
[fibrous layer]

Fig. 18 Synovial joint, exemplified by the shoulder joint.
a Section in the scapular plane
b Structure of the joint capsule

* The joint cavity is illustrated broader to enhance visibility.

Joints

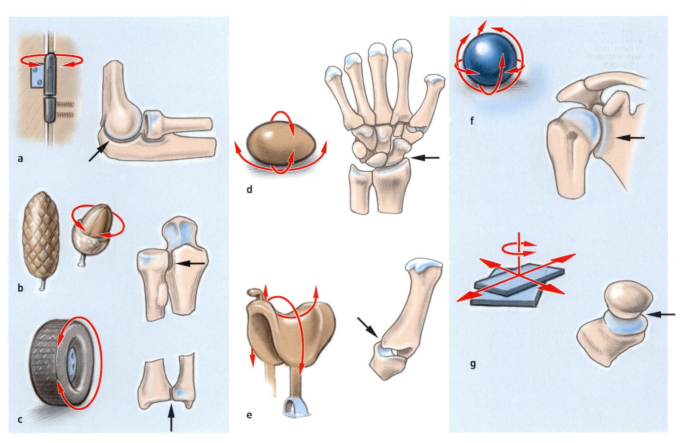

Fig. 19 a–g   Joints.
a   Hinge joint
b   Conoid joint
c   Pivot joint

d   Condylar joint
e   Saddle joint
f   Spheroidal joint
g   Plane joint

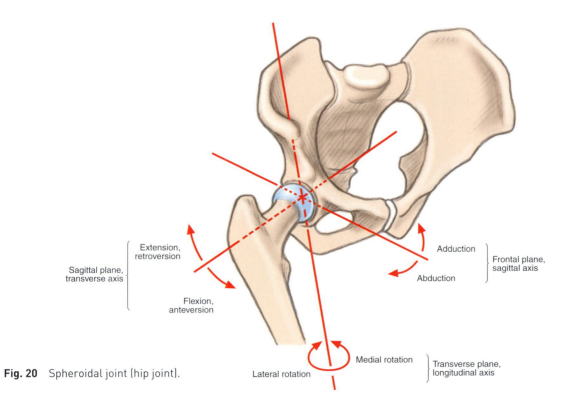

Fig. 20   Spheroidal joint (hip joint).

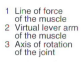

1 Line of force
  of the muscle
2 Virtual lever arm
  of the muscle
3 Axis of rotation
  of the joint

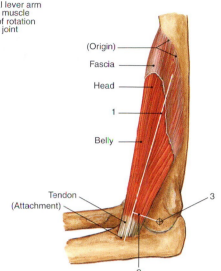

(Origin)

Fascia

Head

1

Belly

Tendon
(Attachment)

3

2

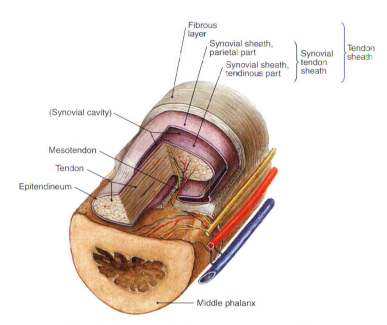

Fibrous
layer

Synovial sheath,
parietal part

Synovial sheath,
tendinous part

Synovial
tendon
sheath

Tendon
sheath

(Synovial cavity)

Mesotendon

Tendon

Epitendineum

Middle phalanx

Fig. 21 Organisation principle of skeletal muscles, exemplified by the brachial muscle.

Fig. 22 Structure of a tendon sheath, exemplified by a finger.

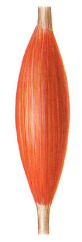

a Fusiform muscle

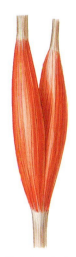

b Two-headed muscle

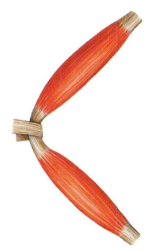

c Two-bellied muscle

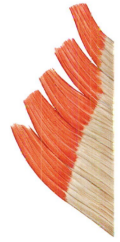

d Flat muscle

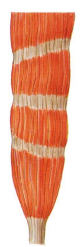

e Intersected muscle

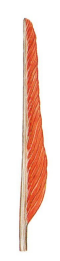

f Semipennate muscle

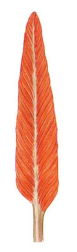

g Pennate muscle

Fig. 23 a–g Types of muscles.
a Single head,
      parallel muscle fibres
b Double head,
      parallel muscle fibres
c Double belly,
      parallel muscle fibres
d Multi-head, flat muscle
e Multi-belly muscle with
      tendinous intersections
f Unipennate muscle
g Bipennate muscle

Skeletal muscles

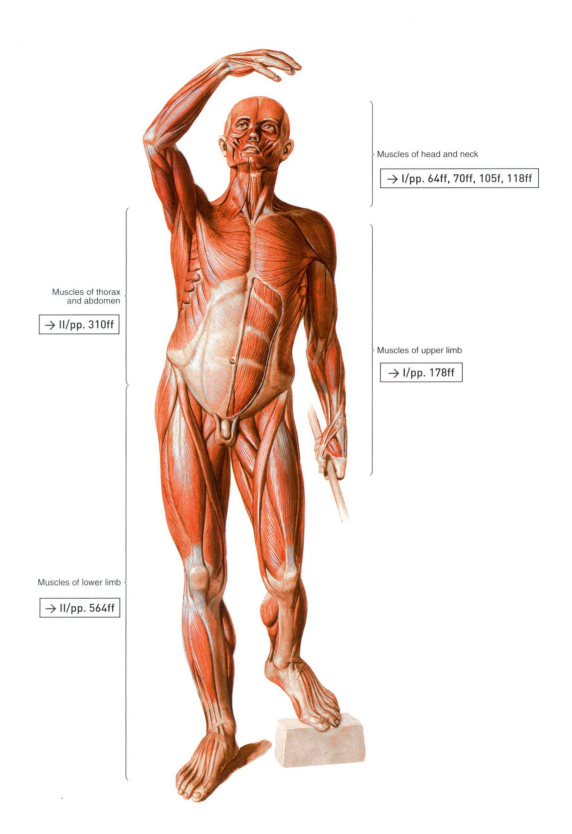

Muscles of head and neck

→ I/pp. 64ff, 70ff, 105f, 118ff

Muscles of thorax
and abdomen

→ II/pp. 310ff

Muscles of upper limb

→ I/pp. 178ff

Muscles of lower limb

→ II/pp. 564ff

Fig. 24 Overview of the skeletal muscles.

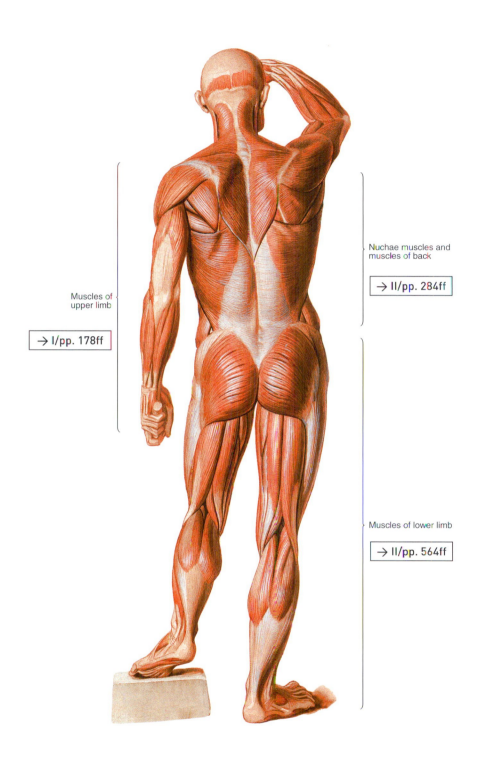

Muscles of
upper limb

→ I/pp. 178ff

Nuchae muscles and
muscles of back

→ II/pp. 284ff

Muscles of lower limb

→ II/pp. 564ff

Fig. 25 Overview of the skeletal muscles.

Digestive and respiratory system

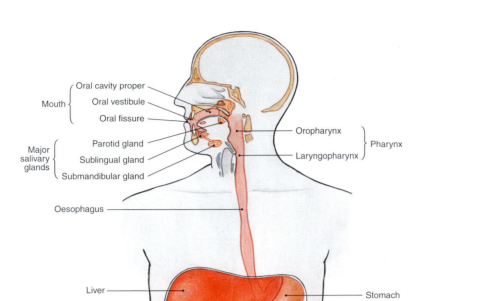

Fig. 26 Overview of the digestive system.

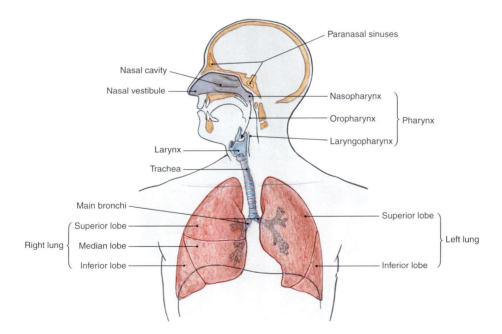

Fig. 27 Overview of the respiratory system.

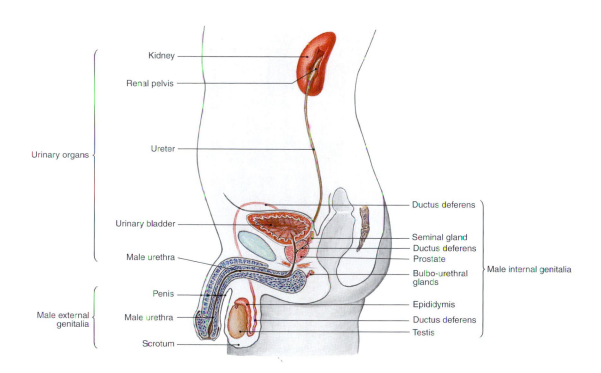

Fig. 28   Overview of the urinary and genital system of the male.

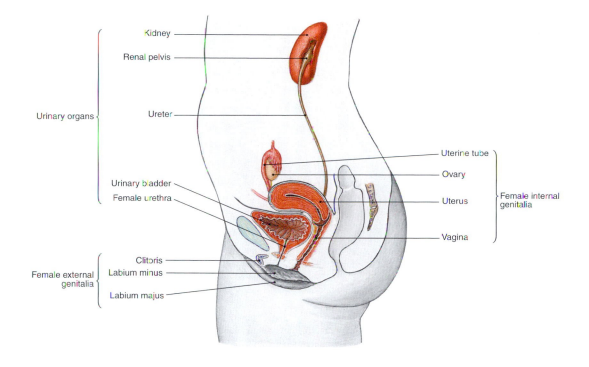

Fig. 29   Overview of the urinary and genital system of the female.

Internal organs, projection

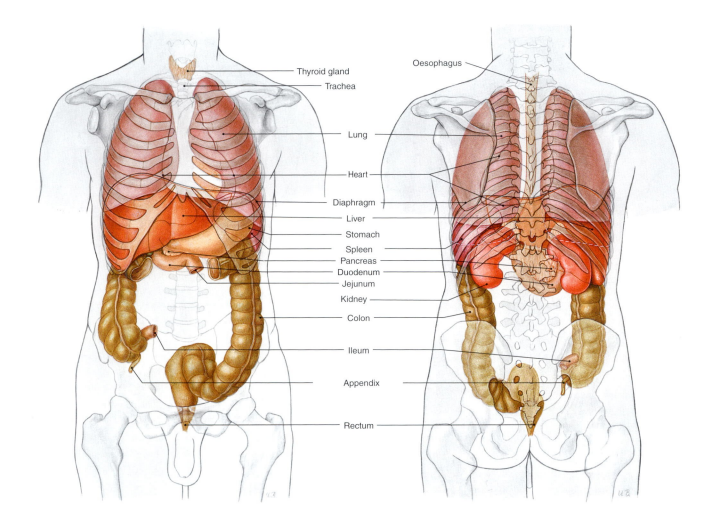

Thyroid gland

Trachea

Oesophagus

Lung

Heart

Diaphragm

Liver

Stomach

Spleen

Pancreas

Duodenum

Jejunum

Kidney

Colon

Ileum

Appendix

Rectum

Fig. 30 Projection of the internal organs onto the surface of the body.

Fig. 31 Projection of the internal organs onto the surface of the body.

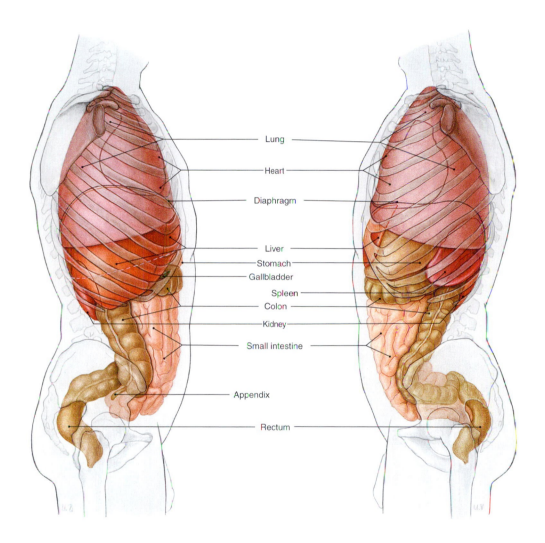

Lung

Heart

Diaphragm

Liver

Stomach

Gallbladder

Spleen

Colon

Kidney

Small intestine

Appendix

Rectum

Fig. 32   Projection of the internal organs onto the surface of the body.

Fig. 33   Projection of the internal organs onto the surface of the body.

Arteries

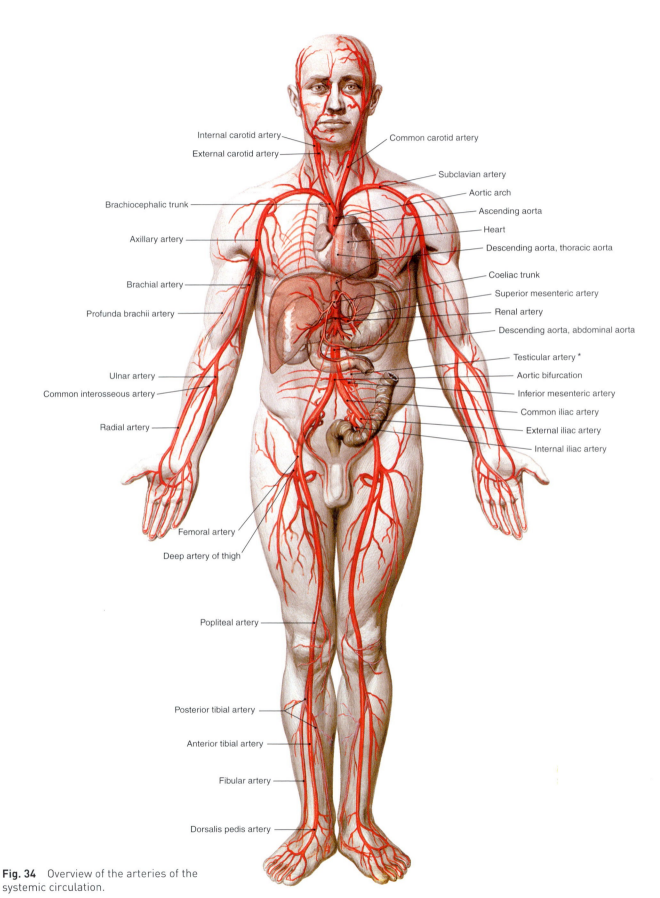

Internal carotid artery

External carotid artery

Brachiocephalic trunk

Axillary artery

Brachial artery

Profunda brachii artery

Ulnar artery

Common interosseous artery

Radial artery

Femoral artery

Deep artery of thigh

Popliteal artery

Posterior tibial artery

Anterior tibial artery

Fibular artery

Dorsalis pedis artery

Common carotid artery

Subclavian artery

Aortic arch

Ascending aorta

Heart

Descending aorta, thoracic aorta

Coeliac trunk

Superior mesenteric artery

Renal artery

Descending aorta, abdominal aorta

Testicular artery *

Aortic bifurcation

Inferior mesenteric artery

Common iliac artery

External iliac artery

Internal iliac artery

Fig. 34   Overview of the arteries of the
systemic circulation.

*   In the female: ovarian artery

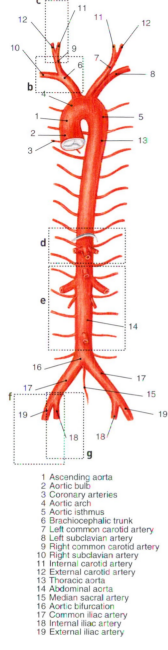

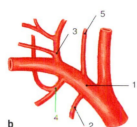

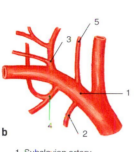

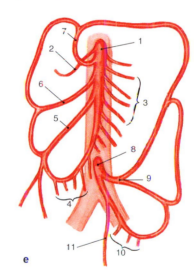

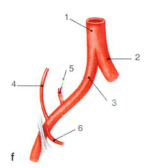

a

1 Ascending aorta
2 Aortic bulb
3 Coronary arteries
4 Aortic arch
5 Aortic isthmus
6 Brachiocephalic trunk
7 Left common carotid artery
8 Left subclavian artery
9 Right common carotid artery
10 Right subclavian artery
11 Internal carotid artery
12 External carotid artery
13 Thoracic aorta
14 Abdominal aorta
15 Median sacral artery
16 Aortic bifurcation
17 Common iliac artery
18 Internal iliac artery
19 External iliac artery

b

1 Subclavian artery
2 Internal thoracic artery
3 Thyrocervical trunk
4 Costocervical trunk
5 Vertebral artery

c

1 Common carotid artery
2 External carotid artery
3 Internal carotid artery
4 Superior thyroid artery
5 Ascending pharyngeal artery
6 Lingual artery
7 Facial artery
8 Occipital artery
9 Posterior auricular artery
10 Superficial temporal artery
11 Maxillary artery

d

1 Coeliac trunk
2 Left gastric artery
3 Common hepatic artery
4 Splenic artery

e

1 Superior mesenteric artery
2 Inferior pancreatico-duodenal artery
3 Jejunal arteries
4 Ileal arteries
5 Ileocolic artery
6 Right colic artery
7 Middle colic artery
8 Inferior mesenteric artery
9 Left colic artery
10 Sigmoid arteries
11 Superior rectal artery

Fig. 35 a–g Aorta and greater arteries; schema of the branching pattern.

a Aorta
b Subclavian artery
c External carotid artery
d Coeliac trunk
e Superior and inferior mesenteric artery
f External iliac artery
g Internal iliac artery

f

1 Common iliac artery
2 Internal iliac artery
3 External iliac artery
4 Inferior epigastric artery
5 Deep circumflex iliac artery
6 Pubic branch

g

1 Common iliac artery
2 External iliac artery
3 Internal iliac artery
4 Obturator artery
5 Internal pudendal artery
6 Inferior gluteal artery
7 Iliolumbar artery
8 Lateral sacral arteries
9 Superior gluteal artery
10 Umbilical artery, patent part
11 Inferior vesical artery
12 Middle rectal artery

Veins

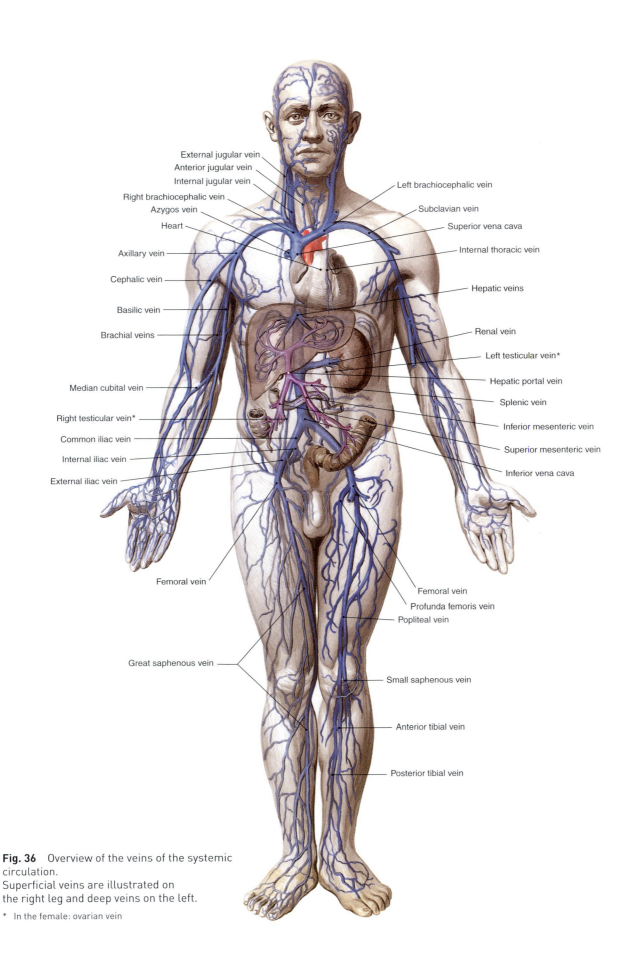

External jugular vein
Anterior jugular vein
Internal jugular vein
Right brachiocephalic vein
Azygos vein
Heart
Axillary vein
Cephalic vein
Basilic vein
Brachial veins
Median cubital vein
Right testicular vein*
Common iliac vein
Internal iliac vein
External iliac vein
Femoral vein
Great saphenous vein

Left brachiocephalic vein
Subclavian vein
Superior vena cava
Internal thoracic vein
Hepatic veins
Renal vein
Left testicular vein*
Hepatic portal vein
Splenic vein
Inferior mesenteric vein
Superior mesenteric vein
Inferior vena cava
Femoral vein
Profunda femoris vein
Popliteal vein
Small saphenous vein
Anterior tibial vein
Posterior tibial vein

Fig. 36   Overview of the veins of the systemic circulation.
Superficial veins are illustrated on the right leg and deep veins on the left.

*   In the female: ovarian vein

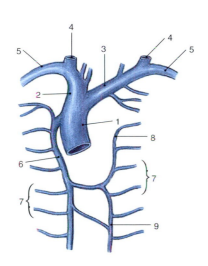

1 Superior vena cava
2 Right brachiocephalic vein
3 Left brachiocephalic vein
4 Internal jugular vein
5 Subclavian vein

6 Azygos vein
7 Posterior intercostal veins
8 Accessory hemi-azygos vein
9 Hemi-azygos vein

Fig. 37 Superior vena cava; schema of the tributaries.

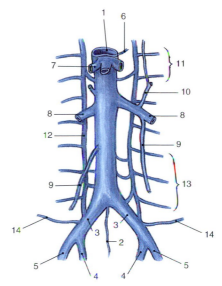

1 Inferior vena cava
2 Median sacral vein
3 Common iliac vein
4 Internal iliac vein
5 External iliac vein
6 Inferior phrenic veins
7 Hepatic veins

8 Renal vein
9 Testicular/ovarian vein
10 Suprarenal vein
11 Posterior intercostal veins
12 Ascending lumbar vein
13 Lumbar veins
14 Iliolumbar vein

Fig. 38 Inferior vena cava; schema of the tributaries.

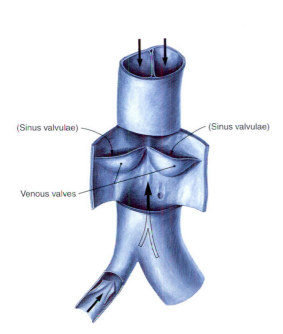

(Sinus valvulae)   (Sinus valvulae)

Venous valves

Fig. 39 Functional principle of venous valves. The arrows pointing upwards indicate the flow of blood. The valves close upon backflow of the blood (arrows pointing downwards).

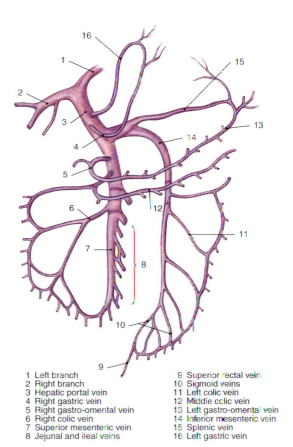

1 Left branch
2 Right branch
3 Hepatic portal vein
4 Right gastric vein
5 Right gastro-omental vein
6 Right colic vein
7 Superior mesenteric vein
8 Jejunal and ileal veins

9 Superior rectal vein
10 Sigmoid veins
11 Left colic vein
12 Middle colic vein
13 Left gastro-omental vein
14 Inferior mesenteric vein
15 Splenic vein
16 Left gastric vein

Fig. 40 Hepatic portal vein.

Foetal circulation

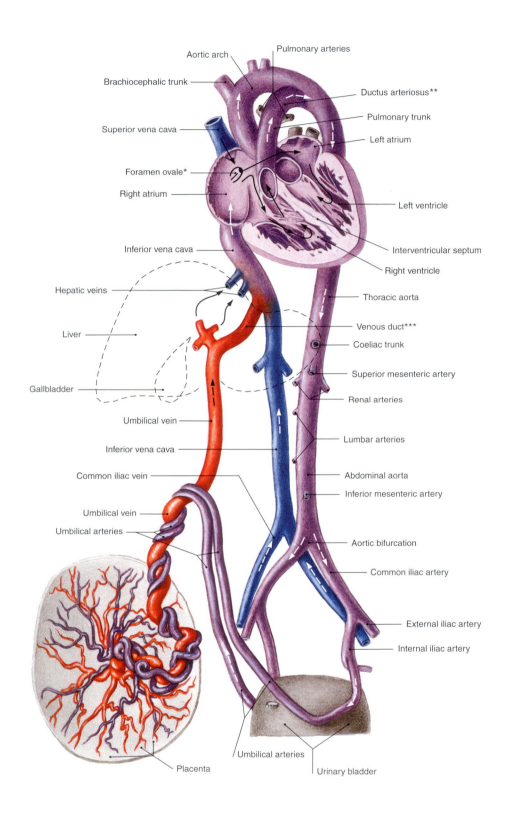

Fig. 41 Schema of foetal circulation.
The different colours indicate the oxygen content in the blood:
red = rich in oxygen,
blue = poor in oxygen,
purple = mixed blood.
Arrows indicate the direction of the blood flow.

*   Short-circuit between the right and the left atrium
** Short-circuit between the pulmonary trunk and the arch of aorta
*** Short-circuit between the umbilical vein and the inferior vena cava

Conversion from foetal to postnatal circulation:

*   The valve-like connection between the right and the left atrium via
    the foramen ovale is passively closed at the onset of respiratory
    activity in the lungs.
** The ductus arteriosus (BOTALLO), on the other hand, closes only
    during the first months of life as its lumen gradually obliterates by
    epithelial proliferation and increased tension of the wall.
*** The ductus venosus (ARANTIUS) obliterates after birth and becomes
    the ligamentum venosum in the portal area of the liver.

Lymphatic system

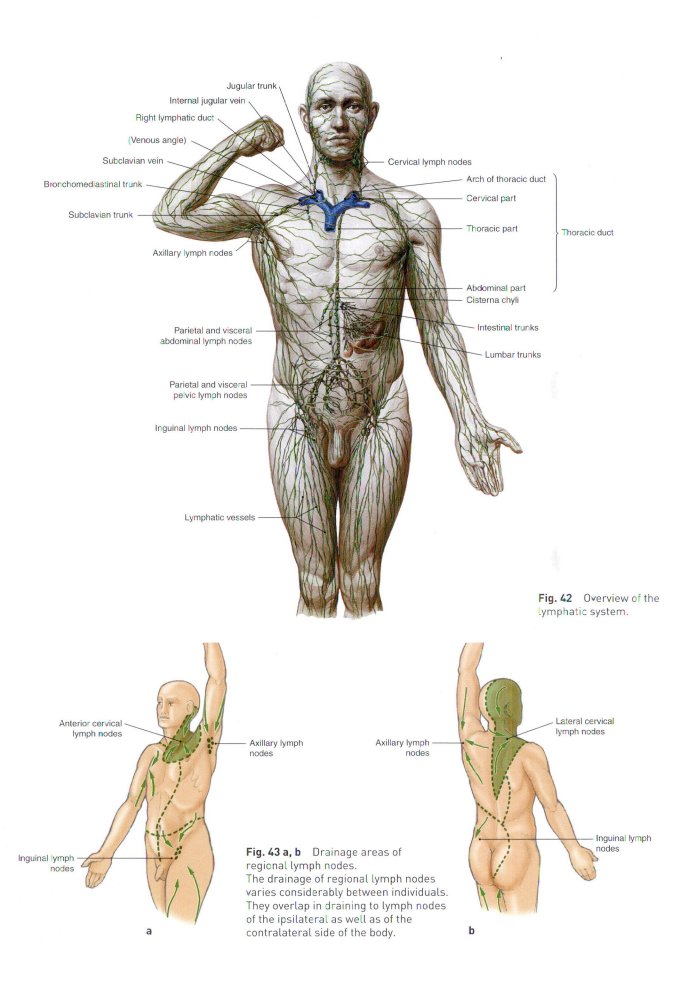

Jugular trunk

Internal jugular vein

Right lymphatic duct

(Venous angle)

Subclavian vein

Bronchomediastinal trunk

Subclavian trunk

Axillary lymph nodes

Parietal and visceral
abdominal lymph nodes

Parietal and visceral
pelvic lymph nodes

Inguinal lymph nodes

Lymphatic vessels

Cervical lymph nodes

Arch of thoracic duct

Cervical part

Thoracic part

Thoracic duct

Abdominal part

Cisterna chyli

Intestinal trunks

Lumbar trunks

Fig. 42 Overview of the
lymphatic system.

Anterior cervical
lymph nodes

Axillary lymph
nodes

Inguinal lymph
nodes

a

Fig. 43 a, b Drainage areas of
regional lymph nodes.
The drainage of regional lymph nodes
varies considerably between individuals.
They overlap in draining to lymph nodes
of the ipsilateral as well as of the
contralateral side of the body.

Lateral cervical
lymph nodes

Axillary lymph
nodes

Inguinal lymph
nodes

b

Central nervous system

Peripheral nervous system

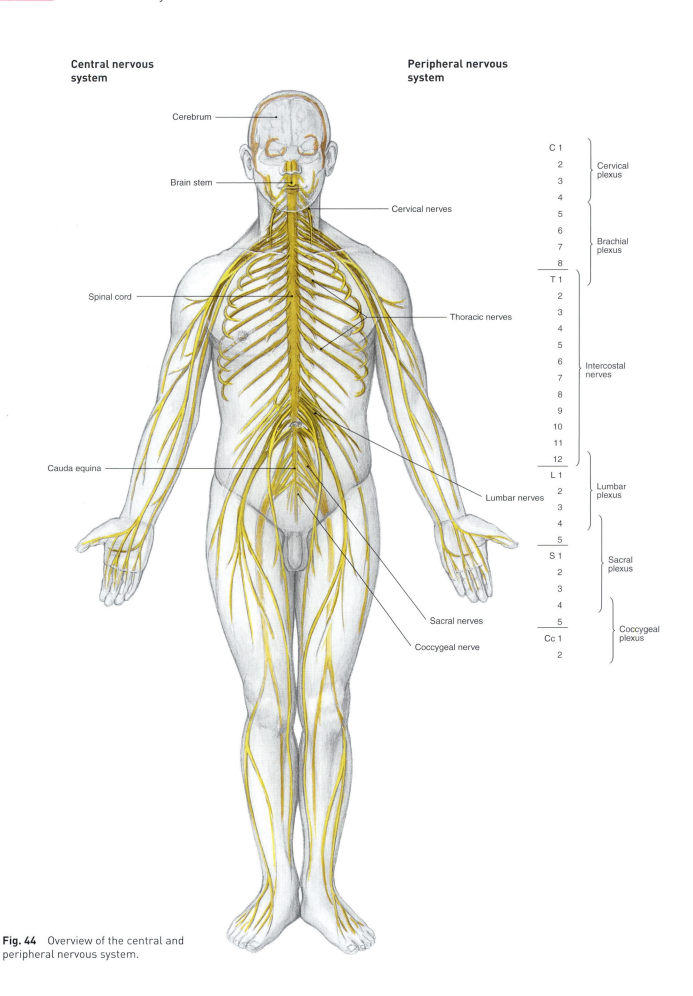

Cerebrum

Brain stem

Cervical nerves

Spinal cord

Thoracic nerves

Cauda equina

Lumbar nerves

Sacral nerves

Coccygeal nerve

C 1
2
3
4

Cervical plexus

5
6
7
8

Brachial plexus

T 1
2
3
4
5
6
7
8
9
10
11

Intercostal nerves

12
L 1
2
3

Lumbar plexus

4
5
S 1
2
3

Sacral plexus

4
5
Cc 1
2

Coccygeal plexus

Fig. 44 Overview of the central and peripheral nervous system.

Periperal nervous system

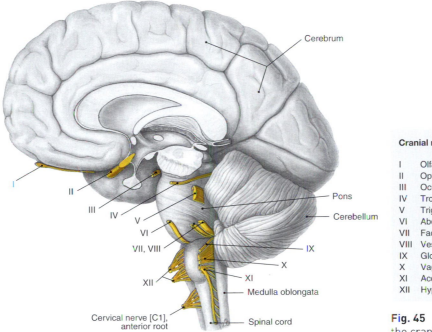

Cranial nerves

I	Olfactory nerves
II	Optic nerve
III	Oculomotor nerve
IV	Trochlear nerve
V	Trigeminal nerve
VI	Abducent nerve
VII	Facial nerve
VIII	Vestibulocochlear nerve
IX	Glossopharyngeal nerve
X	Vagus nerve
XI	Accessory nerve
XII	Hypoglossal nerve

Cerebrum

Pons

Cerebellum

Medulla oblongata

Spinal cord

Cervical nerve [C1], anterior root

Fig. 45 Overview of the brain and the cranial nerves.

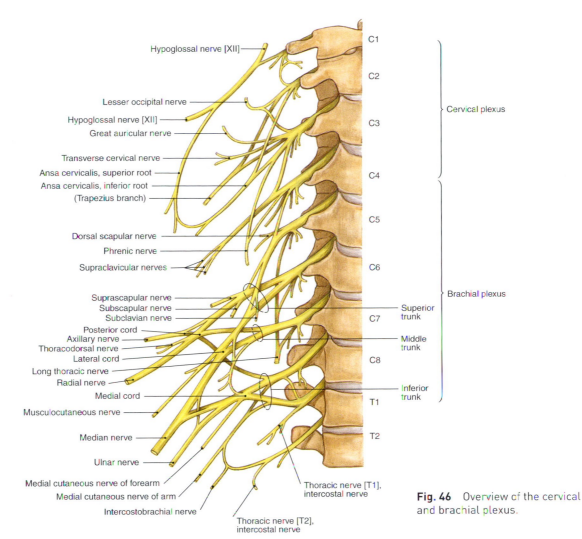

Hypoglossal nerve [XII]

Lesser occipital nerve

Hypoglossal nerve [XII]

Great auricular nerve

Transverse cervical nerve

Ansa cervicalis, superior root

Ansa cervicalis, inferior root

(Trapezius branch)

Dorsal scapular nerve

Phrenic nerve

Supraclavicular nerves

Suprascapular nerve

Subscapular nerve

Subclavian nerve

Posterior cord

Axillary nerve

Thoracodorsal nerve

Lateral cord

Long thoracic nerve

Radial nerve

Medial cord

Musculocutaneous nerve

Median nerve

Ulnar nerve

Medial cutaneous nerve of forearm

Medial cutaneous nerve of arm

Intercostobrachial nerve

C1

C2

C3

C4

C5

C6

C7

C8

T1

T2

Cervical plexus

Brachial plexus

Superior trunk

Middle trunk

Inferior trunk

Thoracic nerve [T1], intercostal nerve

Thoracic nerve [T2], intercostal nerve

Fig. 46 Overview of the cervical and brachial plexus.

Peripheral nervous system

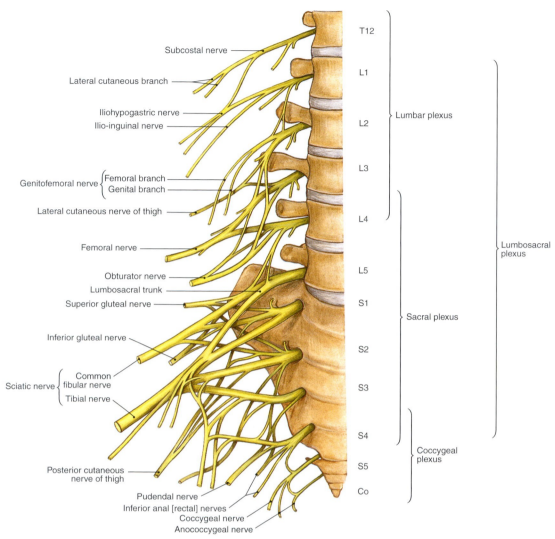

Fig. 47 Overview of the lumbosacral plexus and the coccygeal plexus.

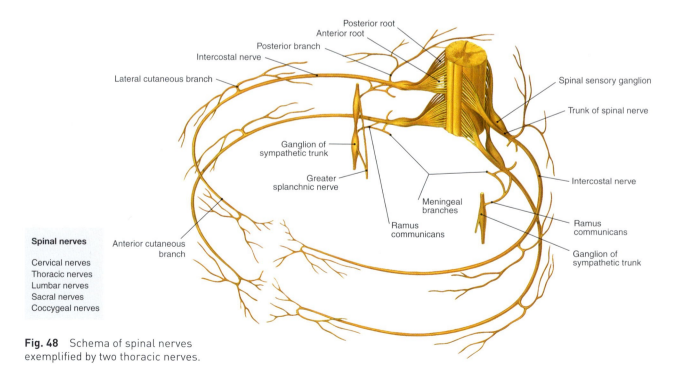

Spinal nerves

Cervical nerves
Thoracic nerves
Lumbar nerves
Sacral nerves
Coccygeal nerves

Fig. 48 Schema of spinal nerves exemplified by two thoracic nerves.

Autonomous nervous system

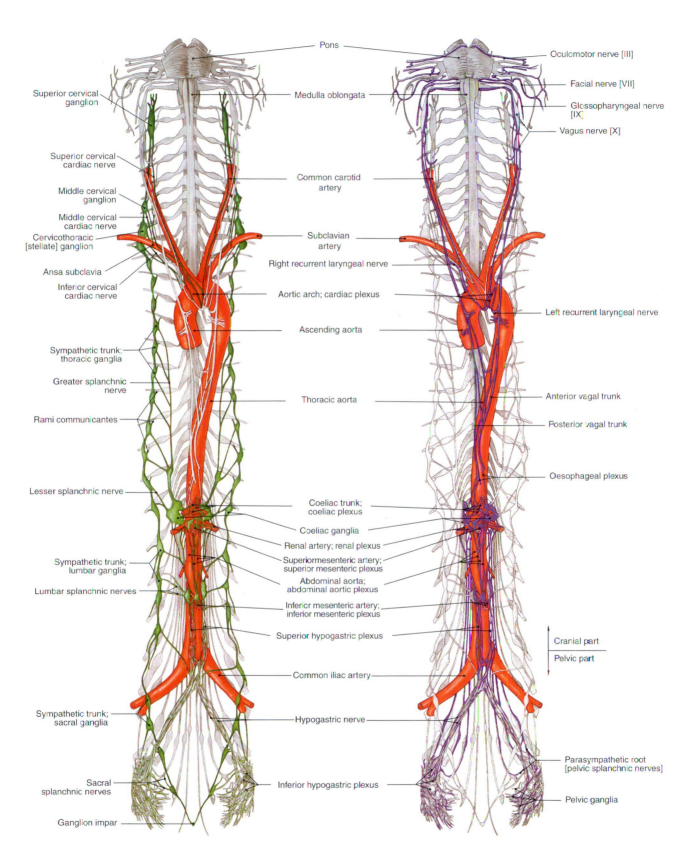

Fig. 49 Sympathetic part of the autonomous nervous system.
The entire system of sympathetic ganglia and their connections located along the vertebral column are referred to as sympathetic trunk (green).

Fig. 50 Parasympathetic part of the autonomous nervous system.
Parasympathetic fibres (violet) usually travel along with other nerve fibres.

Autonomous nervous system

Sympathetic part

Parasympathetic part

Oculomotor nerve [III]

Facial nerve [VII]

Glossopharyngeal nerve [IX]

Vagus nerve [X]

Sympathetic trunk

Coeliac ganglion

Superior mesenteric ganglion

Inferior mesenteric ganglion

Pelvic splanchnic nerves

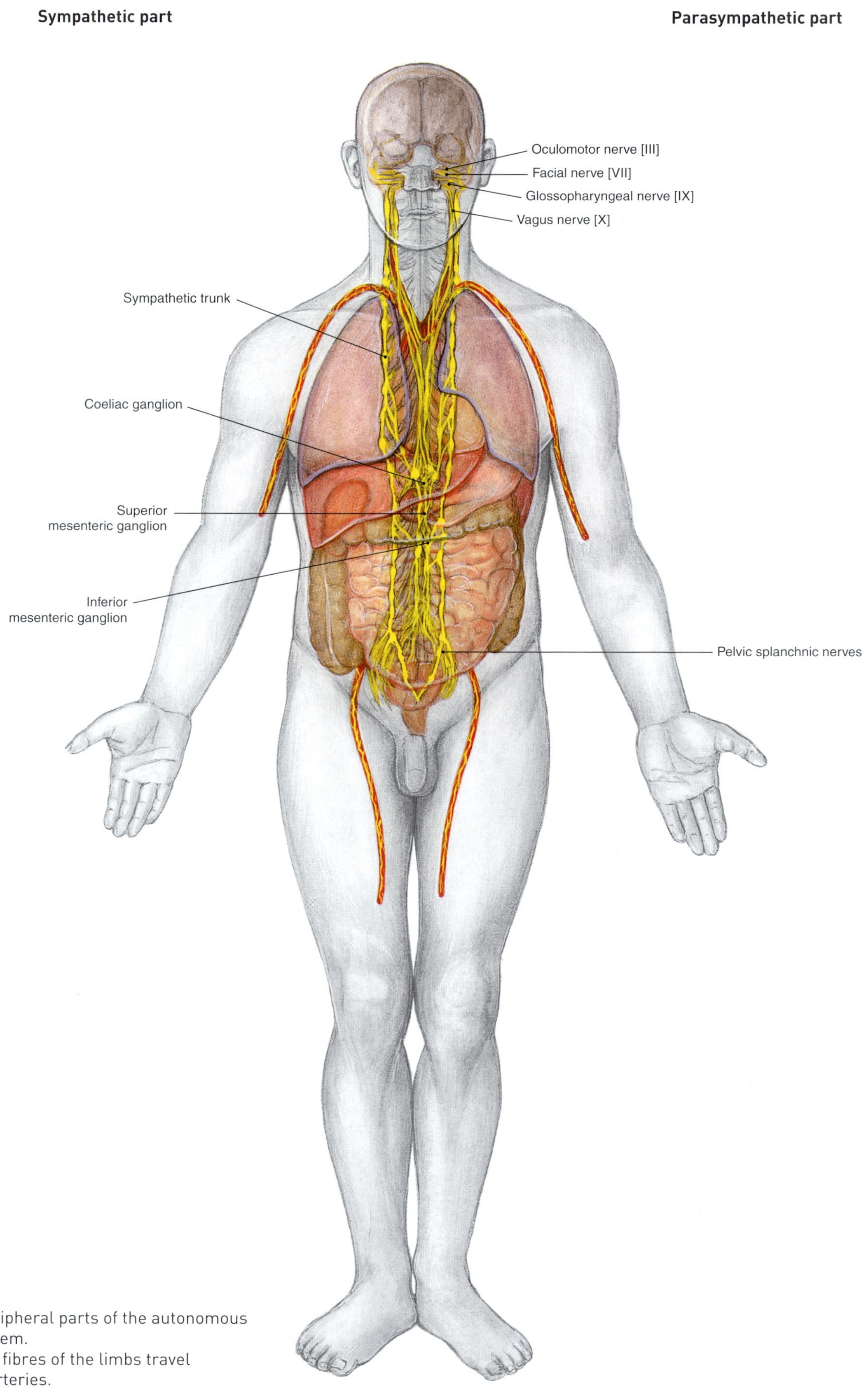

Fig. 51 Peripheral parts of the autonomous nervous system.
Sympathetic fibres of the limbs travel along with arteries.

Autonomous nervous system

Sympathetic part

Parasympathetic part

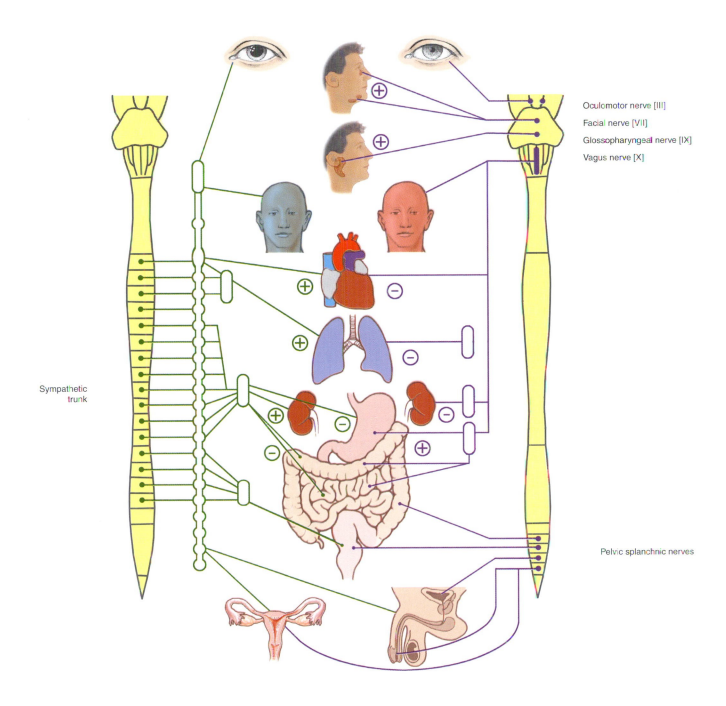

Oculomotor nerve [III]

Facial nerve [VII]

Glossopharyngeal nerve [IX]

Vagus nerve [X]

Sympathetic
trunk

Pelvic splanchnic nerves

Fig. 52 Overview of the functions of the
autonomous nervous system.

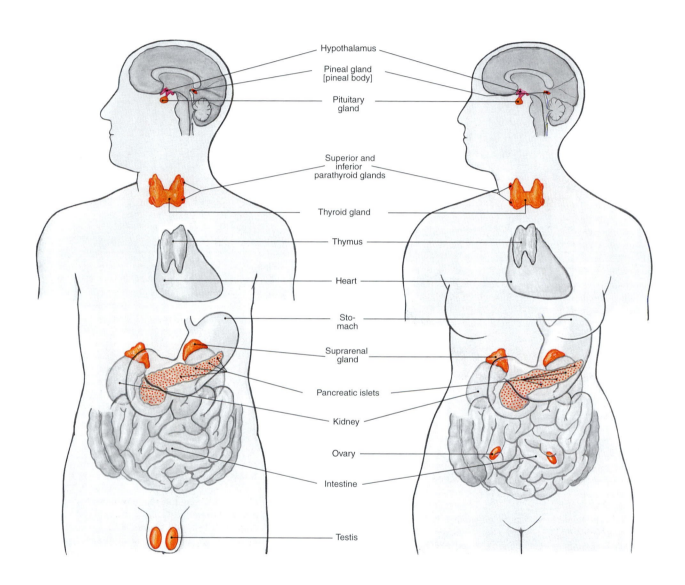

Fig. 53 Endocrine organs of the male.

Fig. 54 Endocrine organs of the female.

Skin and fingernails

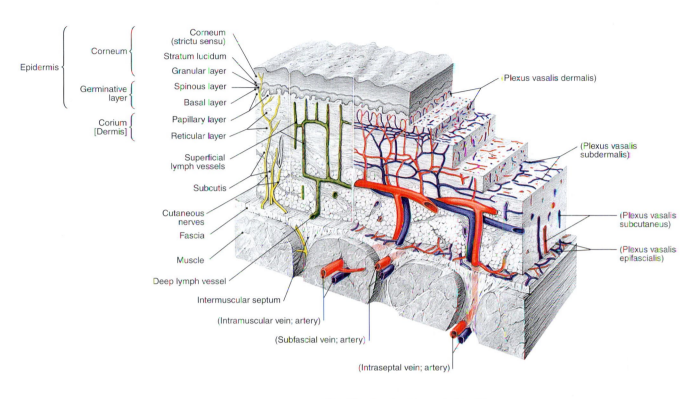

Epidermis
- Corneum
  - Corneum (strictu sensu)
  - Stratum lucidum
  - Granular layer
- Germinative layer
  - Spinous layer
  - Basal layer
Corium [Dermis]
  - Papillary layer
  - Reticular layer

Superficial lymph vessels
Subcutis
Cutaneous nerves
Fascia
Muscle
Deep lymph vessel
Intermuscular septum
(Intramuscular vein; artery)
(Subfascial vein; artery)
(Intraseptal vein; artery)

(Plexus vasalis dermalis)
(Plexus vasalis subdermalis)
(Plexus vasalis subcutaneus)
(Plexus vasalis epifascialis)

Fig. 55 Section through the skin; approximately 11-fold magnification.

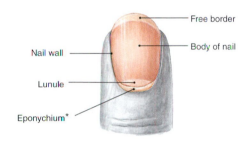

Free border
Body of nail
Nail wall
Lunule
Eponychium*

Fig. 56 Distal phalanx of a digit with fingernail.

* The epidermis of the nail is also known as cuticle.

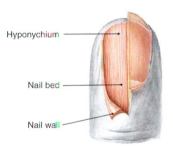

Hyponychium
Nail bed
Nail wall

Fig. 57 Distal phalanx of a digit; the nail has been partly removed.

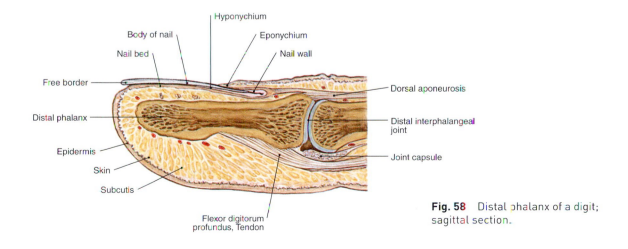

Hyponychium
Body of nail
Eponychium
Nail bed
Nail wall
Free border
Distal phalanx
Epidermis
Skin
Subcutis
Flexor digitorum profundus, Tendon
Dorsal aponeurosis
Distal interphalangeal joint
Joint capsule

Fig. 58 Distal phalanx of a digit; sagittal section.

Regions

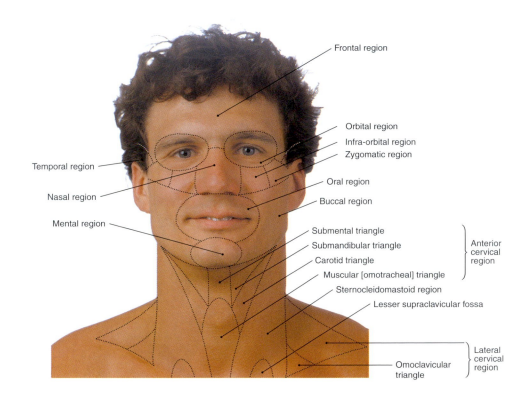

Frontal region

Orbital region
Infra-orbital region
Zygomatic region

Temporal region

Oral region

Nasal region

Buccal region

Mental region

Submental triangle
Submandibular triangle
Carotid triangle
Muscular [omotracheal] triangle
Anterior cervical region

Sternocleidomastoid region

Lesser supraclavicular fossa

Lateral cervical region

Omoclavicular triangle

Fig. 59   Regions of the head and the neck.

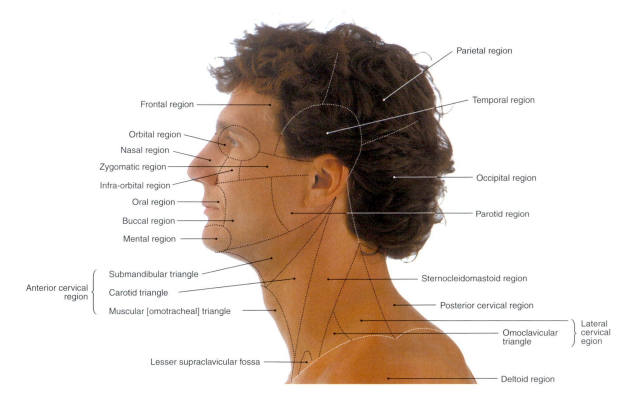

Parietal region

Temporal region

Frontal region

Orbital region

Nasal region

Zygomatic region

Infra-orbital region

Occipital region

Oral region

Buccal region

Parotid region

Mental region

Submandibular triangle

Anterior cervical region

Carotid triangle

Muscular [omotracheal] triangle

Sternocleidomastoid region

Posterior cervical region

Lateral cervical region

Omoclavicular triangle

Lesser supraclavicular fossa

Deltoid region

Fig. 60   Regions of the head and the neck.

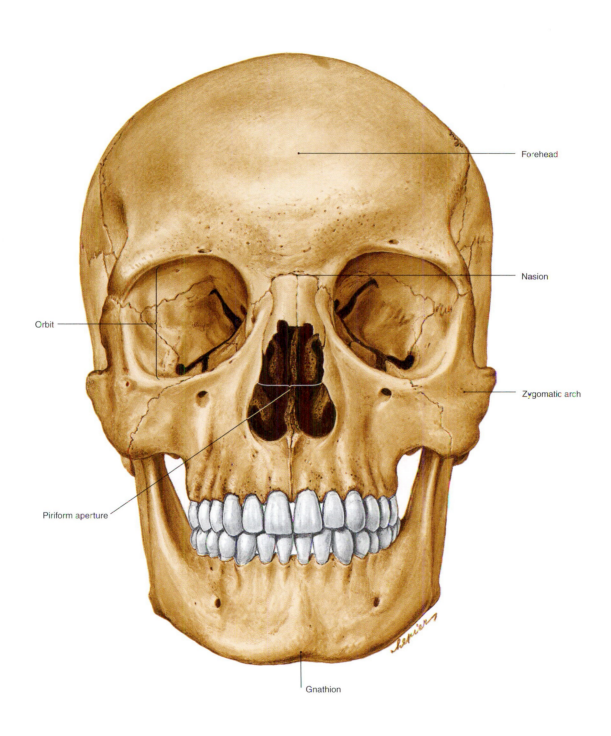

Forehead

Nasion

Orbit

Zygomatic arch

Piriform aperture

Gnathion

Fig. 61   Skull.

Bones of the skull

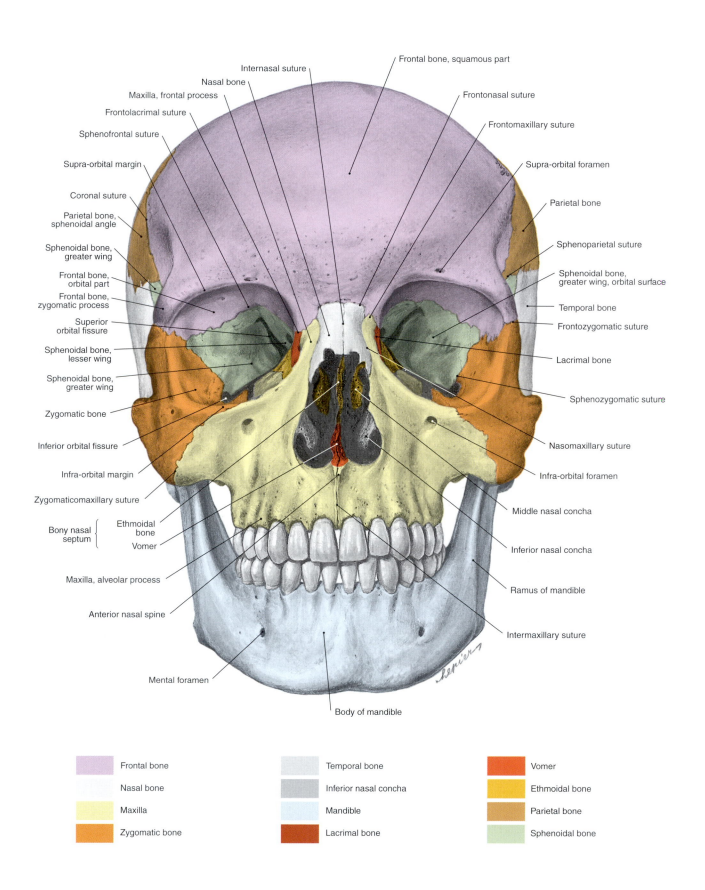

Internasal suture
Nasal bone
Maxilla, frontal process
Frontolacrimal suture
Sphenofrontal suture
Supra-orbital margin
Coronal suture
Parietal bone, sphenoidal angle
Sphenoidal bone, greater wing
Frontal bone, orbital part
Frontal bone, zygomatic process
Superior orbital fissure
Sphenoidal bone, lesser wing
Sphenoidal bone, greater wing
Zygomatic bone
Inferior orbital fissure
Infra-orbital margin
Zygomaticomaxillary suture
Bony nasal septum
Ethmoidal bone
Vomer
Maxilla, alveolar process
Anterior nasal spine
Mental foramen
Body of mandible

Frontal bone, squamous part
Frontonasal suture
Frontomaxillary suture
Supra-orbital foramen
Parietal bone
Sphenoparietal suture
Sphenoidal bone, greater wing, orbital surface
Temporal bone
Frontozygomatic suture
Lacrimal bone
Sphenozygomatic suture
Nasomaxillary suture
Infra-orbital foramen
Middle nasal concha
Inferior nasal concha
Ramus of mandible
Intermaxillary suture

Frontal bone
Nasal bone
Maxilla
Zygomatic bone

Temporal bone
Inferior nasal concha
Mandible
Lacrimal bone

Vomer
Ethmoidal bone
Parietal bone
Sphenoidal bone

Fig. 62 Bones of the skull.

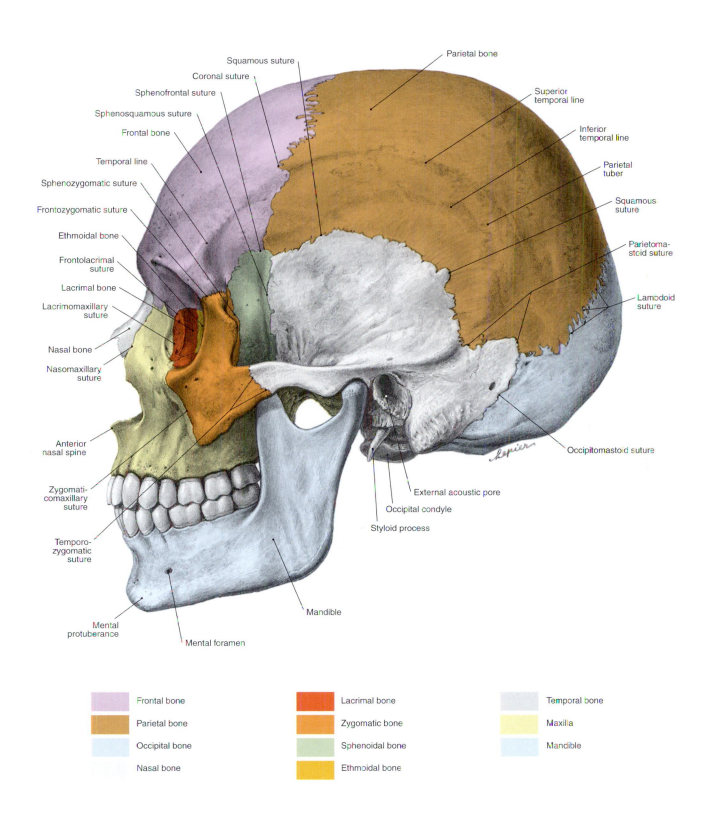

Squamous suture
Coronal suture
Sphenofrontal suture
Sphenosquamous suture
Frontal bone
Temporal line
Sphenozygomatic suture
Frontozygomatic suture
Ethmoidal bone
Frontolacrimal suture
Lacrimal bone
Lacrimomaxillary suture
Nasal bone
Nasomaxillary suture
Anterior nasal spine
Zygomaticomaxillary suture
Temporozygomatic suture
Mental protuberance
Mental foramen

Parietal bone
Superior temporal line
Inferior temporal line
Parietal tuber
Squamous suture
Parietomastoid suture
Lamboid suture
Occipitomastoid suture
External acoustic pore
Occipital condyle
Styloid process
Mandible

Frontal bone
Parietal bone
Occipital bone
Nasal bone
Lacrimal bone
Zygomatic bone
Sphenoidal bone
Ethmoidal bone
Temporal bone
Maxilla
Mandible

Fig. 63 Bones of the skull.

Bones of the skull

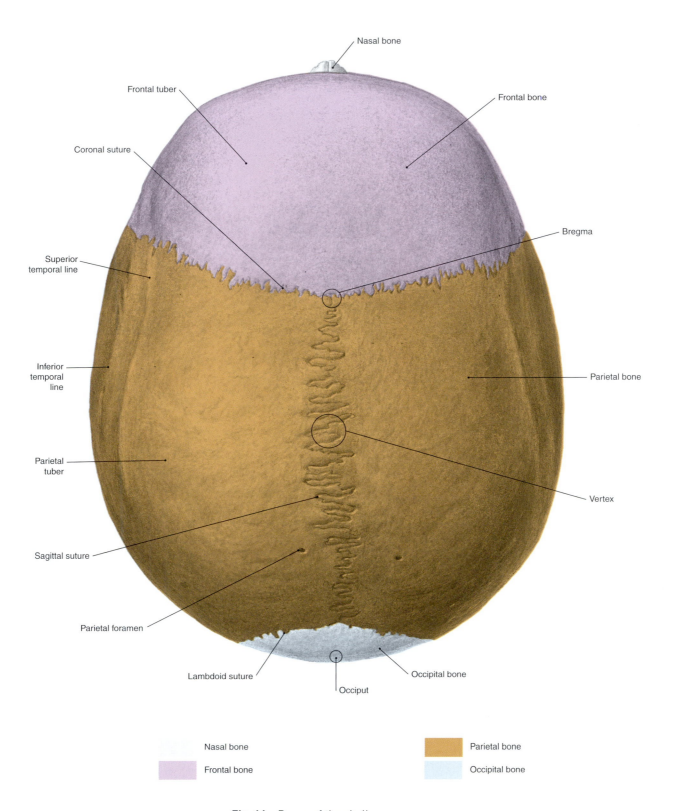

Fig. 64 Bones of the skull;
superior view.

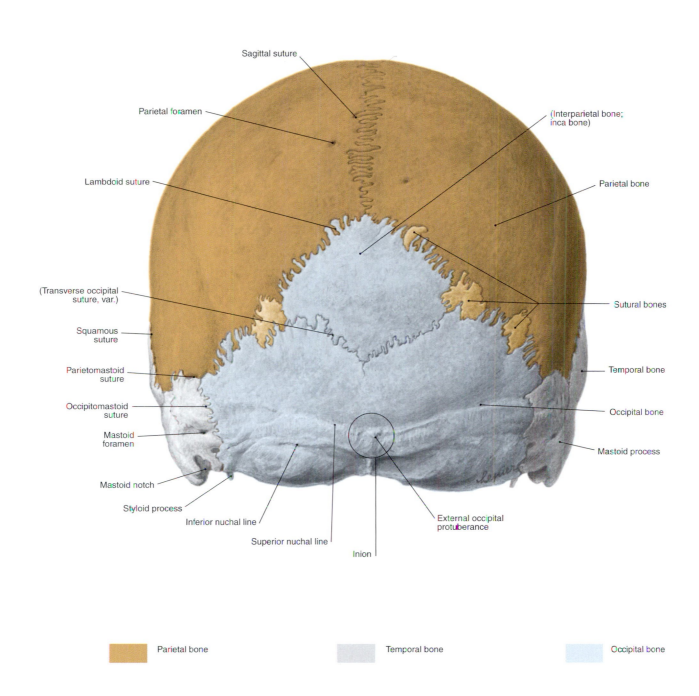

Sagittal suture

Parietal foramen

(Interparietal bone; inca bone)

Lambdoid suture

Parietal bone

(Transverse occipital suture, var.)

Sutural bones

Squamous suture

Parietomastoid suture

Temporal bone

Occipitomastoid suture

Occipital bone

Mastoid foramen

Mastoid process

Mastoid notch

Styloid process

Inferior nuchal line

External occipital protuberance

Superior nuchal line

Inion

Parietal bone

Temporal bone

Occipital bone

Fig. 65 Bones of the skull; posterior view.

Bones of the skull

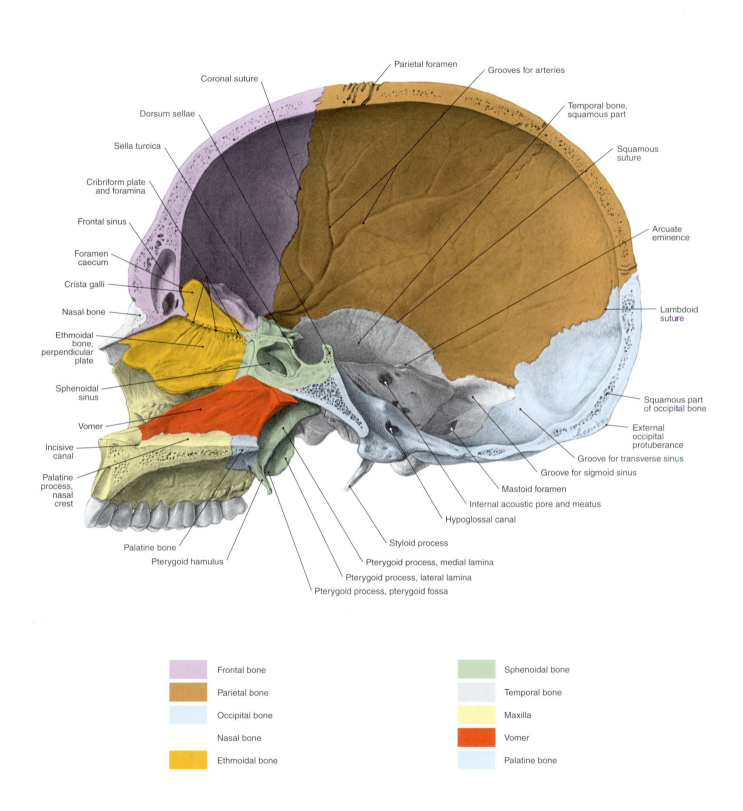

Parietal foramen
Grooves for arteries
Coronal suture
Temporal bone, squamous part
Dorsum sellae
Squamous suture
Sella turcica
Cribriform plate and foramina
Frontal sinus
Arcuate eminence
Foramen caecum
Crista galli
Lambdoid suture
Nasal bone
Ethmoidal bone, perpendicular plate
Sphenoidal sinus
Squamous part of occipital bone
Vomer
External occipital protuberance
Incisive canal
Groove for transverse sinus
Palatine process, nasal crest
Groove for sigmoid sinus
Mastoid foramen
Internal acoustic pore and meatus
Hypoglossal canal
Styloid process
Palatine bone
Pterygoid hamulus
Pterygoid process, medial lamina
Pterygoid process, lateral lamina
Pterygoid process, pterygoid fossa

Frontal bone	Sphenoidal bone
Parietal bone	Temporal bone
Occipital bone	Maxilla
Nasal bone	Vomer
Ethmoidal bone	Palatine bone

Fig. 66 Bones of the skull; medial view.

Bones of the skull

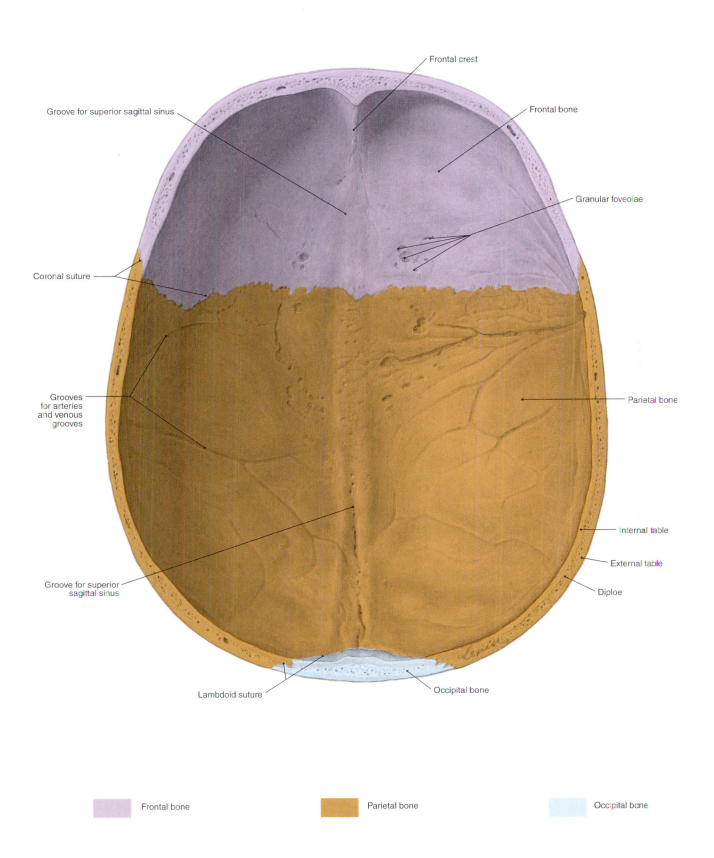

Frontal crest

Groove for superior sagittal sinus

Frontal bone

Granular foveolae

Coronal suture

Grooves for arteries and venous grooves

Parietal bone

Internal table

External table

Diploe

Groove for superior sagittal sinus

Lambdoid suture

Occipital bone

Frontal bone

Parietal bone

Occipital bone

Fig. 67 Calvaria; internal aspect.

Bones of the skull

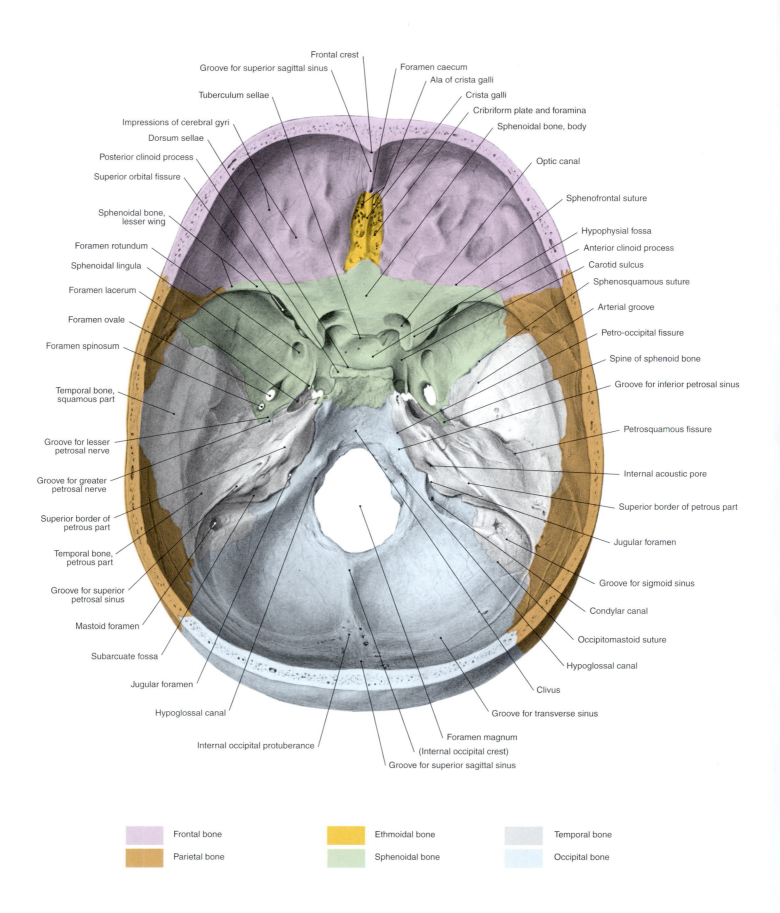

Frontal crest
Groove for superior sagittal sinus
Tuberculum sellae
Impressions of cerebral gyri
Dorsum sellae
Posterior clinoid process
Superior orbital fissure
Sphenoidal bone, lesser wing
Foramen rotundum
Sphenoidal lingula
Foramen lacerum
Foramen ovale
Foramen spinosum
Temporal bone, squamous part
Groove for lesser petrosal nerve
Groove for greater petrosal nerve
Superior border of petrous part
Temporal bone, petrous part
Groove for superior petrosal sinus
Mastoid foramen
Subarcuate fossa
Jugular foramen
Hypoglossal canal
Internal occipital protuberance

Foramen caecum
Ala of crista galli
Crista galli
Cribriform plate and foramina
Sphenoidal bone, body
Optic canal
Sphenofrontal suture
Hypophysial fossa
Anterior clinoid process
Carotid sulcus
Sphenosquamous suture
Arterial groove
Petro-occipital fissure
Spine of sphenoid bone
Groove for inferior petrosal sinus
Petrosquamous fissure
Internal acoustic pore
Superior border of petrous part
Jugular foramen
Groove for sigmoid sinus
Condylar canal
Occipitomastoid suture
Hypoglossal canal
Clivus
Groove for transverse sinus

Foramen magnum
(Internal occipital crest)
Groove for superior sagittal sinus

▉ Frontal bone	▉ Ethmoidal bone	▉ Temporal bone
▉ Parietal bone	▉ Sphenoidal bone	▉ Occipital bone

Fig. 68   Internal surface of the base of the skull.

Bones of the skull

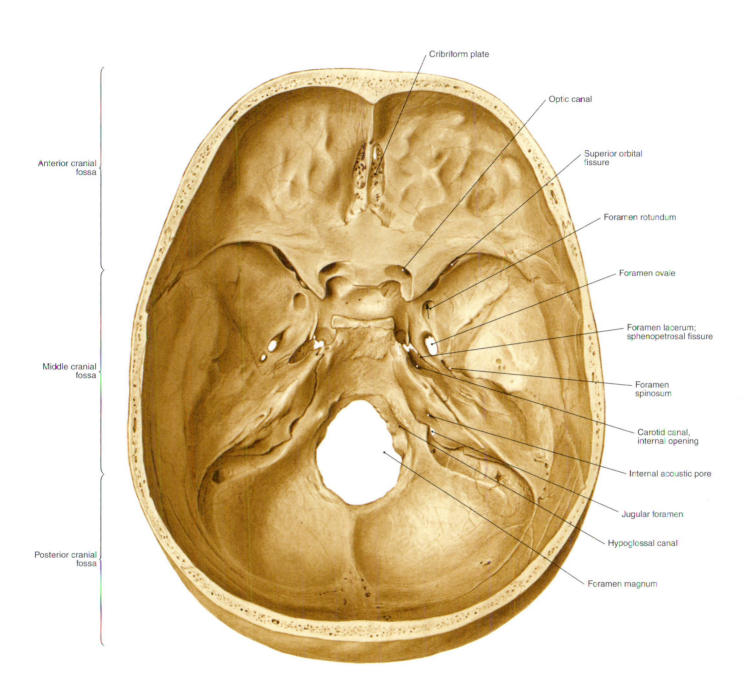

Cribriform plate

Optic canal

Superior orbital fissure

Foramen rotundum

Foramen ovale

Foramen lacerum; sphenopetrosal fissure

Foramen spinosum

Carotid canal, internal opening

Internal acoustic pore

Jugular foramen

Hypoglossal canal

Foramen magnum

Anterior cranial fossa

Middle cranial fossa

Posterior cranial fossa

Fig. 69 Internal surface of the base of the skull and foramina.

→ 1173

Bones of the skull

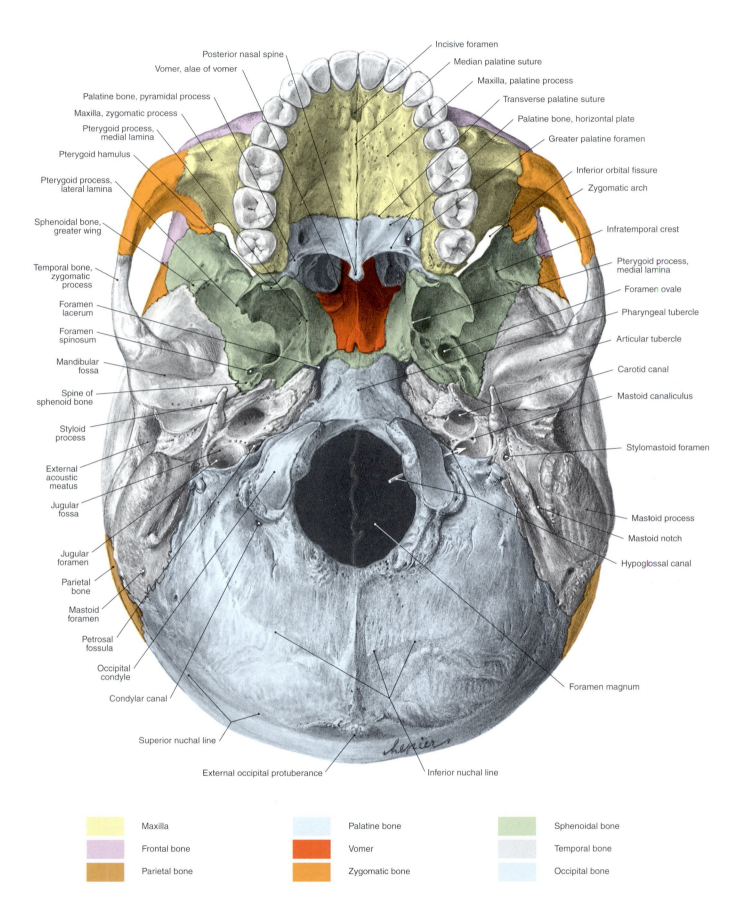

Posterior nasal spine

Vomer, alae of vomer

Palatine bone, pyramidal process

Maxilla, zygomatic process

Pterygoid process, medial lamina

Pterygoid hamulus

Pterygoid process, lateral lamina

Sphenoidal bone, greater wing

Temporal bone, zygomatic process

Foramen lacerum

Foramen spinosum

Mandibular fossa

Spine of sphenoid bone

Styloid process

External acoustic meatus

Jugular fossa

Jugular foramen

Parietal bone

Mastoid foramen

Petrosal fossula

Occipital condyle

Condylar canal

Superior nuchal line

External occipital protuberance

Incisive foramen

Median palatine suture

Maxilla, palatine process

Transverse palatine suture

Palatine bone, horizontal plate

Greater palatine foramen

Inferior orbital fissure

Zygomatic arch

Infratemporal crest

Pterygoid process, medial lamina

Foramen ovale

Pharyngeal tubercle

Articular tubercle

Carotid canal

Mastoid canaliculus

Stylomastoid foramen

Mastoid process

Mastoid notch

Hypoglossal canal

Foramen magnum

Inferior nuchal line

☐ Maxilla	☐ Palatine bone	☐ Sphenoidal bone
☐ Frontal bone	☐ Vomer	☐ Temporal bone
☐ Parietal bone	☐ Zygomatic bone	☐ Occipital bone

Fig. 70   External surface of the base of the skull.

Bones of the skull

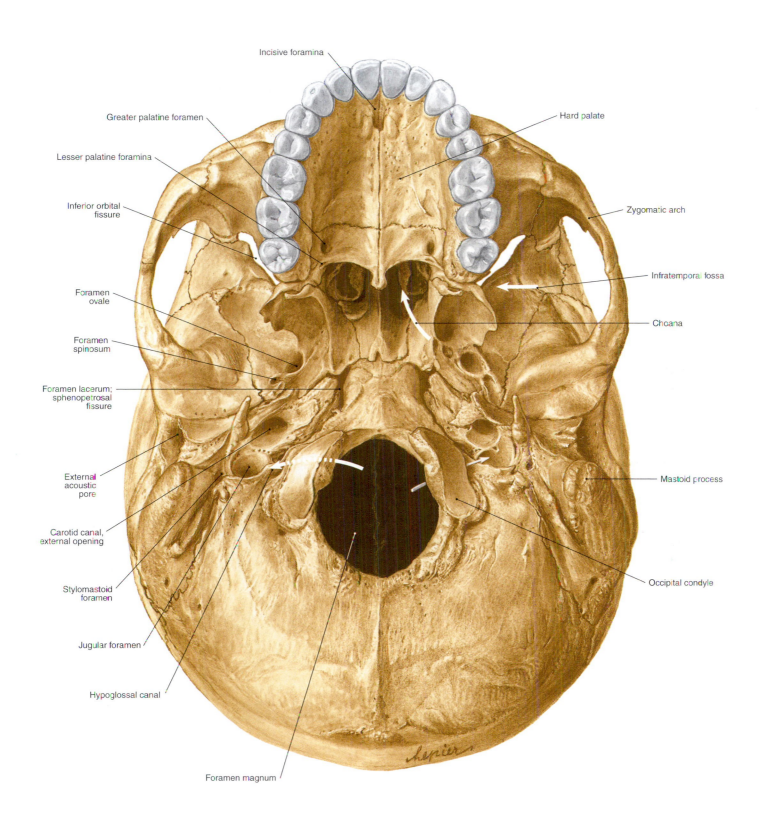

Incisive foramina

Greater palatine foramen

Lesser palatine foramina

Inferior orbital fissure

Foramen ovale

Foramen spinosum

Foramen lacerum; sphenopetrosal fissure

External acoustic pore

Carotid canal, external opening

Stylomastoid foramen

Jugular foramen

Hypoglossal canal

Foramen magnum

Hard palate

Zygomatic arch

Infratemporal fossa

Choana

Mastoid process

Occipital condyle

Fig. 71 External surface of the base of the skull and foramina.

→ 1172

Skull, radiography

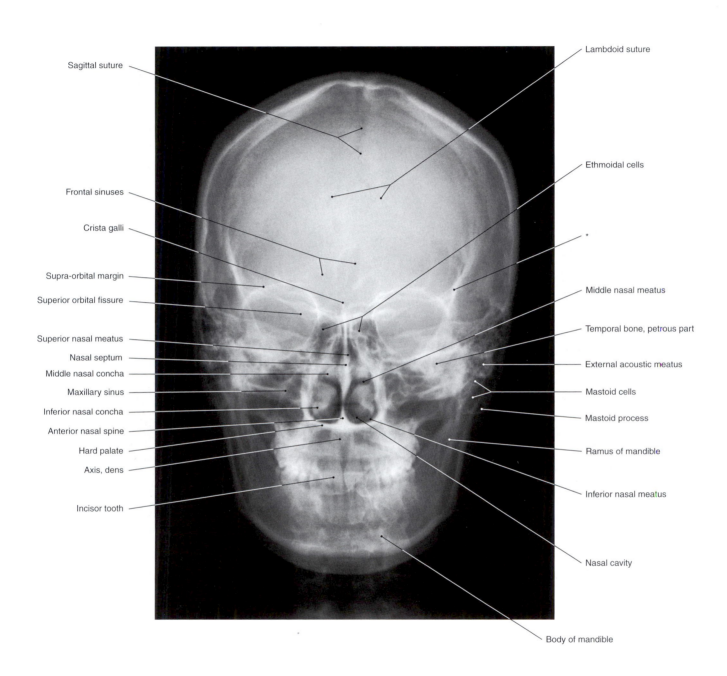

Sagittal suture

Frontal sinuses

Crista galli

Supra-orbital margin

Superior orbital fissure

Superior nasal meatus

Nasal septum

Middle nasal concha

Maxillary sinus

Inferior nasal concha

Anterior nasal spine

Hard palate

Axis, dens

Incisor tooth

Lambdoid suture

Ethmoidal cells

*

Middle nasal meatus

Temporal bone, petrous part

External acoustic meatus

Mastoid cells

Mastoid process

Ramus of mandible

Inferior nasal meatus

Nasal cavity

Body of mandible

Fig. 72   Skull;
AP-teleradiograph.

*   Innominate line, a projection line
without anatomical correlate

Skull, radiography

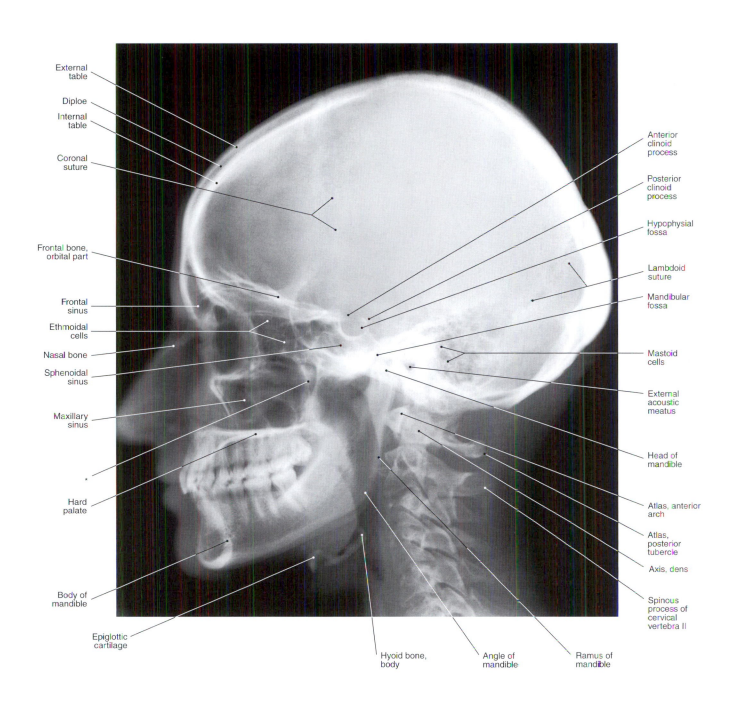

External
table

Diploe

Internal
table

Coronal
suture

Frontal bone,
orbital part

Frontal
sinus

Ethmoidal
cells

Nasal bone

Sphenoidal
sinus

Maxillary
sinus

*

Hard
palate

Body of
mandible

Epiglottic
cartilage

Anterior
clinoid
process

Posterior
clinoid
process

Hypophysial
fossa

Lambdoid
suture

Mandibular
fossa

Mastoid
cells

External
acoustic
meatus

Head of
mandible

Atlas, anterior
arch

Atlas,
posterior
tubercle

Axis, dens

Spinous
process of
cervical
vertebra II

Hyoid bone,
body

Angle of
mandible

Ramus of
mandible

Fig. 73   Skull;
lateral teleradiograph.

*   Posterior wall of the maxillary sinus

Skull, development

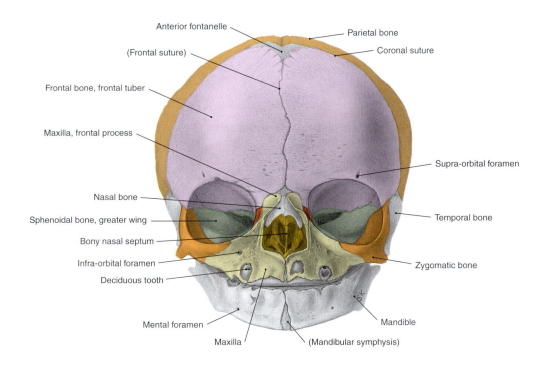

Anterior fontanelle

Parietal bone

(Frontal suture)

Coronal suture

Frontal bone, frontal tuber

Maxilla, frontal process

Supra-orbital foramen

Nasal bone

Sphenoidal bone, greater wing

Temporal bone

Bony nasal septum

Infra-orbital foramen

Zygomatic bone

Deciduous tooth

Mental foramen

Mandible

Maxilla

(Mandibular symphysis)

Fig. 74 Skull of a neonate.

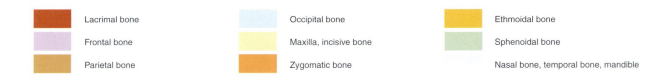

	Lacrimal bone		Occipital bone		Ethmoidal bone
	Frontal bone		Maxilla, incisive bone		Sphenoidal bone
	Parietal bone		Zygomatic bone		Nasal bone, temporal bone, mandible

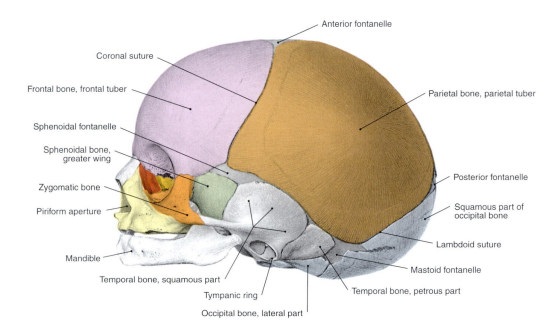

Anterior fontanelle

Coronal suture

Frontal bone, frontal tuber

Parietal bone, parietal tuber

Sphenoidal fontanelle

Sphenoidal bone, greater wing

Zygomatic bone

Posterior fontanelle

Piriform aperture

Squamous part of occipital bone

Lambdoid suture

Mandible

Mastoid fontanelle

Temporal bone, squamous part

Temporal bone, petrous part

Tympanic ring

Occipital bone, lateral part

Fig. 75 Skull of a neonate.

Skull, development

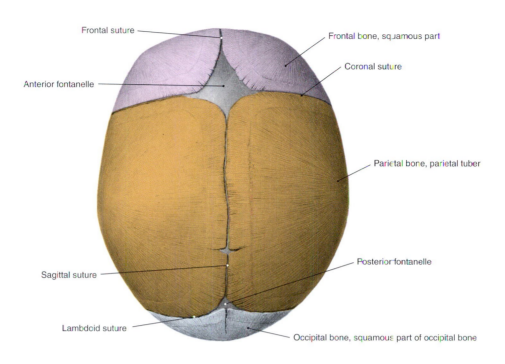

Frontal suture — Frontal bone, squamous part

Coronal suture

Anterior fontanelle

Parietal bone, parietal tuber

Posterior fontanelle

Sagittal suture

Lambdoid suture

Occipital bone, squamous part of occipital bone

Fig. 76 Skull of a neonate.

■	Vomer	■	Occipital bone, palatine bone	■	Maxilla, incisive bone
■	Frontal bone	■	Temporal bone	■	Zygomatic bone
■	Parietal bone	■	Mandible	■	Sphenoidal bone

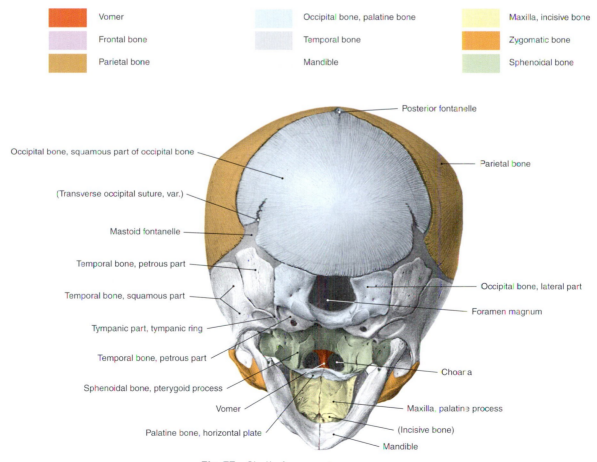

Posterior fontanelle

Occipital bone, squamous part of occipital bone

Parietal bone

(Transverse occipital suture, var.)

Mastoid fontanelle

Temporal bone, petrous part

Temporal bone, squamous part

Occipital bone, lateral part

Foramen magnum

Tympanic part, tympanic ring

Temporal bone, petrous part

Choana

Sphenoidal bone, pterygoid process

Vomer

Maxilla, palatine process

(Incisive bone)

Palatine bone, horizontal plate

Mandible

Fig. 77 Skull of a neonate.

Frontal and ethmoidal bone

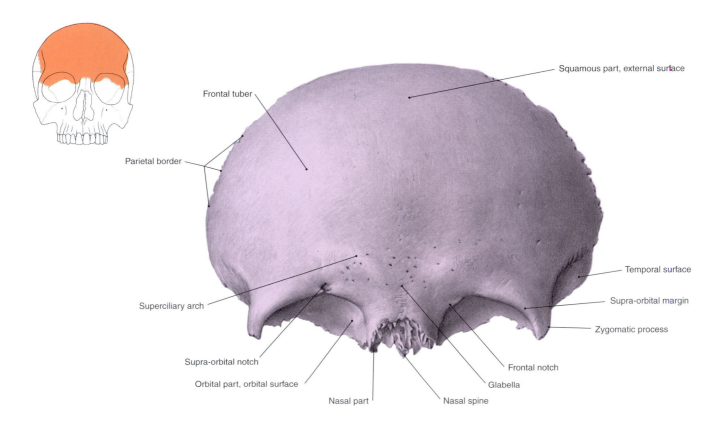

Squamous part, external surface

Frontal tuber

Parietal border

Superciliary arch

Supra-orbital notch

Orbital part, orbital surface

Nasal part

Nasal spine

Glabella

Frontal notch

Zygomatic process

Supra-orbital margin

Temporal surface

Fig. 78 Frontal bone.

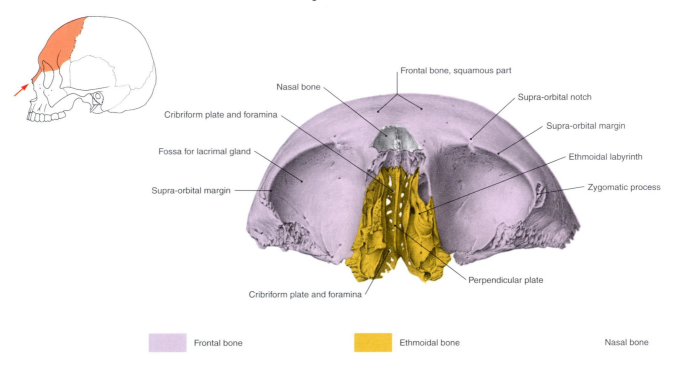

Nasal bone

Frontal bone, squamous part

Cribriform plate and foramina

Supra-orbital notch

Supra-orbital margin

Fossa for lacrimal gland

Ethmoidal labyrinth

Supra-orbital margin

Zygomatic process

Perpendicular plate

Cribriform plate and foramina

	Frontal bone		Ethmoidal bone		Nasal bone

Fig. 79 Frontal bone; ethmoidal bone and nasal bones.

Maxilla and palatine bone

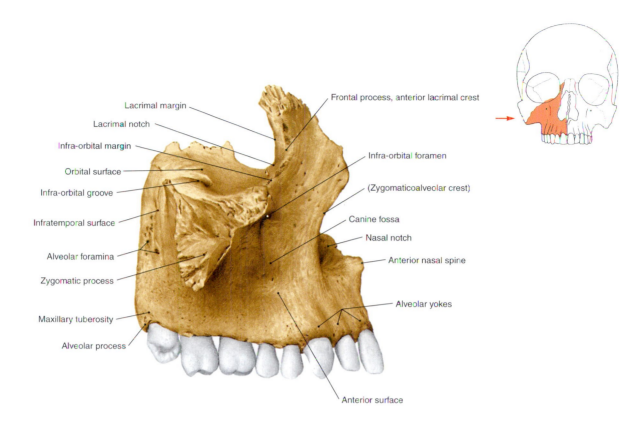

Lacrimal margin

Lacrimal notch

Infra-orbital margin

Orbital surface

Infra-orbital groove

Infratemporal surface

Alveolar foramina

Zygomatic process

Maxillary tuberosity

Alveolar process

Frontal process, anterior lacrimal crest

Infra-orbital foramen

(Zygomaticoalveolar crest)

Canine fossa

Nasal notch

Anterior nasal spine

Alveolar yokes

Anterior surface

Fig. 80 Maxilla.

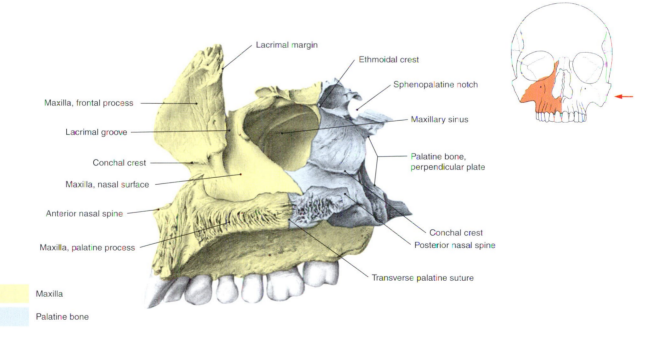

Lacrimal margin

Maxilla, frontal process

Lacrimal groove

Conchal crest

Maxilla, nasal surface

Anterior nasal spine

Maxilla, palatine process

Ethmoidal crest

Sphenopalatine notch

Maxillary sinus

Palatine bone, perpendicular plate

Conchal crest

Posterior nasal spine

Transverse palatine suture

Maxilla

Palatine bone

Fig. 81 Maxilla and palatine bone.

Nasal cavity

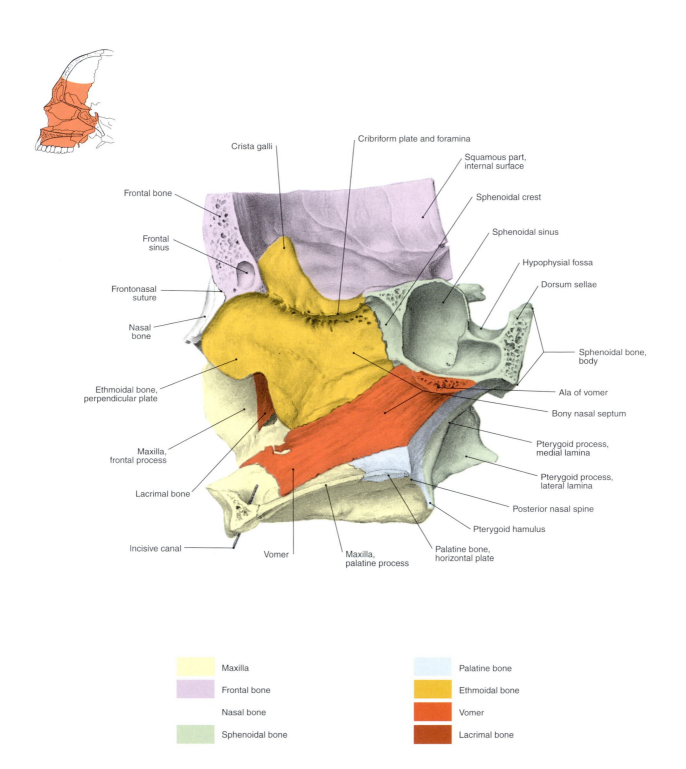

Crista galli

Cribriform plate and foramina

Squamous part, internal surface

Sphenoidal crest

Frontal bone

Frontal sinus

Sphenoidal sinus

Hypophysial fossa

Dorsum sellae

Frontonasal suture

Nasal bone

Sphenoidal bone, body

Ethmoidal bone, perpendicular plate

Ala of vomer

Bony nasal septum

Maxilla, frontal process

Pterygoid process, medial lamina

Pterygoid process, lateral lamina

Lacrimal bone

Posterior nasal spine

Pterygoid hamulus

Incisive canal

Vomer

Maxilla, palatine process

Palatine bone, horizontal plate

	Maxilla		Palatine bone
	Frontal bone		Ethmoidal bone
	Nasal bone		Vomer
	Sphenoidal bone		Lacrimal bone

Fig. 82 Bony nasal septum.

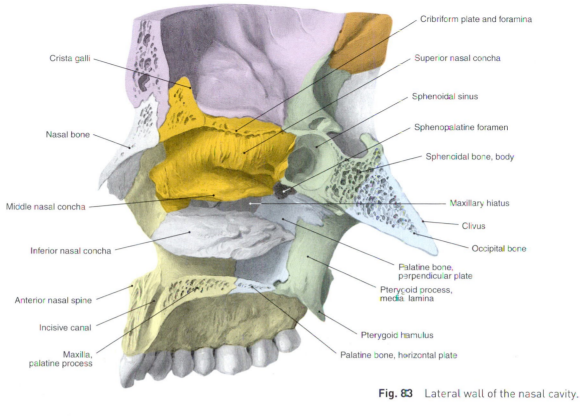

Cribriform plate and foramina
Crista galli
Superior nasal concha
Sphenoidal sinus
Nasal bone
Sphenopalatine foramen
Sphenoidal bone, body
Middle nasal concha
Maxillary hiatus
Clivus
Inferior nasal concha
Occipital bone
Palatine bone, perpendicular plate
Anterior nasal spine
Pterygoid process, medial lamina
Incisive canal
Pterygoid hamulus
Maxilla, palatine process
Palatine bone, horizontal plate

Fig. 83 Lateral wall of the nasal cavity.

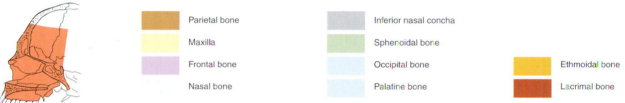

Parietal bone	Inferior nasal concha
Maxilla	Sphenoidal bone
Frontal bone	Occipital bone
Nasal bone	Palatine bone

Ethmoidal bone
Lacrimal bone

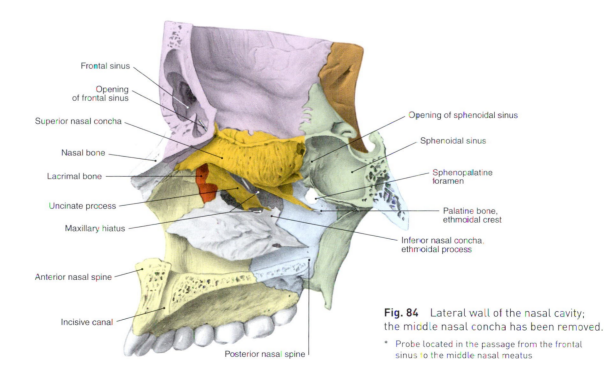

Frontal sinus
Opening of frontal sinus
Superior nasal concha
Opening of sphenoidal sinus
Nasal bone
Sphenoidal sinus
Lacrimal bone
Sphenopalatine foramen
Uncinate process
Maxillary hiatus
Palatine bone, ethmoidal crest
Anterior nasal spine
Inferior nasal concha, ethmoidal process
Incisive canal
Posterior nasal spine

Fig. 84 Lateral wall of the nasal cavity; the middle nasal concha has been removed.

* Probe located in the passage from the frontal sinus to the middle nasal meatus

Hard palate

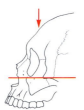

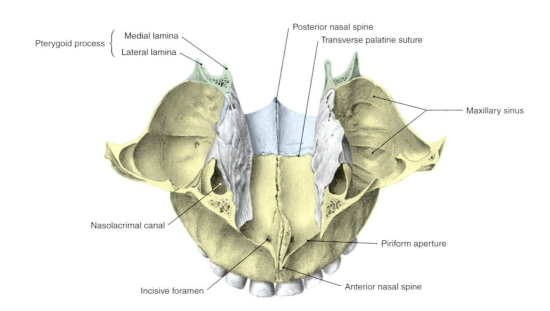

Pterygoid process { Medial lamina / Lateral lamina

Posterior nasal spine

Transverse palatine suture

Maxillary sinus

Nasolacrimal canal

Piriform aperture

Incisive foramen

Anterior nasal spine

Fig. 85 Hard palate; maxillary sinus and inferior nasal concha.

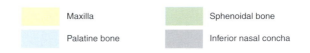

| Maxilla | Sphenoidal bone |
| Palatine bone | Inferior nasal concha |

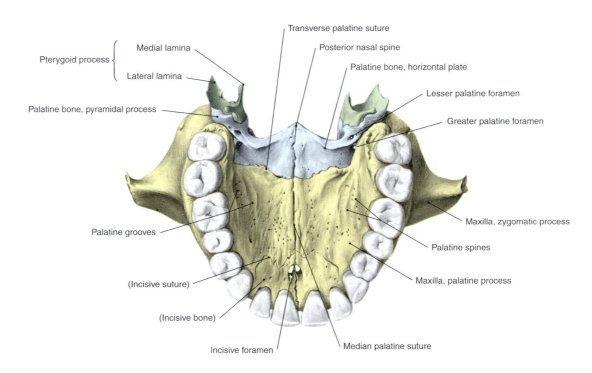

Pterygoid process { Medial lamina / Lateral lamina

Transverse palatine suture

Posterior nasal spine

Palatine bone, horizontal plate

Palatine bone, pyramidal process

Lesser palatine foramen

Greater palatine foramen

Palatine grooves

Maxilla, zygomatic process

Palatine spines

(Incisive suture)

Maxilla, palatine process

(Incisive bone)

Incisive foramen

Median palatine suture

Fig. 86 Hard palate.

Orbit and pterygopalatine fossa

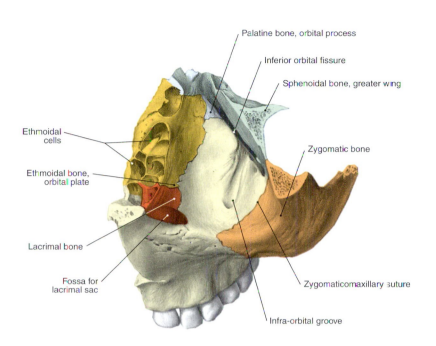

Palatine bone, orbital process

Inferior orbital fissure

Sphenoidal bone, greater wing

Ethmoidal cells

Zygomatic bone

Ethmoidal bone, orbital plate

Lacrimal bone

Fossa for lacrimal sac

Zygomaticomaxillary suture

Infra-orbital groove

Fig. 87 Base of the orbit.

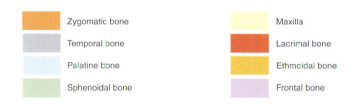

	Zygomatic bone		Maxilla
	Temporal bone		Lacrimal bone
	Palatine bone		Ethmoidal bone
	Sphenoidal bone		Frontal bone

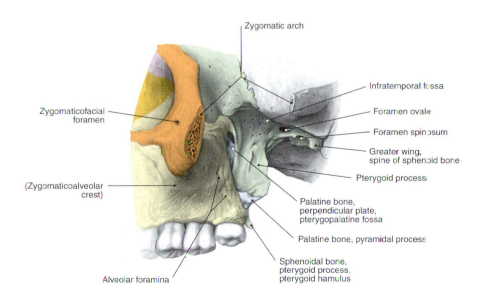

Zygomatic arch

Infratemporal fossa

Zygomaticofacial foramen

Foramen ovale

Foramen spinosum

Greater wing, spine of sphenoid bone

(Zygomaticoalveolar crest)

Pterygoid process

Palatine bone, perpendicular plate, pterygopalatine fossa

Palatine bone, pyramidal process

Sphenoidal bone, pterygoid process, pterygoid hamulus

Alveolar foramina

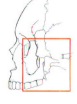

Fig. 88 Pterygopalatine fossa.

Orbit

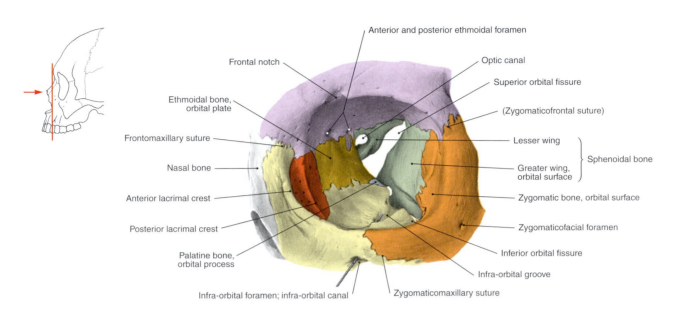

Anterior and posterior ethmoidal foramen

Frontal notch

Optic canal

Superior orbital fissure

Ethmoidal bone, orbital plate

(Zygomaticofrontal suture)

Frontomaxillary suture

Lesser wing

Nasal bone

Greater wing, orbital surface

Sphenoidal bone

Anterior lacrimal crest

Zygomatic bone, orbital surface

Posterior lacrimal crest

Zygomaticofacial foramen

Palatine bone, orbital process

Inferior orbital fissure

Infra-orbital groove

Infra-orbital foramen; infra-orbital canal

Zygomaticomaxillary suture

Fig. 89 Orbit; probe located in the infra-orbital canal.

Nasal bone	Vomer	Temporal bone
Frontal bone	Zygomatic bone	Inferior nasal concha
Palatine bone	Maxilla	Sphenoidal bone
Ethmoidal bone		Lacrimal bone

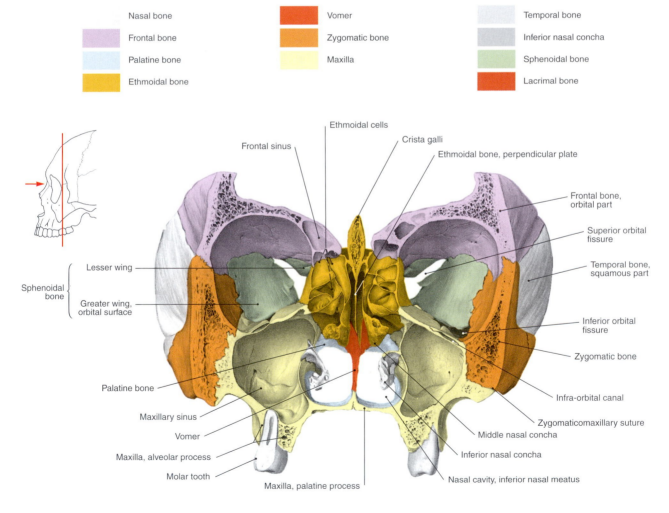

Ethmoidal cells

Frontal sinus

Crista galli

Ethmoidal bone, perpendicular plate

Frontal bone, orbital part

Superior orbital fissure

Lesser wing

Temporal bone, squamous part

Sphenoidal bone

Greater wing, orbital surface

Inferior orbital fissure

Zygomatic bone

Palatine bone

Infra-orbital canal

Maxillary sinus

Zygomaticomaxillary suture

Vomer

Middle nasal concha

Maxilla, alveolar process

Inferior nasal concha

Molar tooth

Nasal cavity, inferior nasal meatus

Maxilla, palatine process

Fig. 90 Facial skeleton; frontal section.

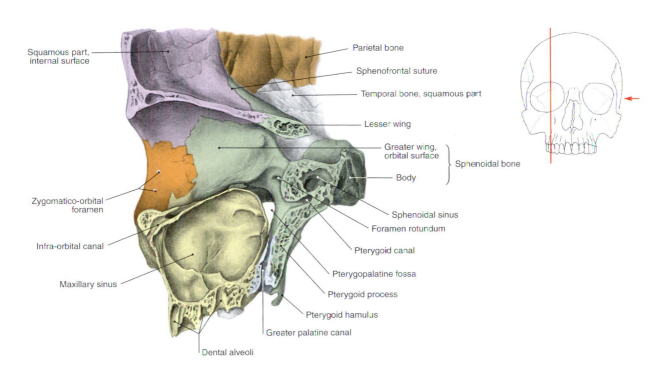

Squamous part, internal surface
Parietal bone
Sphenofrontal suture
Temporal bone, squamous part
Lesser wing
Greater wing, orbital surface
Body
Sphenoidal bone
Sphenoidal sinus
Foramen rotundum
Zygomatico-orbital foramen
Pterygoid canal
Infra-orbital canal
Pterygopalatine fossa
Pterygoid process
Maxillary sinus
Pterygoid hamulus
Greater palatine canal
Dental alveoli

Fig. 91 Orbit; lateral wall.

Frontal bone	Nasal bone	Maxilla
Lacrimal bone	Palatine bone	Temporal bone
Sphenoidal bone	Ethmoidal bone	Zygomatic bone

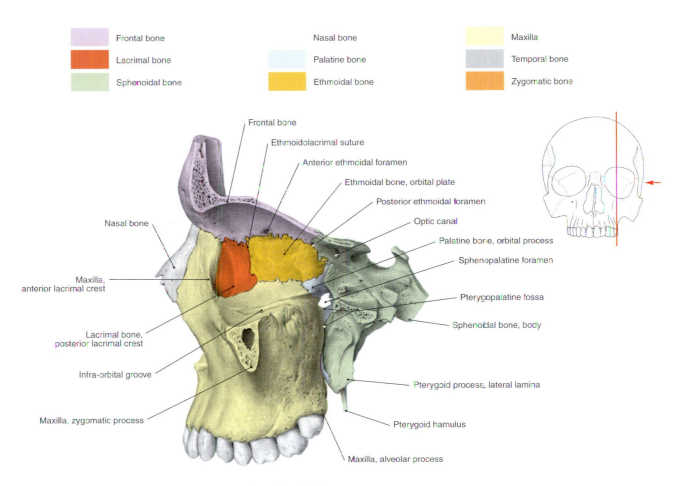

Frontal bone
Ethmoidolacrimal suture
Anterior ethmoidal foramen
Ethmoidal bone, orbital plate
Posterior ethmoidal foramen
Optic canal
Nasal bone
Palatine bone, orbital process
Sphenopalatine foramen
Maxilla, anterior lacrimal crest
Pterygopalatine fossa
Sphenoidal bone, body
Lacrimal bone, posterior lacrimal crest
Infra-orbital groove
Pterygoid process, lateral lamina
Maxilla, zygomatic process
Pterygoid hamulus
Maxilla, alveolar process

Fig. 92 Orbit; medial wall.

Sphenoidal bone

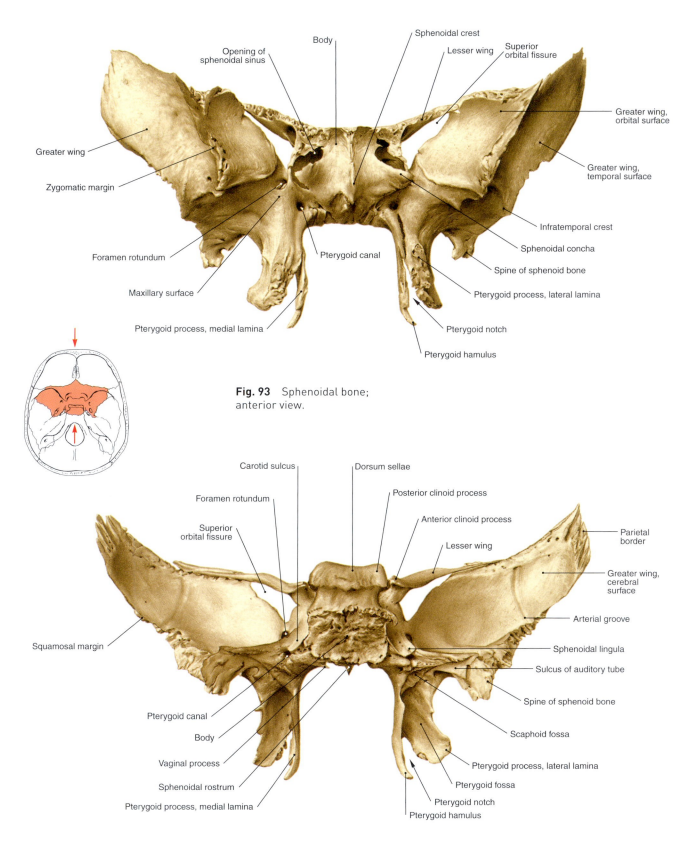

Body
Sphenoidal crest
Opening of sphenoidal sinus
Lesser wing
Superior orbital fissure
Greater wing, orbital surface
Greater wing
Greater wing, temporal surface
Zygomatic margin
Infratemporal crest
Sphenoidal concha
Foramen rotundum
Spine of sphenoid bone
Pterygoid canal
Pterygoid process, lateral lamina
Maxillary surface
Pterygoid notch
Pterygoid process, medial lamina
Pterygoid hamulus

Fig. 93 Sphenoidal bone; anterior view.

Carotid sulcus
Dorsum sellae
Foramen rotundum
Posterior clinoid process
Anterior clinoid process
Superior orbital fissure
Parietal border
Lesser wing
Greater wing, cerebral surface
Arterial groove
Squamosal margin
Sphenoidal lingula
Sulcus of auditory tube
Spine of sphenoid bone
Pterygoid canal
Scaphoid fossa
Body
Vaginal process
Pterygoid process, lateral lamina
Sphenoidal rostrum
Pterygoid fossa
Pterygoid process, medial lamina
Pterygoid notch
Pterygoid hamulus

Fig. 94 Sphenoidal bone; posterior view.

Sphenoidal and occipital bone

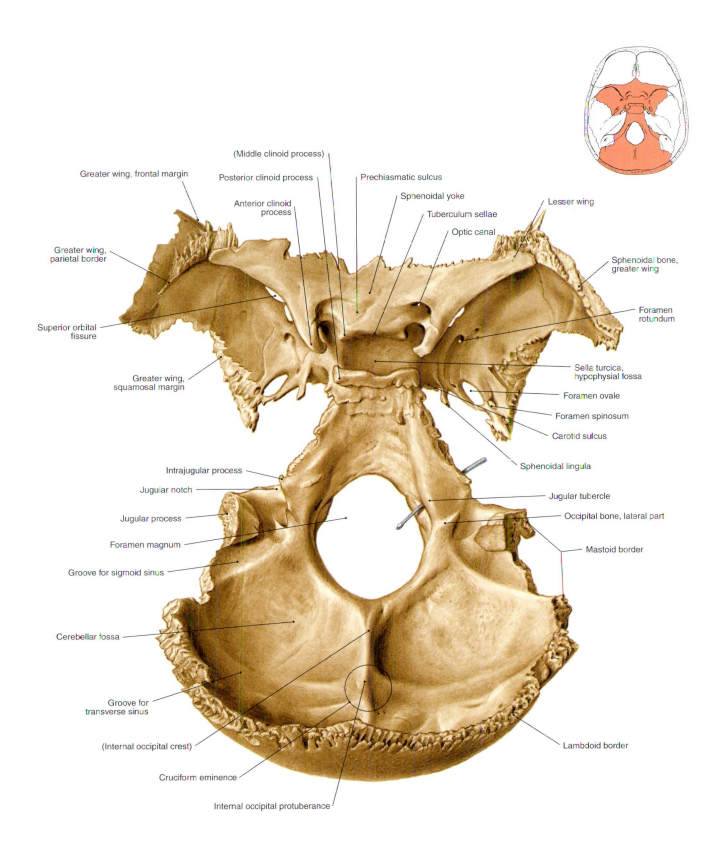

Greater wing, frontal margin

(Middle clinoid process)

Posterior clinoid process

Prechiasmatic sulcus

Sphenoidal yoke

Anterior clinoid process

Tuberculum sellae

Optic canal

Lesser wing

Greater wing, parietal border

Sphenoidal bone, greater wing

Superior orbital fissure

Foramen rotundum

Greater wing, squamosal margin

Sella turcica, hypophysial fossa

Foramen ovale

Foramen spinosum

Carotid sulcus

Sphenoidal lingula

Intrajugular process

Jugular notch

Jugular tubercle

Jugular process

Occipital bone, lateral part

Foramen magnum

Mastoid border

Groove for sigmoid sinus

Cerebellar fossa

Groove for transverse sinus

(Internal occipital crest)

Lambdoid border

Cruciform eminence

Internal occipital protuberance

Fig. 95 Occipital bone and sphenoidal bone.

Temporal bone

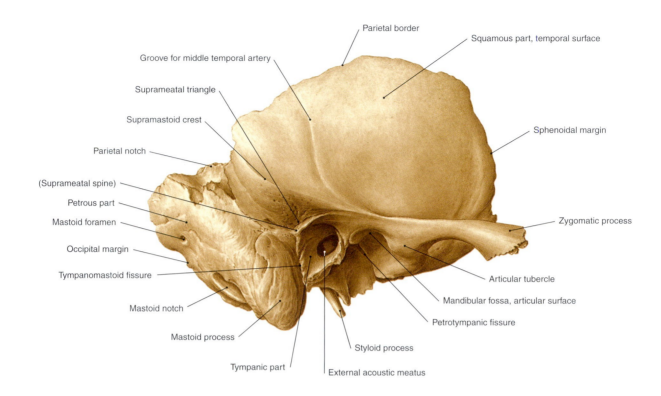

Parietal border

Squamous part, temporal surface

Groove for middle temporal artery

Suprameatal triangle

Supramastoid crest

Sphenoidal margin

Parietal notch

(Suprameatal spine)

Petrous part

Mastoid foramen

Zygomatic process

Occipital margin

Tympanomastoid fissure

Mastoid notch

Articular tubercle

Mandibular fossa, articular surface

Petrotympanic fissure

Mastoid process

Styloid process

Tympanic part

External acoustic meatus

Fig. 96 Temporal bone.

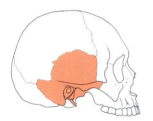

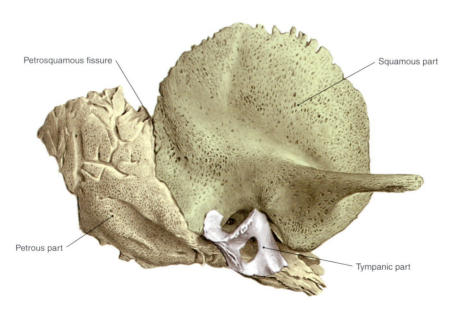

Petrosquamous fissure

Squamous part

Petrous part

Tympanic part

Fig. 97 Temporal bone of a neonate.

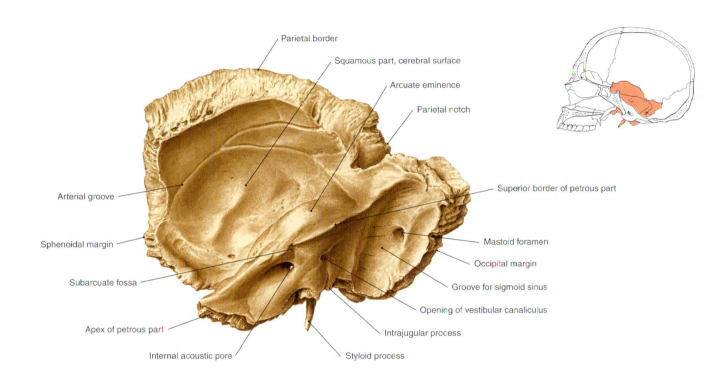

Parietal border
Squamous part, cerebral surface
Arcuate eminence
Parietal notch
Arterial groove
Superior border of petrous part
Sphenoidal margin
Mastoid foramen
Occipital margin
Subarcuate fossa
Groove for sigmoid sinus
Opening of vestibular canaliculus
Apex of petrous part
Intrajugular process
Internal acoustic pore
Styloid process

Fig. 98   Temporal bone.

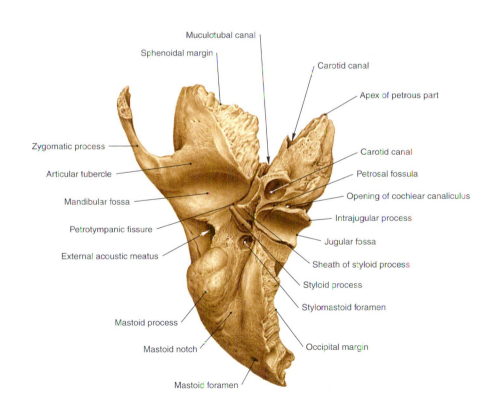
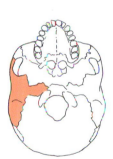

Muculotubal canal
Sphenoidal margin
Carotid canal
Apex of petrous part
Zygomatic process
Carotid canal
Articular tubercle
Petrosal fossula
Mandibular fossa
Opening of cochlear canaliculus
Petrotympanic fissure
Intrajugular process
External acoustic meatus
Jugular fossa
Sheath of styloid process
Styloid process
Stylomastoid foramen
Mastoid process
Occipital margin
Mastoid notch
Mastoid foramen

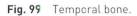

Fig. 99   Temporal bone.

Mandible

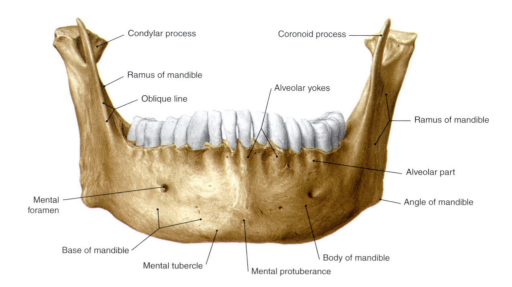

Fig. 100 Mandible.

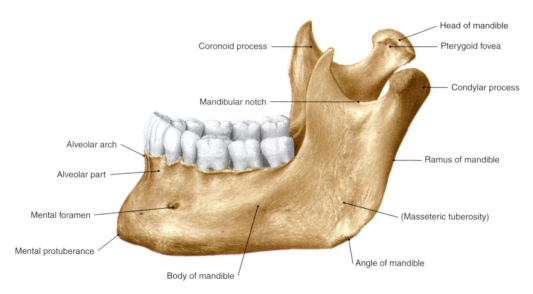

Fig. 101 Mandible.

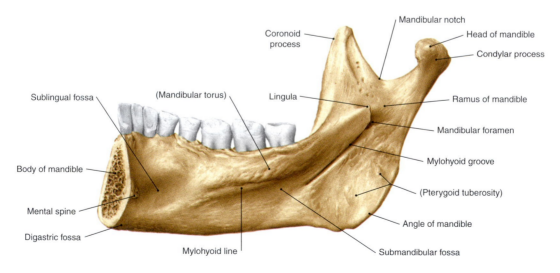

Fig. 102 Mandible.

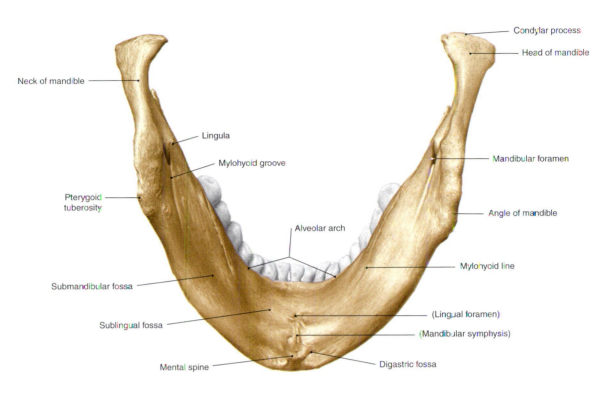

Condylar process

Head of mandible

Neck of mandible

Lingula

Mylohyoid groove

Mandibular foramen

Pterygoid
tuberosity

Angle of mandible

Alveolar arch

Mylohyoid line

Submandibular fossa

(Lingual foramen)

Sublingual fossa

(Mandibular symphysis)

Mental spine

Digastric fossa

Fig. 103 Mandible.

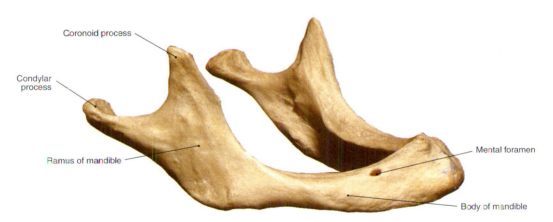

Coronoid process

Condylar
process

Mental foramen

Ramus of mandible

Body of mandible

Fig. 104 Mandible of an elderly individual.

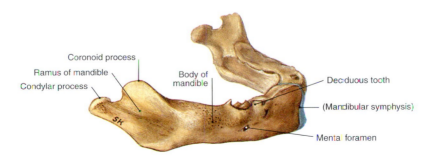

Coronoid process

Ramus of mandible

Condylar process

Body of
mandible

Deciduous tooth

(Mandibular symphysis)

Mental foramen

Fig. 105 Mandible of a neonate.

Temporomandibular joint

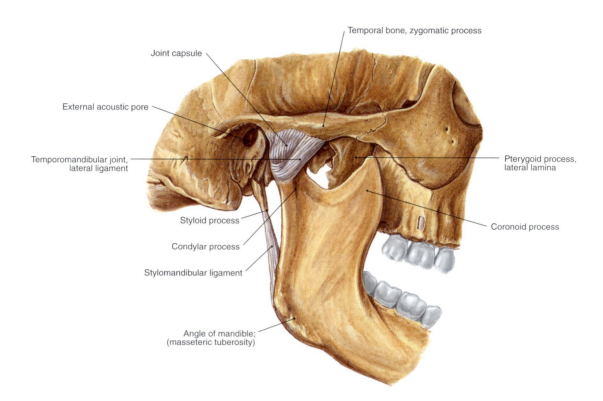

Joint capsule

Temporal bone, zygomatic process

External acoustic pore

Temporomandibular joint, lateral ligament

Pterygoid process, lateral lamina

Styloid process

Coronoid process

Condylar process

Stylomandibular ligament

Angle of mandible; (masseteric tuberosity)

Fig. 106 Temporomandibular joint.

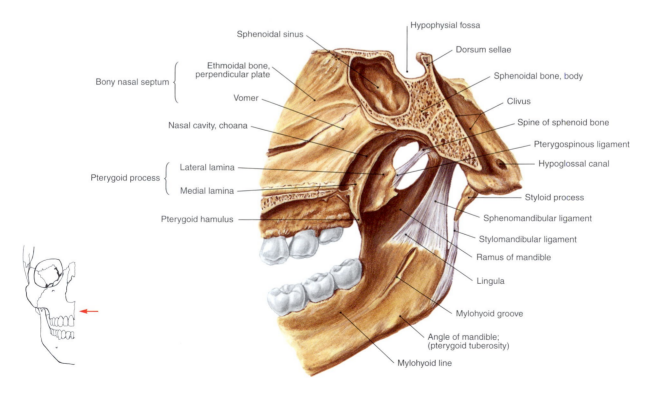

Sphenoidal sinus

Hypophysial fossa

Dorsum sellae

Ethmoidal bone, perpendicular plate

Bony nasal septum

Sphenoidal bone, body

Vomer

Clivus

Nasal cavity, choana

Spine of sphenoid bone

Pterygospinous ligament

Pterygoid process

Lateral lamina

Medial lamina

Hypoglossal canal

Styloid process

Sphenomandibular ligament

Pterygoid hamulus

Stylomandibular ligament

Ramus of mandible

Lingula

Mylohyoid groove

Angle of mandible; (pterygoid tuberosity)

Mylohyoid line

Fig. 107 Pterygospinous and sphenomandibular ligaments.

Temporomandibular joint

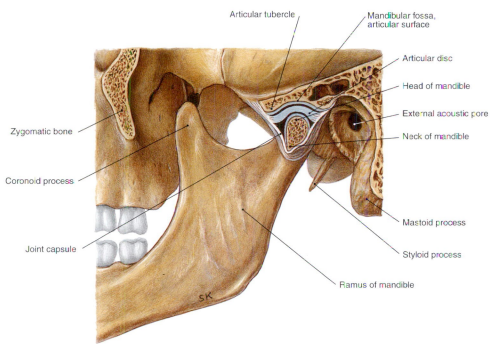

Articular tubercle

Mandibular fossa, articular surface

Articular disc

Head of mandible

External acoustic pore

Neck of mandible

Zygomatic bone

Coronoid process

Mastoid process

Joint capsule

Styloid process

Ramus of mandible

Fig. 108 Temporomandibular joint; sagittal section; mouth almost closed.

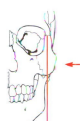

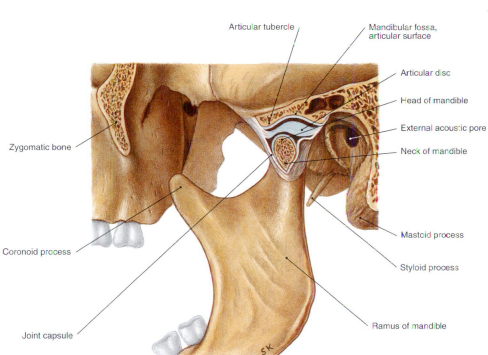

Articular tubercle

Mandibular fossa, articular surface

Articular disc

Head of mandible

External acoustic pore

Neck of mandible

Zygomatic bone

Mastoid process

Coronoid process

Styloid process

Ramus of mandible

Joint capsule

Fig. 109 Temporomandibular joint; sagittal section; mouth opened.

Temporomandibular joint and masticatory muscles

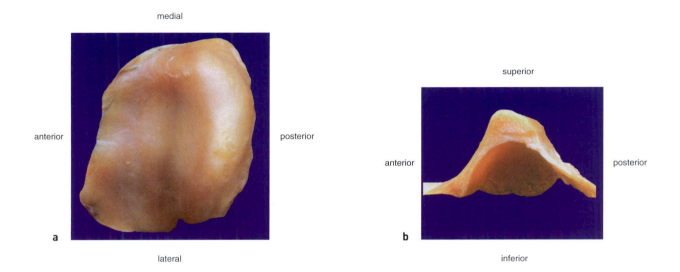

medial

anterior

posterior

lateral

a

superior

anterior

posterior

inferior

b

Fig. 110 a, b Articular disc of the temporomandibular joint.
a Superior view
b Lateral view.

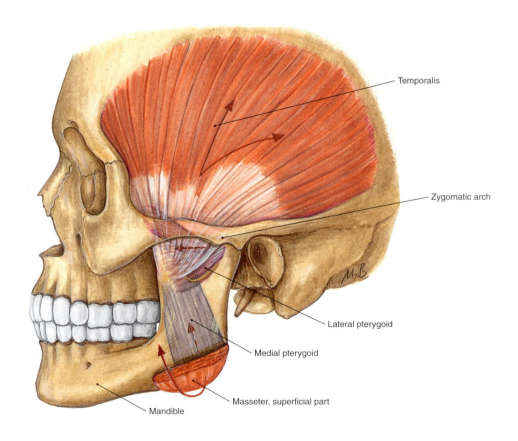

Temporalis

Zygomatic arch

Lateral pterygoid

Medial pterygoid

Masseter, superficial part

Mandible

→ T 4

Fig. 111 Masticatory muscles.
Arrows indicate the direction of muscle traction when closing the mouth.

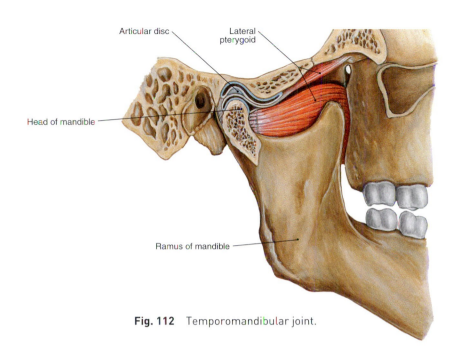

Articular disc
Lateral pterygoid
Head of mandible
Ramus of mandible

Fig. 112   Temporomandibular joint.

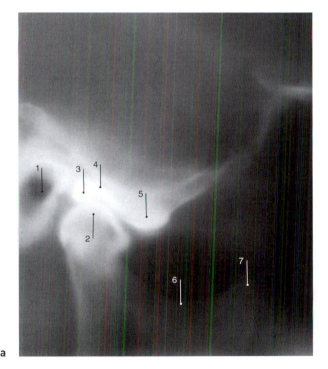

a

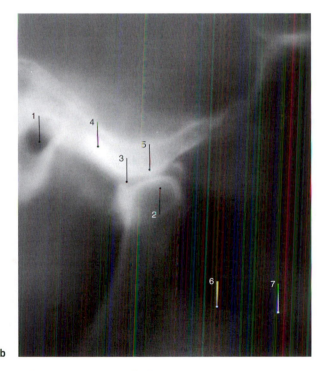

b

1 External acoustic meatus
2 Condylar process
3 Articular disc
4 Temporal bone, mandibular fossa

5 Temporal bone, articular tubercle
6 Mandibular notch
7 Coronoid process

Fig. 113 a, b   Temporomandibular joint;
tomography; lateral projection after injection of a contrast
medium into the joint cavity (arthrography).
a Mouth closed
b Mouth opened

The articular disc shifts forward during opening of the mouth.

→ 108, 109

Masticatory muscles

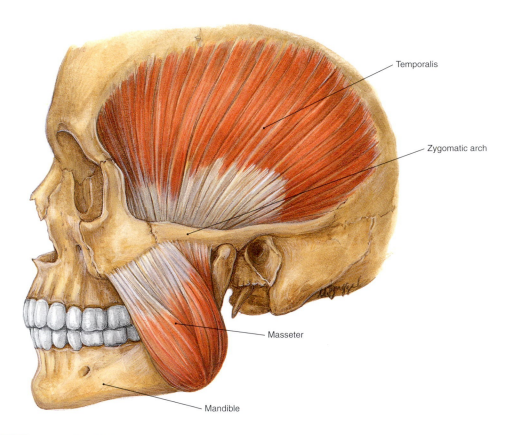

→ T 4

Fig. 114 Masseter and temporal muscle.

Temporalis

Zygomatic arch

Masseter

Mandible

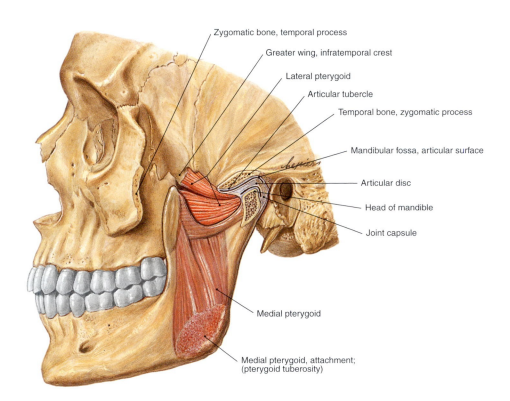

→ T 4

Fig. 115 Temporomandibular joint;
medial and lateral pterygoid muscles.

Zygomatic bone, temporal process

Greater wing, infratemporal crest

Lateral pterygoid

Articular tubercle

Temporal bone, zygomatic process

Mandibular fossa, articular surface

Articular disc

Head of mandible

Joint capsule

Medial pterygoid

Medial pterygoid, attachment;
(pterygoid tuberosity)

Masticatory muscles

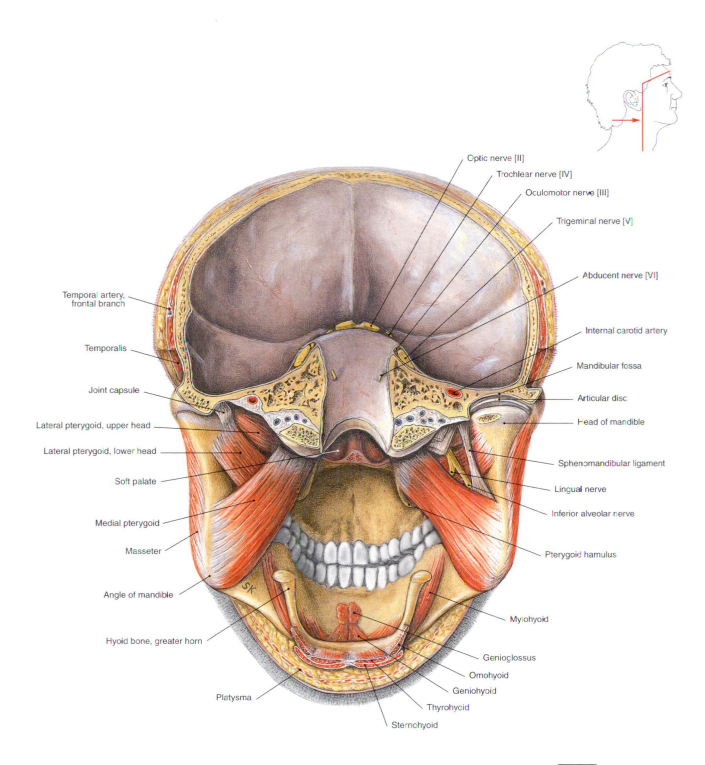

Optic nerve [II]
Trochlear nerve [IV]
Oculomotor nerve [III]
Trigeminal nerve [V]
Abducent nerve [VI]
Internal carotid artery
Mandibular fossa
Articular disc
Head of mandible
Sphenomandibular ligament
Lingual nerve
Inferior alveolar nerve
Pterygoid hamulus
Mylohyoid
Genioglossus
Omohyoid
Geniohyoid
Thyrohyoid
Sternohyoid

Temporal artery, frontal branch
Temporalis
Joint capsule
Lateral pterygoid, upper head
Lateral pterygoid, lower head
Soft palate
Medial pterygoid
Masseter
Angle of mandible
Hyoid bone, greater horn
Platysma

SK

Fig. 116 Masticatory muscles;
frontal section through the temporomandibular joint
and horizontal section through the calvaria;
posterior view.

→ T 4

Masticatory muscles

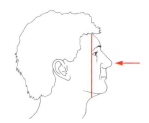

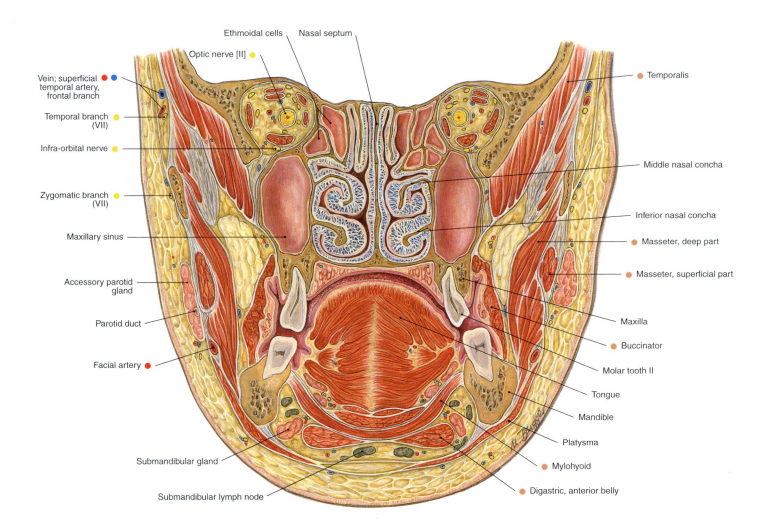

Ethmoidal cells

Nasal septum

Optic nerve [II] ●

Vein; superficial ● ●
temporal artery,
frontal branch

Temporal branch ●
(VII)

Infra-orbital nerve ●

Zygomatic branch ●
(VII)

Maxillary sinus

Accessory parotid
gland

Parotid duct

Facial artery ●

Submandibular gland

Submandibular lymph node

Temporalis ●

Middle nasal concha

Inferior nasal concha

Masseter, deep part ●

Masseter, superficial part ●

Maxilla

Buccinator ●

Molar tooth II

Tongue

Mandible

Platysma

Mylohyoid ●

Digastric, anterior belly ●

→ T 4

Fig. 117 Masticatory muscles;
frontal section;
anterior view.

Masticatory muscles

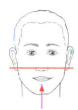

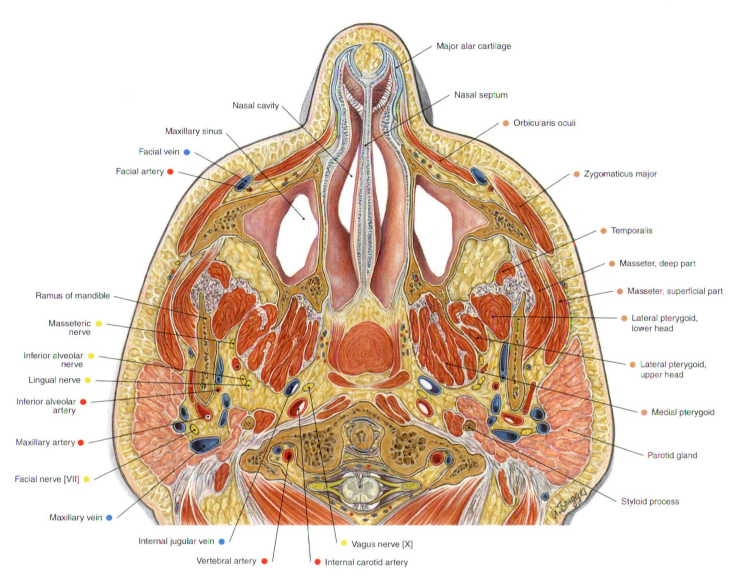

Major alar cartilage

Nasal cavity

Nasal septum

Maxillary sinus

Facial vein ●

Facial artery ●

Orbicularis oculi ●

Zygomaticus major ●

Temporalis ●

Masseter, deep part ●

Masseter, superficial part ●

Lateral pterygoid, lower head ●

Ramus of mandible

Masseteric nerve ●

Inferior alveolar nerve ●

Lingual nerve ●

Inferior alveolar artery ●

Lateral pterygoid, upper head ●

Medial pterygoid ●

Maxillary artery ●

Parotid gland

Facial nerve [VII] ●

Styloid process

Maxillary vein ●

Internal jugular vein ●

Vagus nerve [X] ●

Vertebral artery ●

Internal carotid artery ●

Fig. 118 Masticatory muscles; horizontal section.

 → T 4

Facial and masticatory muscles

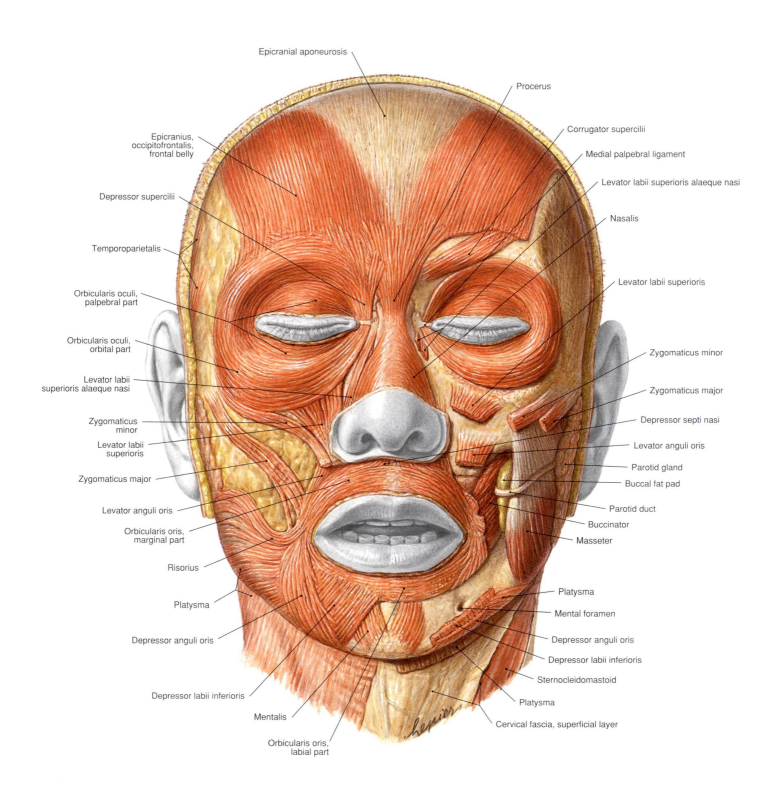

Epicranial aponeurosis

Procerus

Corrugator supercilii

Medial palpebral ligament

Levator labii superioris alaeque nasi

Nasalis

Levator labii superioris

Zygomaticus minor

Zygomaticus major

Depressor septi nasi

Levator anguli oris

Parotid gland

Buccal fat pad

Parotid duct

Buccinator

Masseter

Platysma

Mental foramen

Depressor anguli oris

Depressor labii inferioris

Sternocleidomastoid

Platysma

Cervical fascia, superficial layer

Epicranius, occipitofrontalis, frontal belly

Depressor supercilii

Temporoparietalis

Orbicularis oculi, palpebral part

Orbicularis oculi, orbital part

Levator labii superioris alaeque nasi

Zygomaticus minor

Levator labii superioris

Zygomaticus major

Levator anguli oris

Orbicularis oris, marginal part

Risorius

Platysma

Depressor anguli oris

Depressor labii inferioris

Mentalis

Orbicularis oris, labial part

→ T 1 a, c–f, T 4

Fig. 119 Facial muscles and masticatory muscles.

Facial muscles

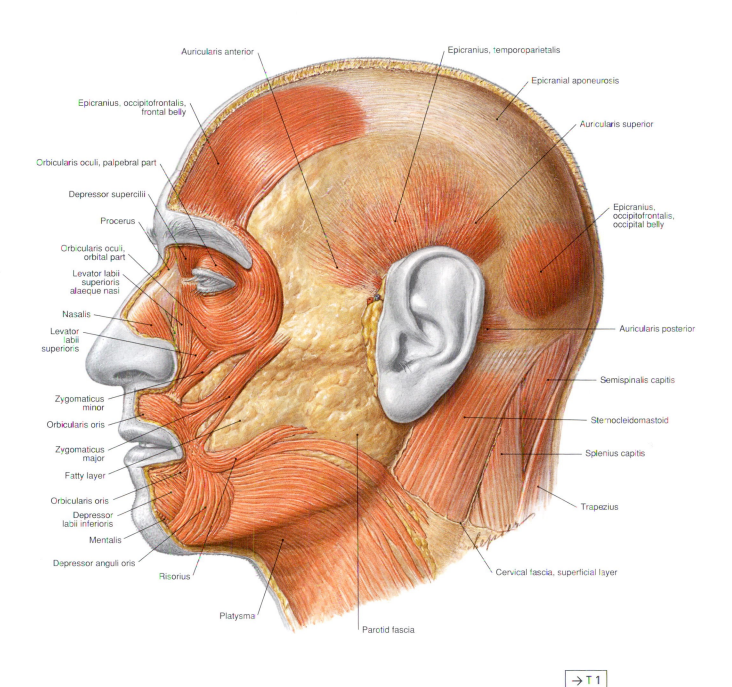

Auricularis anterior

Epicranius, temporoparietalis

Epicranial aponeurosis

Epicranius, occipitofrontalis, frontal belly

Auricularis superior

Orbicularis oculi, palpebral part

Depressor supercilii

Procerus

Epicranius, occipitofrontalis, occipital belly

Orbicularis oculi, orbital part

Levator labii superioris alaeque nasi

Nasalis

Levator labii superioris

Auricularis posterior

Zygomaticus minor

Semispinalis capitis

Orbicularis oris

Sternocleidomastoid

Zygomaticus major

Splenius capitis

Fatty layer

Orbicularis oris

Depressor labii inferioris

Mentalis

Trapezius

Depressor anguli oris

Risorius

Cervical fascia, superficial layer

Platysma

Parotid fascia

→ T 1

121

253

Fig. 120 Facial muscles.

Facial and masticatory muscles

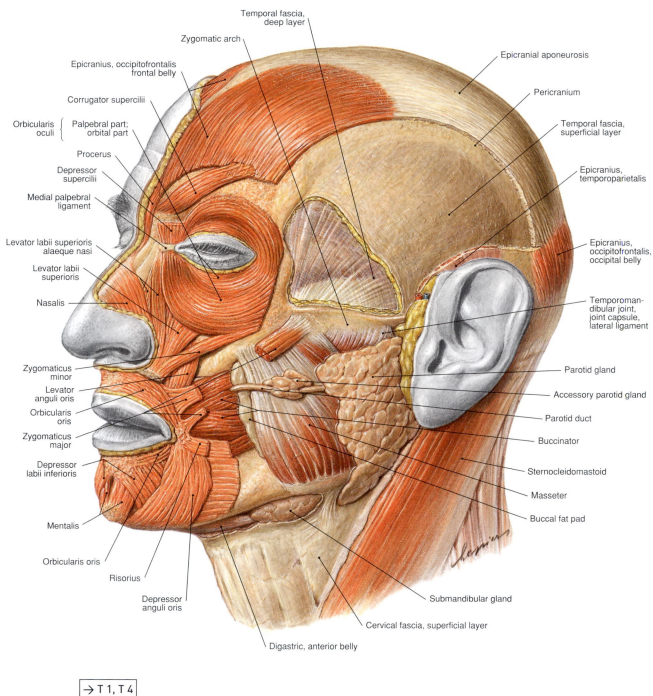

Temporal fascia, deep layer

Zygomatic arch

Epicranius, occipitofrontalis frontal belly

Corrugator supercilii

Orbicularis oculi { Palpebral part; orbital part

Procerus

Depressor supercilii

Medial palpebral ligament

Levator labii superioris alaeque nasi

Levator labii superioris

Nasalis

Zygomaticus minor

Levator anguli oris

Orbicularis oris

Zygomaticus major

Depressor labii inferioris

Mentalis

Orbicularis oris

Risorius

Depressor anguli oris

Digastric, anterior belly

Epicranial aponeurosis

Pericranium

Temporal fascia, superficial layer

Epicranius, temporoparietalis

Epicranius, occipitofrontalis, occipital belly

Temporomandibular joint, joint capsule, lateral ligament

Parotid gland

Accessory parotid gland

Parotid duct

Buccinator

Sternocleidomastoid

Masseter

Buccal fat pad

Submandibular gland

Cervical fascia, superficial layer

→ T 1, T 4

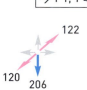

122

120 · 206

Fig. 121 Facial muscles and masticatory muscles.

Facial and masticatory muscles

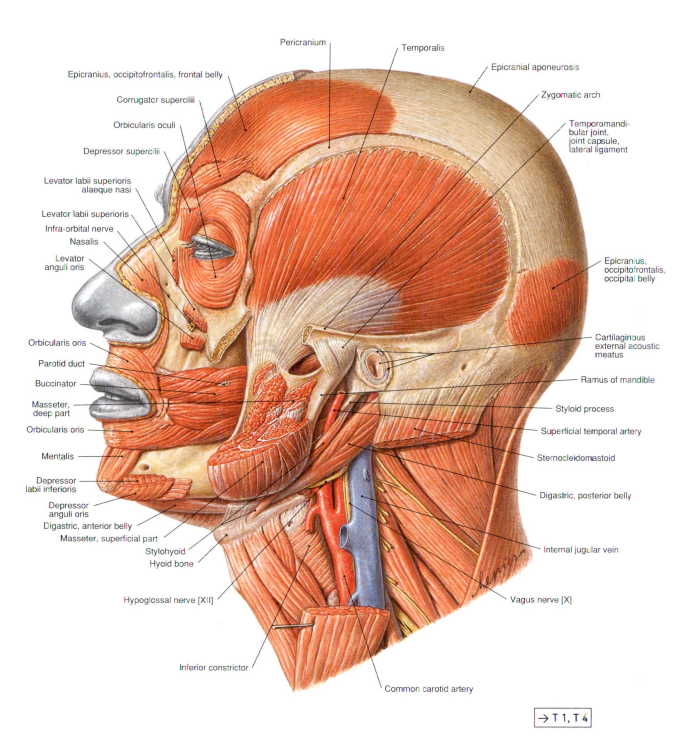

Pericranium

Temporalis

Epicranius, occipitofrontalis, frontal belly

Epicranial aponeurosis

Corrugator supercilii

Zygomatic arch

Orbicularis oculi

Temporomandibular joint, joint capsule, lateral ligament

Depressor supercilii

Levator labii superioris alaeque nasi

Levator labii superioris

Infra-orbital nerve

Nasalis

Levator anguli oris

Epicranius, occipitofrontalis, occipital belly

Orbicularis oris

Parotid duct

Cartilaginous external acoustic meatus

Buccinator

Ramus of mandible

Masseter, deep part

Styloid process

Orbicularis oris

Superficial temporal artery

Mentalis

Sternocleidomastoid

Depressor labii inferioris

Digastric, posterior belly

Depressor anguli oris

Digastric, anterior belly

Masseter, superficial part

Stylohyoid

Hyoid bone

Internal jugular vein

Hypoglossal nerve [XII]

Vagus nerve [X]

Inferior constrictor

Common carotid artery

→ T 1, T 4

Fig. 122 Facial muscles and masticatory muscles.

121

256

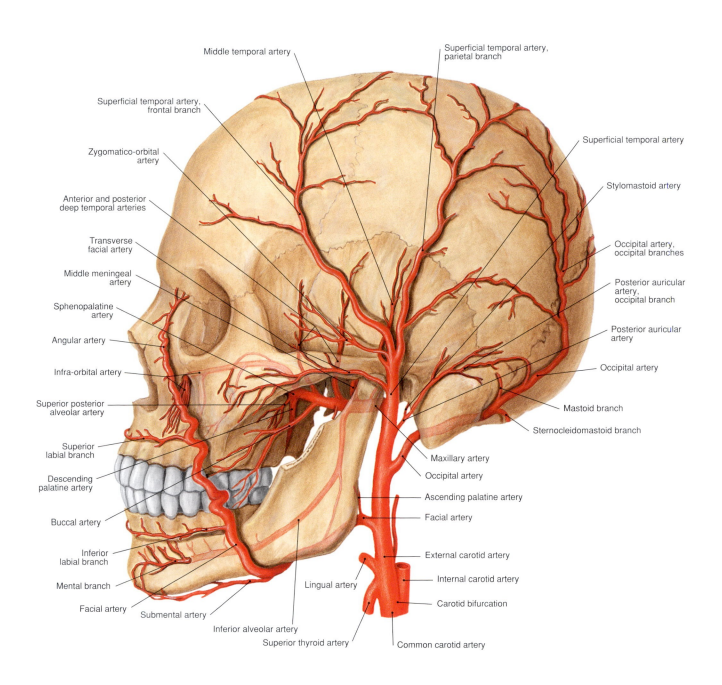

Middle temporal artery

Superficial temporal artery, parietal branch

Superficial temporal artery, frontal branch

Zygomatico-orbital artery

Anterior and posterior deep temporal arteries

Transverse facial artery

Middle meningeal artery

Sphenopalatine artery

Angular artery

Infra-orbital artery

Superior posterior alveolar artery

Superior labial branch

Descending palatine artery

Buccal artery

Inferior labial branch

Mental branch

Facial artery

Submental artery

Inferior alveolar artery

Superior thyroid artery

Lingual artery

Superficial temporal artery

Stylomastoid artery

Occipital artery, occipital branches

Posterior auricular artery, occipital branch

Posterior auricular artery

Occipital artery

Mastoid branch

Sternocleidomastoid branch

Maxillary artery

Occipital artery

Ascending palatine artery

Facial artery

External carotid artery

Internal carotid artery

Carotid bifurcation

Common carotid artery

Fig. 123 External carotid artery.

→ 264

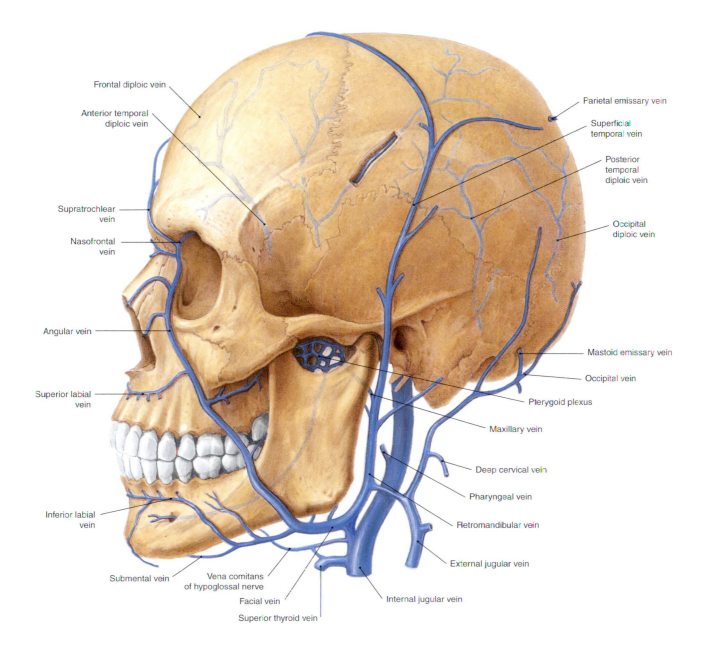

Frontal diploic vein

Anterior temporal diploic vein

Supratrochlear vein

Nasofrontal vein

Angular vein

Superior labial vein

Inferior labial vein

Submental vein

Vena comitans of hypoglossal nerve

Facial vein

Superior thyroid vein

Parietal emissary vein

Superficial temporal vein

Posterior temporal diploic vein

Occipital diploic vein

Mastoid emissary vein

Occipital vein

Pterygoid plexus

Maxillary vein

Deep cervical vein

Pharyngeal vein

Retromandibular vein

External jugular vein

Internal jugular vein

Fig. 124 Internal jugular vein.

→ 259

Lymphatics of the head and the neck

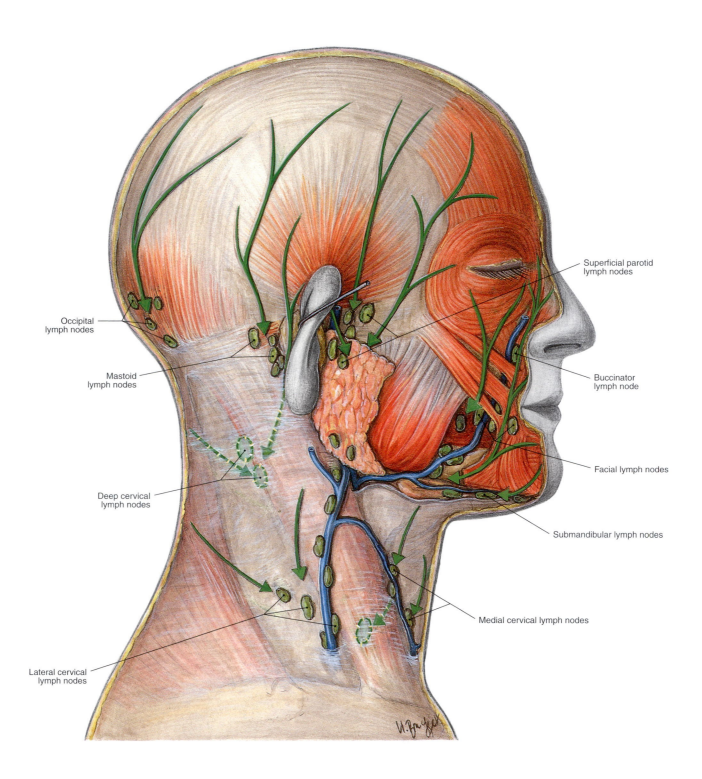

Occipital
lymph nodes

Mastoid
lymph nodes

Deep cervical
lymph nodes

Lateral cervical
lymph nodes

Superficial parotid
lymph nodes

Buccinator
lymph node

Facial lymph nodes

Submandibular lymph nodes

Medial cervical lymph nodes

→ 261, 414

Fig. 125 Lymph nodes and lymphatics
of the head and the neck;
arrows indicate drainage areas.

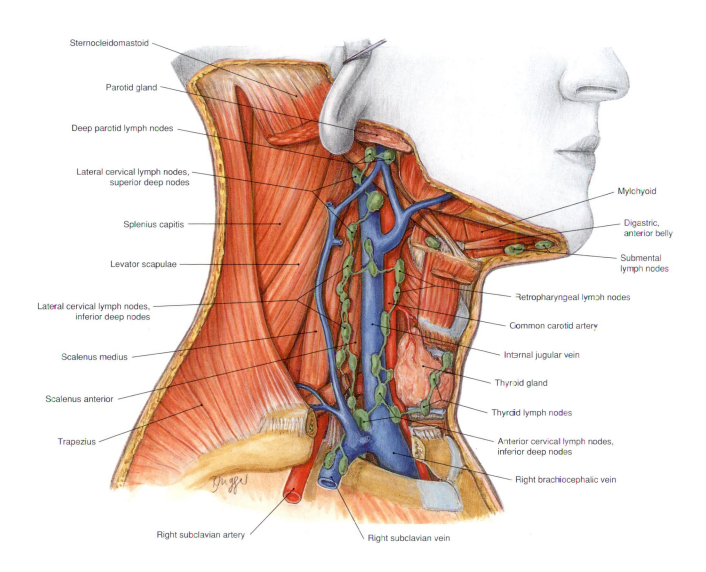

Sternocleidomastoid

Parotid gland

Deep parotid lymph nodes

Lateral cervical lymph nodes, superior deep nodes

Splenius capitis

Levator scapulae

Lateral cervical lymph nodes, inferior deep nodes

Scalenus medius

Scalenus anterior

Trapezius

Right subclavian artery

Right subclavian vein

Mylohyoid

Digastric, anterior belly

Submental lymph nodes

Retropharyngeal lymph nodes

Common carotid artery

Internal jugular vein

Thyroid gland

Thyroid lymph nodes

Anterior cervical lymph nodes, inferior deep nodes

Right brachiocephalic vein

Fig. 126   Deep lymph nodes of the neck.

Facial nerve

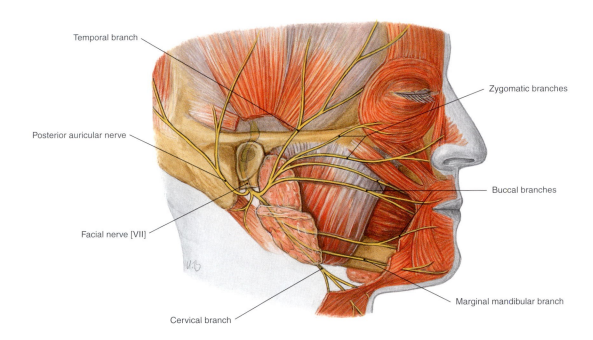

Temporal branch

Posterior auricular nerve

Facial nerve [VII]

Cervical branch

Zygomatic branches

Buccal branches

Marginal mandibular branch

Fig. 127 Facial nerve.

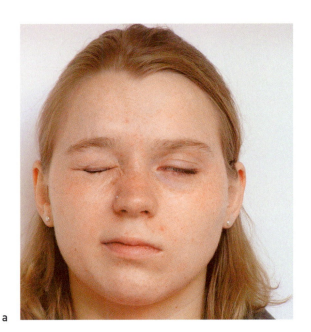

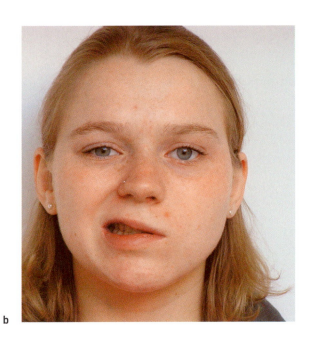

a

b

→ 1182

Fig. 128 a, b Palsy of the left facial nerve.
a The concerned eye cannot be closed upon request (lagophthalmus).
b The teeth of the concerned side cannot be shown upon request.

Cutaneous innervation

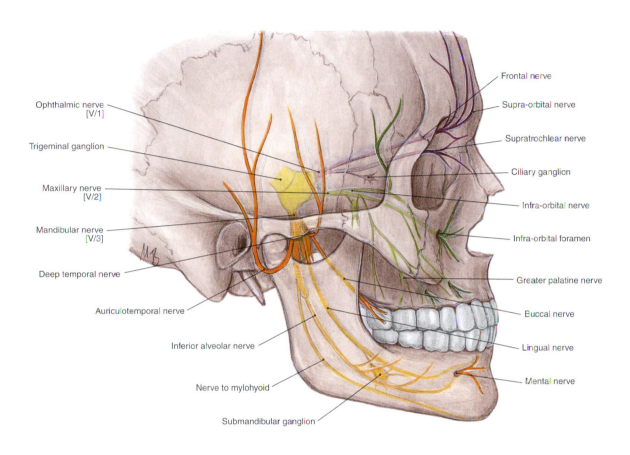

Ophthalmic nerve [V/1]

Trigeminal ganglion

Maxillary nerve [V/2]

Mandibular nerve [V/3]

Deep temporal nerve

Auriculotemporal nerve

Inferior alveolar nerve

Nerve to mylohyoid

Submandibular ganglion

Frontal nerve

Supra-orbital nerve

Supratrochlear nerve

Ciliary ganglion

Infra-orbital nerve

Infra-orbital foramen

Greater palatine nerve

Buccal nerve

Lingual nerve

Mental nerve

Fig. 129 Trigeminal nerve.

→ 472–475

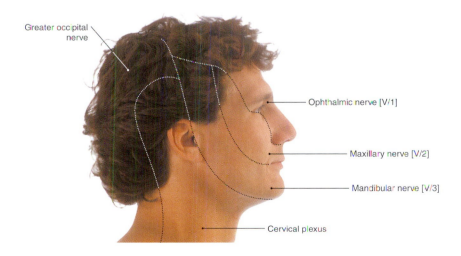

Greater occipital nerve

Ophthalmic nerve [V/1]

Maxillary nerve [V/2]

Mandibular nerve [V/3]

Cervical plexus

Fig. 130 Cutaneous innervation of the head and the neck.

Vessels and nerves of the head and the neck

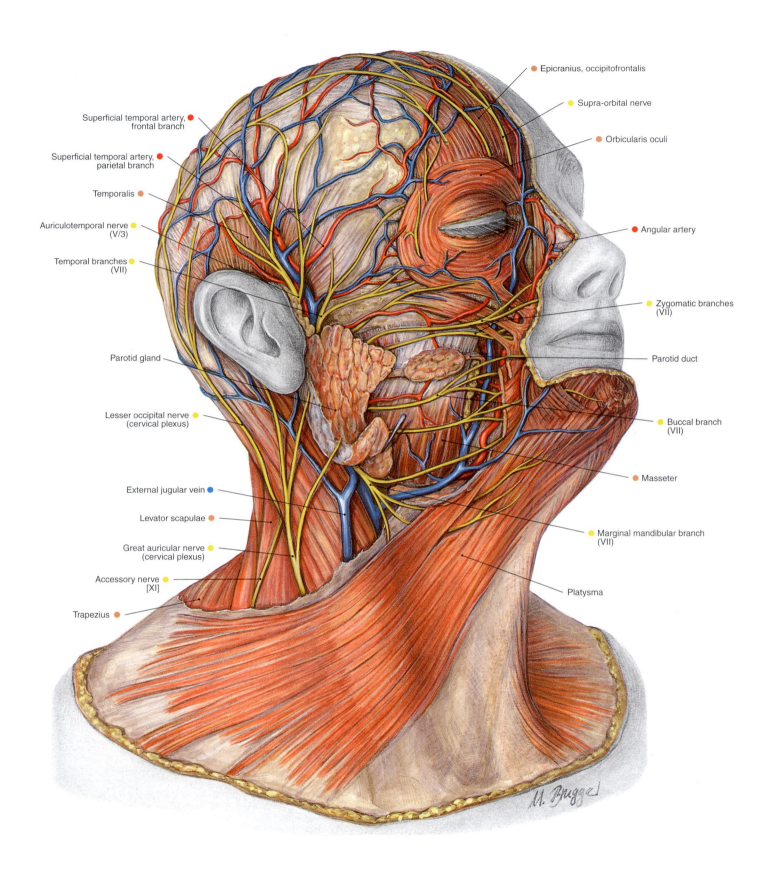

Superficial temporal artery, ● frontal branch

Superficial temporal artery, ● parietal branch

Temporalis ●

Auriculotemporal nerve ● (V/3)

Temporal branches ● (VII)

Parotid gland

Lesser occipital nerve ● (cervical plexus)

External jugular vein ●

Levator scapulae ●

Great auricular nerve ● (cervical plexus)

Accessory nerve ● [XI]

Trapezius ●

● Epicranius, occipitofrontalis

● Supra-orbital nerve

● Orbicularis oculi

● Angular artery

● Zygomatic branches (VII)

Parotid duct

● Buccal branch (VII)

● Masseter

● Marginal mandibular branch (VII)

Platysma

132
254

Fig. 131 Vessels and nerves of the head and the neck; superficial lateral regions.

Vessels and nerves of the head and the neck

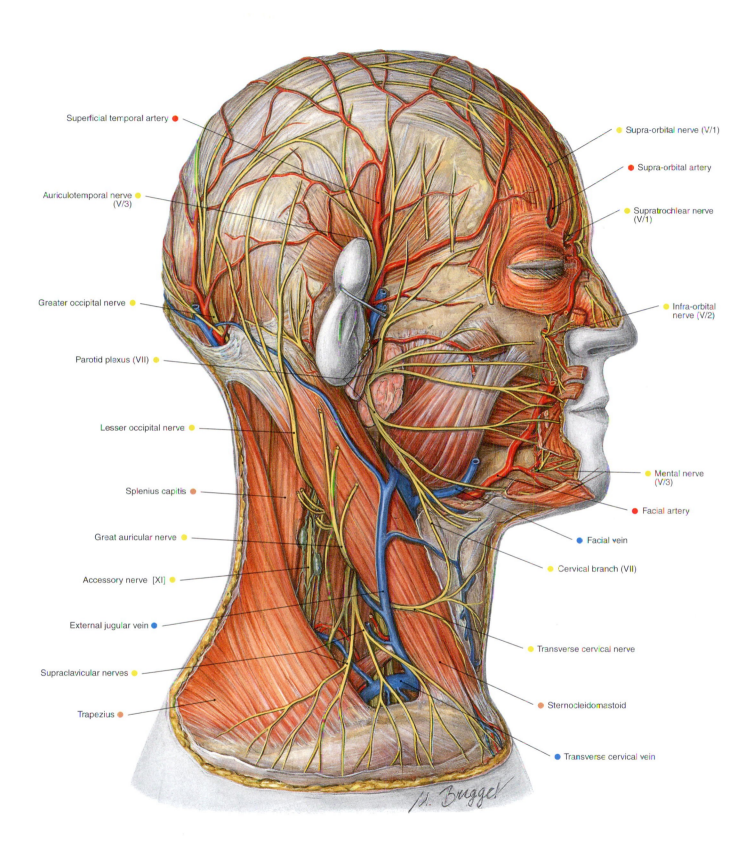

Superficial temporal artery ●

Auriculotemporal nerve ● (V/3)

Greater occipital nerve ●

Parotid plexus (VII) ●

Lesser occipital nerve ●

Splenius capitis ●

Great auricular nerve ●

Accessory nerve [XI] ●

External jugular vein ●

Supraclavicular nerves ●

Trapezius ●

● Supra-orbital nerve (V/1)

● Supra-orbital artery

● Supratrochlear nerve (V/1)

● Infra-orbital nerve (V/2)

● Mental nerve (V/3)

● Facial artery

● Facial vein

● Cervical branch (VII)

● Transverse cervical nerve

● Sternocleidomastoid

● Transverse cervical vein

Fig. 132 Vessels and nerves of the head and the neck; deep lateral regions.

133
256

131

Lateral region of the face

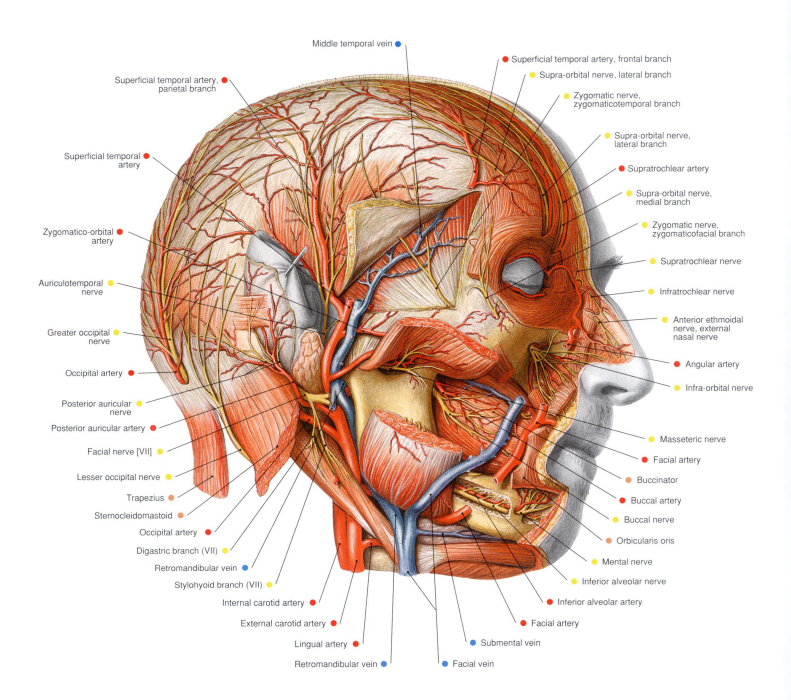

Middle temporal vein ●

Superficial temporal artery, parietal branch ●

Superficial temporal artery ●

Zygomatico-orbital artery ●

Auriculotemporal nerve ●

Greater occipital nerve ●

Occipital artery ●

Posterior auricular nerve ●

Posterior auricular artery ●

Facial nerve [VII] ●

Lesser occipital nerve ●

Trapezius ●

Sternocleidomastoid ●

Occipital artery ●

Digastric branch (VII) ●

Retromandibular vein ●

Stylohyoid branch (VII) ●

Internal carotid artery ●

External carotid artery ●

Lingual artery ●

Retromandibular vein ●

● Superficial temporal artery, frontal branch

● Supra-orbital nerve, lateral branch

● Zygomatic nerve, zygomaticotemporal branch

● Supra-orbital nerve, lateral branch

● Supratrochlear artery

● Supra-orbital nerve, medial branch

● Zygomatic nerve, zygomaticofacial branch

● Supratrochlear nerve

● Infratrochlear nerve

● Anterior ethmoidal nerve, external nasal nerve

● Angular artery

● Infra-orbital nerve

● Masseteric nerve

● Facial artery

● Buccinator

● Buccal artery

● Buccal nerve

● Orbicularis oris

● Mental nerve

● Inferior alveolar nerve

● Inferior alveolar artery

● Facial artery

● Submental vein

● Facial vein

134

132

262

Fig. 133 Vessels and nerves of the head; deep lateral regions.

Maxillary artery

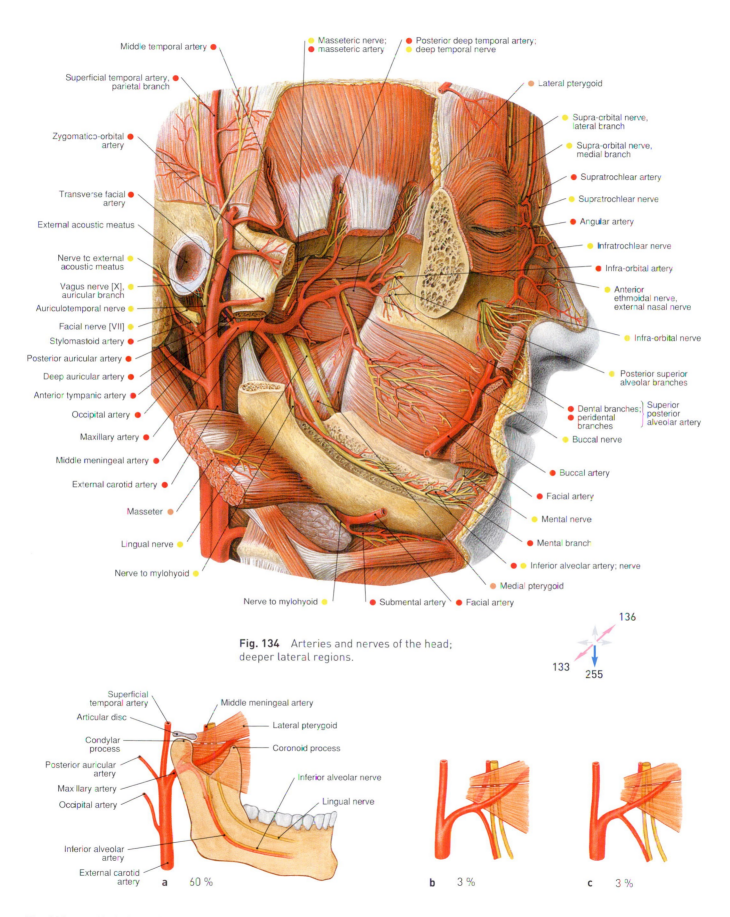

Middle temporal artery ●

Superficial temporal artery, parietal branch

Zygomatico-orbital ● artery

Transverse facial ● artery

External acoustic meatus

Nerve to external acoustic meatus ●

Vagus nerve [X], ● auricular branch

Auriculotemporal nerve ●

Facial nerve [VII] ●

Stylomastoid artery ●

Posterior auricular artery ●

Deep auricular artery ●

Anterior tympanic artery ●

Occipital artery ●

Maxillary artery ●

Middle meningeal artery ●

External carotid artery ●

Masseter ●

Lingual nerve ●

Nerve to mylohyoid ●

Masseteric nerve; ● masseteric artery

Posterior deep temporal artery; ● deep temporal nerve

● Lateral pterygoid

● Supra-orbital nerve, lateral branch

● Supra-orbital nerve, medial branch

● Supratrochlear artery

● Supratrochlear nerve

● Angular artery

● Infratrochlear nerve

● Infra-orbital artery

● Anterior ethmoidal nerve, external nasal nerve

● Infra-orbital nerve

● Posterior superior alveolar branches

● Dental branches; } Superior
● peridental } posterior
branches } alveolar artery

● Buccal nerve

● Buccal artery

● Facial artery

● Mental nerve

● Mental branch

●● Inferior alveolar artery; nerve

● Medial pterygoid

Nerve to mylohyoid ●   ● Submental artery ● Facial artery

Fig. 134 Arteries and nerves of the head; deeper lateral regions.

136
133   255

Superficial temporal artery

Articular disc

Condylar process

Posterior auricular artery

Maxillary artery

Occipital artery

Inferior alveolar artery

External carotid artery

Middle meningeal artery

Lateral pterygoid

Coronoid process

Inferior alveolar nerve

Lingual nerve

a 60 %

b 3 %

c 3 %

Fig. 135 a–c Variations of the middle meningeal artery.

a The middle meningeal artery branches off proximal to the inferior alveolar artery.

b The middle meningeal artery branches off across from the inferior alveolar artery.

c The middle meningeal artery branches off distal to the inferior alveolar artery.

Lateral region of the face

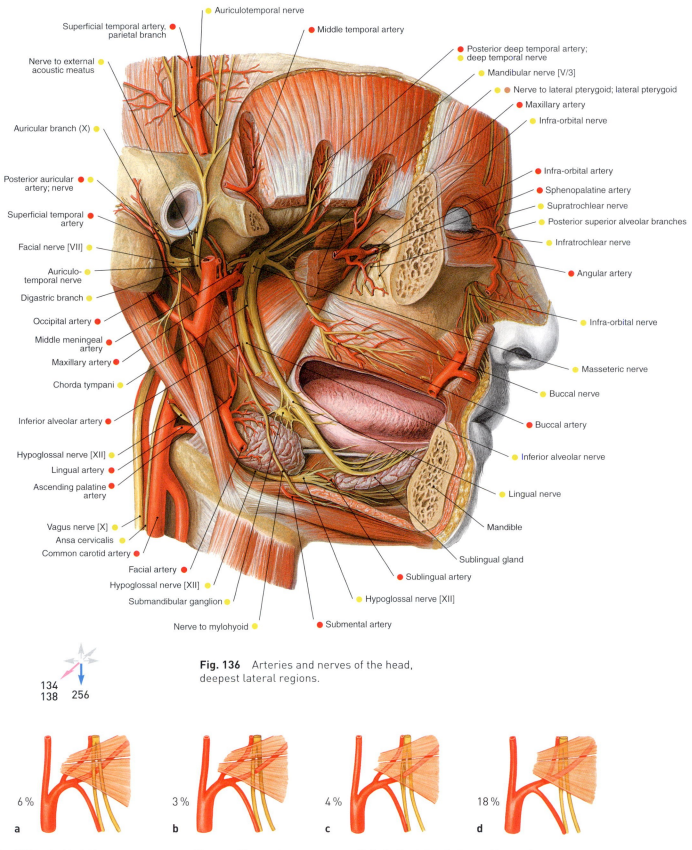

Auriculotemporal nerve

Superficial temporal artery, parietal branch

Middle temporal artery

Posterior deep temporal artery; deep temporal nerve

Nerve to external acoustic meatus

Mandibular nerve [V/3]

Nerve to lateral pterygoid; lateral pterygoid

Maxillary artery

Infra-orbital nerve

Auricular branch (X)

Infra-orbital artery

Sphenopalatine artery

Supratrochlear nerve

Posterior superior alveolar branches

Posterior auricular artery; nerve

Superficial temporal artery

Infratrochlear nerve

Facial nerve [VII]

Angular artery

Auriculo-temporal nerve

Digastric branch

Infra-orbital nerve

Occipital artery

Middle meningeal artery

Maxillary artery

Masseteric nerve

Chorda tympani

Buccal nerve

Inferior alveolar artery

Buccal artery

Inferior alveolar nerve

Hypoglossal nerve [XII]

Lingual artery

Ascending palatine artery

Lingual nerve

Vagus nerve [X]

Ansa cervicalis

Common carotid artery

Mandible

Facial artery

Sublingual gland

Hypoglossal nerve [XII]

Submandibular ganglion

Sublingual artery

Hypoglossal nerve [XII]

Nerve to mylohyoid

Submental artery

134
138

256

Fig. 136 Arteries and nerves of the head, deepest lateral regions.

6 %   3 %   4 %   18 %

a   b   c   d

Fig. 137 a–d Variations in the course of the maxillary artery.

a The maxillary artery passes medially to the lateral pterygoid muscle, the lingual nerve and the inferior alveolar nerve.
b The maxillary artery passes between the lingual nerve and the inferior alveolar nerve.
c The maxillary artery passes through a loop formed by the inferior alveolar nerve.
d The middle meningeal artery branches off distal to the inferior alveolar artery.

Lateral region of the face

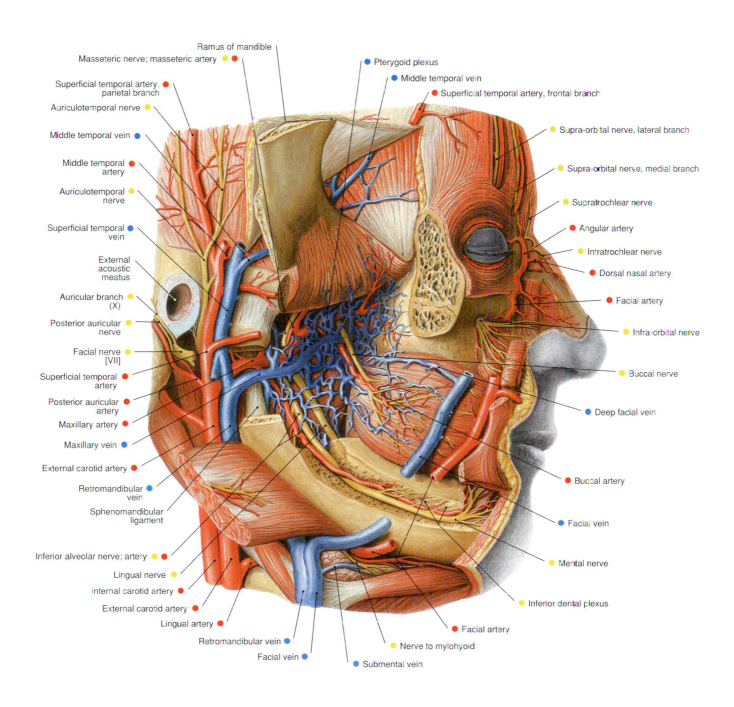

Ramus of mandible

Masseteric nerve; masseteric artery ● ●

Superficial temporal artery, parietal branch ●

Auriculotemporal nerve ●

Middle temporal vein ●

Middle temporal artery ●

Auriculotemporal nerve ●

Superficial temporal vein ●

External acoustic meatus

Auricular branch (X) ●

Posterior auricular nerve ●

Facial nerve [VII] ●

Superficial temporal artery ●

Posterior auricular artery ●

Maxillary artery ●

Maxillary vein ●

External carotid artery ●

Retromandibular vein ●

Sphenomandibular ligament

Inferior alveolar nerve; artery ● ●

Lingual nerve ●

Internal carotid artery ●

External carotid artery ●

Lingual artery ●

Retromandibular vein ●

Facial vein ●

Pterygoid plexus ●

Middle temporal vein ●

Superficial temporal artery, frontal branch ●

Supra-orbital nerve, lateral branch ●

Supra-orbital nerve, medial branch ●

Supratrochlear nerve ●

Angular artery ●

Intratrochlear nerve ●

Dorsal nasal artery ●

Facial artery ●

Infra-orbital nerve ●

Buccal nerve ●

Deep facial vein ●

Buccal artery ●

Facial vein ●

Mental nerve ●

Inferior dental plexus ●

Facial artery ●

Nerve to mylohyoid ●

Submental vein ●

Fig. 138 Vessels and nerves of the head; deeper lateral regions.

136

133 255

Skeleton of the nose

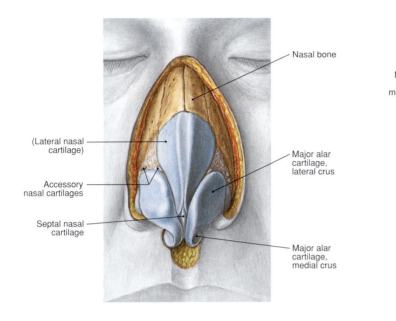

Nasal bone

(Lateral nasal cartilage)

Accessory nasal cartilages

Septal nasal cartilage

Major alar cartilage, lateral crus

Major alar cartilage, medial crus

Fig. 139 Skeleton of the nose.

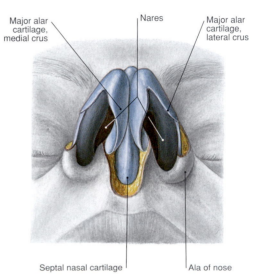

Major alar cartilage, medial crus

Nares

Major alar cartilage, lateral crus

Septal nasal cartilage

Ala of nose

Fig. 140 Nasal cartilages.

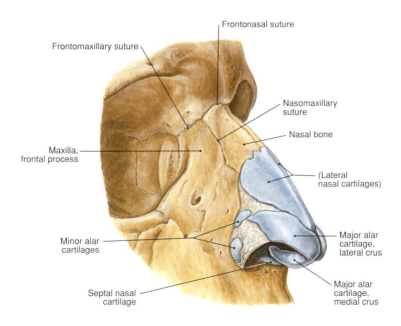

Frontomaxillary suture

Frontonasal suture

Nasomaxillary suture

Nasal bone

Maxilla, frontal process

(Lateral nasal cartilages)

Minor alar cartilages

Major alar cartilage, lateral crus

Septal nasal cartilage

Major alar cartilage, medial crus

Fig. 141 Skeleton of the nose.

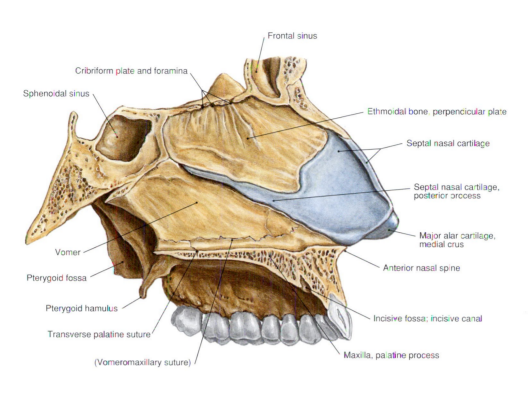

Frontal sinus

Cribriform plate and foramina

Sphenoidal sinus

Ethmoidal bone, perpencicular plate

Septal nasal cartilage

Septal nasal cartilage, posterior prccess

Major alar cartilage, medial crus

Vomer

Anterior nasal spine

Pterygoid fossa

Pterygoid hamulus

Incisive fossa; incisive canal

Transverse palatine suture

(Vomeromaxillary suture)

Maxilla, palatine process

Fig. 142   Nasal septum.

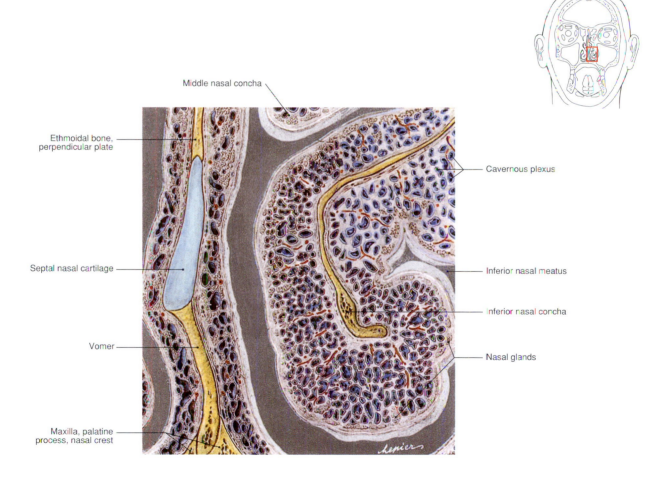

Middle nasal concha

Ethmoidal bone, perpendicular plate

Cavernous plexus

Septal nasal cartilage

Inferior nasal meatus

Inferior nasal concha

Vomer

Nasal glands

Maxilla, palatine process, nasal crest

Fig. 143   Inferior nasal concha.

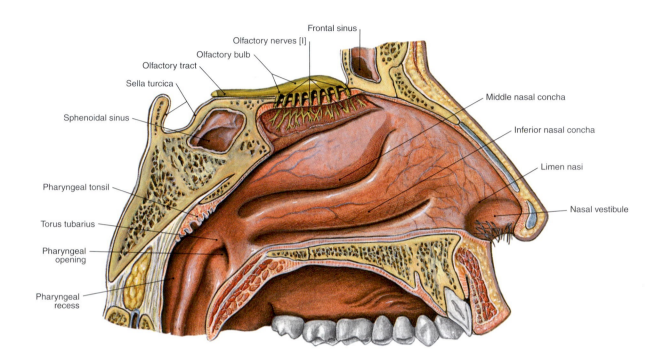

Frontal sinus
Olfactory nerves [I]
Olfactory bulb
Olfactory tract
Sella turcica
Sphenoidal sinus
Pharyngeal tonsil
Torus tubarius
Pharyngeal opening
Pharyngeal recess

Middle nasal concha
Inferior nasal concha
Limen nasi
Nasal vestibule

Fig. 144 Lateral wall of the nasal cavity.

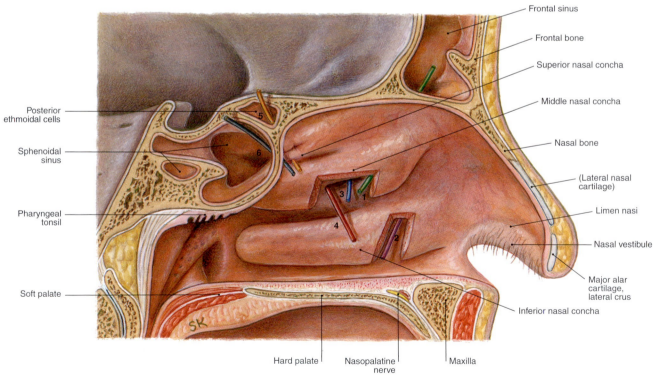

Posterior ethmoidal cells
Sphenoidal sinus
Pharyngeal tonsil
Soft palate

Frontal sinus
Frontal bone
Superior nasal concha
Middle nasal concha
Nasal bone
(Lateral nasal cartilage)
Limen nasi
Nasal vestibule
Major alar cartilage, lateral crus
Inferior nasal concha

Hard palate
Nasopalatine nerve
Maxilla

Openings of:
1 Sinus frontalis
2 Nasolacrimal duct
3 Anterior ethmoidal cells
4 Maxillary sinus
5 Posterior ethmoidal cells
6 Sphenoidal sinus

Fig. 145 Nasal cavity and openings of the paranasal sinuses.

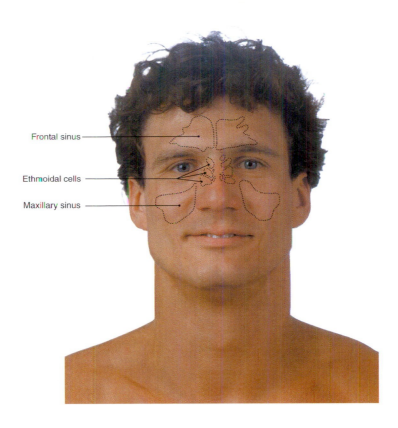

Fig. 146   Projection of the paranasal sinuses.

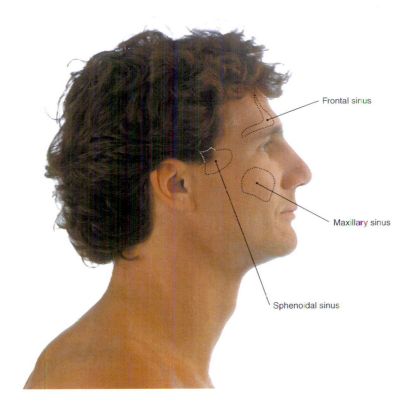

Fig. 147   Projection of the paranasal sinuses.

Paranasal sinuses

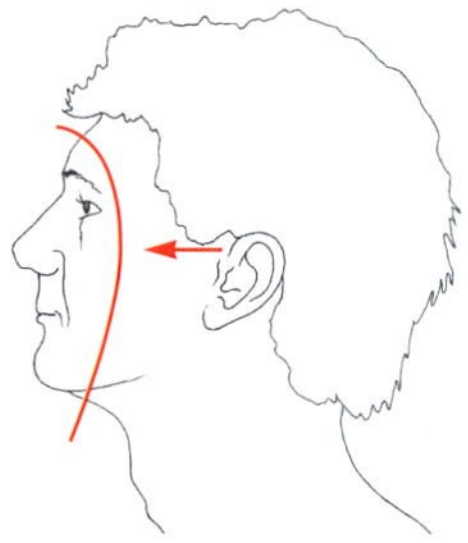

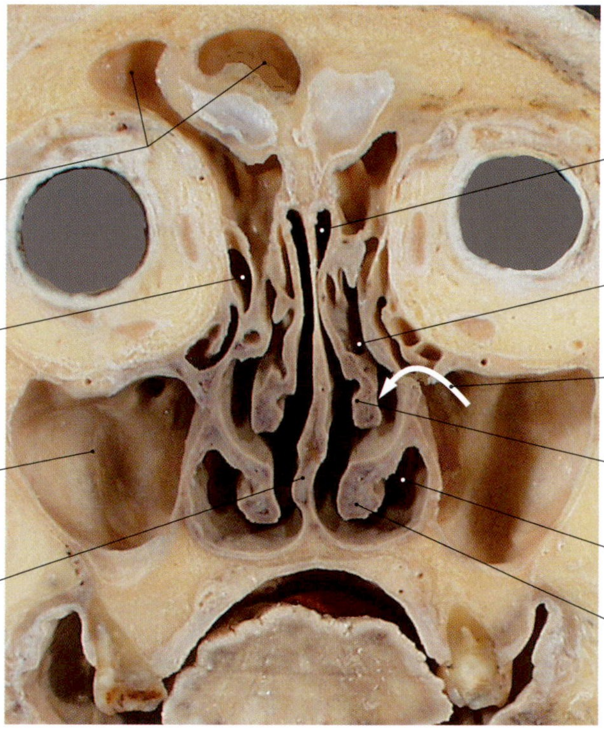

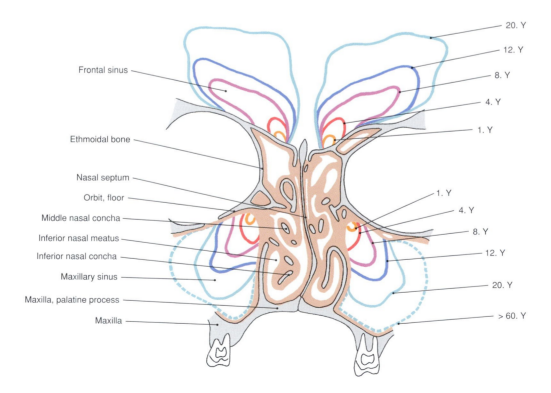

Frontal sinus

Ethmoidal cells

Maxillary sinus

Nasal septum

Superior nasal meatus

Middle nasal meatus

Semilunaris hiatus

Middle nasal concha

Inferior nasal meatus

Inferior nasal concha

Fig. 148 Paranasal sinuses.

Frontal sinus

Ethmoidal bone

Nasal septum

Orbit, floor

Middle nasal concha

Inferior nasal meatus

Inferior nasal concha

Maxillary sinus

Maxilla, palatine process

Maxilla

20. Y

12. Y

8. Y

4. Y

1. Y

1. Y

4. Y

8. Y

12. Y

20. Y

> 60. Y

Fig. 149 Development of the maxillary and frontal sinuses.
Y – year of life

Parasanal sinuses, radiography

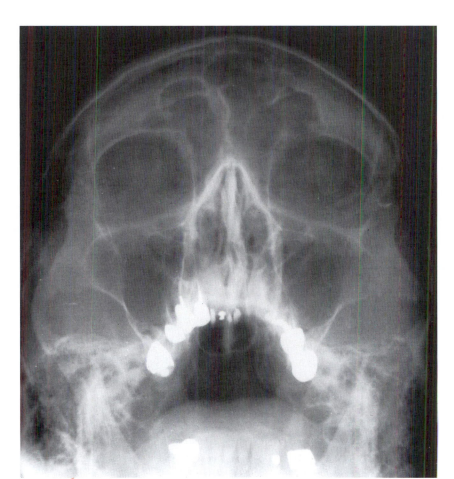

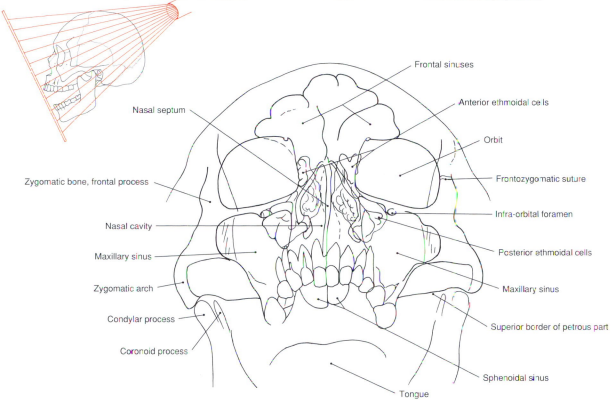

Frontal sinuses

Anterior ethmoidal cells

Orbit

Frontozygomatic suture

Infra-orbital foramen

Posterior ethmoidal cells

Maxillary sinus

Superior border of petrous part

Sphenoidal sinus

Nasal septum

Zygomatic bone, frontal process

Nasal cavity

Maxillary sinus

Zygomatic arch

Condylar process

Coronoid process

Tongue

Fig. 150   Paranasal sinuses;
PA-radiograph.

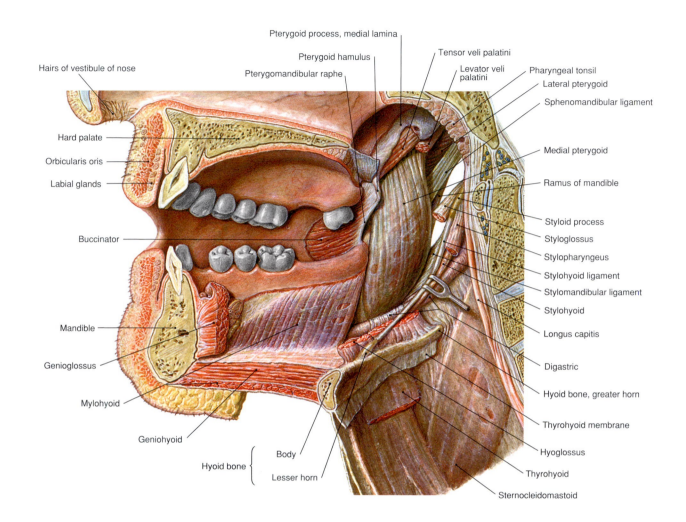

Fig. 151 Oral cavity.

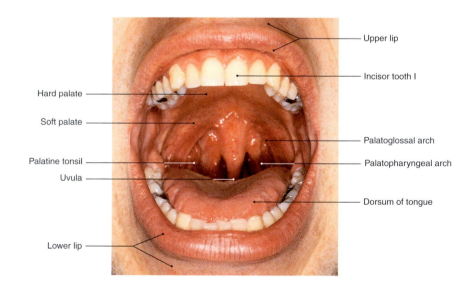

Fig. 152 Oral cavity.

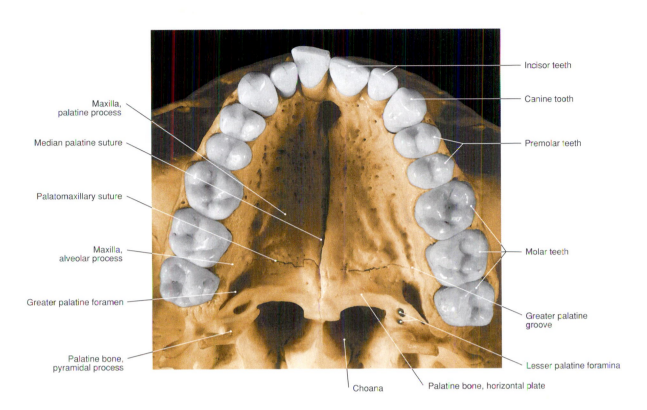

Maxilla, palatine process

Median palatine suture

Palatomaxillary suture

Maxilla, alveolar process

Greater palatine foramen

Palatine bone, pyramidal process

Incisor teeth

Canine tooth

Premolar teeth

Molar teeth

Greater palatine groove

Lesser palatine foramina

Choana

Palatine bone, horizontal plate

Fig. 153   Upper dental arcade and bony palate.

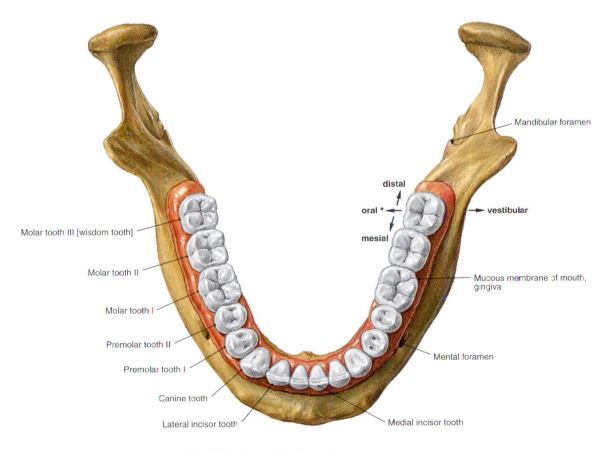

Mandibular foramen

distal

oral *

vestibular

mesial

Molar tooth III [wisdom tooth]

Molar tooth II

Molar tooth I

Premolar tooth II

Premolar tooth I

Canine tooth

Lateral incisor tooth

Mucous membrane of mouth, gingiva

Mental foramen

Medial incisor tooth

Fig. 154   Lower dental arcade.

* In the mandible oral is synonymous with lingual, and in the maxilla it is synonymous with palatinal.

Teeth, structure

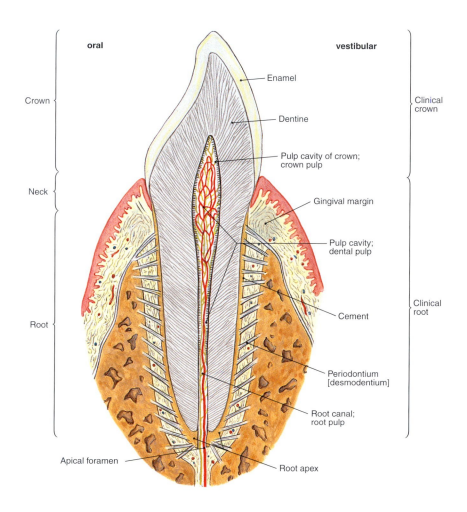

oral

vestibular

Crown

Enamel

Dentine

Clinical crown

Pulp cavity of crown; crown pulp

Neck

Gingival margin

Pulp cavity; dental pulp

Clinical root

Root

Cement

Periodontium [desmodentium]

Root canal; root pulp

Apical foramen

Root apex

Fig. 155 Incisor tooth.

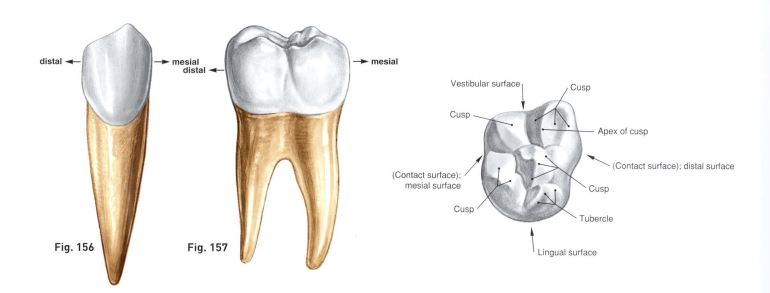

distal ← → mesial

mesial
distal ← → distal

→ mesial

Vestibular surface

Cusp

Cusp

Apex of cusp

(Contact surface); mesial surface

(Contact surface); distal surface

Cusp

Cusp

Tubercle

Lingual surface

Fig. 156

Fig. 157

Fig. 156 ► Permanent lower canine tooth.

Fig. 157 ► Deciduous second molar tooth.

Fig. 158 Permanent upper first molar tooth.

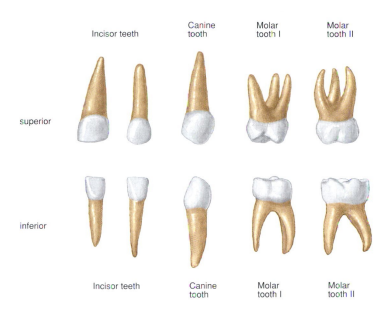

Incisor teeth   Canine tooth   Molar tooth I   Molar tooth II

superior

inferior

Incisor teeth   Canine tooth   Molar tooth I   Molar tooth II

Fig. 159   Deciduous teeth of a 3-year-old child; vestibular view.

			Maxilla					

right 55 54 53 52 51 | 61 62 63 64 65 left
85 84 83 82 81 | 71 72 73 74 75

Mandible

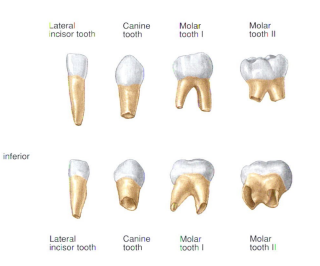

Lateral incisor tooth   Canine tooth   Molar tooth I   Molar tooth II

inferior

Lateral incisor tooth   Canine tooth   Molar tooth I   Molar tooth II

Fig. 160   Deciduous teeth of a 2-year-old child;
top row viewed from vestibular;
bottom row viewed obliquely from inferior.

Teeth

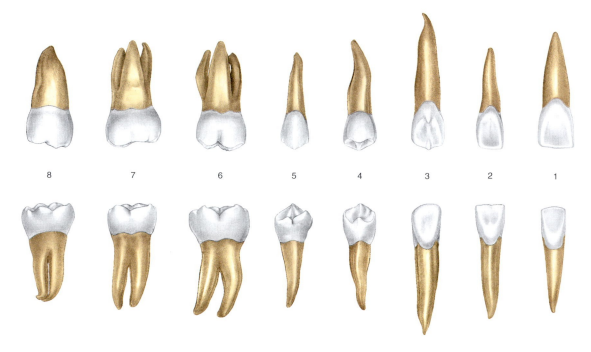

8   7   6   5   4   3   2   1

Fig. 161 Permanent teeth;
oral view.
(See p. 97 for identification of the numbers.)

Maxilla

right	18	17	16	15	14	13	12	11	21	22	23	24	25	26	27	28	left
	48	47	46	45	44	43	42	41	31	32	33	34	35	36	37	38	

Mandible

Adult dentition

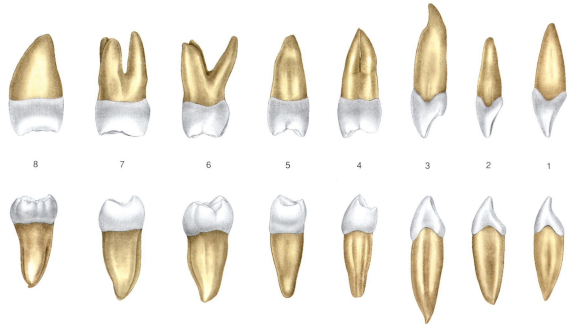

8   7   6   5   4   3   2   1

Fig. 162 Permanent teeth;
distal view.
(See p. 97 for identification of the numbers.)

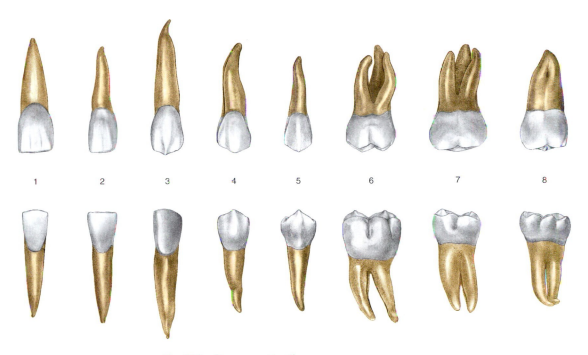

Fig. 163 Permanent teeth;
vestibular view.

1 Incisor tooth I
2 Incisor tooth II
3 Canine tooth
4 Premolar tooth I

5 Premolar tooth II
6 Molar tooth I
7 Molar tooth II
8 Molar tooth III
  [wisdom tooth]

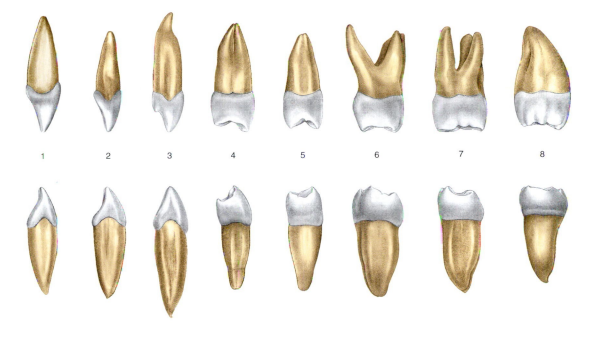

Fig. 164 Permanent teeth;
mesial view.

Teeth, development

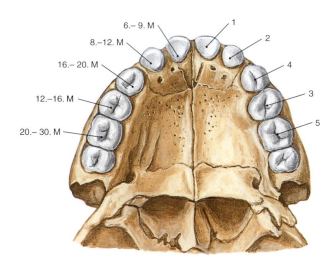

6.– 9. M
8.–12. M
16.– 20. M
12.–16. M
20.– 30. M
1
2
4
3
5

Fig. 165 Maxilla with deciduous teeth and the
first permanent tooth;
left: median time of eruption in months (M);
right: order of eruption.

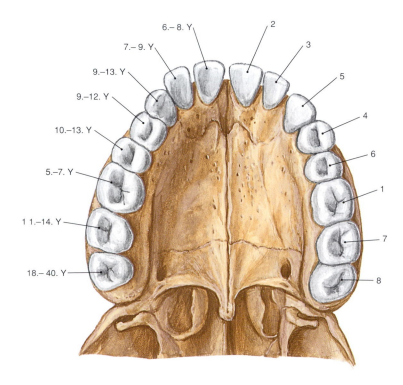

6.– 8. Y
7.– 9. Y
9.–13. Y
9.–12. Y
10.–13. Y
5.–7. Y
1 1.–14. Y
18.– 40. Y
2
3
5
4
6
1
7
8

Fig. 166 Maxilla with permanent teeth;
left: median time of eruption in years (Y);
right: order of eruption.

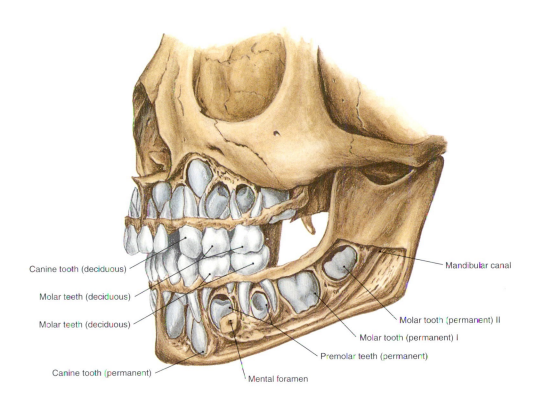

Canine tooth (deciduous)

Molar teeth (deciduous)

Molar teeth (deciduous)

Canine tooth (permanent)

Mandibular canal

Molar tooth (permanent) II

Molar tooth (permanent) I

Premolar teeth (permanent)

Mental foramen

Fig. 167   Maxilla and mandible
of a 5-year-old child;
deciduous teeth and anlage of permanent teeth.

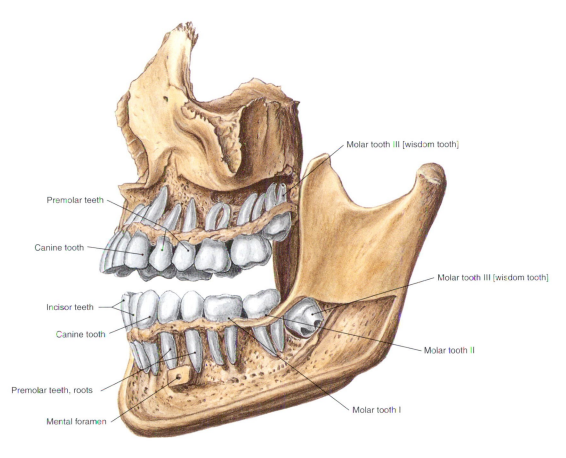

Premolar teeth

Canine tooth

Incisor teeth

Canine tooth

Premolar teeth, roots

Mental foramen

Molar tooth III [wisdom tooth]

Molar tooth III [wisdom tooth]

Molar tooth II

Molar tooth I

Fig. 168   Maxilla and mandible
of a 20-year-old male.

Teeth, radiography

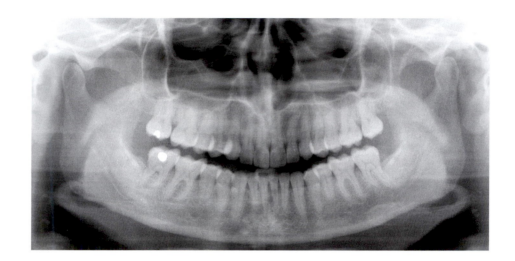

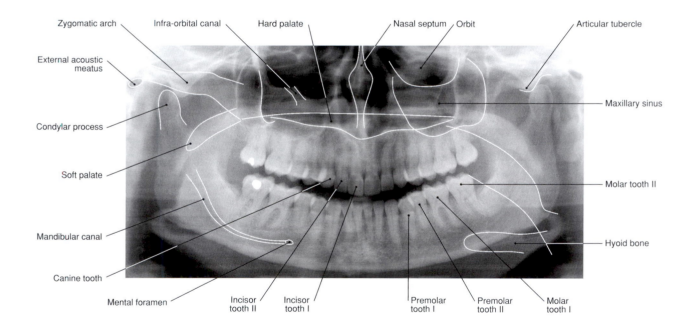

Fig. 169 Maxilla and mandible;
panoramic radiograph;
without wisdom teeth.

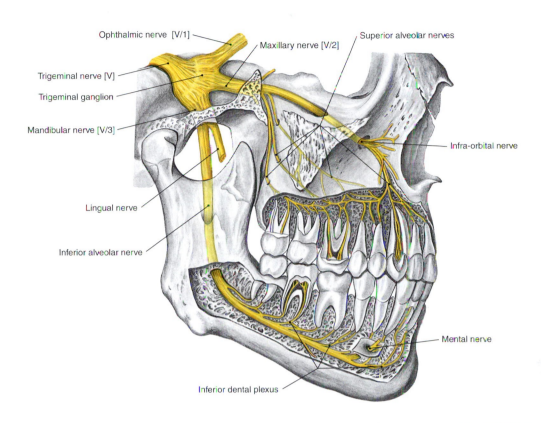

Ophthalmic nerve [V/1]
Maxillary nerve [V/2]
Superior alveolar nerves
Trigeminal nerve [V]
Trigeminal ganglion
Mandibular nerve [V/3]
Infra-orbital nerve
Lingual nerve
Inferior alveolar nerve
Mental nerve
Inferior dental plexus

Fig. 170   Maxillary and mandibular nerve.

→ 1178, 1179

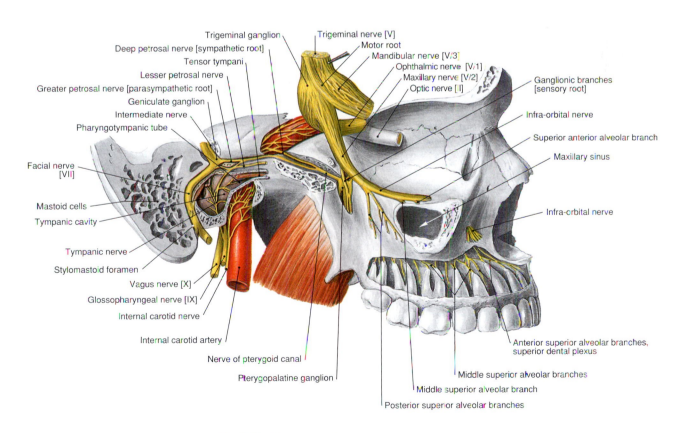

Trigeminal ganglion
Deep petrosal nerve [sympathetic root]
Tensor tympani
Lesser petrosal nerve
Greater petrosal nerve [parasympathetic root]
Geniculate ganglion
Intermediate nerve
Pharyngotympanic tube
Facial nerve [VII]
Mastoid cells
Tympanic cavity
Tympanic nerve
Stylomastoid foramen
Vagus nerve [X]
Glossopharyngeal nerve [IX]
Internal carotid nerve
Internal carotid artery
Nerve of pterygoid canal
Pterygopalatine ganglion

Trigeminal nerve [V]
Motor root
Mandibular nerve [V/3]
Ophthalmic nerve [V/1]
Maxillary nerve [V/2]
Optic nerve [II]
Ganglionic branches [sensory root]
Infra-orbital nerve
Superior anterior alveolar branch
Maxillary sinus
Infra-orbital nerve
Anterior superior alveolar branches, superior dental plexus
Middle superior alveolar branches
Middle superior alveolar branch
Posterior superior alveolar branches

Fig. 171   Pterygopalatine ganglion.

Palate

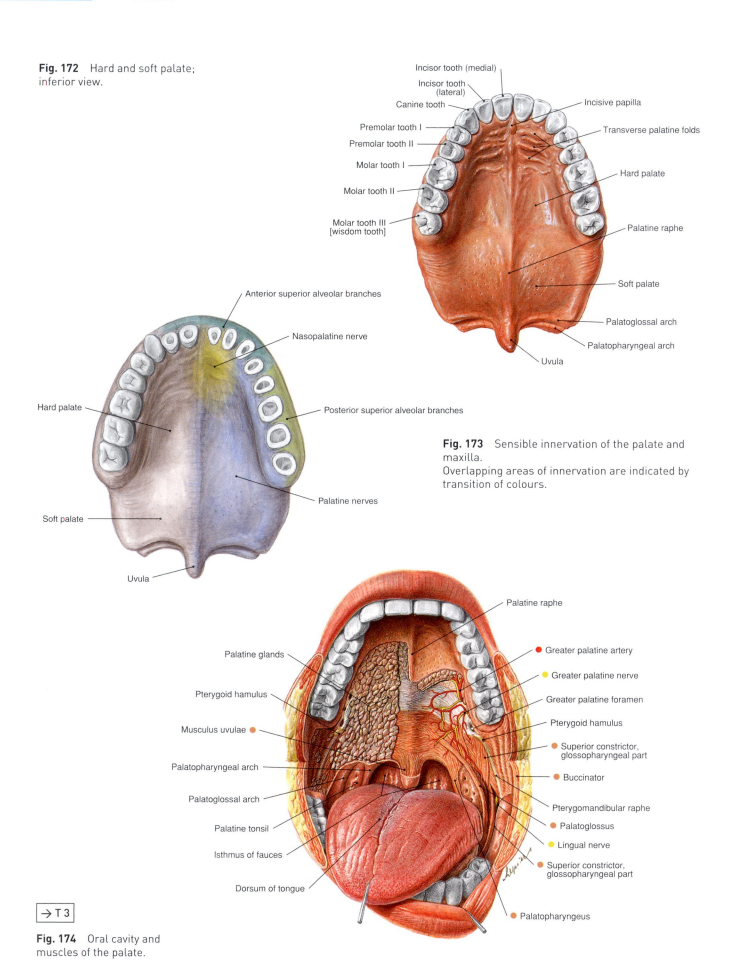

Fig. 172 Hard and soft palate; inferior view.

Incisor tooth (medial)
Incisor tooth (lateral)
Canine tooth
Premolar tooth I
Premolar tooth II
Molar tooth I
Molar tooth II
Molar tooth III [wisdom tooth]

Incisive papilla
Transverse palatine folds
Hard palate
Palatine raphe
Soft palate
Palatoglossal arch
Palatopharyngeal arch
Uvula

Anterior superior alveolar branches
Nasopalatine nerve
Hard palate
Posterior superior alveolar branches
Soft palate
Palatine nerves
Uvula

Fig. 173 Sensible innervation of the palate and maxilla.
Overlapping areas of innervation are indicated by transition of colours.

Palatine raphe
Palatine glands
Pterygoid hamulus
Musculus uvulae ●
Palatophyryngeal arch
Palatoglossal arch
Palatine tonsil
Isthmus of fauces
Dorsum of tongue

Greater palatine artery
Greater palatine nerve
Greater palatine foramen
Pterygoid hamulus
● Superior constrictor, glossopharyngeal part
● Buccinator
Pterygomandibular raphe
● Palatoglossus
● Lingual nerve
● Superior constrictor, glossopharyngeal part
● Palatopharyngeus

→ T 3

Fig. 174 Oral cavity and muscles of the palate.

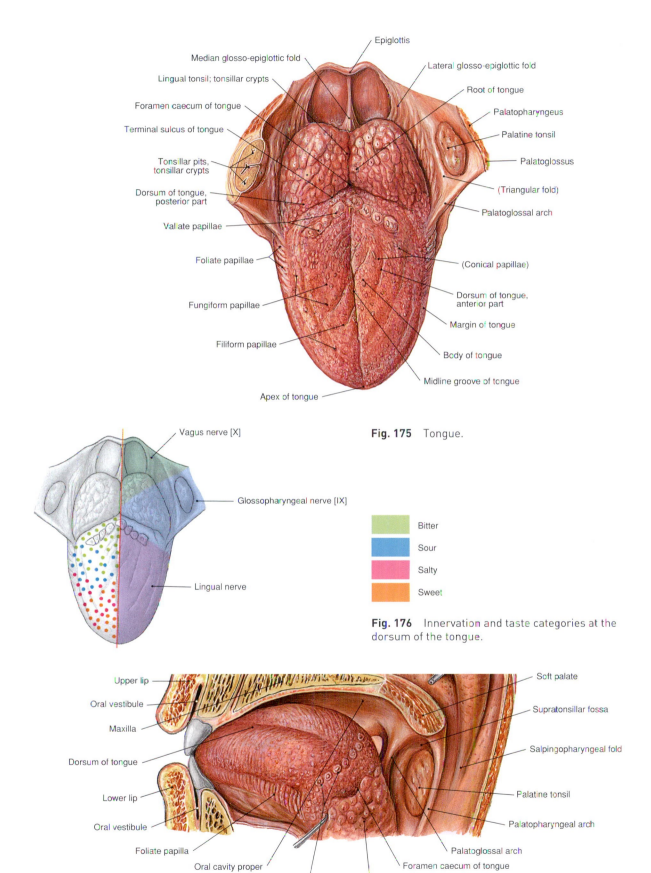

Epiglottis

Median glosso-epiglottic fold

Lateral glosso-epiglottic fold

Lingual tonsil; tonsillar crypts

Root of tongue

Foramen caecum of tongue

Palatopharyngeus

Terminal sulcus of tongue

Palatine tonsil

Tonsillar pits, tonsillar crypts

Palatoglossus

Dorsum of tongue, posterior part

(Triangular fold)

Palatoglossal arch

Vallate papillae

Foliate papillae

(Conical papillae)

Dorsum of tongue, anterior part

Fungiform papillae

Margin of tongue

Filiform papillae

Body of tongue

Midline groove of tongue

Apex of tongue

Fig. 175   Tongue.

Vagus nerve [X]

Glossopharyngeal nerve [IX]

Lingual nerve

Bitter
Sour
Salty
Sweet

Fig. 176   Innervation and taste categories at the dorsum of the tongue.

Upper lip

Soft palate

Oral vestibule

Supratonsillar fossa

Maxilla

Salpingopharyngeal fold

Dorsum of tongue

Lower lip

Palatine tonsil

Oral vestibule

Palatopharyngeal arch

Foliate papilla

Palatoglossal arch

Oral cavity proper

Foramen caecum of tongue

Vallate papillae

Lingual tonsil

Fig. 177   Oral cavity.

Muscles of the tongue

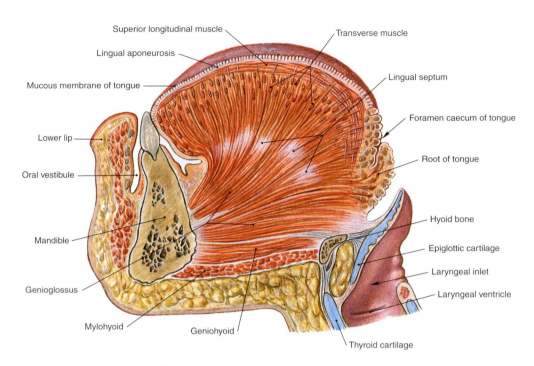

→ T 2a **Fig. 178** Tongue and muscles of the tongue; median section.

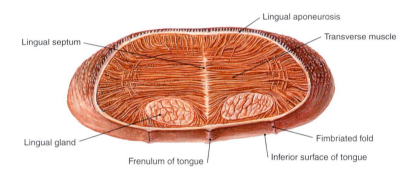

→ T 2a **Fig. 179** Tongue and muscles of the tongue; cross-section through the tip of the tongue.

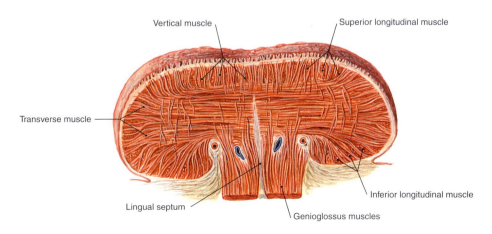

→ T 2a **Fig. 180** Tongue, and muscles of the tongue; cross-section at the level of the middle of the tongue.

Hyoid bone and infra- and suprahyoid muscles

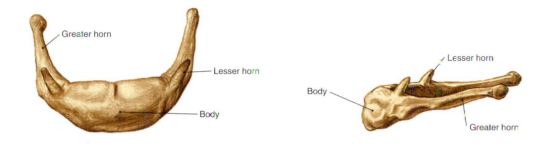

Fig. 181   Hyoid bone.

Fig. 182   Hyoid bone.

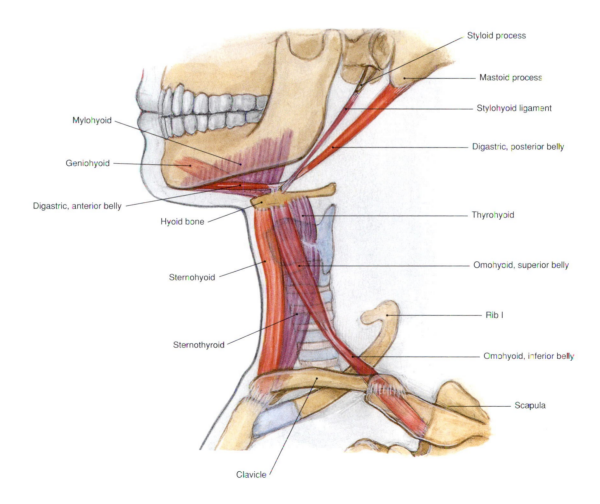

Fig. 183   Muscular suspension of the hyoid bone.

→ T 9, T 10

Suprahyoid muscles

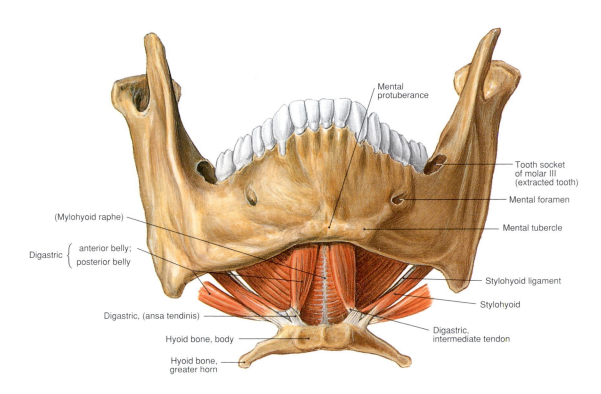

Mental
protuberance

Tooth socket
of molar III
(extracted tooth)

Mental foramen

Mental tubercle

(Mylohyoid raphe)

Digastric { anterior belly;
posterior belly

Stylohyoid ligament

Stylohyoid

Digastric, (ansa tendinis)

Digastric,
intermediate tendon

Hyoid bone, body

Hyoid bone,
greater horn

→ T 9

Fig. 184   Mandible and suprahyoid muscles.

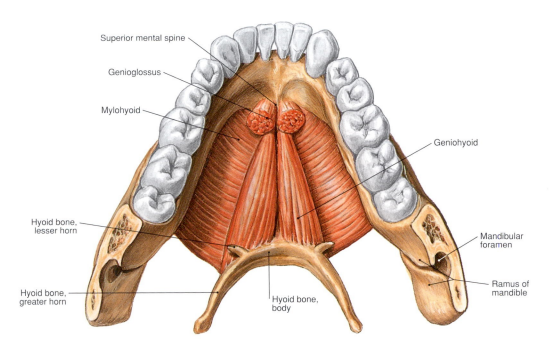

Superior mental spine

Genioglossus

Mylohyoid

Geniohyoid

Hyoid bone,
lesser horn

Mandibular
foramen

Hyoid bone,
greater horn

Hyoid bone,
body

Ramus of
mandible

→ T 9

Fig. 185   Mandible; suprahyoid muscles
and hyoid bone.

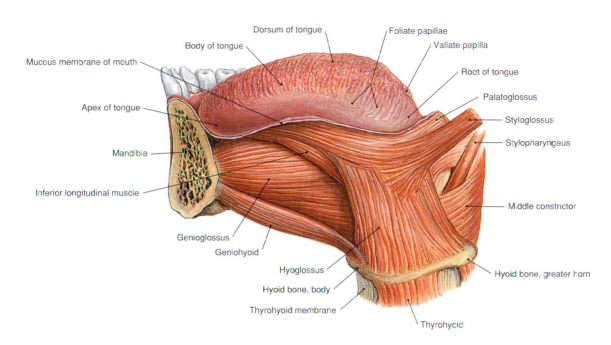

Fig. 187   Tongue and muscles of the tongue.

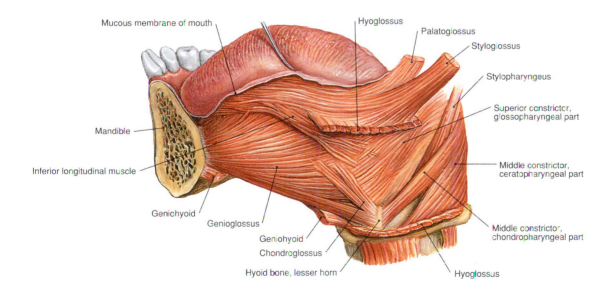

Fig. 187   Tongue and muscles of the tongue.

→ T 2b

Muscles of the tongue and the pharynx

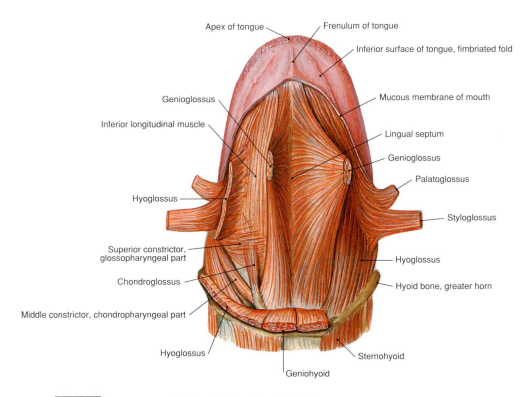

→ T 2b

Fig. 188 Muscles of the tongue.

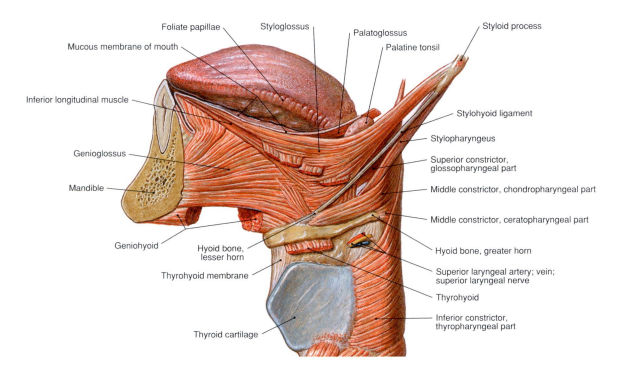

→ T 2b, T 5

Fig. 189 Muscles of the tongue and
muscles of the pharynx.

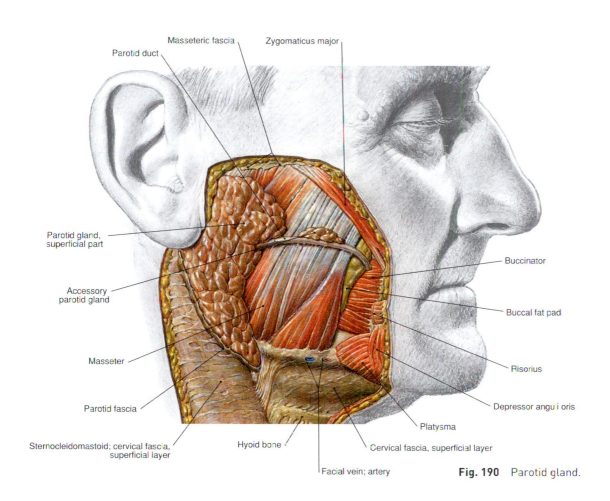

Masseteric fascia

Zygomaticus major

Parotid duct

Parotid gland, superficial part

Accessory parotid gland

Masseter

Parotid fascia

Sternocleidomastoid; cervical fascia, superficial layer

Hyoid bone

Facial vein; artery

Buccinator

Buccal fat pad

Risorius

Depressor anguli oris

Platysma

Cervical fascia, superficial layer

Fig. 190   Parotid gland.

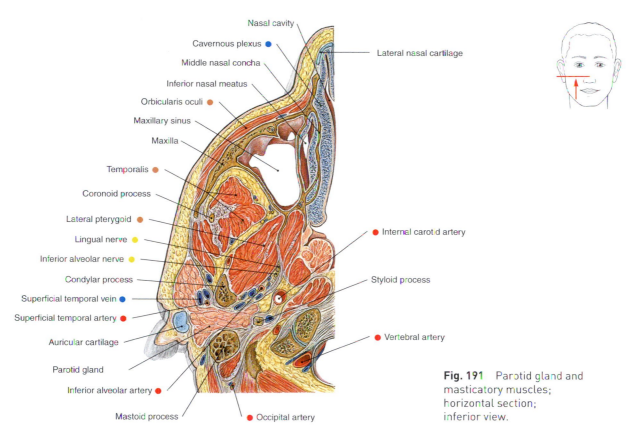

Nasal cavity

Cavernous plexus ●

Middle nasal concha

Inferior nasal meatus

Orbicularis oculi ●

Maxillary sinus

Maxilla

Temporalis ●

Coronoid process

Lateral pterygoid ●

Lingual nerve ●

Inferior alveolar nerve ●

Condylar process

Superficial temporal vein ●

Superficial temporal artery ●

Auricular cartilage

Parotid gland

Inferior alveolar artery ●

Mastoid process

● Occipital artery

Lateral nasal cartilage

● Internal carotid artery

Styloid process

● Vertebral artery

Fig. 191   Parotid gland and masticatory muscles; horizontal section; inferior view.

Submandibular gland

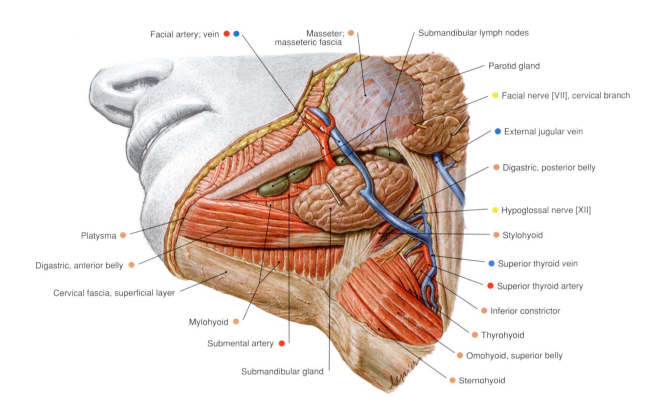

Facial artery; vein ● ●
Masseter; masseteric fascia ●
Submandibular lymph nodes
Parotid gland
● Facial nerve [VII], cervical branch
● External jugular vein
● Digastric, posterior belly
● Hypoglossal nerve [XII]
Platysma ●
● Stylohyoid
Digastric, anterior belly ●
● Superior thyroid vein
Cervical fascia, superficial layer
● Superior thyroid artery
● Inferior constrictor
Mylohyoid ●
● Thyrohyoid
Submental artery ●
● Omohyoid, superior belly
Submandibular gland
● Sternohyoid

Fig. 192 Submandibular gland.

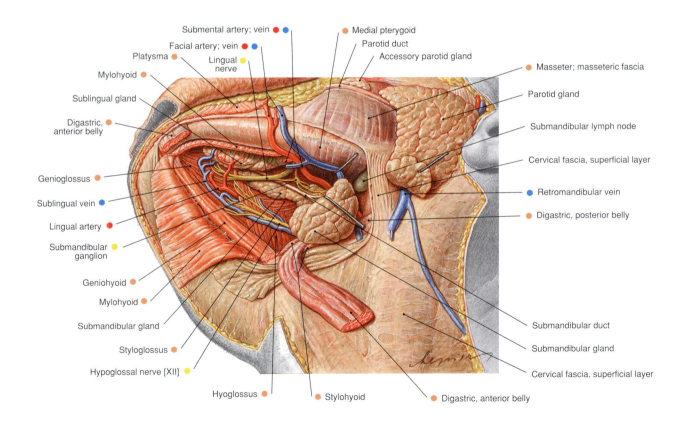

Submental artery; vein ● ●
Medial pterygoid ●
Parotid duct
Facial artery; vein ● ●
Accessory parotid gland
Platysma ●
Lingual nerve ●
Mylohyoid ●
● Masseter; masseteric fascia
Parotid gland
Sublingual gland ●
Digastric, anterior belly ●
Submandibular lymph node
Cervical fascia, superficial layer
Genioglossus ●
● Retromandibular vein
Sublingual vein ●
● Digastric, posterior belly
Lingual artery ●
Submandibular ganglion ●
Geniohyoid ●
Mylohyoid ●
Submandibular gland
Submandibular duct
Styloglossus ●
Submandibular gland
Hypoglossal nerve [XII] ●
Cervical fascia, superficial layer
Hyoglossus ●
Stylohyoid ●
Digastric, anterior belly ●

Fig. 193 Major salivary glands; inferolateral view.

Submandibular and sublingual gland

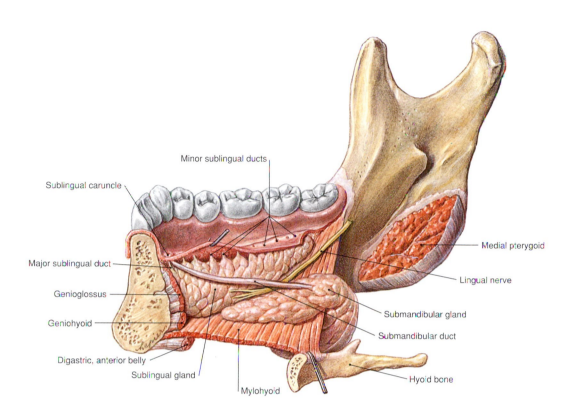

Fig. 194 Submandibular gland and sublingual gland.

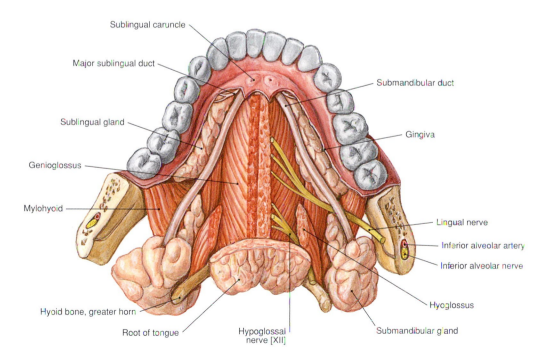

Fig. 195 Sublingual gland and submandibular gland; superior view.

Openings of the salivary glands

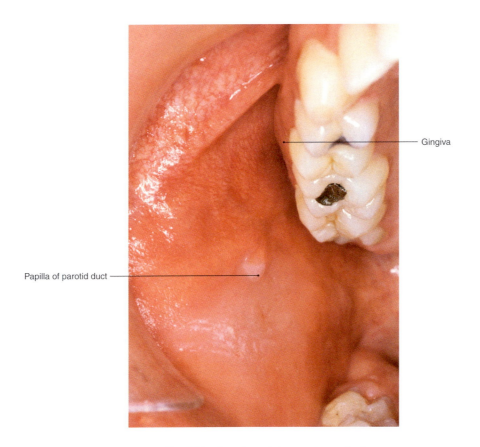

Gingiva

Papilla of parotid duct

Fig. 196 Opening of the excretory duct
of the parotid gland.

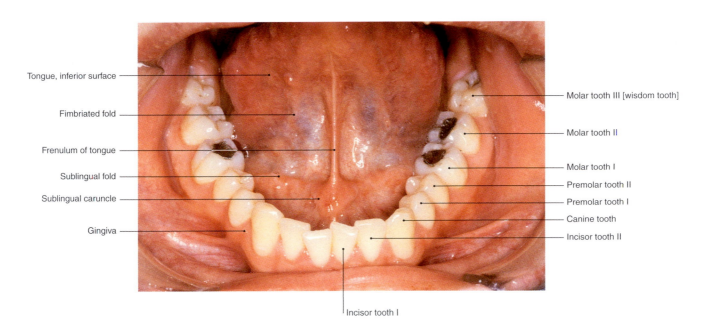

Tongue, inferior surface

Fimbriated fold

Frenulum of tongue

Sublingual fold

Sublingual caruncle

Gingiva

Molar tooth III [wisdom tooth]

Molar tooth II

Molar tooth I

Premolar tooth II

Premolar tooth I

Canine tooth

Incisor tooth II

Incisor tooth I

→ 154

Fig. 197 Opening of the excretory duct
of the submandibular gland.

Arteries and nerves of the oral cavity

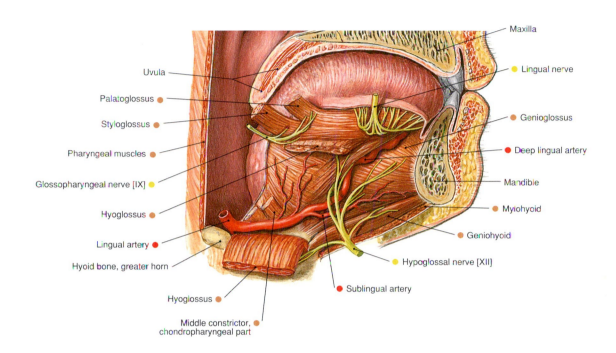

Maxilla

Uvula

Palatoglossus ●

Styloglossus ●

Pharyngeal muscles ●

Glossopharyngeal nerve [IX] ●

Hyoglossus ●

Lingual artery ●

Hyoid bone, greater horn

Hyoglossus ●

Middle constrictor, ● chondropharyngeal part

Lingual nerve ●

Genioglossus ●

Deep lingual artery ●

Mandible

Myiohyoid ●

Geniohyoid ●

Hypoglossal nerve [XII] ●

Sublingual artery ●

Fig. 198   Arteries and nerves of the tongue; medial view.

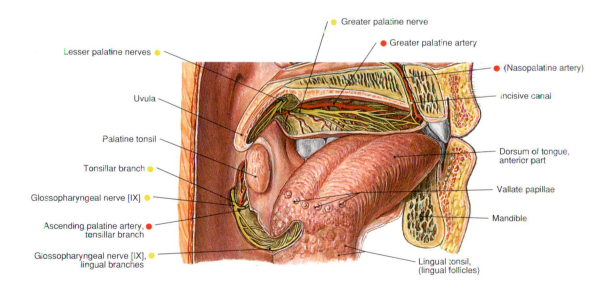

Greater palatine nerve ●

Greater palatine artery ●

Lesser palatine nerves ●

Uvula

Palatine tonsil

Tonsillar branch ●

Glossopharyngeal nerve [IX] ●

Ascending palatine artery, ● tonsillar branch

Glossopharyngeal nerve [IX], ● lingual branches

(Nasopalatine artery) ●

incisive canal

Dorsum of tongue, anterior part

Vallate papillae

Mandible

Lingual tonsil, (lingual follicles)

Fig. 199   Arteries and nerves of the palate and the root of the tongue; medial view.

Vessels and nerves of the tongue and the larynx

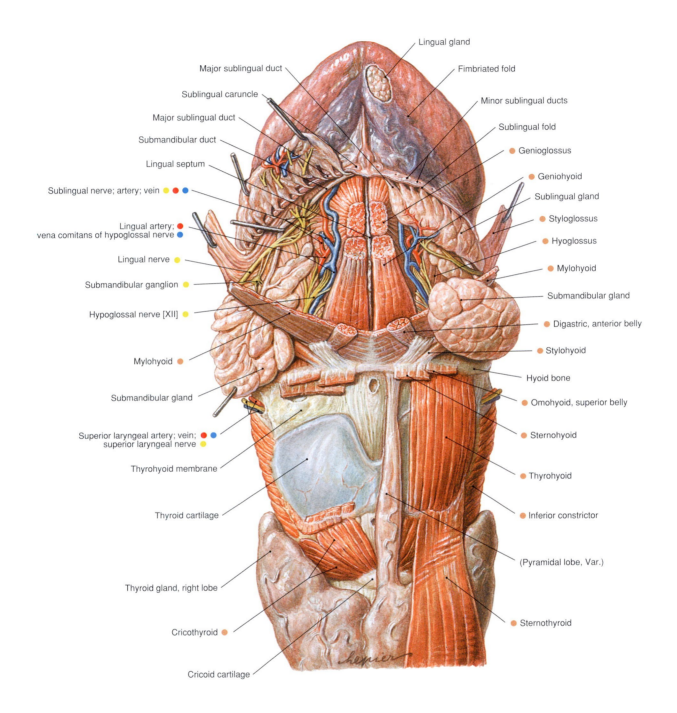

Lingual gland

Major sublingual duct

Sublingual caruncle

Major sublingual duct

Submandibular duct

Lingual septum

Sublingual nerve; artery; vein ● ● ●

Lingual artery; ●
vena comitans of hypoglossal nerve ●

Lingual nerve ●

Submandibular ganglion ●

Hypoglossal nerve [XII] ●

Mylohyoid ●

Submandibular gland

Superior laryngeal artery; vein; ● ●
superior laryngeal nerve ●

Thyrohyoid membrane

Thyroid cartilage

Thyroid gland, right lobe

Cricothyroid ●

Cricoid cartilage

Fimbriated fold

Minor sublingual ducts

Sublingual fold

● Genioglossus

● Geniohyoid

Sublingual gland

● Styloglossus

● Hyoglossus

● Mylohyoid

Submandibular gland

● Digastric, anterior belly

● Stylohyoid

Hyoid bone

● Omohyoid, superior belly

● Sternohyoid

● Thyrohyoid

● Inferior constrictor

(Pyramidal lobe, Var.)

● Sternothyroid

→ 204, 218, 234, 237

Fig. 200 Vessels and nerves of the tongue; major
salivary glands and larynx; anterior-inferior view.

Vessels and nerves of the tongue and the thyroid gland

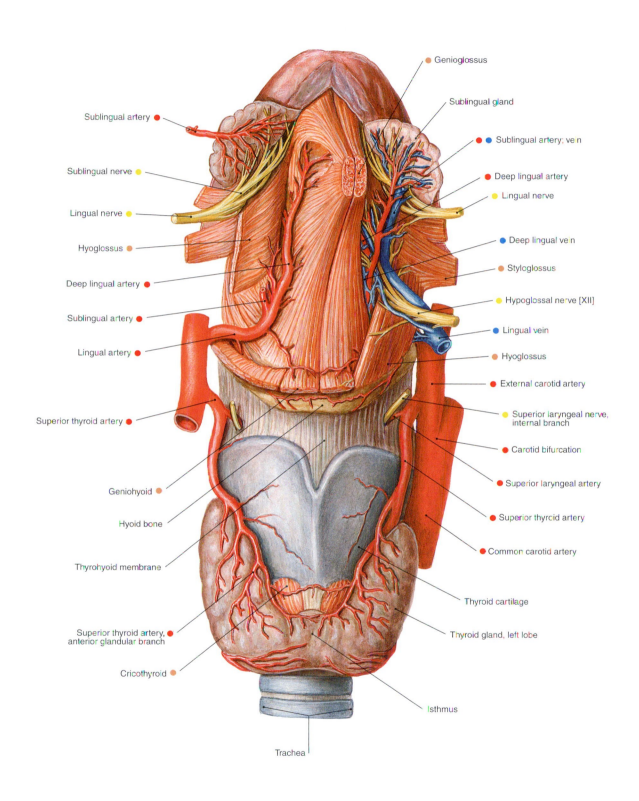

Genioglossus

Sublingual gland

● Sublingual artery; vein

● Deep lingual artery

● Lingual nerve

● Deep lingual vein

● Styloglossus

● Hypoglossal nerve [XII]

● Lingual vein

● Hyoglossus

● External carotid artery

● Superior laryngeal nerve, internal branch

● Carotid bifurcation

● Superior laryngeal artery

● Superior thyroid artery

● Common carotid artery

Thyroid cartilage

Thyroid gland, left lobe

Isthmus

Sublingual artery ●

Sublingual nerve ●

Lingual nerve ●

Hyoglossus ●

Deep lingual artery ●

Sublingual artery ●

Lingual artery ●

Superior thyroid artery ●

Geniohyoid ●

Hyoid bone

Thyrohyoid membrane

Superior thyroid artery, ●
anterior glandular branch

Cricothyroid ●

Trachea

Fig. 201 Vessels and nerves of the tongue and the
thyroid gland; anterior-inferior view.

→ 238, 264

Head, frontal section

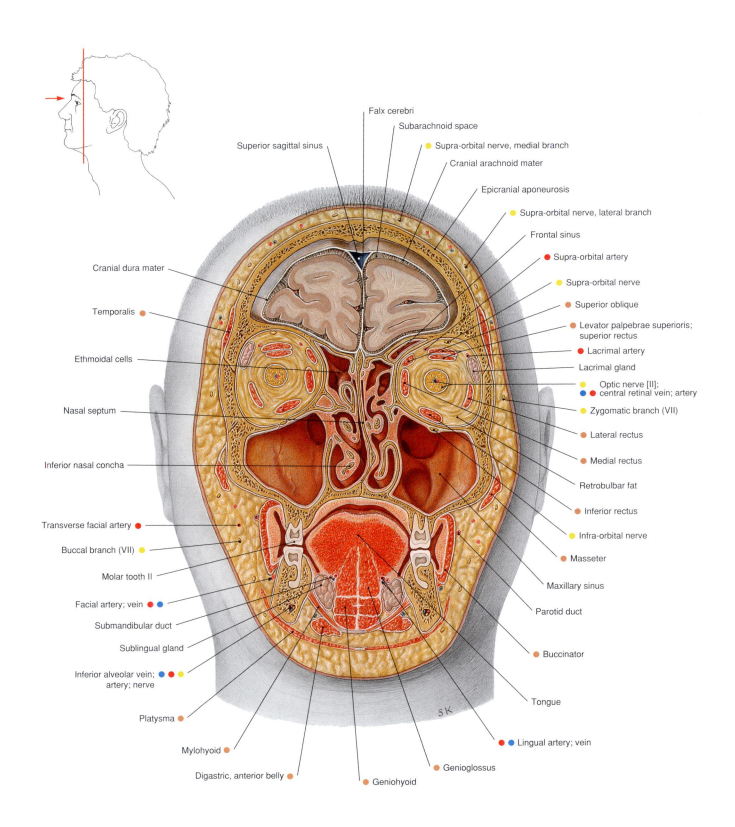

Falx cerebri

Subarachnoid space

● Supra-orbital nerve, medial branch

Cranial arachnoid mater

Superior sagittal sinus

Epicranial aponeurosis

● Supra-orbital nerve, lateral branch

Frontal sinus

● Supra-orbital artery

Cranial dura mater

● Supra-orbital nerve

● Superior oblique

Temporalis ●

● Levator palpebrae superioris; superior rectus

● Lacrimal artery

Ethmoidal cells

Lacrimal gland

● Optic nerve [II];
● ● central retinal vein; artery

Nasal septum

● Zygomatic branch (VII)

● Lateral rectus

● Medial rectus

Inferior nasal concha

Retrobulbar fat

● Inferior rectus

● Infra-orbital nerve

Transverse facial artery ●

● Masseter

Buccal branch (VII) ●

Molar tooth II ●

Maxillary sinus

Facial artery; vein ● ●

Parotid duct

Submandibular duct

Sublingual gland

● Buccinator

Inferior alveolar vein; ● ● ●
artery; nerve

Tongue

Platysma ●

● ● Lingual artery; vein

Mylohyoid ●

● Genioglossus

Digastric, anterior belly ●

● Geniohyoid

S K

Fig. 202 Frontal section through the head of a 48-year-old male
at the level of the second upper molar tooth;
anterior view.

Head, frontal section

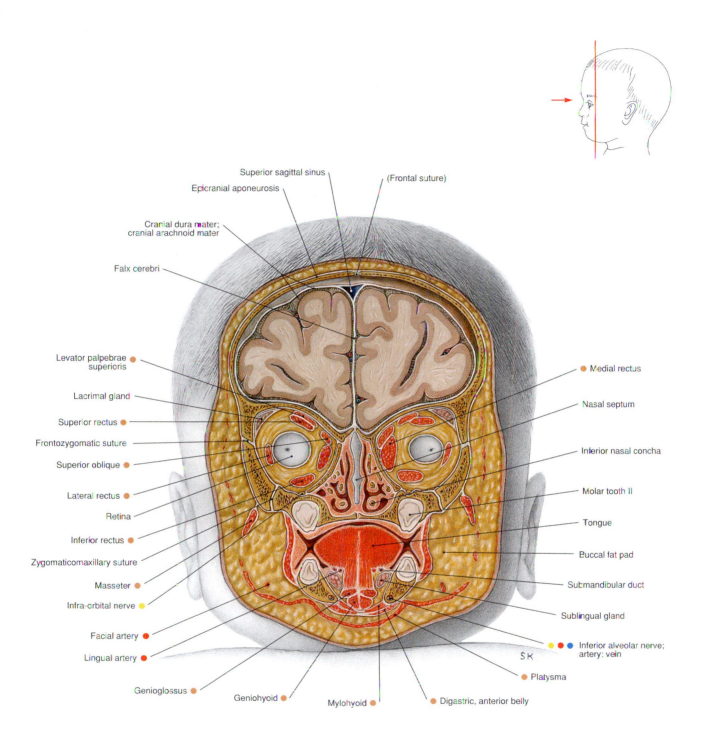

Superior sagittal sinus

Epicranial aponeurosis

(Frontal suture)

Cranial dura mater;
cranial arachnoid mater

Falx cerebri

Levator palpebrae
superioris

Medial rectus

Lacrimal gland

Nasal septum

Superior rectus

Frontozygomatic suture

Inferior nasal concha

Superior oblique

Molar tooth II

Lateral rectus

Retina

Tongue

Inferior rectus

Buccal fat pad

Zygomaticomaxillary suture

Submandibular duct

Masseter

Sublingual gland

Infra-orbital nerve

Facial artery

Inferior alveolar nerve;
artery; vein

Lingual artery

SK

Platysma

Genioglossus

Digastric, anterior belly

Geniohyoid

Mylohyoid

Fig. 203 Frontal section through the head of a neonate
at the level of the second upper molar tooth;
anterior view.
Note the absence of the maxillary sinus and the close proximity
of the tooth anlage to the orbit.

Muscles of the neck and tracheotomy

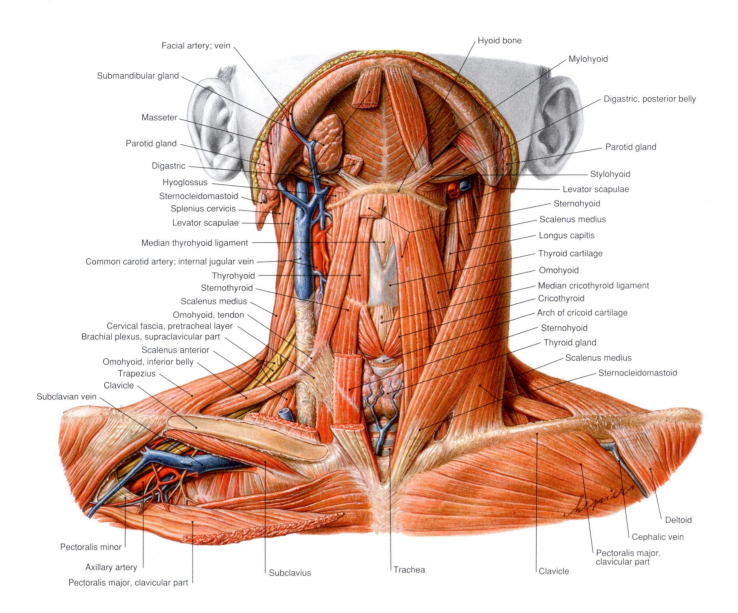

Facial artery; vein

Submandibular gland

Masseter

Parotid gland

Digastric

Hyoglossus

Sternocleidomastoid

Splenius cervicis

Levator scapulae

Median thyrohyoid ligament

Common carotid artery; internal jugular vein

Thyrohyoid

Sternothyroid

Scalenus medius

Omohyoid, tendon

Cervical fascia, pretracheal layer

Brachial plexus, supraclavicular part

Scalenus anterior

Omohyoid, inferior belly

Trapezius

Clavicle

Subclavian vein

Pectoralis minor

Axillary artery

Pectoralis major, clavicular part

Subclavius

Trachea

Hyoid bone

Mylohyoid

Digastric, posterior belly

Parotid gland

Stylohyoid

Levator scapulae

Sternohyoid

Scalenus medius

Longus capitis

Thyroid cartilage

Omohyoid

Median cricothyroid ligament

Cricothyroid

Arch of cricoid cartilage

Sternohyoid

Thyroid gland

Scalenus medius

Sternocleidomastoid

Deltoid

Cephalic vein

Pectoralis major, clavicular part

Clavicle

→ T 8, T 9, T 10, T 11

Fig. 204   Muscles of the neck.

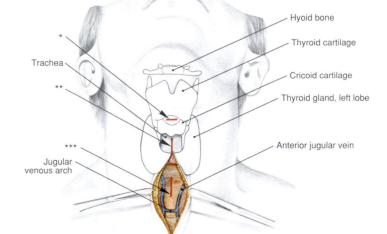

Fig. 205   Surgical access to the trachea
with the neck hyperextended.

*   Coniotomy
**   Upper tracheotomy (above the isthmus of the thyroid gland)
*** Lower tracheotomy (below the isthmus of the thyroid gland)

Trachea

Jugular
venous arch

Hyoid bone

Thyroid cartilage

Cricoid cartilage

Thyroid gland, left lobe

Anterior jugular vein

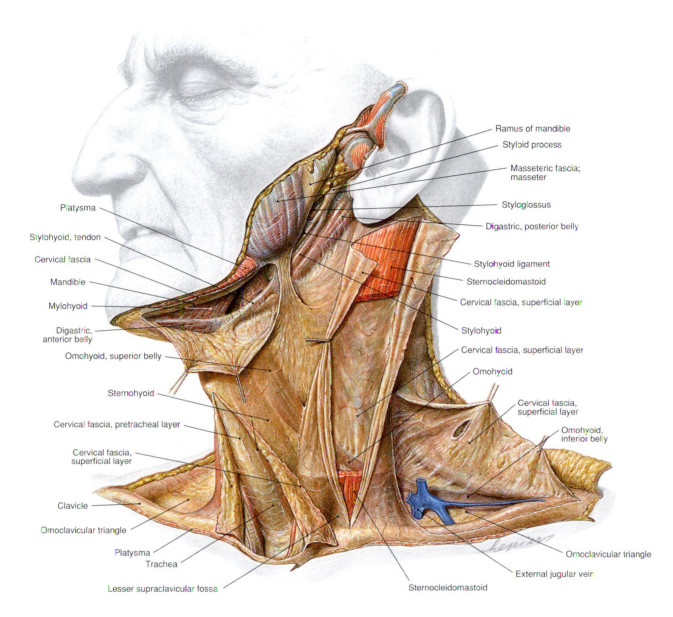

Ramus of mandible

Styloid process

Masseteric fascia; masseter

Styloglossus

Digastric, posterior belly

Stylohyoid ligament

Sternocleidomastoid

Cervical fascia, superficial layer

Stylohyoid

Cervical fascia, superficial layer

Omohyoid

Cervical fascia, superficial layer

Omohyoid, inferior belly

Omoclavicular triangle

External jugular vein

Sternocleidomastoid

Platysma

Stylohyoid, tendon

Cervical fascia

Mandible

Mylohyoid

Digastric, anterior belly

Omohyoid, superior belly

Sternohyoid

Cervical fascia, pretracheal layer

Cervical fascia, superficial layer

Clavicle

Omoclavicular triangle

Platysma

Trachea

Lesser supraclavicular fossa

Fig. 206 Cervical fascia.

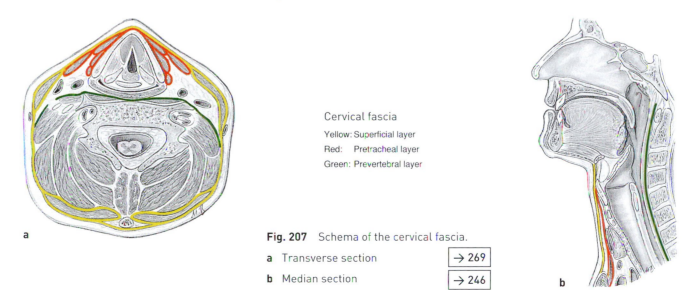

Cervical fascia

Yellow: Superficial layer
Red: Pretracheal layer
Green: Prevertebral layer

Fig. 207 Schema of the cervical fascia.

a Transverse section   → 269

b Median section   → 246

a

b

Muscles of the neck

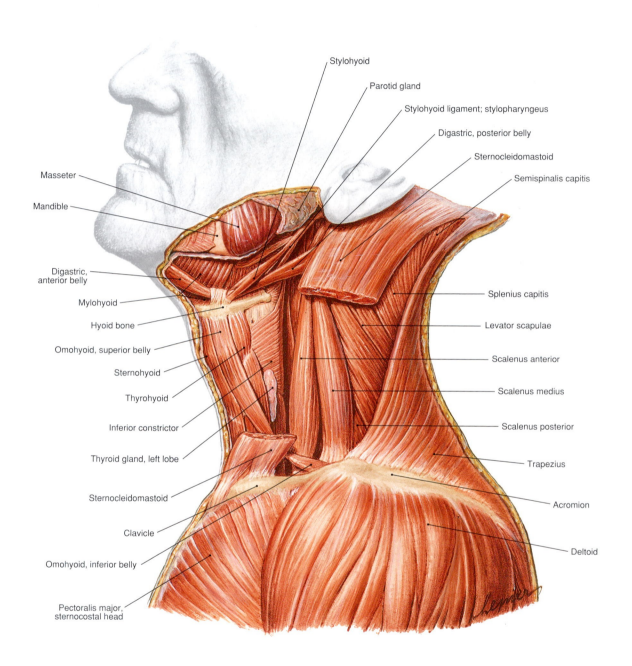

Stylohyoid

Parotid gland

Stylohyoid ligament; stylopharyngeus

Digastric, posterior belly

Sternocleidomastoid

Semispinalis capitis

Masseter

Mandible

Digastric, anterior belly

Mylohyoid

Hyoid bone

Omohyoid, superior belly

Sternohyoid

Thyrohyoid

Inferior constrictor

Thyroid gland, left lobe

Sternocleidomastoid

Clavicle

Omohyoid, inferior belly

Pectoralis major, sternocostal head

Splenius capitis

Levator scapulae

Scalenus anterior

Scalenus medius

Scalenus posterior

Trapezius

Acromion

Deltoid

→ T 8, T 9, T 10, T 11

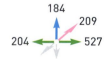

Fig. 208 Muscles of the neck.

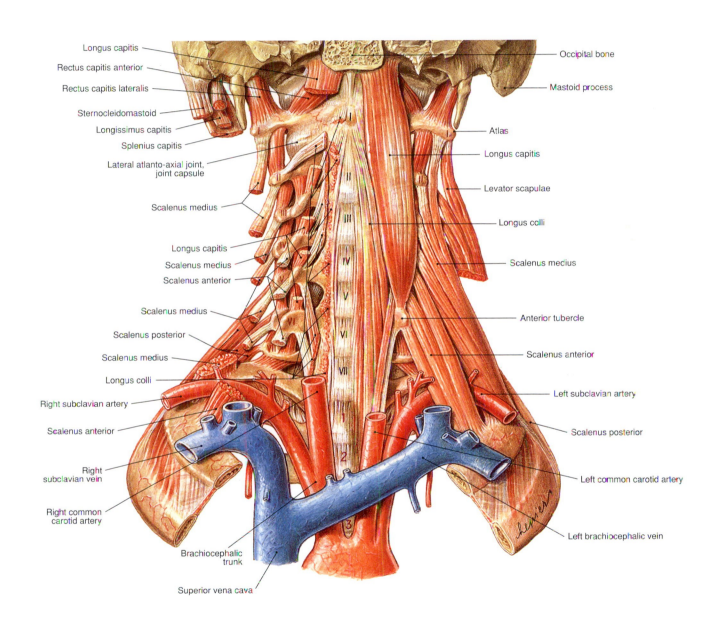

Longus capitis

Rectus capitis anterior

Rectus capitis lateralis

Sternocleidomastoid

Longissimus capitis

Splenius capitis

Lateral atlanto-axial joint, joint capsule

Scalenus medius

Longus capitis

Scalenus medius

Scalenus anterior

Scalenus medius

Scalenus posterior

Scalenus medius

Longus colli

Right subclavian artery

Scalenus anterior

Right subclavian vein

Right common carotid artery

Brachiocephalic trunk

Superior vena cava

Occipital bone

Mastoid process

Atlas

Longus capitis

Levator scapulae

Longus colli

Scalenus medius

Anterior tubercle

Scalenus anterior

Left subclavian artery

Scalenus posterior

Left common carotid artery

Left brachiocephalic vein

Fig. 209   Prevertebral muscles and scalenus muscles.
I – VII = First to seventh cervical vertebra
1 – 3 = First to third thoracic vertebra

→ T 11, T 12

Skeleton of the larynx

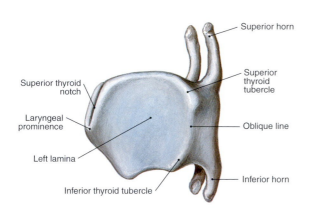

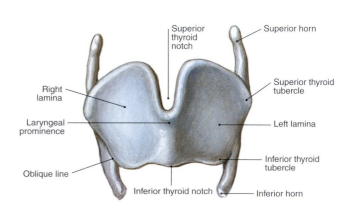

Fig. 210 Thyroid cartilage; viewed from the left.

Fig. 211 Thyroid cartilage; ventral view.

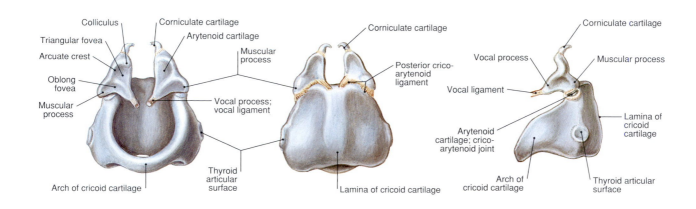

Fig. 212 Cartilages of the larynx; ventrosuperior view.

Fig. 213 Cartilages of the larynx; dorsal view.

Fig. 214 Cartilages of the larynx; viewed from the left.

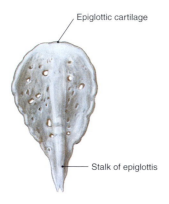

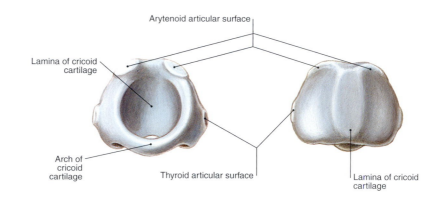

Fig. 215 Epiglottic cartilage; dorsal view.

Fig. 216 Cricoid cartilage; ventrosuperior view.

Fig. 217 Cricoid cartilage; dorsal view.

Hyoid bone and skeleton of the larynx

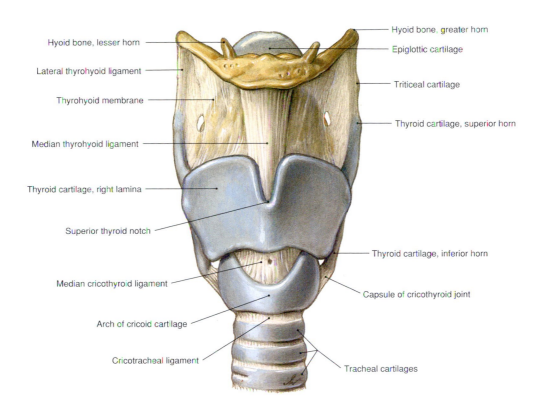

Hyoid bone, lesser horn

Lateral thyrohyoid ligament

Thyrohyoid membrane

Median thyrohyoid ligament

Thyroid cartilage, right lamina

Superior thyroid notch

Median cricothyroid ligament

Arch of cricoid cartilage

Cricotracheal ligament

Hyoid bone, greater horn

Epiglottic cartilage

Triticeal cartilage

Thyroid cartilage, superior horn

Thyroid cartilage, inferior horn

Capsule of cricothyroid joint

Tracheal cartilages

Fig. 218 Larynx and hyoid bone; ventral view.

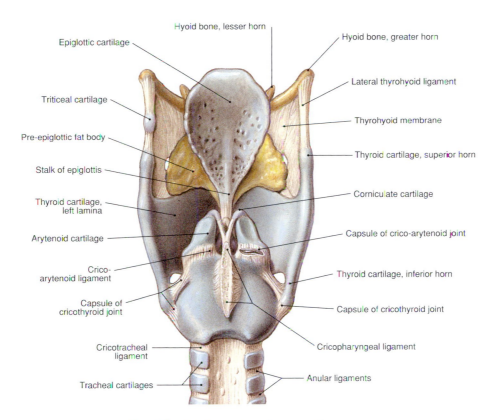

Hyoid bone, lesser horn

Epiglottic cartilage

Triticeal cartilage

Pre-epiglottic fat body

Stalk of epiglottis

Thyroid cartilage, left lamina

Arytenoid cartilage

Crico-arytenoid ligament

Capsule of cricothyroid joint

Cricotracheal ligament

Tracheal cartilages

Hyoid bone, greater horn

Lateral thyrohyoid ligament

Thyrohyoid membrane

Thyroid cartilage, superior horn

Corniculate cartilage

Capsule of crico-arytenoid joint

Thyroid cartilage, inferior horn

Capsule of cricothyroid joint

Cricopharyngeal ligament

Anular ligaments

Fig. 219 Cartilages of the larynx and hyoid bone; dorsal view.

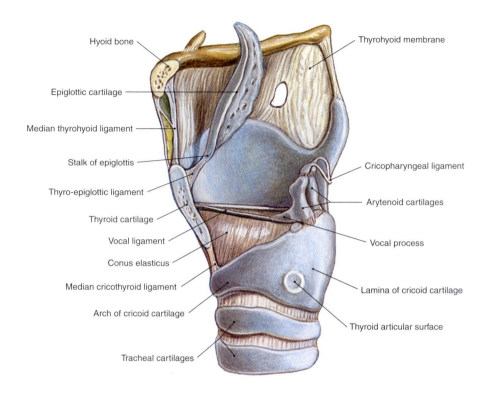

Hyoid bone

Epiglottic cartilage

Median thyrohyoid ligament

Stalk of epiglottis

Thyro-epiglottic ligament

Thyroid cartilage

Vocal ligament

Conus elasticus

Median cricothyroid ligament

Arch of cricoid cartilage

Tracheal cartilages

Thyrohyoid membrane

Cricopharyngeal ligament

Arytenoid cartilages

Vocal process

Lamina of cricoid cartilage

Thyroid articular surface

Fig. 220   Larynx and hyoid bone;
viewed from the left.

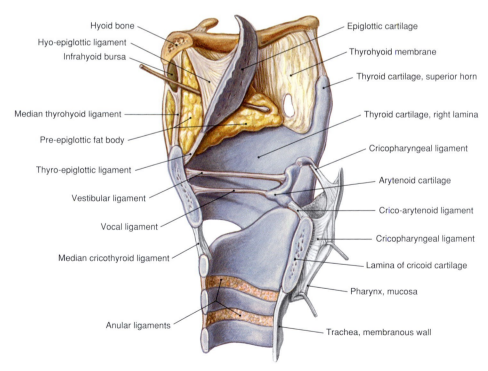

Hyoid bone

Hyo-epiglottic ligament

Infrahyoid bursa

Median thyrohyoid ligament

Pre-epiglottic fat body

Thyro-epiglottic ligament

Vestibular ligament

Vocal ligament

Median cricothyroid ligament

Anular ligaments

Epiglottic cartilage

Thyrohyoid membrane

Thyroid cartilage, superior horn

Thyroid cartilage, right lamina

Cricopharyngeal ligament

Arytenoid cartilage

Crico-arytenoid ligament

Cricopharyngeal ligament

Lamina of cricoid cartilage

Pharynx, mucosa

Trachea, membranous wall

Fig. 221   Larynx and hyoid bone;
median section;
medial view.

Laryngeal muscles

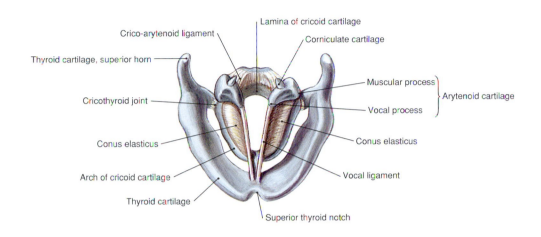

Fig. 222 Cartilages of the larynx and vocal ligament; ventrosuperior view.

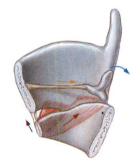

a Cricothyroid muscle

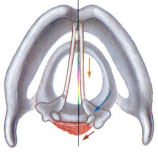

b Oblique and transverse arytenoid muscles

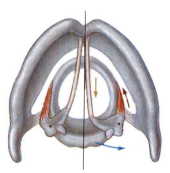

c Lateral crico-arytenoid muscle

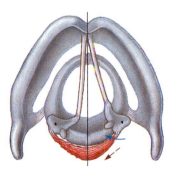

d Posterior crico-arytenoid muscle

Fig. 223 a–d Schema showing the functions of the laryngeal muscles;
yellow arrows: tension of the vocal ligament;
red arrows: muscle contraction;
blue arrows: direction of rotation;

the muscles on the left are relaxed; those on the right are contracted;
superior view.

Hyoid bone and skeleton of the larynx

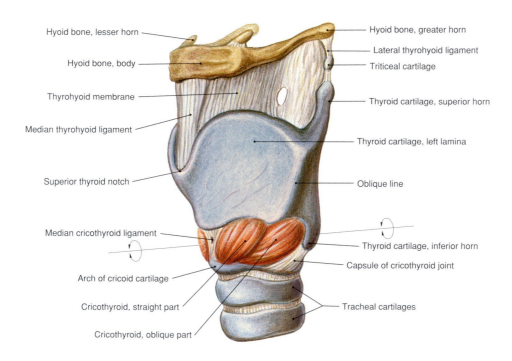

Hyoid bone, lesser horn

Hyoid bone, body

Thyrohyoid membrane

Median thyrohyoid ligament

Superior thyroid notch

Median cricothyroid ligament

Arch of cricoid cartilage

Cricothyroid, straight part

Cricothyroid, oblique part

Hyoid bone, greater horn

Lateral thyrohyoid ligament

Triticeal cartilage

Thyroid cartilage, superior horn

Thyroid cartilage, left lamina

Oblique line

Thyroid cartilage, inferior horn

Capsule of cricothyroid joint

Tracheal cartilages

→ T 6

Fig. 224   Cricothyroid muscle;
ventral view from the left.

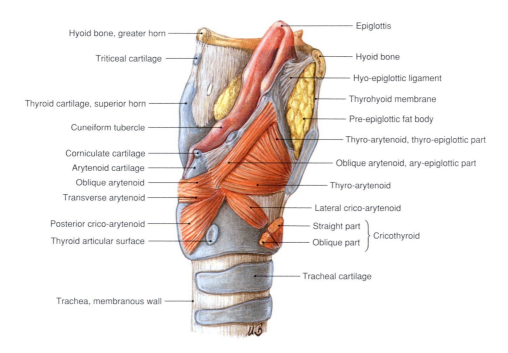

Hyoid bone, greater horn

Triticeal cartilage

Thyroid cartilage, superior horn

Cuneiform tubercle

Corniculate cartilage

Arytenoid cartilage

Oblique arytenoid

Transverse arytenoid

Posterior crico-arytenoid

Thyroid articular surface

Trachea, membranous wall

Epiglottis

Hyoid bone

Hyo-epiglottic ligament

Thyrohyoid membrane

Pre-epiglottic fat body

Thyro-arytenoid, thyro-epiglottic part

Oblique arytenoid, ary-epiglottic part

Thyro-arytenoid

Lateral crico-arytenoid

Straight part ⎫
Oblique part ⎬ Cricothyroid
⎭

Tracheal cartilage

→ T 6

Fig. 225   Laryngeal muscles;
dorsal view from the right.

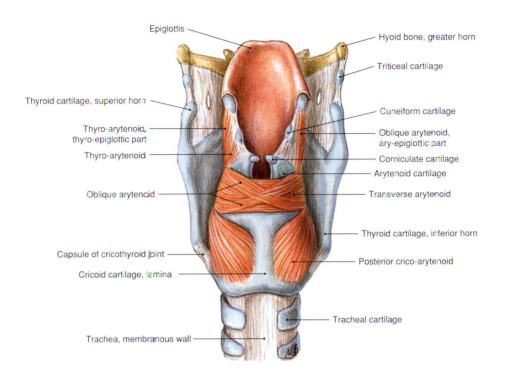

Epiglottis

Hyoid bone, greater horn

Triticeal cartilage

Thyroid cartilage, superior horn

Cuneiform cartilage

Thyro-arytenoid, thyro-epiglottic part

Oblique arytenoid, ary-epiglottic part

Thyro-arytenoid

Corniculate cartilage

Arytenoid cartilage

Oblique arytenoid

Transverse arytenoid

Thyroid cartilage, inferior horn

Capsule of cricothyroid joint

Posterior crico-arytenoid

Cricoid cartilage, lamina

Tracheal cartilage

Trachea, membranous wall

Fig. 226 Laryngeal muscles; dorsal view.

→ T 6

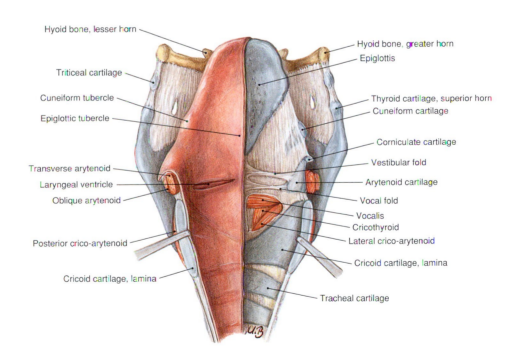

Hyoid bone, lesser horn

Hyoid bone, greater horn

Epiglottis

Triticeal cartilage

Cuneiform tubercle

Thyroid cartilage, superior horn

Cuneiform cartilage

Epiglottic tubercle

Corniculate cartilage

Transverse arytenoid

Vestibular fold

Laryngeal ventricle

Arytenoid cartilage

Oblique arytenoid

Vocal fold

Vocalis

Cricothyroid

Posterior crico-arytenoid

Lateral crico-arytenoid

Cricoid cartilage, lamina

Cricoid cartilage, lamina

Tracheal cartilage

Fig. 227 Larynx; sectioned from dorsal in the median plane and separated with hooks; dorsal view.

→ T 6

Fig. 228 a, b Laryngoscopy.
a Indirect laryngoscopy
b Direct, endoscopic laryngoscopy

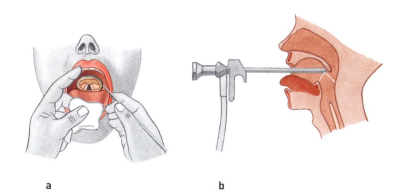

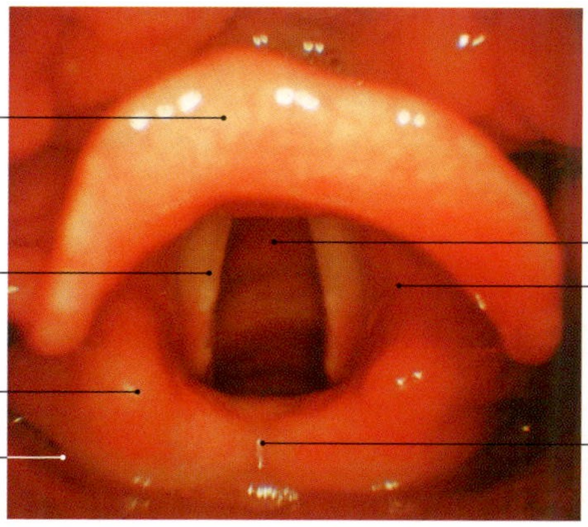

a   b

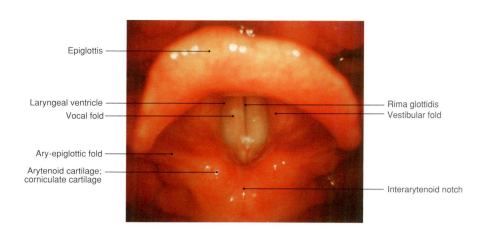

Epiglottis

Vocal fold

Rima glottidis

Vestibular fold

Arytenoid cartilage;
corniculate cartilage

Piriform fossa

Interarytenoid notch

Fig. 229 Direct laryngoscopy;
respiratory position.

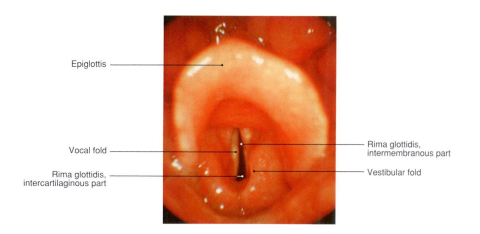

Epiglottis

Laryngeal ventricle
Vocal fold

Rima glottidis
Vestibular fold

Ary-epiglottic fold

Arytenoid cartilage;
corniculate cartilage

Interarytenoid notch

Fig. 230 Direct laryngoscopy;
phonation position.

Epiglottis

Vocal fold

Rima glottidis,
intermembranous part

Rima glottidis,
intercartilaginous part

Vestibular fold

Fig. 231 Direct laryngoscopy;
whispering position.

Inner contour of the larynx

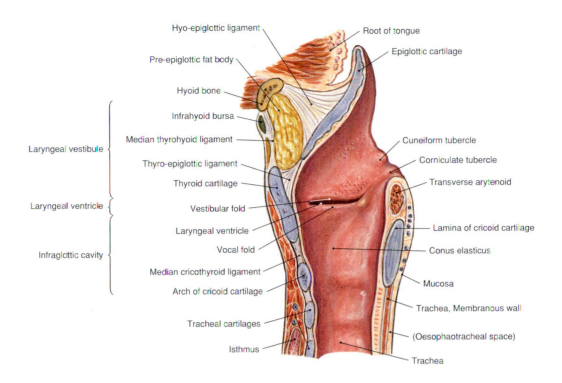

Hyo-epiglottic ligament
Pre-epiglottic fat body
Hyoid bone
Infrahyoid bursa
Median thyrohyoid ligament
Thyro-epiglottic ligament
Thyroid cartilage
Vestibular fold
Laryngeal ventricle
Vocal fold
Median cricothyroid ligament
Arch of cricoid cartilage
Tracheal cartilages
Isthmus

Root of tongue
Epiglottic cartilage
Cuneiform tubercle
Corniculate tubercle
Transverse arytenoid
Lamina of cricoid cartilage
Conus elasticus
Mucosa
Trachea, Membranous wall
(Oesophaotracheal space)
Trachea

Laryngeal vestibule
Laryngeal ventricle
Infraglottic cavity

Fig. 232   Larynx.

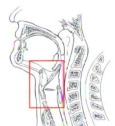

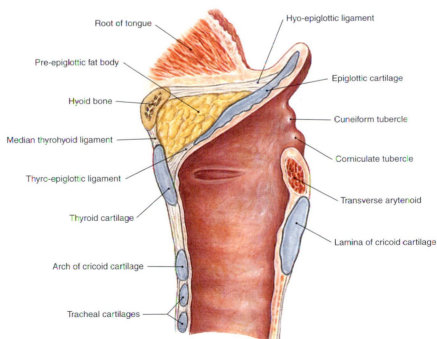

Root of tongue
Pre-epiglottic fat body
Hyoid bone
Median thyrohyoid ligament
Thyro-epiglottic ligament
Thyroid cartilage
Arch of cricoid cartilage
Tracheal cartilages

Hyo-epiglottic ligament
Epiglottic cartilage
Cuneiform tubercle
Corniculate tubercle
Transverse arytenoid
Lamina of cricoid cartilage

Fig. 233   Larynx;
position of the epiglottis during swallowing.

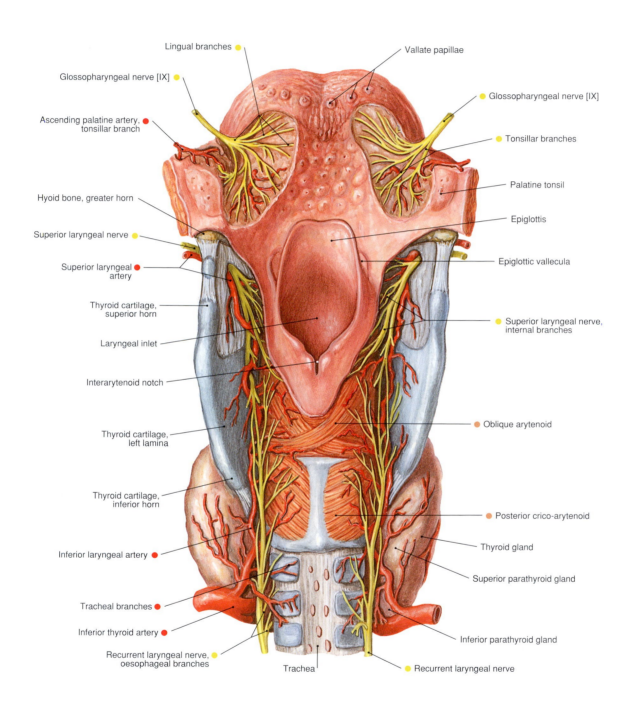

Lingual branches

Glossopharyngeal nerve [IX]

Ascending palatine artery, tonsillar branch

Hyoid bone, greater horn

Superior laryngeal nerve

Superior laryngeal artery

Thyroid cartilage, superior horn

Laryngeal inlet

Interarytenoid notch

Thyroid cartilage, left lamina

Thyroid cartilage, inferior horn

Inferior laryngeal artery

Tracheal branches

Inferior thyroid artery

Recurrent laryngeal nerve, oesophageal branches

Vallate papillae

Glossopharyngeal nerve [IX]

Tonsillar branches

Palatine tonsil

Epiglottis

Epiglottic vallecula

Superior laryngeal nerve, internal branches

Oblique arytenoid

Posterior crico-arytenoid

Thyroid gland

Superior parathyroid gland

Inferior parathyroid gland

Trachea

Recurrent laryngeal nerve

→ 252

Fig. 234 Arteries and nerves of the larynx and the root of the tongue.

Larynx, transverse sections

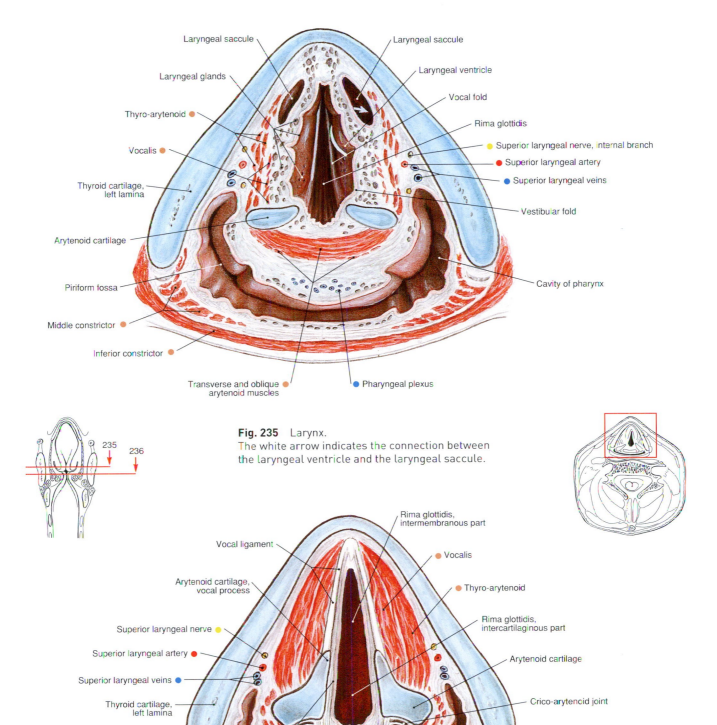

Laryngeal saccule

Laryngeal saccule

Laryngeal glands

Laryngeal ventricle

Thyro-arytenoid ●

Vocal fold

Rima glottidis

Vocalis ●

● Superior laryngeal nerve, internal branch

● Superior laryngeal artery

Thyroid cartilage, left lamina

● Superior laryngeal veins

Arytenoid cartilage

Vestibular fold

Piriform fossa

Cavity of pharynx

Middle constrictor ●

Inferior constrictor ●

Transverse and oblique ● arytenoid muscles

● Pharyngeal plexus

Fig. 235 Larynx.
The white arrow indicates the connection between the laryngeal ventricle and the laryngeal saccule.

235   236

Vocal ligament

Rima glottidis, intermembranous part

● Vocalis

Arytenoid cartilage, vocal process

● Thyro-arytenoid

Superior laryngeal nerve ●

Rima glottidis, intercartilaginous part

Superior laryngeal artery ●

Arytenoid cartilage

Superior laryngeal veins ●

Crico-arytenoid joint

Thyroid cartilage, left lamina

Cavity of pharynx

Piriform fossa

Mucosa

Posterior crico-arytenoid ●

● Inferior constrictor

Mucosa

Lamina of cricoid cartilage

Fig. 236 Larynx.

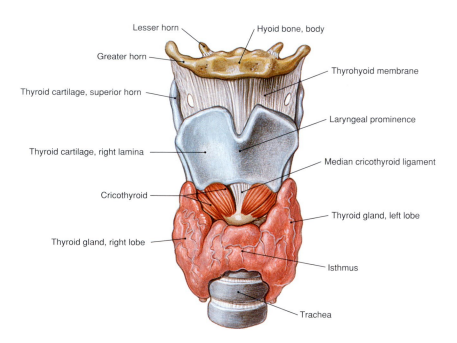

→ 205

Fig. 237   Thyroid gland and larynx.

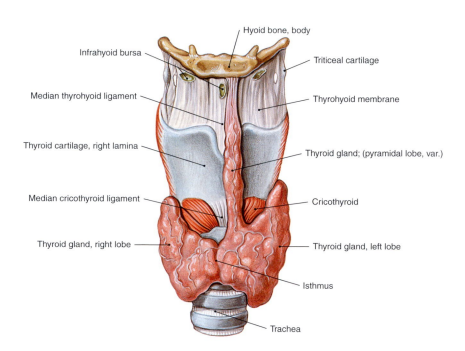

Fig. 238   Thyroid gland and larynx.

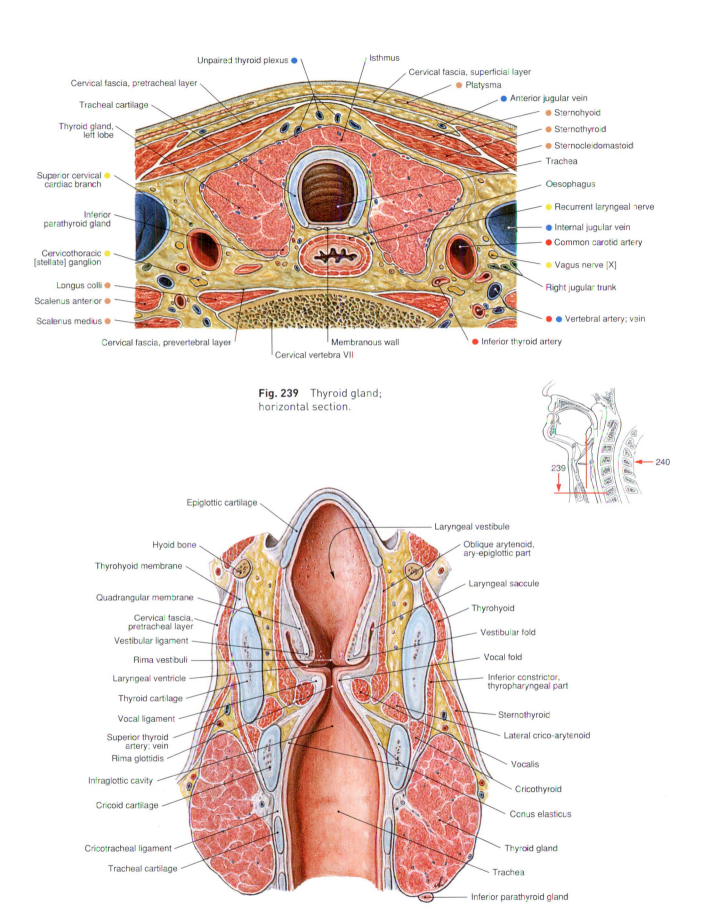

Unpaired thyroid plexus ●
Isthmus
Cervical fascia, superficial layer
Cervical fascia, pretracheal layer
● Platysma
Tracheal cartilage
● Anterior jugular vein
Thyroid gland, left lobe
● Sternohyoid
● Sternothyroid
● Sternocleidomastoid
Trachea
Superior cervical cardiac branch ●
Oesophagus
● Recurrent laryngeal nerve
Inferior parathyroid gland
● Internal jugular vein
● Common carotid artery
Cervicothoracic [stellate] ganglion ●
● Vagus nerve [X]
Right jugular trunk
Longus colli ●
Scalenus anterior ●
Scalenus medius ●
● ● Vertebral artery; vein
Cervical fascia, prevertebral layer
Membranous wall
● Inferior thyroid artery
Cervical vertebra VII

Fig. 239 Thyroid gland; horizontal section.

239
240

Epiglottic cartilage
Laryngeal vestibule
Hyoid bone
Oblique arytenoid, ary-epiglottic part
Thyrohyoid membrane
Laryngeal saccule
Quadrangular membrane
Thyrohyoid
Cervical fascia, pretracheal layer
Vestibular fold
Vestibular ligament
Vocal fold
Rima vestibuli
Laryngeal ventricle
Inferior constrictor, thyropharyngeal part
Thyroid cartilage
Vocal ligament
Sternothyroid
Superior thyroid artery; vein
Lateral crico-arytenoid
Rima glottidis
Vocalis
Infraglottic cavity
Cricothyroid
Cricoid cartilage
Conus elasticus
Cricotracheal ligament
Thyroid gland
Tracheal cartilage
Trachea
Inferior parathyroid gland

Fig. 240 Thyroid gland; frontal section.

Arterial supply of the thyroid gland

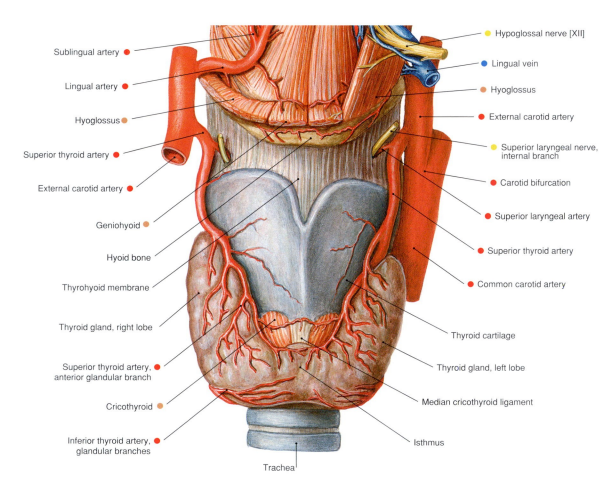

Sublingual artery ●

Lingual artery ●

Hyoglossus ●

Superior thyroid artery ●

External carotid artery ●

Geniohyoid ●

Hyoid bone

Thyrohyoid membrane

Thyroid gland, right lobe

Superior thyroid artery, anterior glandular branch ●

Cricothyroid ●

Inferior thyroid artery, glandular branches ●

Trachea

Hypoglossal nerve [XII] ●

Lingual vein ●

Hyoglossus ●

External carotid artery ●

Superior laryngeal nerve, internal branch ●

Carotid bifurcation ●

Superior laryngeal artery ●

Superior thyroid artery ●

Common carotid artery ●

Thyroid cartilage

Thyroid gland, left lobe

Median cricothyroid ligament

Isthmus

Fig. 241 Vessels and nerves of the thyroid gland and the larynx.

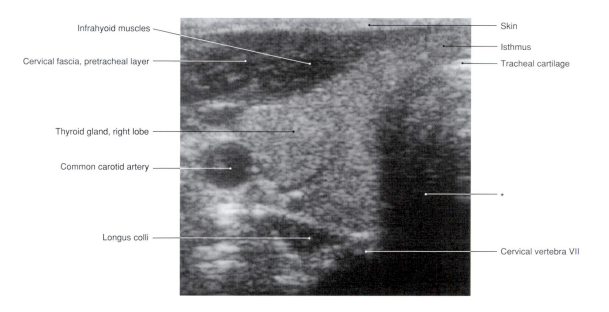

Infrahyoid muscles

Cervical fascia, pretracheal layer

Thyroid gland, right lobe

Common carotid artery

Longus colli

Skin

Isthmus

Tracheal cartilage

*

Cervical vertebra VII

Fig. 242 Thyroid gland; oblique ultrasound image in ventrodorsal direction; inferior view (right, 200%).

* Ultrasound shadow of the trachea

Pathological enlargement of the thyroid gland

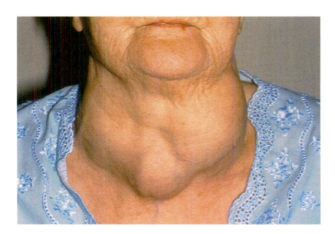

Fig. 243 Thyroid gland;
enlargement of the thyroid gland with three obvious nodes, Struma nodosa.

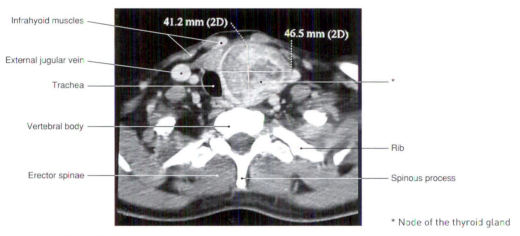

Infrahyoid muscles

External jugular vein

Trachea

Vertebral body

Erector spinae

41.2 mm (2D)

46.5 mm (2D)

*

Rib

Spinous process

* Node of the thyroid gland

Fig. 244 Neck;
computed tomographic (CT) section;
inferior view.
The trachea is displaced towards the right by a pathologically enlarged
node of the thyroid gland.

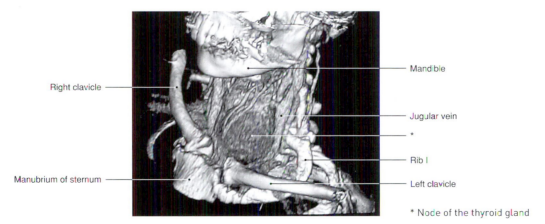

Right clavicle

Manubrium of sternum

Mandible

Jugular vein

*

Rib I

Left clavicle

* Node of the thyroid gland

Fig. 245 Neck;
3-dimensional reconstruction from computed tomographic (CT) sections
showing a heavily enlarged left lobe of the thyroid gland;
same patient as in Fig. 244.

Nasal and pharyngeal cavity, paramedian section

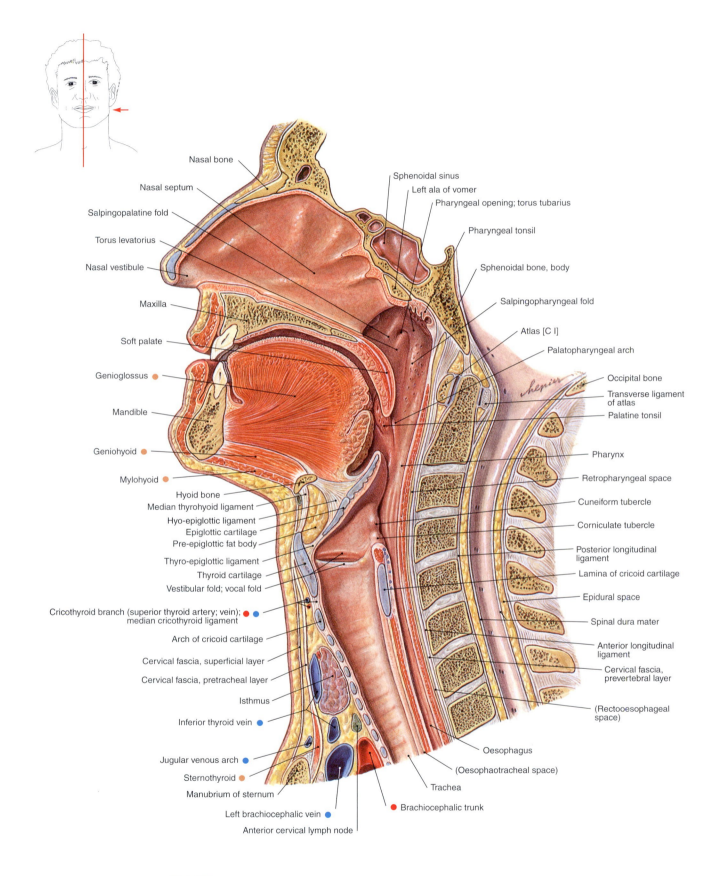

Nasal bone

Nasal septum

Salpingopalatine fold

Torus levatorius

Nasal vestibule

Maxilla

Soft palate

Genioglossus

Mandible

Geniohyoid

Mylohyoid

Hyoid bone

Median thyrohyoid ligament

Hyo-epiglottic ligament

Epiglottic cartilage

Pre-epiglottic fat body

Thyro-epiglottic ligament

Thyroid cartilage

Vestibular fold; vocal fold

Cricothyroid branch (superior thyroid artery; vein);
median cricothyroid ligament

Arch of cricoid cartilage

Cervical fascia, superficial layer

Cervical fascia, pretracheal layer

Isthmus

Inferior thyroid vein

Jugular venous arch

Sternothyroid

Manubrium of sternum

Left brachiocephalic vein

Anterior cervical lymph node

Sphenoidal sinus

Left ala of vomer

Pharyngeal opening; torus tubarius

Pharyngeal tonsil

Sphenoidal bone, body

Salpingopharyngeal fold

Atlas [C I]

Palatopharyngeal arch

Occipital bone

Transverse ligament of atlas

Palatine tonsil

Pharynx

Retropharyngeal space

Cuneiform tubercle

Corniculate tubercle

Posterior longitudinal ligament

Lamina of cricoid cartilage

Epidural space

Spinal dura mater

Anterior longitudinal ligament

Cervical fascia, prevertebral layer

(Rectooesophageal space)

Oesophagus

(Oesophaotracheal space)

Trachea

Brachiocephalic trunk

→ 271

Fig. 246 Nasal cavity;
oral cavity; pharynx and larynx;
paramedian section.

Pharyngeal muscles

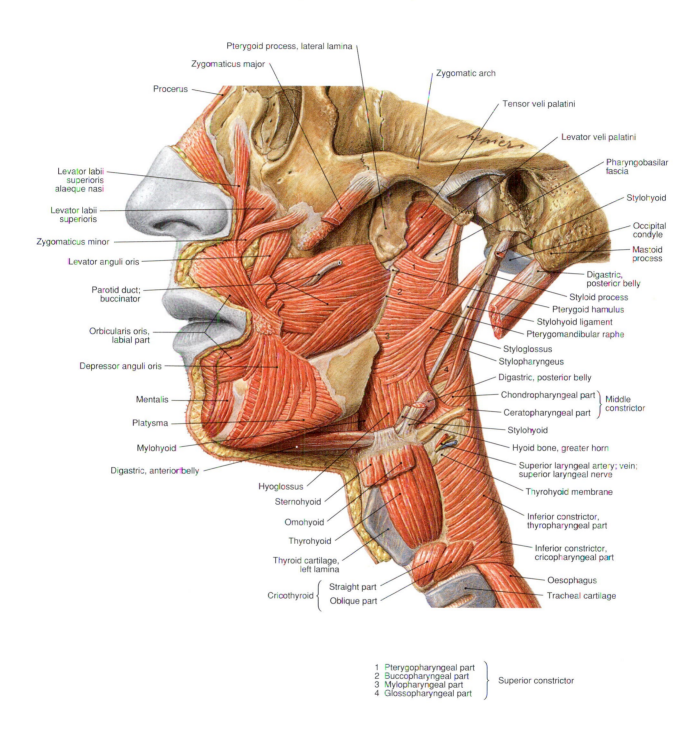

Pterygoid process, lateral lamina
Zygomaticus major
Procerus
Zygomatic arch
Tensor veli palatini
Levator veli palatini
Levator labii superioris alaeque nasi
Pharyngobasilar fascia
Levator labii superioris
Stylohyoid
Zygomaticus minor
Occipital condyle
Levator anguli oris
Mastoid process
Parotid duct; buccinator
Digastric, posterior belly
Styloid process
Pterygoid hamulus
Orbicularis oris, labial part
Stylohyoid ligament
Pterygomandibular raphe
Depressor anguli oris
Styloglossus
Stylopharyngeus
Digastric, posterior belly
Mentalis
Chondropharyngeal part — Middle constrictor
Platysma
Ceratopharyngeal part
Stylohyoid
Mylohyoid
Hyoid bone, greater horn
Digastric, anterior belly
Superior laryngeal artery; vein; superior laryngeal nerve
Hyoglossus
Thyrohyoid membrane
Sternohyoid
Inferior constrictor, thyropharyngeal part
Omohyoid
Inferior constrictor, cricopharyngeal part
Thyrohyoid
Thyroid cartilage, left lamina
Oesophagus
Tracheal cartilage
Cricothyroid { Straight part / Oblique part }

1 Pterygopharyngeal part
2 Buccopharyngeal part — Superior constrictor
3 Mylopharyngeal part
4 Glossopharyngeal part

Fig. 247 Pharyngeal muscles and facial muscles.

→ T 1e, f, T 5

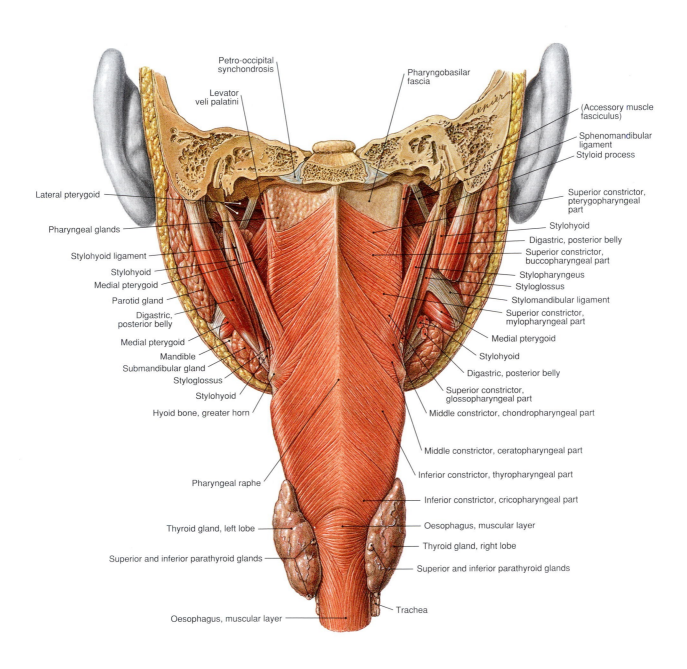

Petro-occipital synchondrosis

Levator veli palatini

Pharyngobasilar fascia

(Accessory muscle fasciculus)

Sphenomandibular ligament

Styloid process

Lateral pterygoid

Pharyngeal glands

Stylohyoid ligament

Stylohyoid

Medial pterygoid

Parotid gland

Digastric, posterior belly

Medial pterygoid

Mandible

Submandibular gland

Styloglossus

Stylohyoid

Hyoid bone, greater horn

Pharyngeal raphe

Thyroid gland, left lobe

Superior and inferior parathyroid glands

Oesophagus, muscular layer

Superior constrictor, pterygopharyngeal part

Stylohyoid

Digastric, posterior belly

Superior constrictor, buccopharyngeal part

Stylopharyngeus

Styloglossus

Stylomandibular ligament

Superior constrictor, mylopharyngeal part

Medial pterygoid

Stylohyoid

Digastric, posterior belly

Superior constrictor, glossopharyngeal part

Middle constrictor, chondropharyngeal part

Middle constrictor, ceratopharyngeal part

Inferior constrictor, thyropharyngeal part

Inferior constrictor, cricopharyngeal part

Oesophagus, muscular layer

Thyroid gland, right lobe

Superior and inferior parathyroid glands

Trachea

→ T 5

Fig. 248 Pharyngeal muscles.

Inner contour of the pharynx

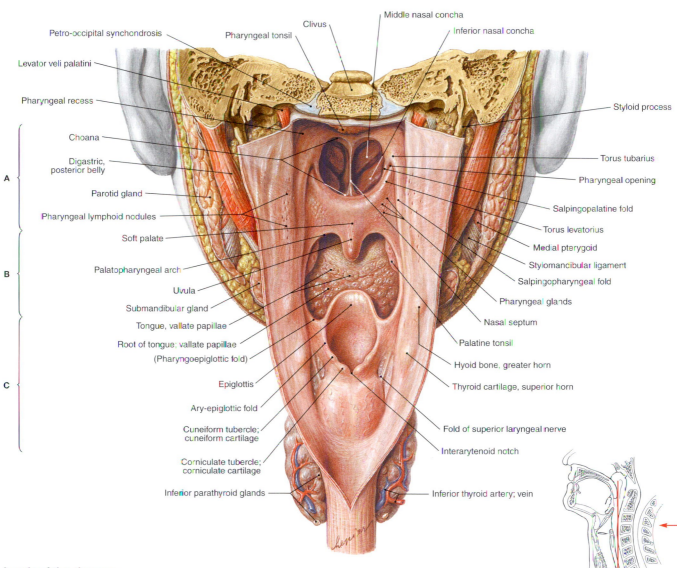

Petro-occipital synchondrosis
Levator veli palatini
Pharyngeal recess
Choana
Digastric, posterior belly
Parotid gland
Pharyngeal lymphoid nodules
Soft palate
Palatopharyngeal arch
Uvula
Submandibular gland
Tongue, vallate papillae
Root of tongue; vallate papillae
(Pharyngoepiglottic fold)
Epiglottis
Ary-epiglottic fold
Cuneiform tubercle; cuneiform cartilage
Corniculate tubercle; corniculate cartilage
Inferior parathyroid glands

Clivus
Pharyngeal tonsil
Middle nasal concha
Inferior nasal concha
Styloid process
Torus tubarius
Pharyngeal opening
Salpingopalatine fold
Torus levatorius
Medial pterygoid
Stylomandibular ligament
Salpingopharyngeal fold
Pharyngeal glands
Nasal septum
Palatine tonsil
Hyoid bone, greater horn
Thyroid cartilage, superior horn
Fold of superior laryngeal nerve
Interarytenoid notch
Inferior thyroid artery; vein

A
B
C

Levels of the pharynx:
A Nasopharynx
B Oropharynx
C Laryngopharynx, hypopharynx

Fig. 249 Pharynx.

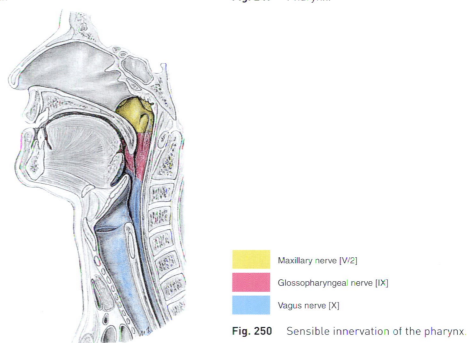

Maxillary nerve [V/2]
Glossopharyngeal nerve [IX]
Vagus nerve [X]

Fig. 250 Sensible innervation of the pharynx.

Vessels and nerves of the parapharyngeal space

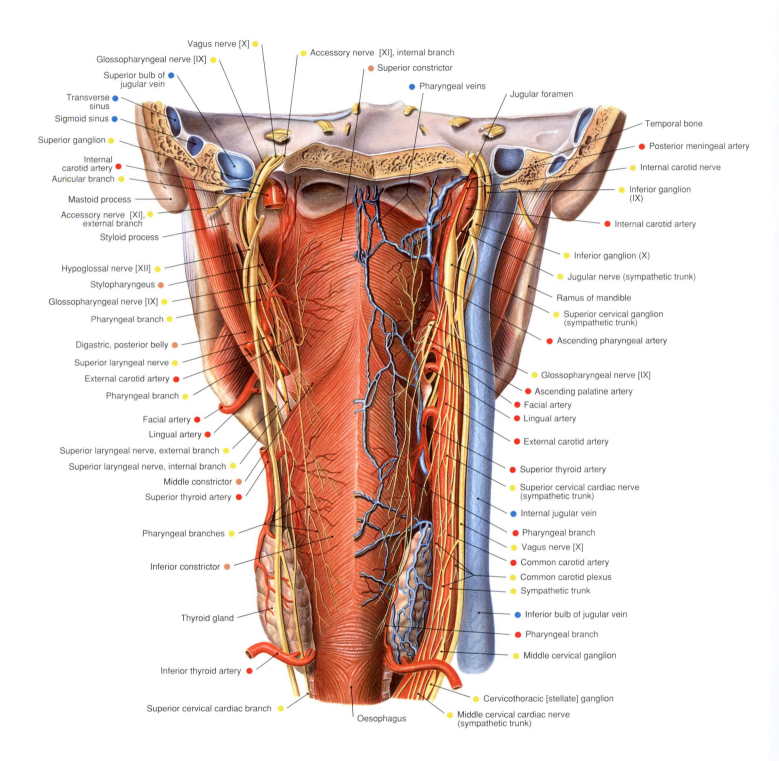

Vagus nerve [X] ●
Glossopharyngeal nerve [IX] ●
Superior bulb of jugular vein ●
Transverse sinus ●
Sigmoid sinus ●
Superior ganglion ●
Internal carotid artery ●
Auricular branch ●
Mastoid process
Accessory nerve [XI], external branch
Styloid process
Hypoglossal nerve [XII] ●
Stylopharyngeus ●
Glossopharyngeal nerve [IX] ●
Pharyngeal branch ●
Digastric, posterior belly ●
Superior laryngeal nerve ●
External carotid artery ●
Pharyngeal branch ●
Facial artery ●
Lingual artery ●
Superior laryngeal nerve, external branch
Superior laryngeal nerve, internal branch
Middle constrictor ●
Superior thyroid artery ●
Pharyngeal branches ●
Inferior constrictor ●
Thyroid gland
Inferior thyroid artery ●
Superior cervical cardiac branch

Accessory nerve [XI], internal branch ●
Superior constrictor ●
Pharyngeal veins ●
Jugular foramen
Temporal bone
Posterior meningeal artery ●
Internal carotid nerve ●
Inferior ganglion (IX) ●
Internal carotid artery ●
Inferior ganglion (X) ●
Jugular nerve (sympathetic trunk) ●
Ramus of mandible
Superior cervical ganglion (sympathetic trunk) ●
Ascending pharyngeal artery ●
Glossopharyngeal nerve [IX] ●
Ascending palatine artery ●
Facial artery ●
Lingual artery ●
External carotid artery ●
Superior thyroid artery ●
Superior cervical cardiac nerve (sympathetic trunk) ●
Internal jugular vein ●
Pharyngeal branch ●
Vagus nerve [X] ●
Common carotid artery ●
Common carotid plexus ●
Sympathetic trunk ●
Inferior bulb of jugular vein ●
Pharyngeal branch ●
Middle cervical ganglion ●
Cervicothoracic [stellate] ganglion ●
Middle cervical cardiac nerve (sympathetic trunk) ●
Oesophagus

Fig. 251   Vessels and nerves of the pharynx and the parapharyngeal space.

252

669

Vessels and nerves of the parapharyngeal space

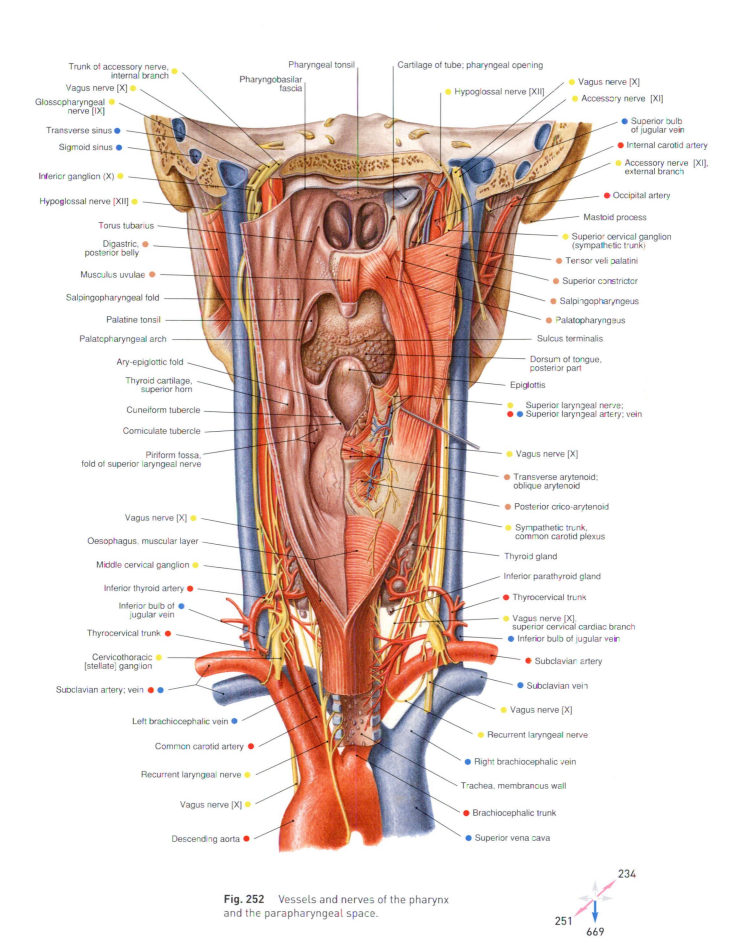

Trunk of accessory nerve, internal branch
Vagus nerve [X]
Glossopharyngeal nerve [IX]
Transverse sinus
Sigmoid sinus
Inferior ganglion (X)
Hypoglossal nerve [XII]
Torus tubarius
Digastric, posterior belly
Musculus uvulae
Salpingopharyngeal fold
Palatine tonsil
Palatopharyngeal arch
Ary-epiglottic fold
Thyroid cartilage, superior horn
Cuneiform tubercle
Corniculate tubercle
Piriform fossa, fold of superior laryngeal nerve
Vagus nerve [X]
Oesophagus, muscular layer
Middle cervical ganglion
Inferior thyroid artery
Inferior bulb of jugular vein
Thyrocervical trunk
Cervicothoracic [stellate] ganglion
Subclavian artery; vein
Left brachiocephalic vein
Common carotid artery
Recurrent laryngeal nerve
Vagus nerve [X]
Descending aorta

Pharyngeal tonsil
Pharyngobasilar fascia
Cartilage of tube; pharyngeal opening

Vagus nerve [X]
Hypoglossal nerve [XII]
Accessory nerve [XI]
Superior bulb of jugular vein
Internal carotid artery
Accessory nerve [XI], external branch
Occipital artery
Mastoid process
Superior cervical ganglion (sympathetic trunk)
Tensor veli palatini
Superior constrictor
Salpingopharyngeus
Palatopharyngeus
Sulcus terminalis
Dorsum of tongue, posterior part
Epiglottis
Superior laryngeal nerve;
Superior laryngeal artery; vein
Vagus nerve [X]
Transverse arytenoid; oblique arytenoid
Posterior crico-arytenoid
Sympathetic trunk, common carotid plexus
Thyroid gland
Inferior parathyroid gland
Thyrocervical trunk
Vagus nerve [X], superior cervical cardiac branch
Inferior bulb of jugular vein
Subclavian artery
Subclavian vein
Vagus nerve [X]
Recurrent laryngeal nerve
Right brachiocephalic vein
Trachea, membranous wall
Brachiocephalic trunk
Superior vena cava

Fig. 252 Vessels and nerves of the pharynx and the parapharyngeal space.

234
251
669

Vessels and nerves of the neck

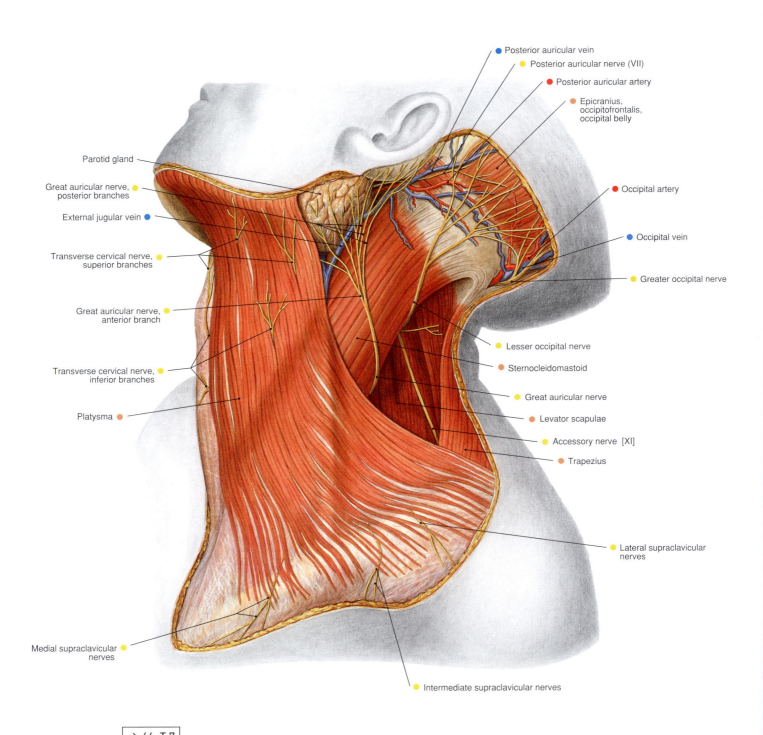

Posterior auricular vein

Posterior auricular nerve (VII)

Posterior auricular artery

Epicranius, occipitofrontalis, occipital belly

Parotid gland

Great auricular nerve, posterior branches

External jugular vein

Occipital artery

Transverse cervical nerve, superior branches

Occipital vein

Great auricular nerve, anterior branch

Greater occipital nerve

Lesser occipital nerve

Sternocleidomastoid

Transverse cervical nerve, inferior branches

Great auricular nerve

Platysma

Levator scapulae

Accessory nerve [XI]

Trapezius

Lateral supraclavicular nerves

Medial supraclavicular nerves

Intermediate supraclavicular nerves

→ 46, T 7

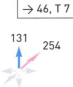

131

254

Fig. 253 Vessels and nerves of the anterior and the lateral region of the neck; superficial layer.

Vessels and nerves of the neck

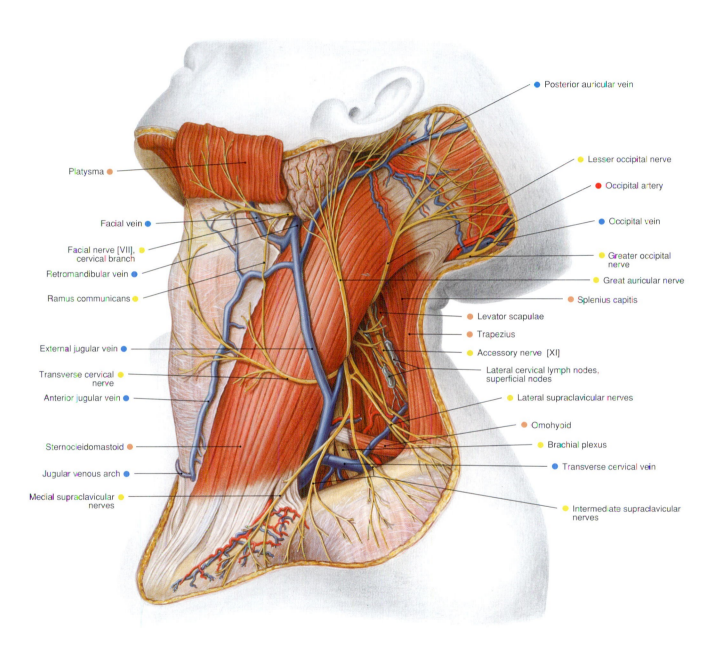

Posterior auricular vein

Platysma ●

Lesser occipital nerve

Occipital artery

Facial vein ●

Occipital vein

Facial nerve [VII], ● cervical branch

Greater occipital nerve

Retromandibular vein ●

Great auricular nerve

Ramus communicans ●

Splenius capitis

Levator scapulae

Trapezius

External jugular vein ●

Accessory nerve [XI]

Lateral cervical lymph nodes, superficial nodes

Transverse cervical ● nerve

Anterior jugular vein ●

Lateral supraclavicular nerves

Omohyoid

Sternocleidomastoid ●

Brachial plexus

Jugular venous arch ●

Transverse cervical vein

Medial supraclavicular ● nerves

Intermediate supraclavicular nerves

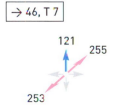

→ 46, T 7

121

255

253

Fig. 254 Vessels and nerves of the lateral region of the neck; parts of the platysma have been reflected cranially and the superficial layer of the cervical fascia has been largely removed.

Vessels and nerves of the neck

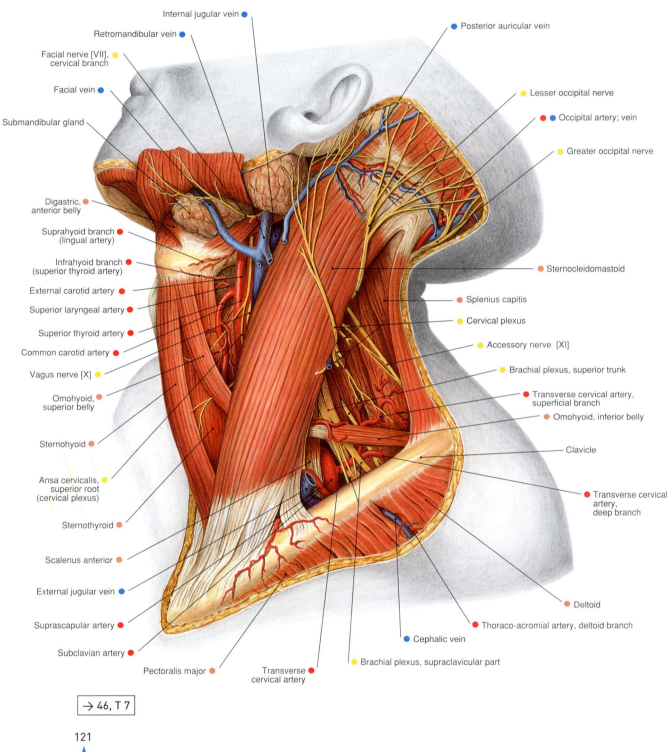

Internal jugular vein

Retromandibular vein

Facial nerve [VII], cervical branch

Facial vein

Submandibular gland

Digastric, anterior belly

Suprahyoid branch (lingual artery)

Infrahyoid branch (superior thyroid artery)

External carotid artery

Superior laryngeal artery

Superior thyroid artery

Common carotid artery

Vagus nerve [X]

Omohyoid, superior belly

Sternohyoid

Ansa cervicalis, superior root (cervical plexus)

Sternothyroid

Scalenus anterior

External jugular vein

Suprascapular artery

Subclavian artery

Pectoralis major

Transverse cervical artery

Posterior auricular vein

Lesser occipital nerve

Occipital artery; vein

Greater occipital nerve

Sternocleidomastoid

Splenius capitis

Cervical plexus

Accessory nerve [XI]

Brachial plexus, superior trunk

Transverse cervical artery, superficial branch

Omohyoid, inferior belly

Clavicle

Transverse cervical artery, deep branch

Deltoid

Thoraco-acromial artery, deltoid branch

Cephalic vein

Brachial plexus, supraclavicular part

→ 46, T 7

121

254

Fig. 255 Vessels and nerves of the anterior and the lateral region of the neck; the superficial and the middle layer of the cervical fascia have been removed.

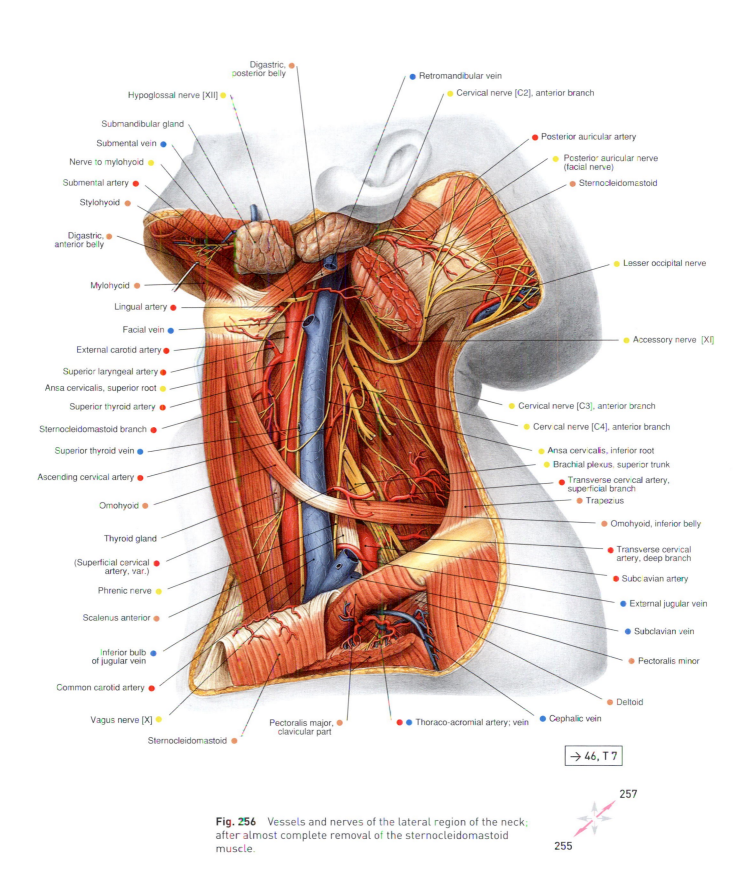

Digastric, posterior belly

Hypoglossal nerve [XII]

Submandibular gland

Submental vein

Nerve to mylohyoid

Submental artery

Stylohyoid

Digastric, anterior belly

Mylohyoid

Lingual artery

Facial vein

External carotid artery

Superior laryngeal artery

Ansa cervicalis, superior root

Superior thyroid artery

Sternocleidomastoid branch

Superior thyroid vein

Ascending cervical artery

Omohyoid

Thyroid gland

(Superficial cervical artery, var.)

Phrenic nerve

Scalenus anterior

Inferior bulb of jugular vein

Common carotid artery

Vagus nerve [X]

Pectoralis major, clavicular part

Sternocleidomastoid

Retromandibular vein

Cervical nerve [C2], anterior branch

Posterior auricular artery

Posterior auricular nerve (facial nerve)

Sternocleidomastoid

Lesser occipital nerve

Accessory nerve [XI]

Cervical nerve [C3], anterior branch

Cervical nerve [C4], anterior branch

Ansa cervicalis, inferior root

Brachial plexus, superior trunk

Transverse cervical artery, superficial branch

Trapezius

Omohyoid, inferior belly

Transverse cervical artery, deep branch

Subclavian artery

External jugular vein

Subclavian vein

Pectoralis minor

Deltoid

Thoraco-acromial artery; vein

Cephalic vein

→ 46, T 7

257

Fig. 256 Vessels and nerves of the lateral region of the neck; after almost complete removal of the sternocleidomastoid muscle.

255

Vessels and nerves of the neck

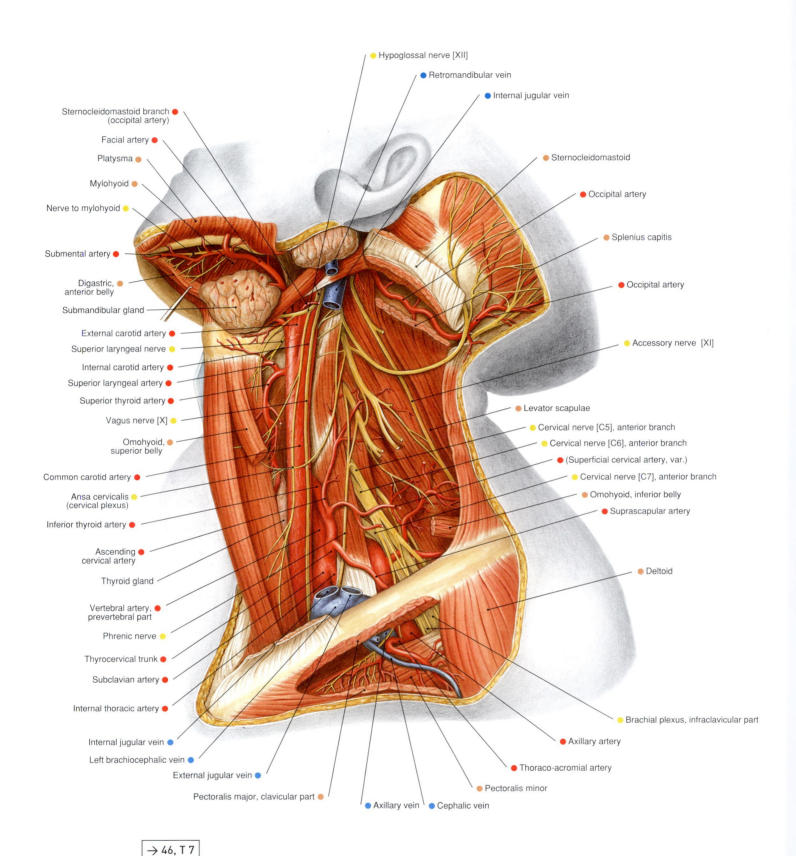

Hypoglossal nerve [XII]

Retromandibular vein

Internal jugular vein

Sternocleidomastoid branch (occipital artery)

Facial artery

Platysma

Mylohyoid

Nerve to mylohyoid

Submental artery

Digastric, anterior belly

Submandibular gland

External carotid artery

Superior laryngeal nerve

Internal carotid artery

Superior laryngeal artery

Superior thyroid artery

Vagus nerve [X]

Omohyoid, superior belly

Common carotid artery

Ansa cervicalis (cervical plexus)

Inferior thyroid artery

Ascending cervical artery

Thyroid gland

Vertebral artery, prevertebral part

Phrenic nerve

Thyrocervical trunk

Subclavian artery

Internal thoracic artery

Internal jugular vein

Left brachiocephalic vein

External jugular vein

Pectoralis major, clavicular part

Axillary vein

Cephalic vein

Sternocleidomastoid

Occipital artery

Splenius capitis

Occipital artery

Accessory nerve [XI]

Levator scapulae

Cervical nerve [C5], anterior branch

Cervical nerve [C6], anterior branch

(Superficial cervical artery, var.)

Cervical nerve [C7], anterior branch

Omohyoid, inferior belly

Suprascapular artery

Deltoid

Brachial plexus, infraclavicular part

Axillary artery

Thoraco-acromial artery

Pectoralis minor

→ 46, T 7

256 258

Fig. 257 Vessels and nerves of the lateral region of the neck; deep layer.

Vessels and nerves of the neck and the axilla

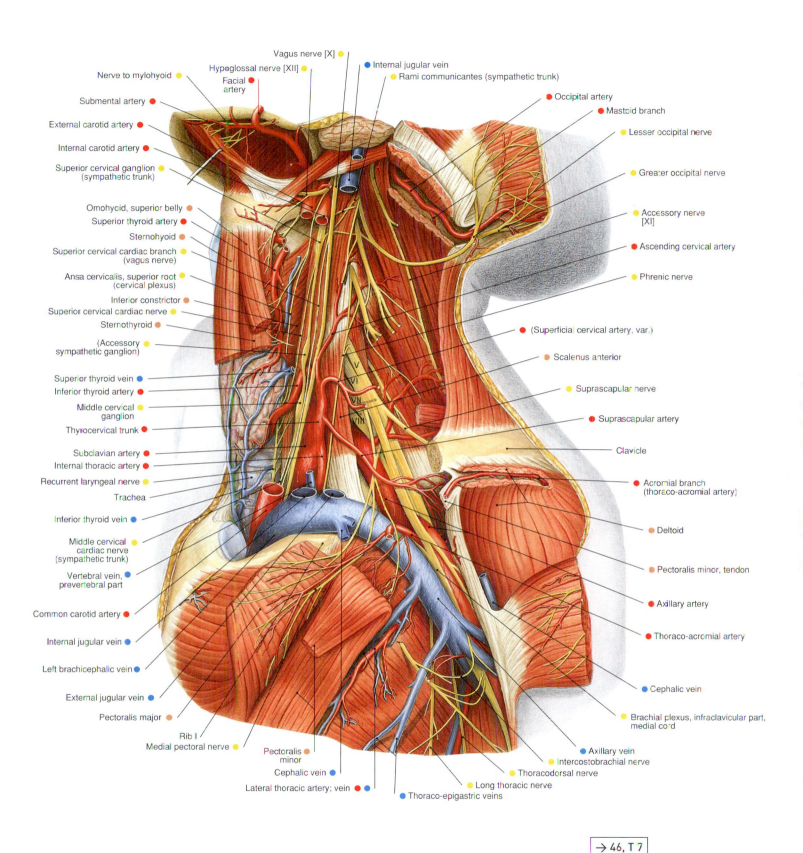

Vagus nerve [X] ●
Hypoglossal nerve [XII] ●
Nerve to mylohyoid
Facial ● artery
Submental artery ●
External carotid artery ●
Internal carotid artery ●
Superior cervical ganglion ●
(sympathetic trunk)
Omohyoid, superior belly ●
Superior thyroid artery ●
Sternohyoid ●
Superior cervical cardiac branch ●
(vagus nerve)
Ansa cervicalis, superior root ●
(cervical plexus)
Inferior constrictor ●
Superior cervical cardiac nerve ●
Sternothyroid ●
(Accessory ●
sympathetic ganglion)
Superior thyroid vein ●
Inferior thyroid artery ●
Middle cervical ●
ganglion
Thyrocervical trunk ●
Subclavian artery ●
Internal thoracic artery ●
Recurrent laryngeal nerve ●
Trachea
Inferior thyroid vein ●
Middle cervical ●
cardiac nerve
(sympathetic trunk)
Vertebral vein, ●
prevertebral part
Common carotid artery ●
Internal jugular vein ●
Left brachiocephalic vein ●
External jugular vein ●
Pectoralis major ●
Rib I
Medial pectoral nerve ●
Pectoralis ● minor
Cephalic vein ●
Lateral thoracic artery; vein ● ●

● Internal jugular vein
● Rami communicantes (sympathetic trunk)
● Occipital artery
● Mastoid branch
● Lesser occipital nerve
● Greater occipital nerve
● Accessory nerve [XI]
● Ascending cervical artery
● Phrenic nerve
● (Superficial cervical artery, var.)
● Scalenus anterior
● Suprascapular nerve
● Suprascapular artery
Clavicle
● Acromial branch (thoraco-acromial artery)
● Deltoid
● Pectoralis minor, tendon
● Axillary artery
● Thoraco-acromial artery
● Cephalic vein
● Brachial plexus, infraclavicular part, medial cord
● Axillary vein
● Intercostobrachial nerve
● Thoracodorsal nerve
● Long thoracic nerve
● Thoraco-epigastric veins

V
VI
VII
VIII

→ 46, T 7

Fig. 258 Vessels and nerves of the lateral region of the neck and the axillary region.
The numbers V–VIII indicate ventral branches of the corresponding cervical nerves.

257
413

Veins of the neck

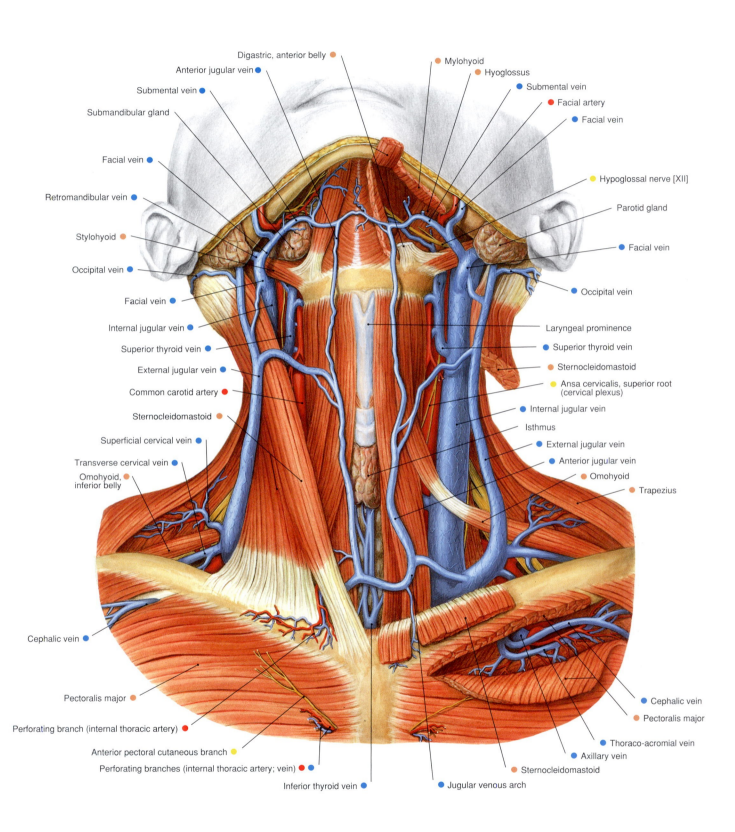

Digastric, anterior belly ●
Anterior jugular vein ●
Submental vein ●
Submandibular gland
Facial vein ●
Retromandibular vein ●
Stylohyoid ●
Occipital vein ●
Facial vein ●
Internal jugular vein ●
Superior thyroid vein ●
External jugular vein ●
Common carotid artery ●
Sternocleidomastoid ●
Superficial cervical vein ●
Transverse cervical vein ●
Omohyoid, inferior belly ●
Cephalic vein ●
Pectoralis major ●
Perforating branch (internal thoracic artery) ●
Anterior pectoral cutaneous branch ●
Perforating branches (internal thoracic artery; vein) ● ●
Inferior thyroid vein ●

Mylohyoid ●
Hyoglossus ●
● Submental vein
● Facial artery
● Facial vein
● Hypoglossal nerve [XII]
Parotid gland
● Facial vein
● Occipital vein
Laryngeal prominence
● Superior thyroid vein
● Sternocleidomastoid
● Ansa cervicalis, superior root (cervical plexus)
● Internal jugular vein
Isthmus
● External jugular vein
● Anterior jugular vein
● Omohyoid
● Trapezius
● Cephalic vein
● Pectoralis major
● Thoraco-acromial vein
Axillary vein
● Sternocleidomastoid
Jugular venous arch ●

Fig. 259 Veins of the neck.

Vessels and nerves of the upper thoracic aperture

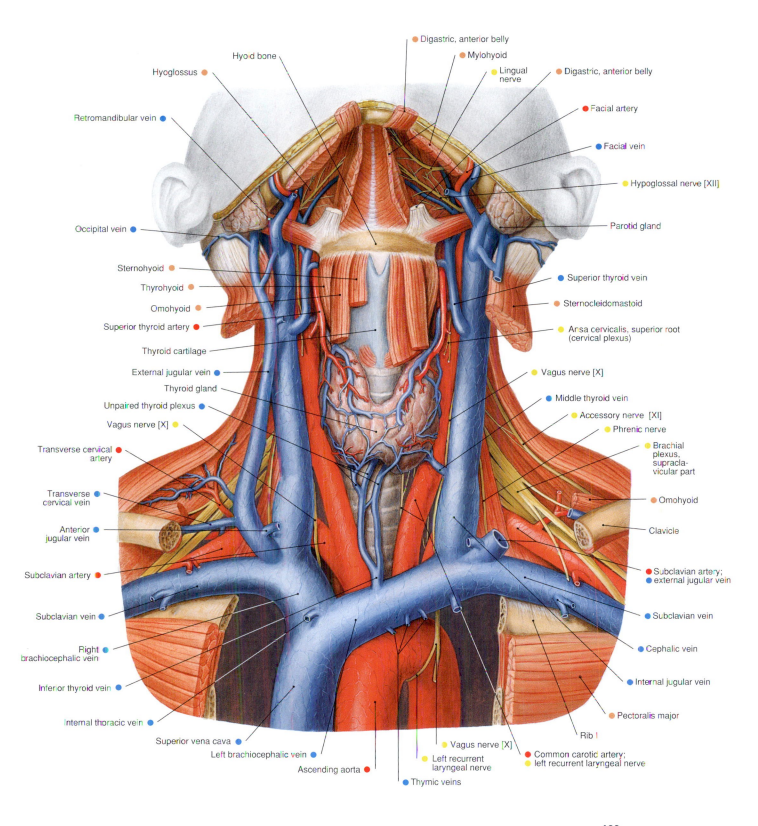

- Digastric, anterior belly
- Mylohyoid
- Lingual nerve
- Digastric, anterior belly
- Facial artery
- Facial vein
- Hypoglossal nerve [XII]
- Parotid gland
- Superior thyroid vein
- Sternocleidomastoid
- Ansa cervicalis, superior root (cervical plexus)
- Vagus nerve [X]
- Middle thyroid vein
- Accessory nerve [XI]
- Phrenic nerve
- Brachial plexus, supraclavicular part
- Omohyoid
- Clavicle
- Subclavian artery; external jugular vein
- Subclavian vein
- Cephalic vein
- Internal jugular vein
- Pectoralis major
- Rib I
- Common carotid artery; left recurrent laryngeal nerve

Hyoid bone
Hyoglossus
Retromandibular vein
Occipital vein
Sternohyoid
Thyrohyoid
Omohyoid
Superior thyroid artery
Thyroid cartilage
External jugular vein
Thyroid gland
Unpaired thyroid plexus
Vagus nerve [X]
Transverse cervical artery
Transverse cervical vein
Anterior jugular vein
Subclavian artery
Subclavian vein
Right brachiocephalic vein
Inferior thyroid vein
Internal thoracic vein
Superior vena cava
Left brachiocephalic vein
Ascending aorta

Vagus nerve [X]
Left recurrent laryngeal nerve
Thymic veins

Fig. 260 Vessels and nerves of the neck and the upper thoracic aperture.

133
258
259

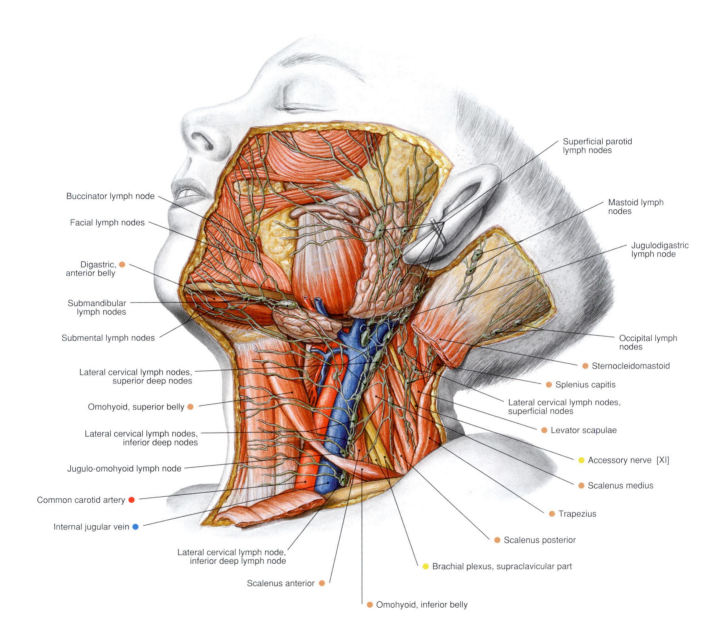

Buccinator lymph node

Facial lymph nodes

Digastric, anterior belly ●

Submandibular lymph nodes

Submental lymph nodes

Lateral cervical lymph nodes, superior deep nodes

Omohyoid, superior belly ●

Lateral cervical lymph nodes, inferior deep nodes

Jugulo-omohyoid lymph node

Common carotid artery ●

Internal jugular vein ●

Lateral cervical lymph node, inferior deep lymph node

Scalenus anterior ●

Omohyoid, inferior belly ●

Superficial parotid lymph nodes

Mastoid lymph nodes

Jugulodigastric lymph node

Occipital lymph nodes

Sternocleidomastoid ●

Splenius capitis ●

Lateral cervical lymph nodes, superficial nodes

Levator scapulae ●

Accessory nerve [XI] ●

Scalenus medius ●

Trapezius ●

Scalenus posterior ●

Brachial plexus, supraclavicular part ●

→ 125, 126

Fig. 261 Superficial lymphatics and lymph nodes of the head and the neck of an 8-year-old child.

Vessels and nerves of the submandibular triangle

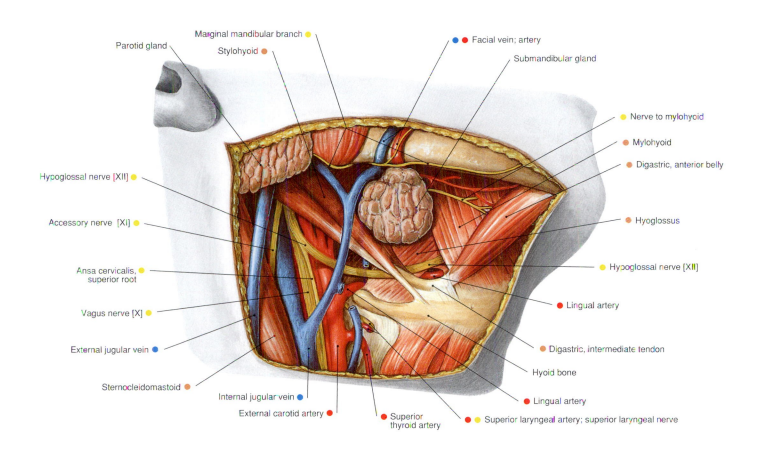

Marginal mandibular branch ●
Stylohyoid ●
Parotid gland
● ● Facial vein; artery
Submandibular gland
Nerve to mylohyoid ●
Mylohyoid ●
Digastric, anterior belly ●
Hypoglossal nerve [XII] ●
Hyoglossus ●
Accessory nerve [XI] ●
Hypoglossal nerve [XII] ●
Ansa cervicalis, superior root ●
Lingual artery ●
Vagus nerve [X] ●
Digastric, intermediate tendon ●
External jugular vein ●
Hyoid bone
Sternocleidomastoid ●
Lingual artery ●
Internal jugular vein ●
External carotid artery ●
Superior thyroid artery ●
● ● Superior laryngeal artery; superior laryngeal nerve

Fig. 262 Vessels and nerves of the submandibular triangle.

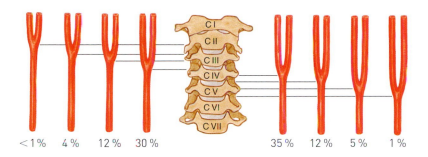

| C I |
| C II |
| C III |
| C IV |
| C V |
| C VI |
| C VII |

<1 % 4 % 12 % 30 %   35 % 12 % 5 % 1 %

Fig. 263 Level of the bifurcation of the common carotid artery in relation to the cervical vertebrae.

Subclavian artery

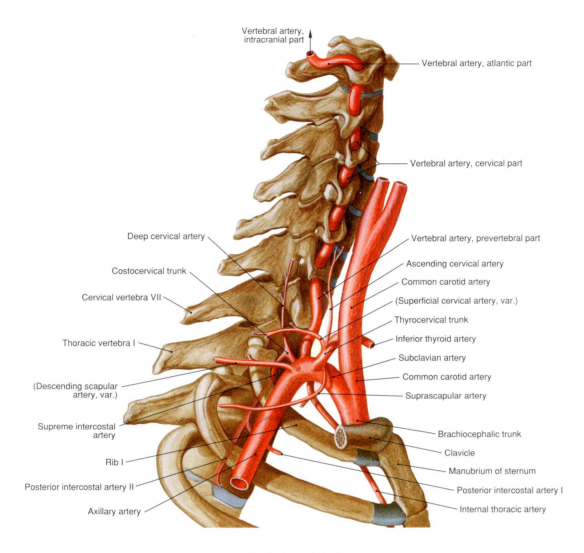

Vertebral artery, intracranial part

Vertebral artery, atlantic part

Vertebral artery, cervical part

Deep cervical artery

Costocervical trunk

Cervical vertebra VII

Thoracic vertebra I

(Descending scapular artery, var.)

Supreme intercostal artery

Rib I

Posterior intercostal artery II

Axillary artery

Vertebral artery, prevertebral part

Ascending cervical artery

Common carotid artery

(Superficial cervical artery, var.)

Thyrocervical trunk

Inferior thyroid artery

Subclavian artery

Common carotid artery

Suprascapular artery

Brachiocephalic trunk

Clavicle

Manubrium of sternum

Posterior intercostal artery I

Internal thoracic artery

Fig. 264   Subclavian artery.

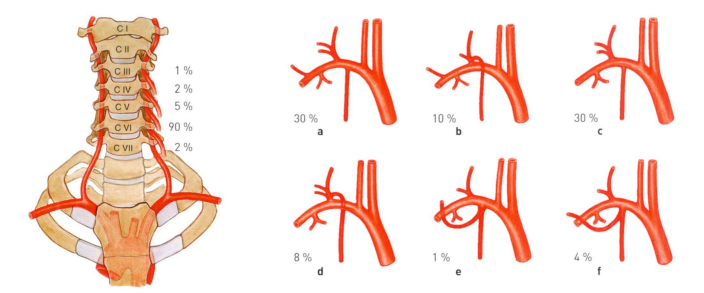

C I
C II
C III   1 %
C IV   2 %
C V   5 %
C VI   90 %
C VII   2 %

30 %   10 %   30 %
a   b   c

8 %   1 %   4 %
d   e   f

Fig. 265   Level of the entry of the vertebral artery into the transverse foramina.

Fig. 266 a–f   Variations in the truncus formed by the inferior thyroid artery, the suprascapular artery, the transverse cervical artery and the internal thoracic artery, when the vertebral artery branches off separately from the costocervical truncus.

Vessels and nerves of the neck and the uper thoracic aperture

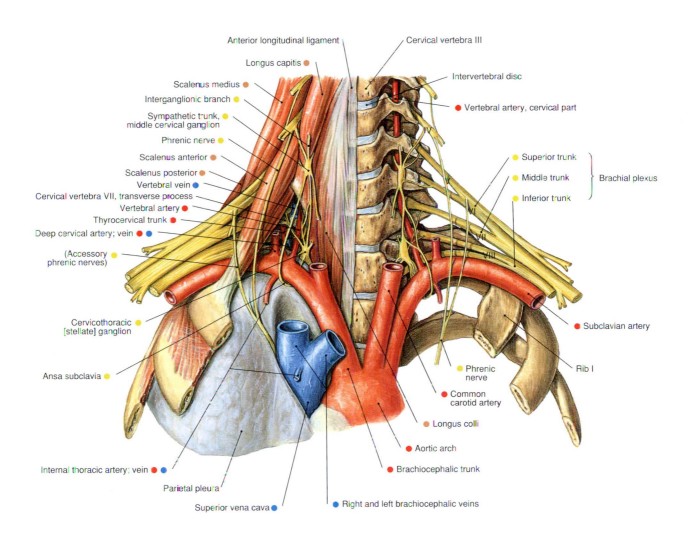

Anterior longitudinal ligament
Cervical vertebra III
Longus capitis ●
Scalenus medius ●
Interganglionic branch ●
Sympathetic trunk, middle cervical ganglion ●
Phrenic nerve ●
Scalenus anterior ●
Scalenus posterior ●
Vertebral vein ●
Cervical vertebra VII, transverse process
Vertebral artery ●
Thyrocervical trunk ●
Deep cervical artery; vein ● ●
(Accessory phrenic nerves) ●
Cervicothoracic [stellate] ganglion ●
Ansa subclavia ●
Internal thoracic artery; vein ● ●
Parietal pleura
Superior vena cava ●

Intervertebral disc
● Vertebral artery, cervical part
● Superior trunk
● Middle trunk } Brachial plexus
● Inferior trunk
● Subclavian artery
Rib I
● Phrenic nerve
● Common carotid artery
● Longus colli
● Aortic arch
● Brachiocephalic trunk
● Right and left brachiocephalic veins

Fig. 267 Vessels and nerves at the transition from the neck to the thorax.
The numbers IV–VIII indicate ventral branches of the corresponding spinal nerves.

→ 46, 386, T 7, T 24

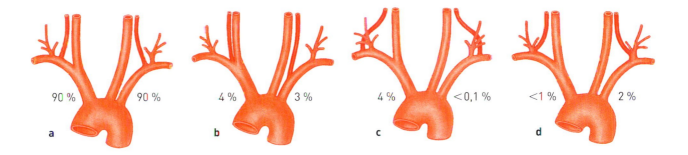

90 % 90 % 4 % 3 % 4 % <0,1 % <1 % 2 %
a b c d

Fig. 268 a–d Variations in the origin of the vertebral artery.

Neck, transverse section

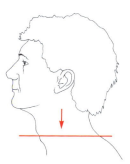

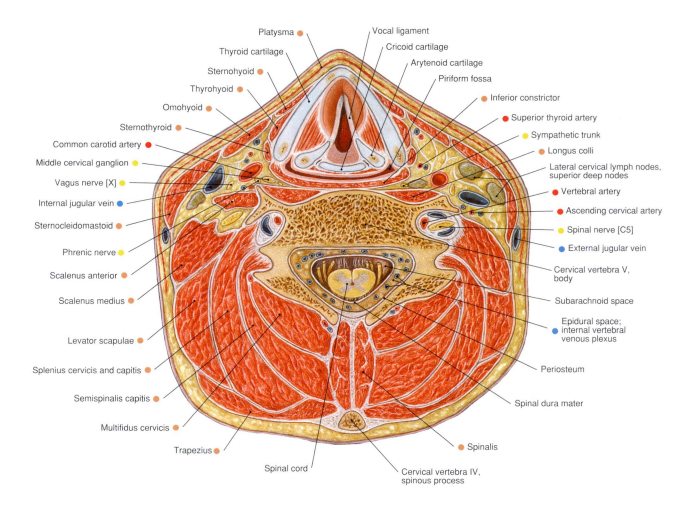

Platysma ●
Thyroid cartilage ●
Sternohyoid ●
Thyrohyoid ●
Omohyoid ●
Sternothyroid ●
Common carotid artery ●
Middle cervical ganglion ●
Vagus nerve [X] ●
Internal jugular vein ●
Sternocleidomastoid ●
Phrenic nerve ●
Scalenus anterior ●
Scalenus medius ●
Levator scapulae ●
Splenius cervicis and capitis ●
Semispinalis capitis ●
Multifidus cervicis ●
Trapezius ●
Spinal cord
Cervical vertebra IV, spinous process

Vocal ligament
Cricoid cartilage
Arytenoid cartilage
Piriform fossa
● Inferior constrictor
● Superior thyroid artery
● Sympathetic trunk
● Longus colli
Lateral cervical lymph nodes, superior deep nodes
● Vertebral artery
● Ascending cervical artery
● Spinal nerve [C5]
● External jugular vein
Cervical vertebra V, body
Subarachnoid space
● Epidural space; internal vertebral venous plexus
Periosteum
Spinal dura mater
● Spinalis

→ 236

Fig. 269 Neck;
transverse section at the level of the vocal cord.

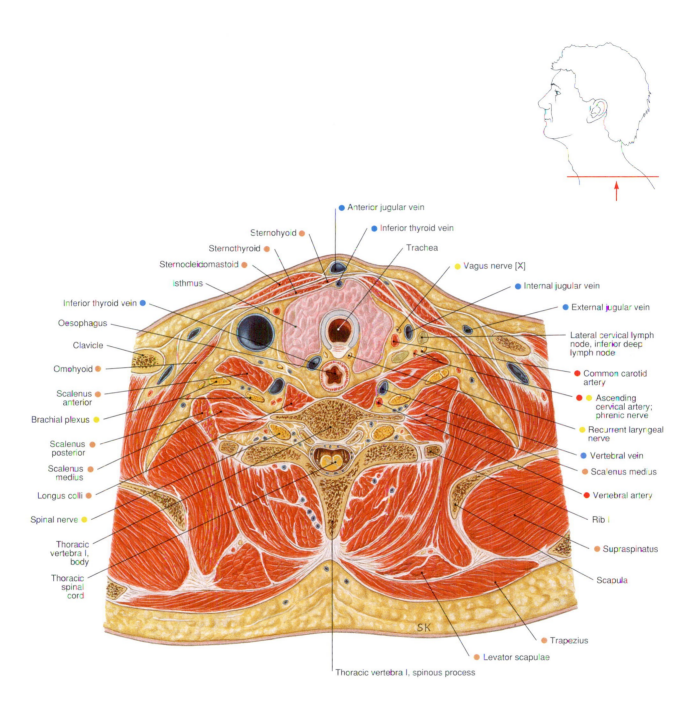

Anterior jugular vein

Sternohyoid ●

Inferior thyroid vein ●

Sternothyroid ●

Trachea

Sternocleidomastoid ●

Vagus nerve [X] ●

isthmus

Internal jugular vein ●

Inferior thyroid vein ●

External jugular vein ●

Oesophagus

Lateral cervical lymph node, inferior deep lymph node

Clavicle

Omohyoid ●

Common carotid artery ●

Scalenus anterior ●

Ascending cervical artery; phrenic nerve ● ●

Brachial plexus ●

Recurrent laryngeal nerve ●

Scalenus posterior ●

Vertebral vein ●

Scalenus medius ●

Scalenus medius ●

Longus colli ●

Vertebral artery ●

Spinal nerve ● ●

Rib I

Thoracic vertebra I, body

Supraspinatus ●

Thoracic spinal cord

Scapula

SK

Trapezius ●

Levator scapulae ●

Thoracic vertebra I, spinous process

Fig. 270 Neck; transverse section at the level of the first thoracic vertebra.

→ 239

Oral cavity and pharynx, median section

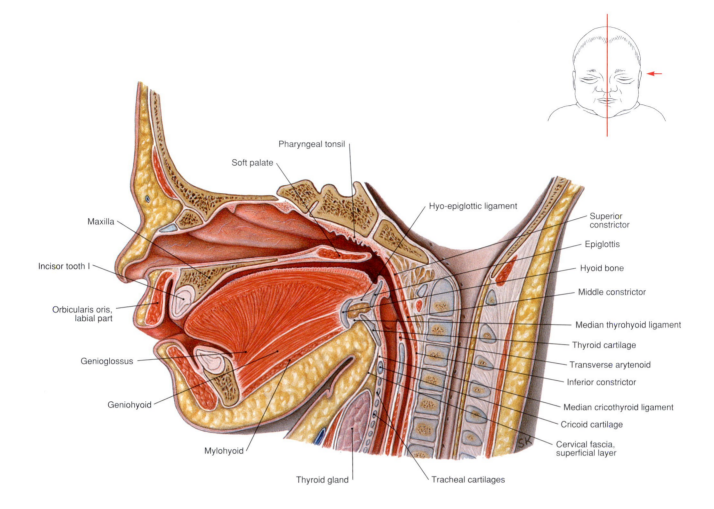

Pharyngeal tonsil

Soft palate

Hyo-epiglottic ligament

Maxilla

Incisor tooth I

Orbicularis oris, labial part

Genioglossus

Geniohyoid

Mylohyoid

Thyroid gland

Tracheal cartilages

Superior constrictor

Epiglottis

Hyoid bone

Middle constrictor

Median thyrohyoid ligament

Thyroid cartilage

Transverse arytenoid

Inferior constrictor

Median cricothyroid ligament

Cricoid cartilage

Cervical fascia, superficial layer

→ 246

Fig. 271 Facial part of the head and neck; median section through the head of a neonate.

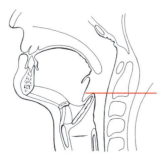

Fig. 272 Schema illustrating the distance between the root of the tongue and the epiglottis in the adult.

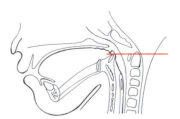

Fig. 273 Schema illustrating that the larynx in the neonate is positioned considerably higher than in the adult.

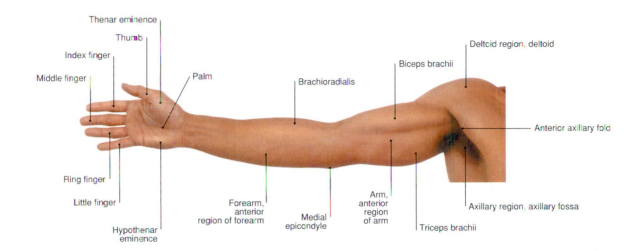

Thenar eminence

Thumb

Index finger

Middle finger

Palm

Brachioradialis

Biceps brachii

Deltoid region, deltoid

Anterior axillary fold

Ring finger

Little finger

Hypothenar eminence

Forearm, anterior region of forearm

Medial epicondyle

Arm, anterior region of arm

Triceps brachii

Axillary region, axillary fossa

Fig. 274   Upper limb.

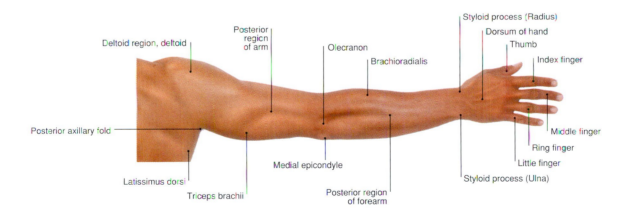

Deltoid region, deltoid

Posterior region of arm

Olecranon

Brachioradialis

Styloid process (Radius)

Dorsum of hand

Thumb

Index finger

Posterior axillary fold

Middle finger

Ring finger

Little finger

Styloid process (Ulna)

Latissimus dorsi

Triceps brachii

Medial epicondyle

Posterior region of forearm

Fig. 275   Upper limb.

Skeleton of the upper limb

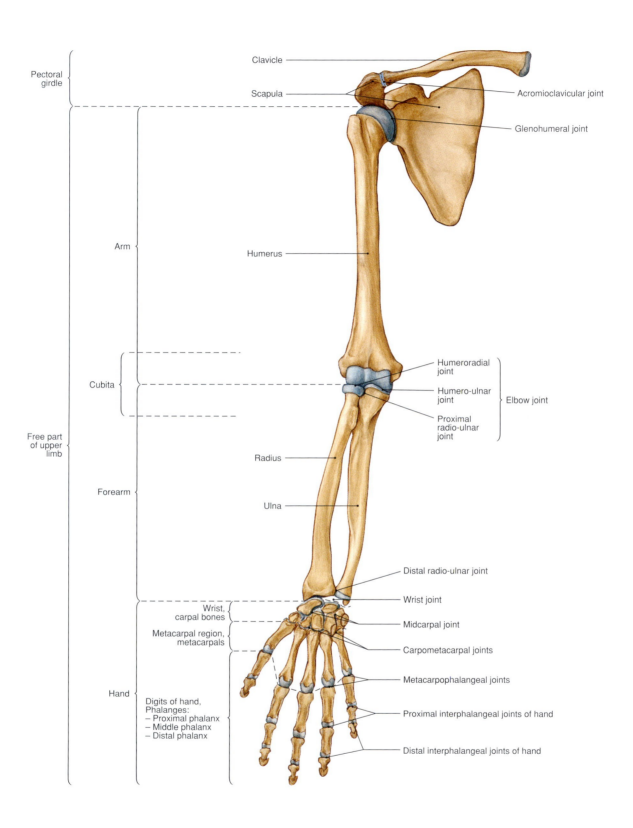

Clavicle

Scapula

Acromioclavicular joint

Glenohumeral joint

Pectoral girdle

Arm

Humerus

Humeroradial joint

Humero-ulnar joint

Proximal radio-ulnar joint

Elbow joint

Cubita

Free part of upper limb

Radius

Forearm

Ulna

Distal radio-ulnar joint

Wrist joint

Wrist, carpal bones

Midcarpal joint

Metacarpal region, metacarpals

Carpometacarpal joints

Metacarpophalangeal joints

Hand

Digits of hand, Phalanges:
– Proximal phalanx
– Middle phalanx
– Distal phalanx

Proximal interphalangeal joints of hand

Distal interphalangeal joints of hand

Fig. 276 Upper limb; overview, bones and joints.

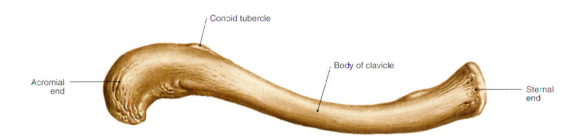

Fig. 277   Clavicle;
superior view.

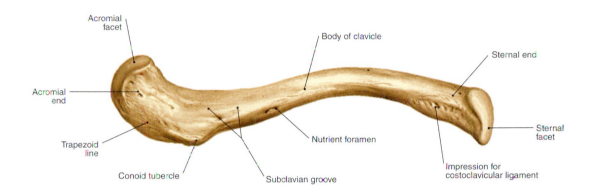

Fig. 278   Clavicle;
inferior view.

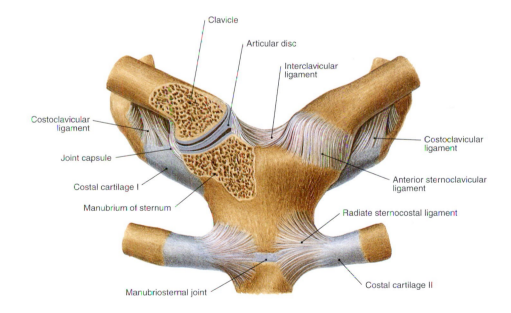

Fig. 279   Sternoclavicular joint;
ventral view.

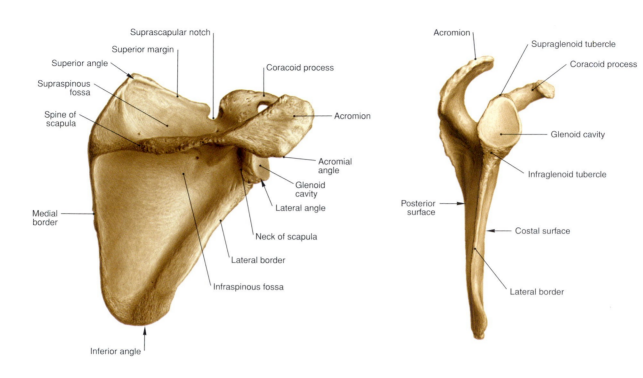

Fig. 280 Scapula;
dorsal view.

Fig. 281 Scapula;
lateral view.

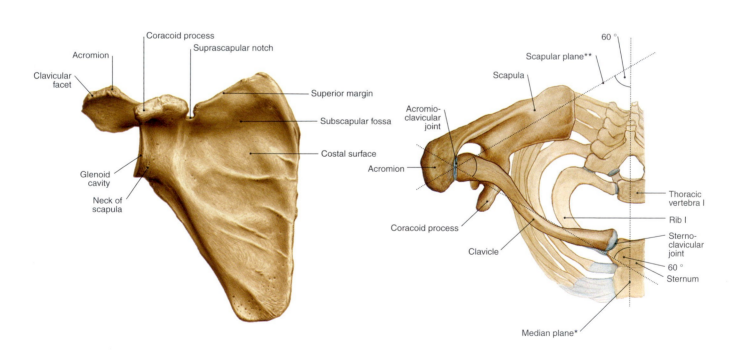

Fig. 282 Scapula;
ventral view.

Fig. 283 Shoulder girdle; superior view.
The angles refer to the average relations in the adult.

* Median plane
** Scapular plane

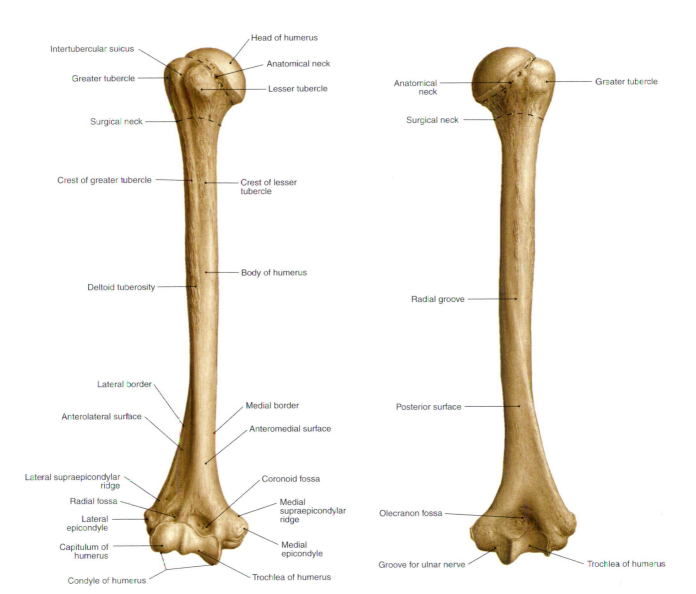

Head of humerus

Intertubercular sulcus

Anatomical neck

Greater tubercle

Lesser tubercle

Surgical neck

Crest of greater tubercle

Crest of lesser tubercle

Body of humerus

Deltoid tuberosity

Lateral border

Medial border

Anterolateral surface

Anteromedial surface

Lateral supraepicondylar ridge

Coronoid fossa

Radial fossa

Medial supraepicondylar ridge

Lateral epicondyle

Capitulum of humerus

Medial epicondyle

Condyle of humerus

Trochlea of humerus

Anatomical neck

Greater tubercle

Surgical neck

Radial groove

Posterior surface

Olecranon fossa

Groove for ulnar nerve

Trochlea of humerus

Fig. 284   Humerus;
ventral view.

Fig. 285   Humerus;
dorsal view.

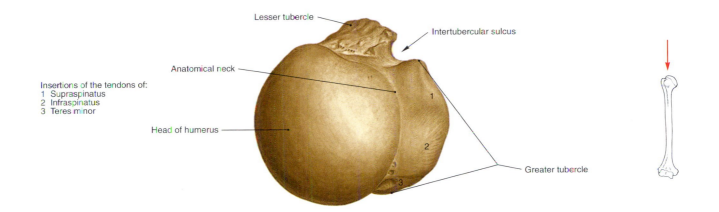

Lesser tubercle

Intertubercular sulcus

Anatomical neck

Insertions of the tendons of:
1 Supraspinatus
2 Infraspinatus
3 Teres minor

Head of humerus

Greater tubercle

Fig. 286   Humerus;
proximal view.

Shoulder joint

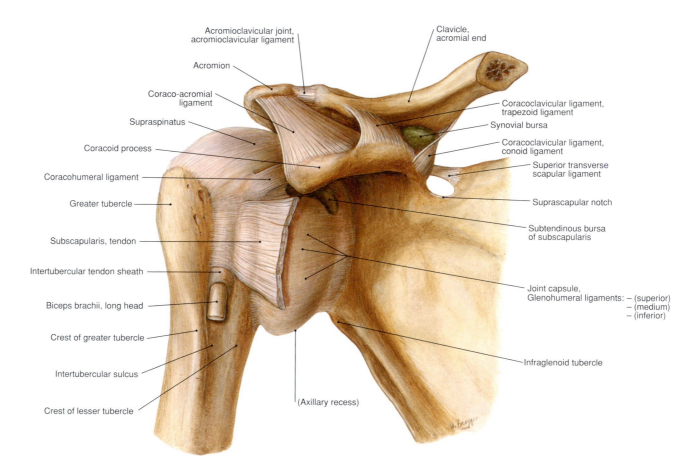

Acromioclavicular joint, acromioclavicular ligament

Acromion

Coraco-acromial ligament

Supraspinatus

Coracoid process

Coracohumeral ligament

Greater tubercle

Subscapularis, tendon

Intertubercular tendon sheath

Biceps brachii, long head

Crest of greater tubercle

Intertubercular sulcus

Crest of lesser tubercle

Clavicle, acromial end

Coracoclavicular ligament, trapezoid ligament

Synovial bursa

Coracoclavicular ligament, conoid ligament

Superior transverse scapular ligament

Suprascapular notch

Subtendinous bursa of subscapularis

Joint capsule, Glenohumeral ligaments: – (superior) – (medium) – (inferior)

Infraglenoid tubercle

(Axillary recess)

Fig. 287 Shoulder joint; ventral view.

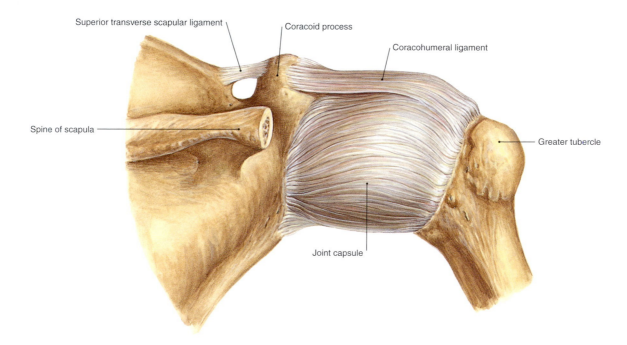

Superior transverse scapular ligament

Coracoid process

Coracohumeral ligament

Spine of scapula

Greater tubercle

Joint capsule

Fig. 288 Shoulder joint; the acromion has been removed; dorsal view.

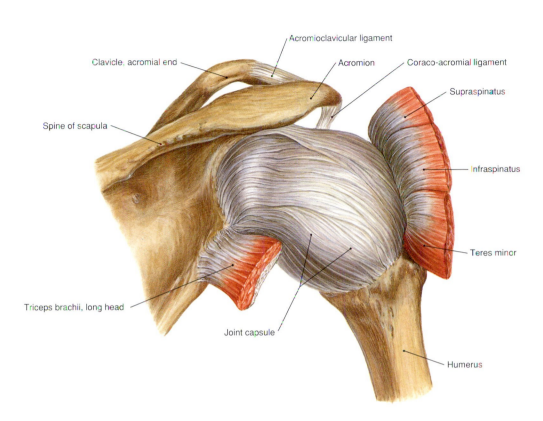

Acromioclavicular ligament

Clavicle, acromial end

Acromion

Coraco-acromial ligament

Supraspinatus

Spine of scapula

Infraspinatus

Teres minor

Triceps brachii, long head

Joint capsule

Humerus

Fig. 289 Shoulder joint;
dorsal view.

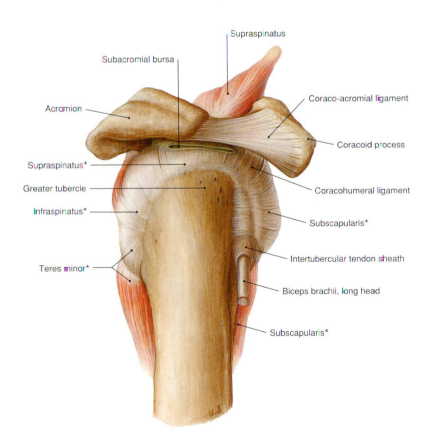

Supraspinatus

Subacromial bursa

Acromion

Coraco-acromial ligament

Coracoid process

Supraspinatus*

Greater tubercle

Coracohumeral ligament

Infraspinatus*

Subscapularis*

Intertubercular tendon sheath

Teres minor*

Biceps brachii, long head

Subscapularis*

Fig. 290 Shoulder joint;
lateral view.

Together, the muscle tendons marked with * form the so-called
rotator cuff.

Shoulder joint

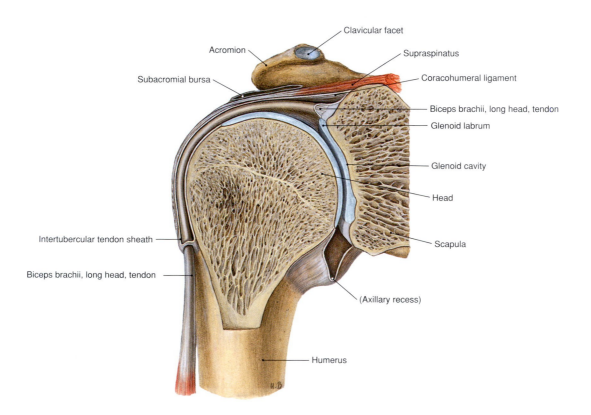

Fig. 291 Shoulder joint;
section at the level of the scapula;
ventral view.

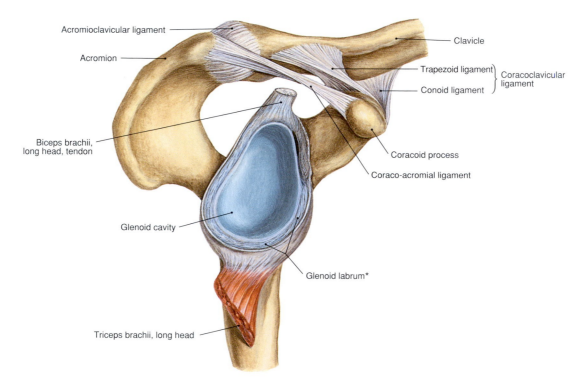

Fig. 292 Shoulder joint; lateral view.
Next to its origin at the supraglenoidal tubercle, the tendon of the biceps
muscle is predominantly attached to the glenoid labrum.

* It forms a fibrocartilaginous collar around the glenoid cavity.

Shoulder joint, radiography

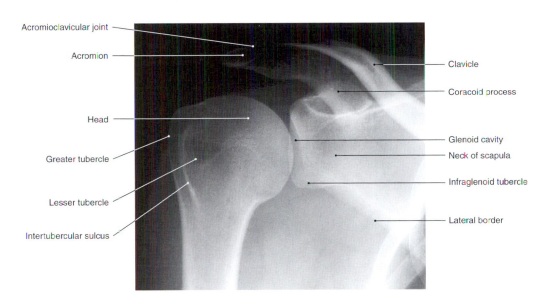

Acromioclavicular joint

Acromion

Head

Greater tubercle

Lesser tubercle

Intertubercular sulcus

Clavicle

Coracoid process

Glenoid cavity

Neck of scapula

Infraglenoid tubercle

Lateral border

Fig. 293 Shoulder joint;
AP-radiograph.

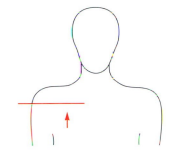

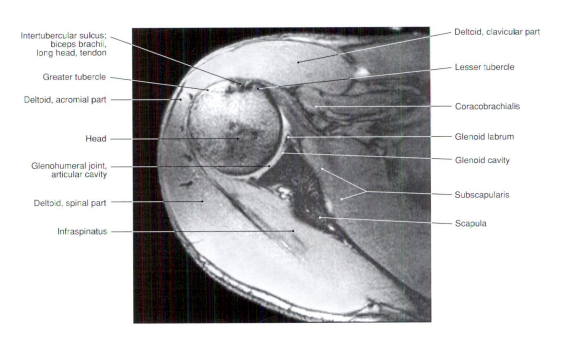

Intertubercular sulcus;
biceps brachii,
long head, tendon

Greater tubercle

Deltoid, acromial part

Head

Glenohumeral joint,
articular cavity

Deltoid, spinal part

Infraspinatus

Deltoid, clavicular part

Lesser tubercle

Coracobrachialis

Glenoid labrum

Glenoid cavity

Subscapularis

Scapula

Fig. 294 Shoulder joint;
computed tomographic (CT) cross-section;
the joint cavity is filled with air (pneumo-CT);
inferior view.

Ulna

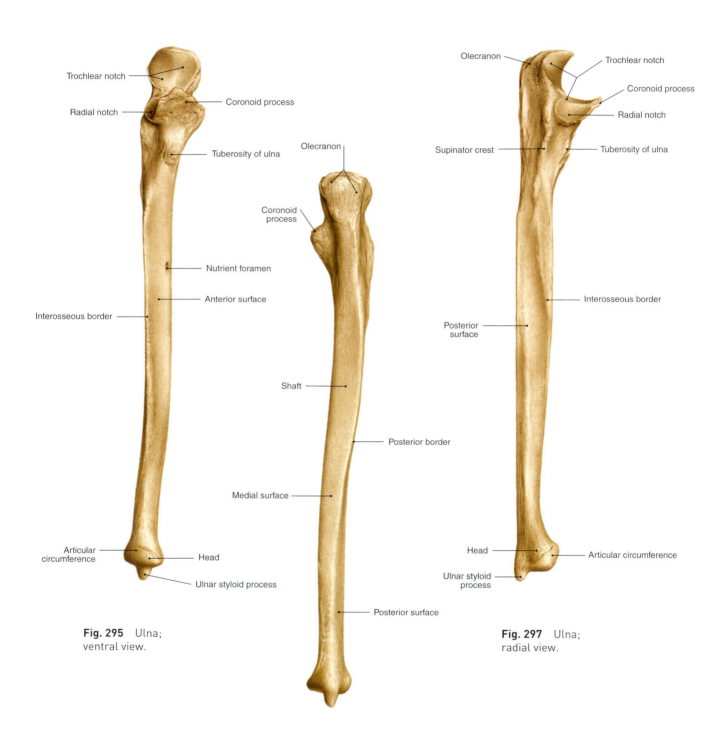

Trochlear notch

Radial notch

Coronoid process

Tuberosity of ulna

Nutrient foramen

Anterior surface

Interosseous border

Articular circumference

Head

Ulnar styloid process

Fig. 295 Ulna; ventral view.

Olecranon

Coronoid process

Shaft

Posterior border

Medial surface

Posterior surface

Fig. 296 Ulna; dorsal view.

Olecranon

Trochlear notch

Coronoid process

Radial notch

Supinator crest

Tuberosity of ulna

Interosseous border

Posterior surface

Head

Articular circumference

Ulnar styloid process

Fig. 297 Ulna; radial view.

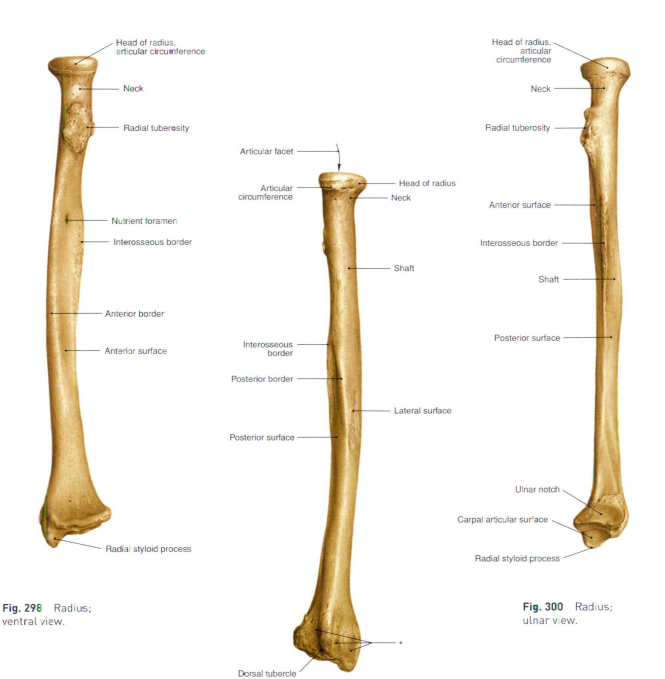

Head of radius,
articular circumference

Neck

Radial tuberosity

Nutrient foramen

Interosseous border

Anterior border

Anterior surface

Radial styloid process

Fig. 298 Radius;
ventral view.

Articular facet

Articular
circumference

Head of radius

Neck

Shaft

Interosseous
border

Posterior border

Lateral surface

Posterior surface

Dorsal tubercle

*

Fig. 299 Radius;
dorsal view.

* Grooves and crests for the
attachment of the extensor
tendons

Head of radius,
articular
circumference

Neck

Radial tuberosity

Anterior surface

Interosseous border

Shaft

Posterior surface

Ulnar notch

Carpal articular surface

Radial styloid process

Fig. 300 Radius;
ulnar view.

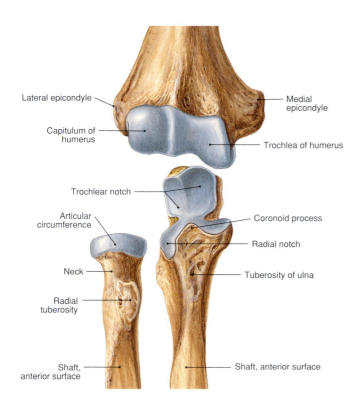

Fig. 301   Elbow joint;
ventral view.

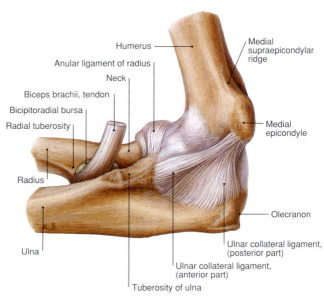

Fig. 302   Elbow joint
in 90° flexion and 90° supination;
medial view.

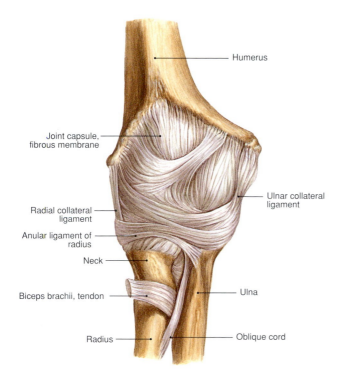

Fig. 303   Elbow joint;
ventral view.

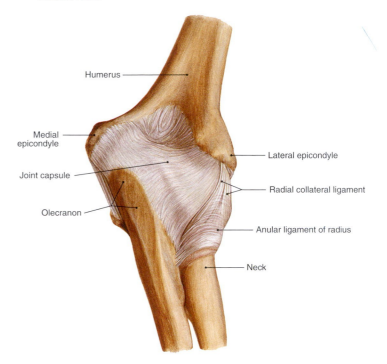

Fig. 304   Elbow joint;
dorsal view.

Junctions of the bones of the forearm

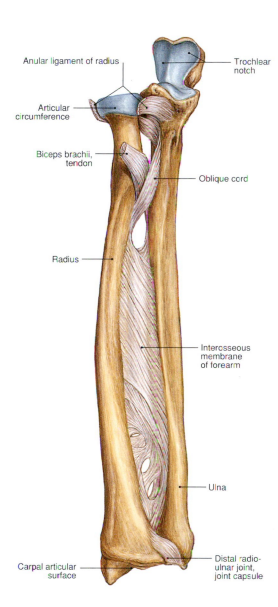

Anular ligament of radius

Trochlear notch

Articular circumference

Biceps brachii, tendon

Oblique cord

Radius

Interosseous membrane of forearm

Ulna

Carpal articular surface

Distal radio-ulnar joint, joint capsule

Fig. 305   Junctions of the bones of the forearm; in supination; ventral view.

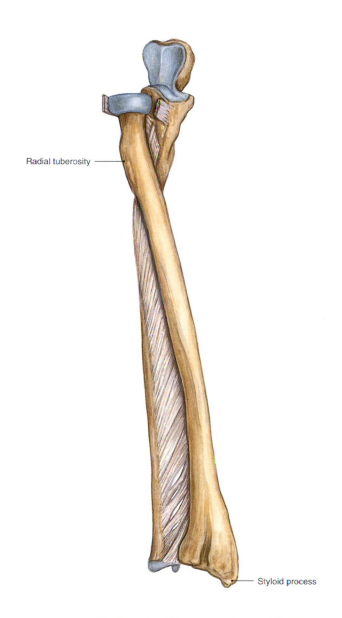

Radial tuberosity

Styloid process

Fig. 306   Junctions of the bones of the forearm; in pronation; ventral view of the ulna, dorsal view of the radius.

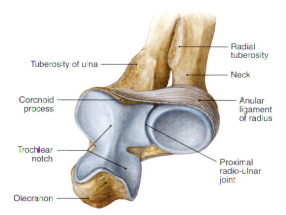

Tuberosity of ulna

Radial tuberosity

Neck

Coronoid process

Anular ligament of radius

Trochlear notch

Proximal radio-ulnar joint

Olecranon

Fig. 307   Proximal radio-ulnar joint; ventroproximal view.

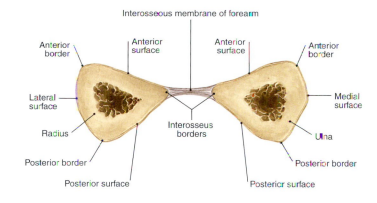

Interosseous membrane of forearm

Anterior border

Anterior surface

Anterior surface

Anterior border

Lateral surface

Medial surface

Radius

Interosseus borders

Ulna

Posterior border

Posterior border

Posterior surface

Posterior surface

Fig. 308   Cross-section through the bones of the forearm; distal view.

Elbow joint, sections and radiography

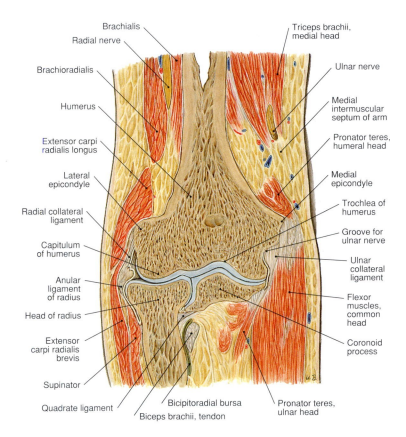

Fig. 309 Elbow joint; frontal section.

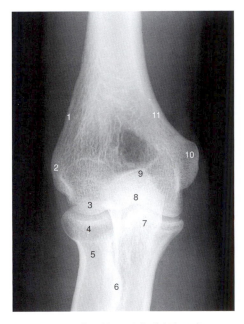

1 Lateral supraepicondylar ridge	6 Radial tuberosity
2 Lateral epicondyle	7 Coronoid process
3 Capitulum of humerus	8 Trochlea of humerus
4 Head of radius	9 Olecranon
5 Neck	10 Medial epicondyle
	11 Medial supraepicondylar ridge

Fig. 310 Elbow joint; AP-radiograph.

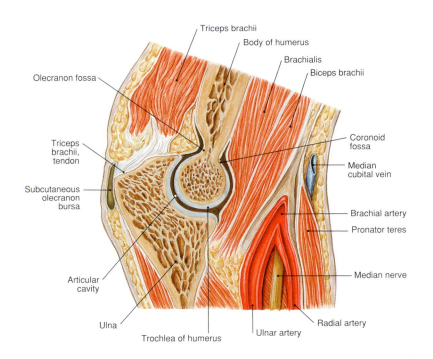

Fig. 311 Elbow joint; sagittal section.

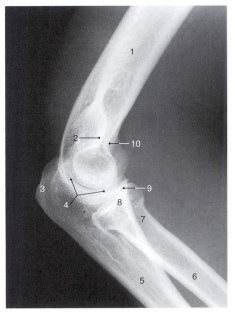

1 Humerus	6 Radius
2 Olecranon fossa	7 Neck
3 Olecranon	8 Head of radius
4 Trochlear notch	9 Coronoid process
5 Ulna	10 Coronoid fossa

Fig. 312 Elbow joint; lateral radiograph.

Skeleton of the hand

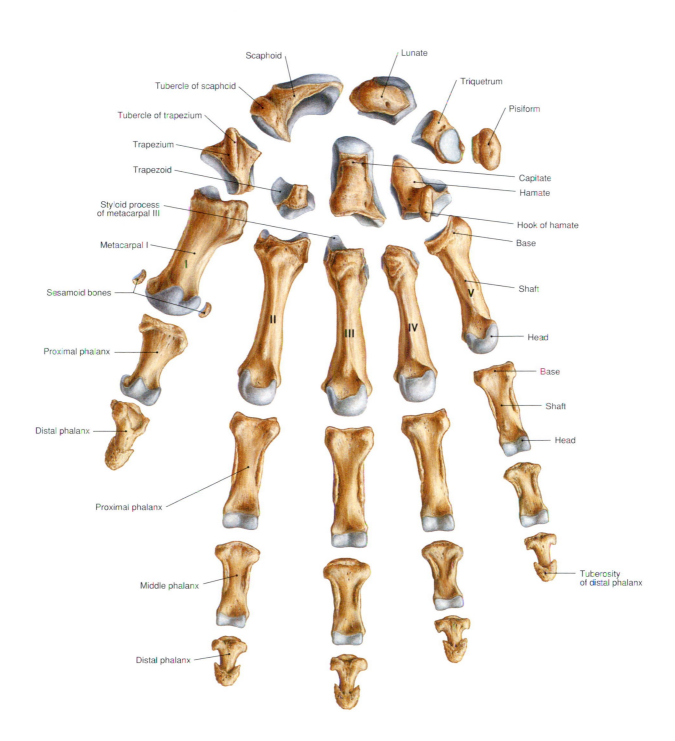

Scaphoid

Lunate

Tubercle of scaphoid

Triquetrum

Tubercle of trapezium

Pisiform

Trapezium

Trapezoid

Capitate

Hamate

Styloid process
of metacarpal III

Hook of hamate

Metacarpal I

Base

Sesamoid bones

Shaft

Proximal phalanx

Head

Base

Shaft

Distal phalanx

Head

Proximal phalanx

Tuberosity
of distal phalanx

Middle phalanx

Distal phalanx

I   Thumb
II   Index finger
III Middle finger
IV   Ring finger
V   Little finger

Fig. 313   Bones of the hand;
palmar view.

Skeleton of the hand

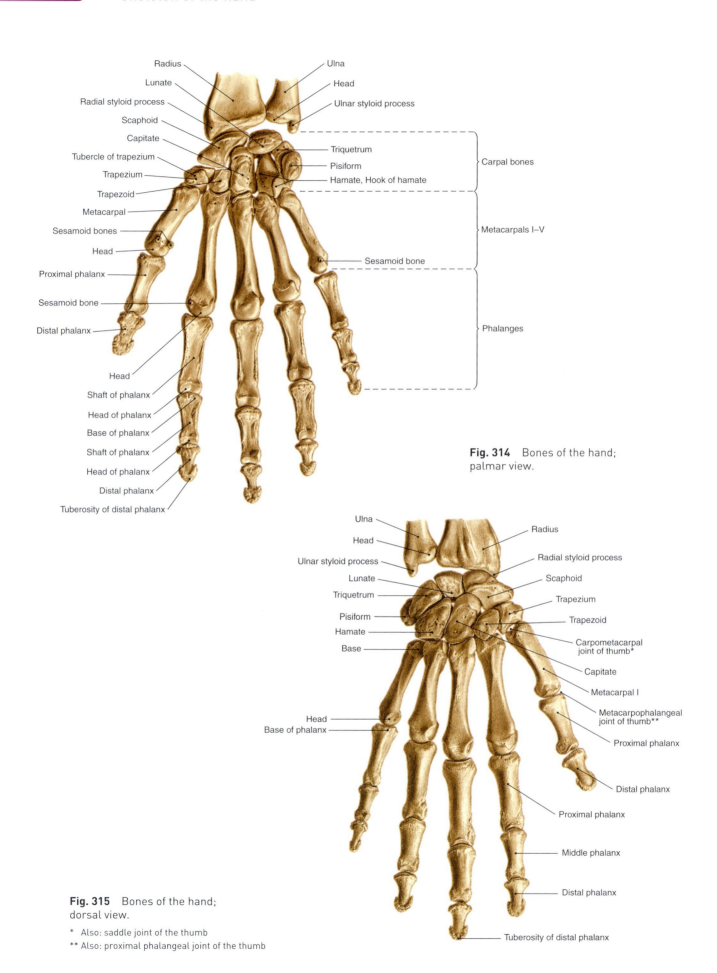

Radius
Lunate
Radial styloid process
Scaphoid
Capitate
Tubercle of trapezium
Trapezium
Trapezoid
Metacarpal
Sesamoid bones
Head
Proximal phalanx
Sesamoid bone
Distal phalanx
Head
Shaft of phalanx
Head of phalanx
Base of phalanx
Shaft of phalanx
Head of phalanx
Distal phalanx
Tuberosity of distal phalanx

Ulna
Head
Ulnar styloid process
Triquetrum
Pisiform
Hamate, Hook of hamate
Sesamoid bone
Carpal bones
Metacarpals I–V
Phalanges

Fig. 314 Bones of the hand; palmar view.

Ulna
Head
Ulnar styloid process
Lunate
Triquetrum
Pisiform
Hamate
Base
Head
Base of phalanx

Radius
Radial styloid process
Scaphoid
Trapezium
Trapezoid
Carpometacarpal joint of thumb*
Capitate
Metacarpal I
Metacarpophalangeal joint of thumb**
Proximal phalanx
Distal phalanx
Proximal phalanx
Middle phalanx
Distal phalanx
Tuberosity of distal phalanx

Fig. 315 ▶ Bones of the hand; dorsal view.

* Also: saddle joint of the thumb
** Also: proximal phalangeal joint of the thumb

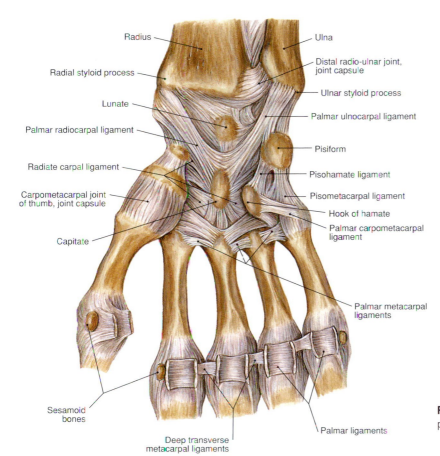

Radius

Radial styloid process

Lunate

Palmar radiocarpal ligament

Radiate carpal ligament

Carpometacarpal joint
of thumb, joint capsule

Capitate

Ulna

Distal radio-ulnar joint,
joint capsule

Ulnar styloid process

Palmar ulnocarpal ligament

Pisiform

Pisohamate ligament

Pisometacarpal ligament

Hook of hamate

Palmar carpometacarpal
ligament

Palmar metacarpal
ligaments

Sesamoid
bones

Deep transverse
metacarpal ligaments

Palmar ligaments

Fig. 316   Joints and ligaments of the hand;
palmar view.

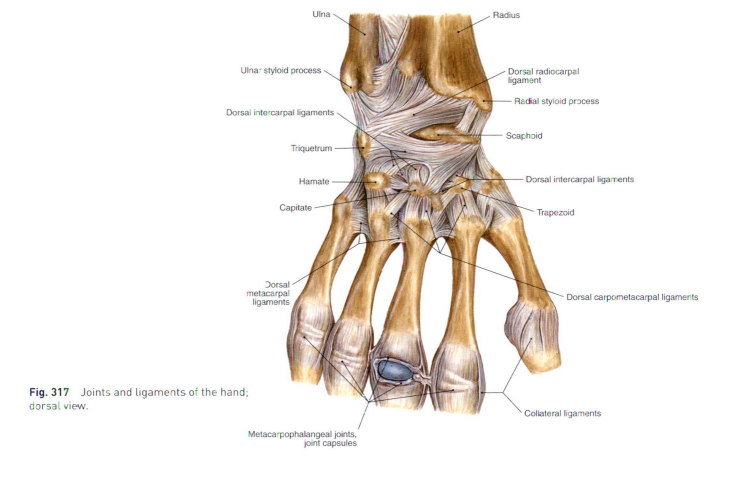

Ulna

Ulnar styloid process

Dorsal intercarpal ligaments

Triquetrum

Hamate

Capitate

Dorsal
metacarpal
ligaments

Radius

Dorsal radiocarpal
ligament

Radial styloid process

Scaphoid

Dorsal intercarpal ligaments

Trapezoid

Dorsal carpometacarpal ligaments

Collateral ligaments

Metacarpophalangeal joints,
joint capsules

Fig. 317   Joints and ligaments of the hand;
dorsal view.

Joints of the hand

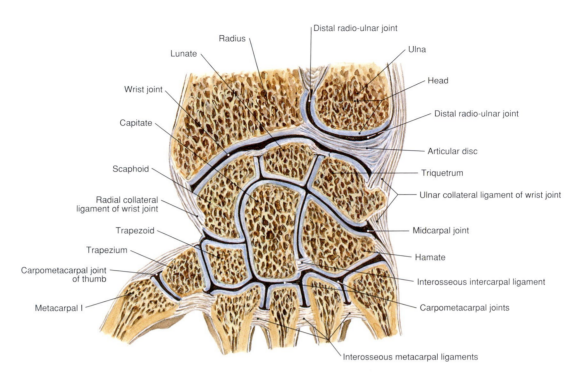

Fig. 318 Carpal joints;
longitudinal section parallel to the dorsum of the hand.

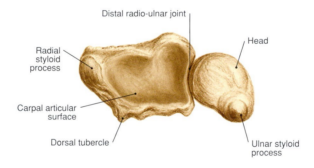

Fig. 319 Ulna and radius;
distal view.

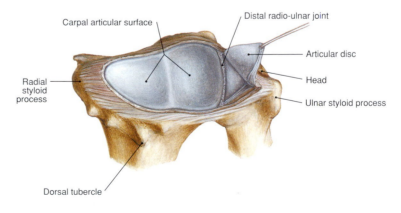

Fig. 320 Distal radio-ulnar joint;
distal-dorsal view.

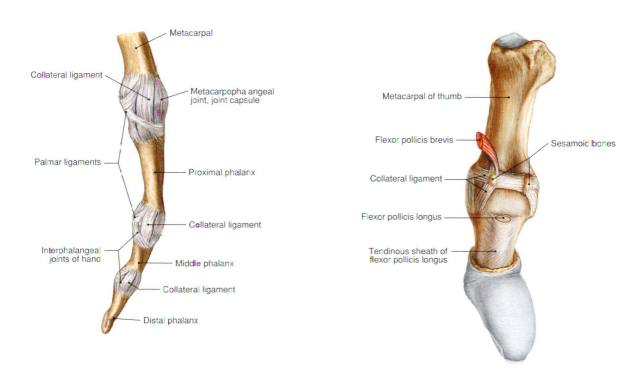

Fig. 321 Finger joints;
lateral view.

Fig. 322 Metacarpophalangeal joint of
the thumb; radial-palmar view.

Labels in Fig. 321:
Metacarpal
Collateral ligament
Metacarpophalangeal joint, joint capsule
Palmar ligaments
Proximal phalanx
Collateral ligament
Interphalangeal joints of hand
Middle phalanx
Collateral ligament
Distal phalanx

Labels in Fig. 322:
Metacarpal of thumb
Flexor pollicis brevis
Sesamoid bones
Collateral ligament
Flexor pollicis longus
Tendinous sheath of flexor pollicis longus

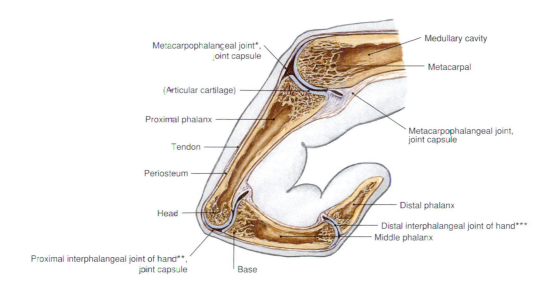

Labels in Fig. 323:
Metacarpophalangeal joint*, joint capsule
Medullary cavity
(Articular cartilage)
Metacarpal
Proximal phalanx
Tendon
Metacarpophalangeal joint, joint capsule
Periosteum
Head
Distal phalanx
Distal interphalangeal joint of hand***
Middle phalanx
Proximal interphalangeal joint of hand**, joint capsule
Base

Fig. 323 Finger joints;
sagittal section;
lateral view.

*   Clinical term: **MP** (= **m**etacarpophalangeal joint)
**   Clinical term: **PIP** (= **p**roximal **i**nter**p**halangeal joint)
*** Clinical term: **DIP** (= **d**istal **i**nter**p**halangeal joint)

Wrist, radiography

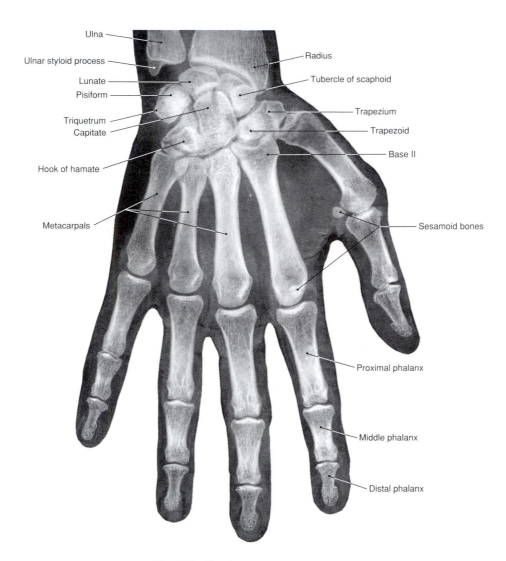

Ulna
Ulnar styloid process
Lunate
Pisiform
Triquetrum
Capitate
Hook of hamate
Metacarpals

Radius
Tubercle of scaphoid
Trapezium
Trapezoid
Base II
Sesamoid bones
Proximal phalanx
Middle phalanx
Distal phalanx

Fig. 324 Hand;
PA-radiograph.
Note: The pisiform bone is projected onto
the triquetral bone.

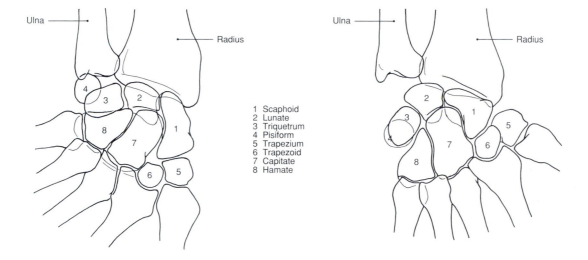

Ulna
Radius

1 Scaphoid
2 Lunate
3 Triquetrum
4 Pisiform
5 Trapezium
6 Trapezoid
7 Capitate
8 Hamate

Ulna
Radius

Fig. 325 Ulnar abduction of the hand;
schema of a PA-radiograph.

Fig. 326 Radial abduction of the hand;
schema of a PA-radiograph.

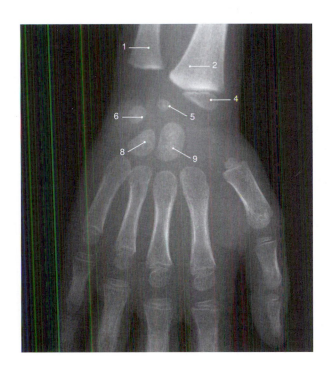

Fig. 327   PA-radiograph of the hand of a 4½-year-old boy.

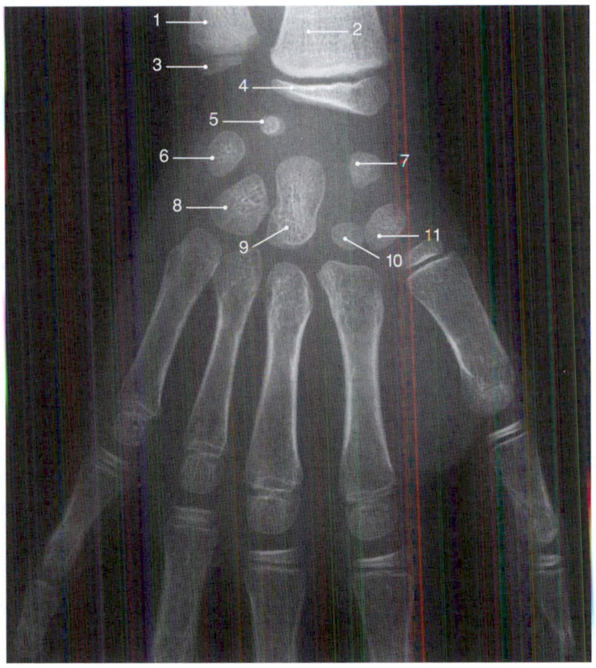

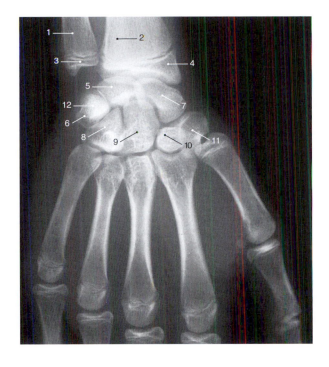

Fig. 328   PA-radiograph of the hand of a 7-year-old boy.

1 Ulna, diaphysis	4 Radius, distal epiphysis	7 Scaphoid	10 Trapezoid
2 Radius, diaphysis	5 Lunate	8 Hamate	11 Trapezium
3 Ulna, distal epiphysis	6 Triquetrum	9 Capitate	12 Pisiform

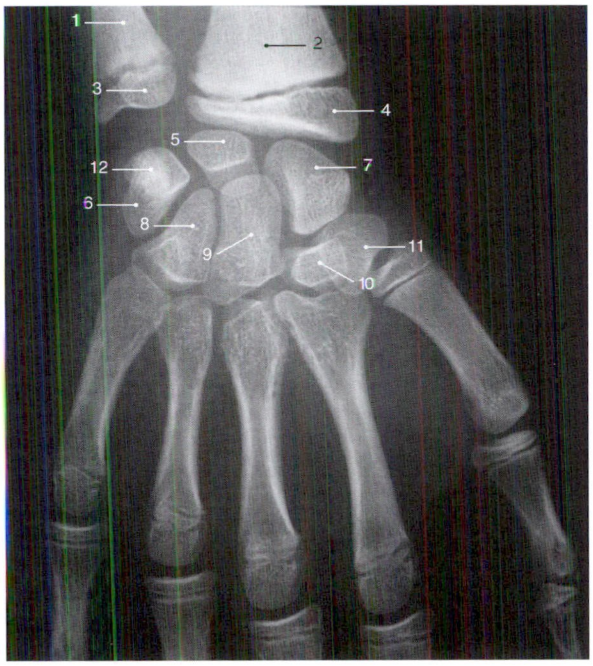

Fig. 329   PA-radiograph of the hand of an 11-year-old boy.

Fig. 330   PA-radiograph of the hand of a 13-year-old boy.

Fascia of the upper limb

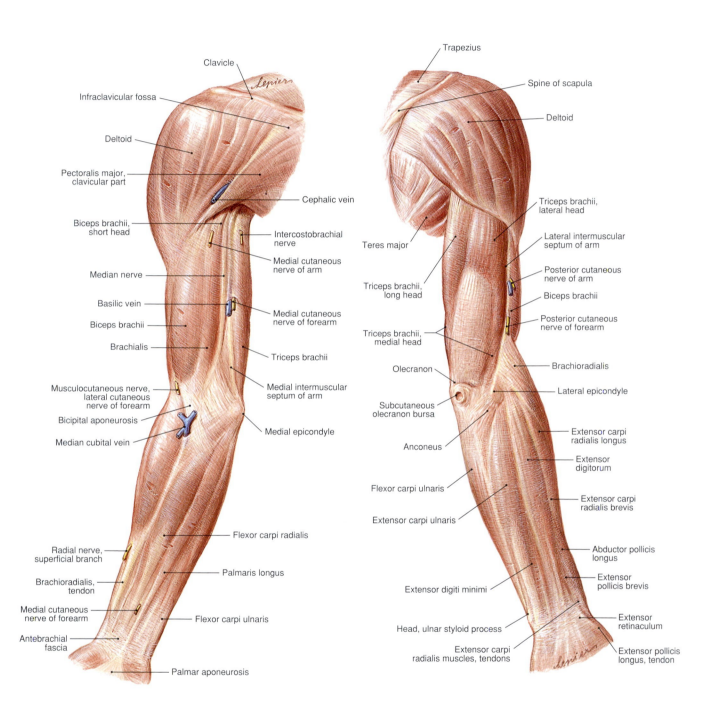

Clavicle

Infraclavicular fossa

Deltoid

Pectoralis major, clavicular part

Biceps brachii, short head

Median nerve

Basilic vein

Biceps brachii

Brachialis

Musculocutaneous nerve, lateral cutaneous nerve of forearm

Bicipital aponeurosis

Median cubital vein

Radial nerve, superficial branch

Brachioradialis, tendon

Medial cutaneous nerve of forearm

Antebrachial fascia

Palmar aponeurosis

Cephalic vein

Intercostobrachial nerve

Medial cutaneous nerve of arm

Medial cutaneous nerve of forearm

Triceps brachii

Medial intermuscular septum of arm

Medial epicondyle

Flexor carpi radialis

Palmaris longus

Flexor carpi ulnaris

Trapezius

Spine of scapula

Deltoid

Triceps brachii, lateral head

Teres major

Lateral intermuscular septum of arm

Posterior cutaneous nerve of arm

Triceps brachii, long head

Biceps brachii

Posterior cutaneous nerve of forearm

Triceps brachii, medial head

Brachioradialis

Olecranon

Lateral epicondyle

Subcutaneous olecranon bursa

Anconeus

Extensor carpi radialis longus

Extensor digitorum

Flexor carpi ulnaris

Extensor carpi radialis brevis

Extensor carpi ulnaris

Abductor pollicis longus

Extensor digiti minimi

Extensor pollicis brevis

Extensor retinaculum

Head, ulnar styloid process

Extensor carpi radialis muscles, tendons

Extensor pollicis longus, tendon

Fig. 331   Fascia of the flexor aspect of the upper limb.

Fig. 332   Fascia of the extensor aspect of the upper limb.

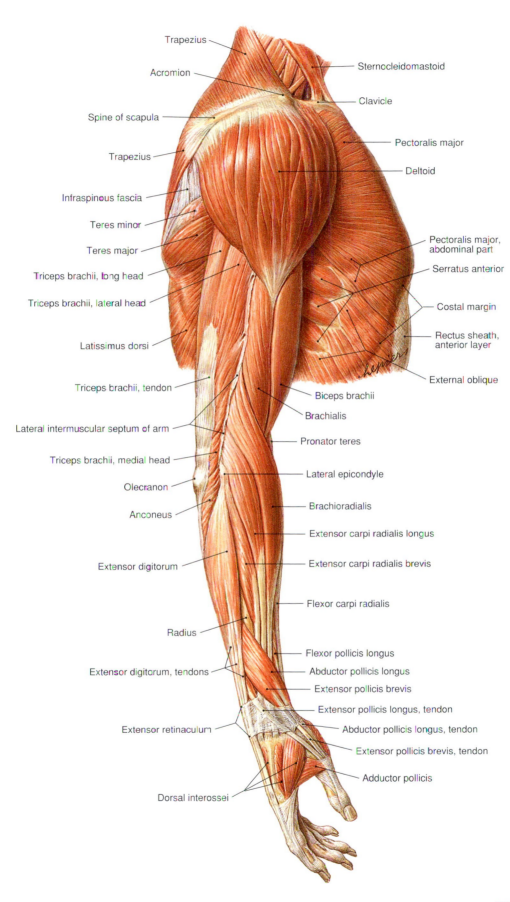

Trapezius
Acromion
Spine of scapula
Trapezius
Infraspinous fascia
Teres minor
Teres major
Triceps brachii, long head
Triceps brachii, lateral head
Latissimus dorsi
Triceps brachii, tendon
Lateral intermuscular septum of arm
Triceps brachii, medial head
Olecranon
Anconeus
Extensor digitorum
Radius
Extensor digitorum, tendons
Extensor retinaculum
Dorsal interossei

Sternocleidomastoid
Clavicle
Pectoralis major
Deltoid
Pectoralis major, abdominal part
Serratus anterior
Costal margin
Rectus sheath, anterior layer
External oblique
Biceps brachii
Brachialis
Pronator teres
Lateral epicondyle
Brachioradialis
Extensor carpi radialis longus
Extensor carpi radialis brevis
Flexor carpi radialis
Flexor pollicis longus
Abductor pollicis longus
Extensor pollicis brevis
Extensor pollicis longus, tendon
Abductor pollicis longus, tendon
Extensor pollicis brevis, tendon
Adductor pollicis

Fig. 333   Muscles of the upper limb, the thorax and the inferior region of the neck.

→ T 26–T 38

Muscles of the upper limb

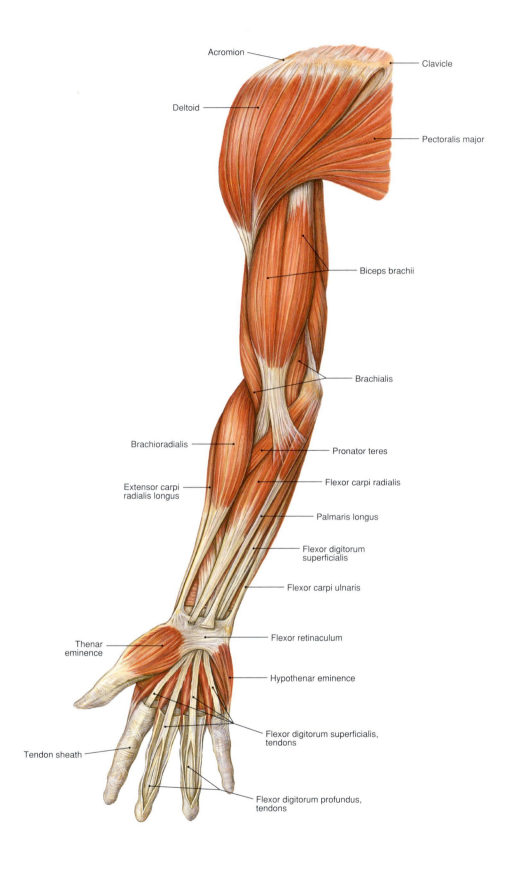

Acromion

Clavicle

Deltoid

Pectoralis major

Biceps brachii

Brachialis

Brachioradialis

Pronator teres

Extensor carpi radialis longus

Flexor carpi radialis

Palmaris longus

Flexor digitorum superficialis

Flexor carpi ulnaris

Thenar eminence

Flexor retinaculum

Hypothenar eminence

Flexor digitorum superficialis, tendons

Tendon sheath

Flexor digitorum profundus, tendons

→ T 26–T 38

Fig. 334   Muscles of the flexor aspect of the upper limb.

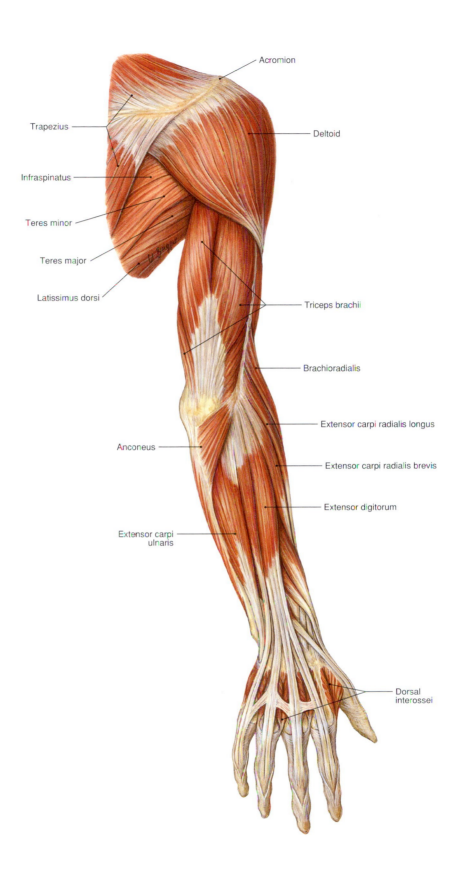

Acromion

Trapezius

Deltoid

Infraspinatus

Teres minor

Teres major

Triceps brachii

Latissimus dorsi

Brachioradialis

Extensor carpi radialis longus

Anconeus

Extensor carpi radialis brevis

Extensor digitorum

Extensor carpi ulnaris

Dorsal interossei

Fig. 335   Muscles of the extensor aspect of the upper limb.

→ T 26–T 38

Muscles of the shoulder

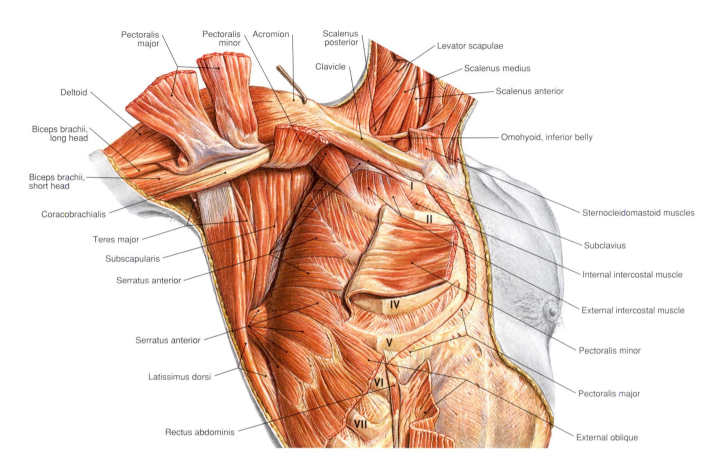

Pectoralis major
Pectoralis minor
Acromion
Scalenus posterior
Clavicle
Levator scapulae
Scalenus medius
Scalenus anterior
Deltoid
Biceps brachii, long head
Omohyoid, inferior belly
Biceps brachii, short head
Coracobrachialis
Teres major
Subscapularis
Serratus anterior
Sternocleidomastoid muscles
Subclavius
Internal intercostal muscle
I
II
IV
V
VI
VII
Serratus anterior
Latissimus dorsi
External intercostal muscle
Pectoralis minor
Pectoralis major
Rectus abdominis
External oblique

→ 204, 570, 571

Fig. 336 Muscles of the arm, the thorax and the inferior region of the neck.
I, II, IV–VII indicate the corresponding ribs.

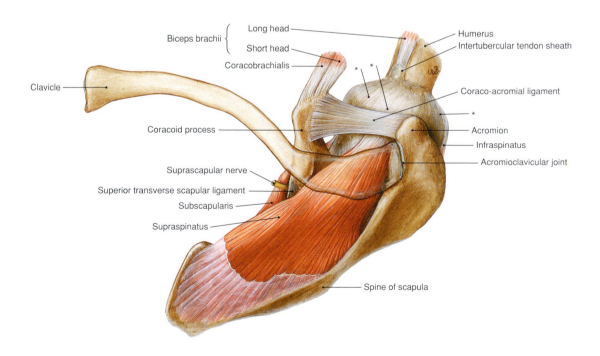

Biceps brachii { Long head / Short head
Coracobrachialis
Clavicle
Humerus
Intertubercular tendon sheath
Coraco-acromial ligament
Acromion
Infraspinatus
Acromioclavicular joint
Coracoid process
Suprascapular nerve
Superior transverse scapular ligament
Subscapularis
Supraspinatus
Spine of scapula

→ T 27

Fig. 337 Shoulder and muscles of the shoulder.
Together, the muscle tendons marked with * form the so-called rotator cuff.

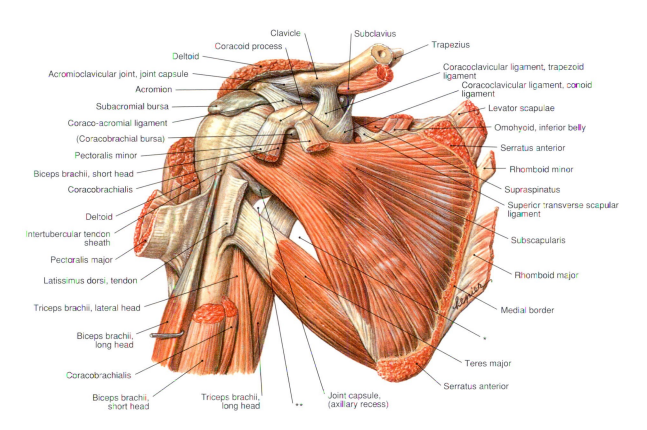

Clavicle
Subclavius
Coracoid process
Deltoid
Trapezius
Acromioclavicular joint, joint capsule
Coracoclavicular ligament, trapezoid ligament
Acromion
Coracoclavicular ligament, conoid ligament
Subacromial bursa
Levator scapulae
Coraco-acromial ligament
Omohyoid, inferior belly
(Coracobrachial bursa)
Serratus anterior
Pectoralis minor
Rhomboid minor
Biceps brachii, short head
Supraspinatus
Coracobrachialis
Superior transverse scapular ligament
Deltoid
Intertubercular tendon sheath
Subscapularis
Pectoralis major
Latissimus dorsi, tendon
Rhomboid major
Triceps brachii, lateral head
Medial border
Biceps brachii, long head
*
Coracobrachialis
Teres major
Biceps brachii, short head
Triceps brachii, long head
**
Joint capsule, (axillary recess)
Serratus anterior

Fig. 338   Shoulder and muscles of the shoulder.

→ T 26

*   Triangular space
** Quadrangular space

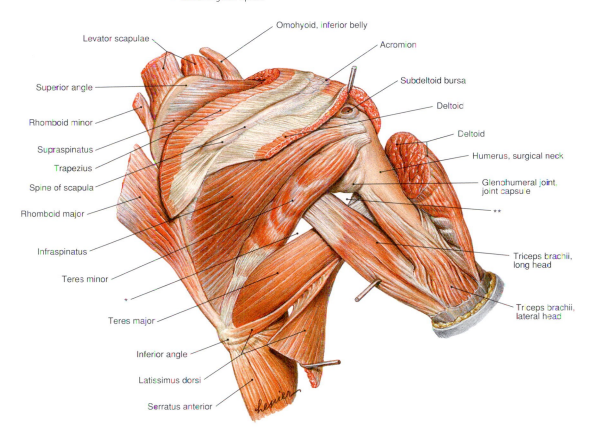

Omohyoid, inferior belly
Levator scapulae
Acromion
Superior angle
Subdeltoid bursa
Rhomboid minor
Deltoid
Supraspinatus
Deltoid
Trapezius
Humerus, surgical neck
Spine of scapula
Glenohumeral joint, joint capsule
Rhomboid major
**
Infraspinatus
Triceps brachii, long head
Teres minor
*
Teres major
Triceps brachii, lateral head
Inferior angle
Latissimus dorsi
Serratus anterior

Fig. 339   Shoulder and muscles of the shoulder.

→ T 28

*   Triangular space
** Quadrangular space

Muscles of the shoulder

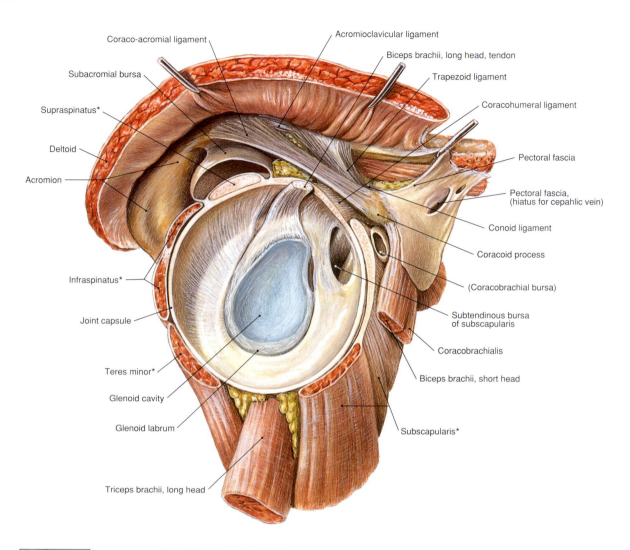

Coraco-acromial ligament
Subacromial bursa
Supraspinatus*
Deltoid
Acromion
Infraspinatus*
Joint capsule
Teres minor*
Glenoid cavity
Glenoid labrum
Triceps brachii, long head

Acromioclavicular ligament
Biceps brachii, long head, tendon
Trapezoid ligament
Coracohumeral ligament
Pectoral fascia
Pectoral fascia, (hiatus for cepahlic vein)
Conoid ligament
Coracoid process
(Coracobrachial bursa)
Subtendinous bursa of subscapularis
Coracobrachialis
Biceps brachii, short head
Subscapularis*

→ T 26–T 28

Fig. 340 Shoulder joint; lateral view.
Together, the muscle tendons marked with * form the so-called rotator cuff.

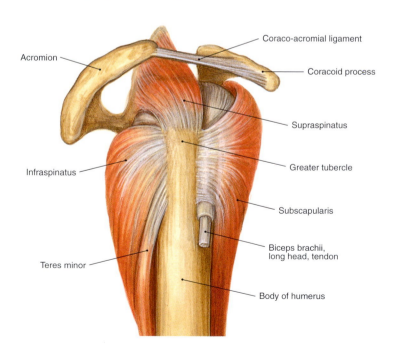

Acromion
Infraspinatus
Teres minor

Coraco-acromial ligament
Coracoid process
Supraspinatus
Greater tubercle
Subscapularis
Biceps brachii, long head, tendon
Body of humerus

→ T 26–T 28

Fig. 341 Muscles of the so-called rotator cuff; lateral view.

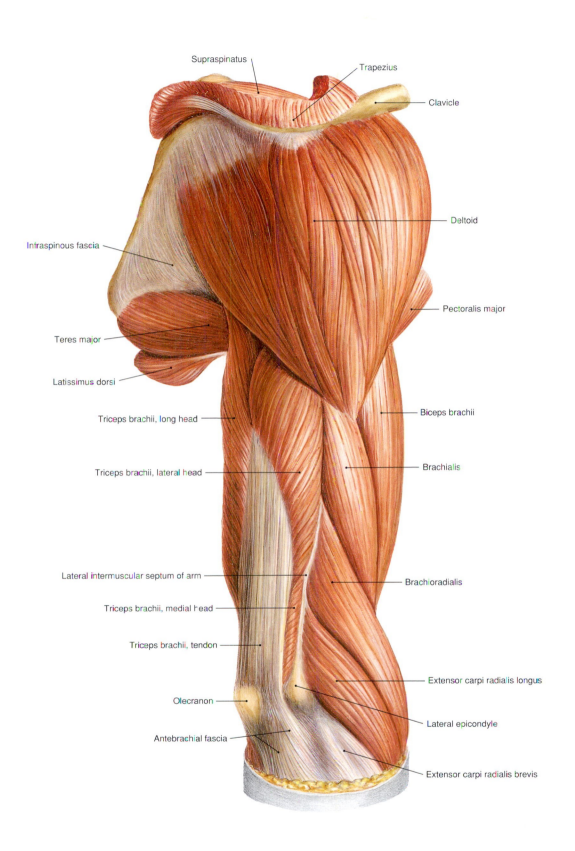

Supraspinatus

Trapezius

Clavicle

Deltoid

Intraspinous fascia

Pectoralis major

Teres major

Latissimus dorsi

Biceps brachii

Triceps brachii, long head

Brachialis

Triceps brachii, lateral head

Lateral intermuscular septum of arm

Brachioradialis

Triceps brachii, medial head

Triceps brachii, tendon

Extensor carpi radialis longus

Olecranon

Lateral epicondyle

Antebrachial fascia

Extensor carpi radialis brevis

Fig. 342   Muscles of the arm;
superficial layer;
dorsolateral view.

→ T 27, T 30

Origins and insertions of the muscles of the shoulder and the arm

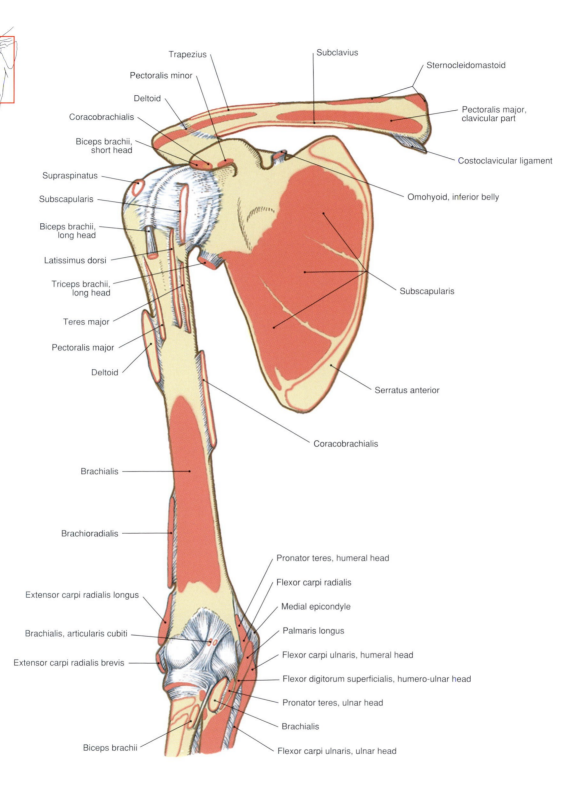

Trapezius
Subclavius
Sternocleidomastoid
Pectoralis minor
Deltoid
Pectoralis major, clavicular part
Coracobrachialis
Costoclavicular ligament
Biceps brachii, short head
Omohyoid, inferior belly
Supraspinatus
Subscapularis
Biceps brachii, long head
Latissimus dorsi
Subscapularis
Triceps brachii, long head
Teres major
Pectoralis major
Deltoid
Serratus anterior
Coracobrachialis
Brachialis
Brachioradialis
Pronator teres, humeral head
Flexor carpi radialis
Medial epicondyle
Extensor carpi radialis longus
Palmaris longus
Brachialis, articularis cubiti
Flexor carpi ulnaris, humeral head
Extensor carpi radialis brevis
Flexor digitorum superficialis, humero-ulnar head
Pronator teres, ulnar head
Brachialis
Biceps brachii
Flexor carpi ulnaris, ulnar head

→ T 26–T 30

Fig. 343   Origins and insertions of the muscles at the clavicle, the scapula and the humerus (as well as ulnar origins of multi-head muscles).

Origins and insertions of the muscles of the shoulder and the arm

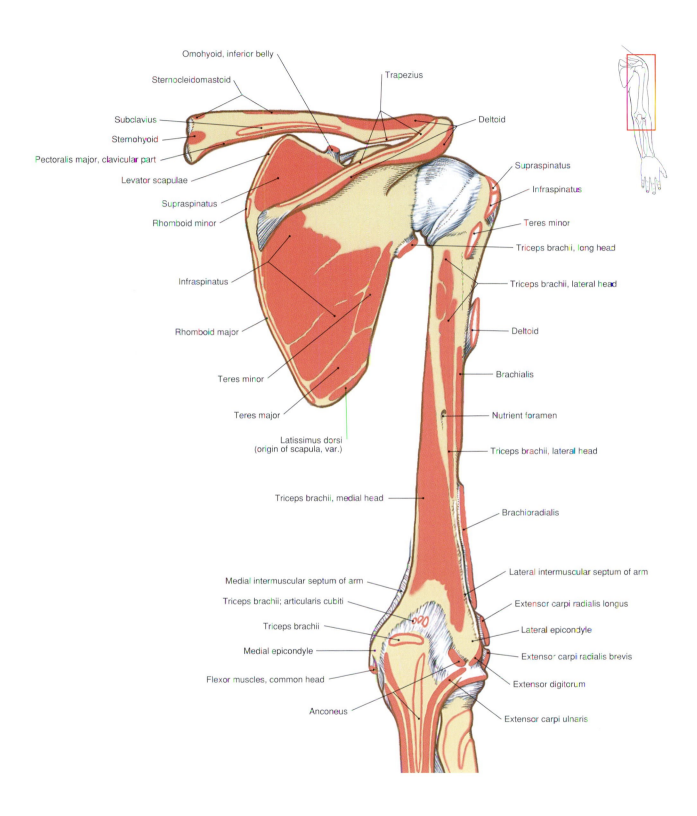

Omohyoid, inferior belly

Sternocleidomastoid

Subclavius

Sternohyoid

Pectoralis major, clavicular part

Levator scapulae

Supraspinatus

Rhomboid minor

Infraspinatus

Rhomboid major

Teres minor

Teres major

Latissimus dorsi
(origin of scapula, var.)

Triceps brachii, medial head

Medial intermuscular septum of arm

Triceps brachii; articularis cubiti

Triceps brachii

Medial epicondyle

Flexor muscles, common head

Anconeus

Trapezius

Deltoid

Supraspinatus

Infraspinatus

Teres minor

Triceps brachii, long head

Triceps brachii, lateral head

Deltoid

Brachialis

Nutrient foramen

Triceps brachii, lateral head

Brachioradialis

Lateral intermuscular septum of arm

Extensor carpi radialis longus

Lateral epicondyle

Extensor carpi radialis brevis

Extensor digitorum

Extensor carpi ulnaris

Fig. 344   Origins and insertions of the muscles at the clavicle,
the scapula and the humerus (as well as ulnar origins of
multi-head muscles).

→ T 26–T 30

Muscles of the arm

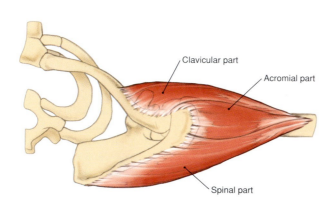

Fig. 345 Deltoid muscle.

→ T 27

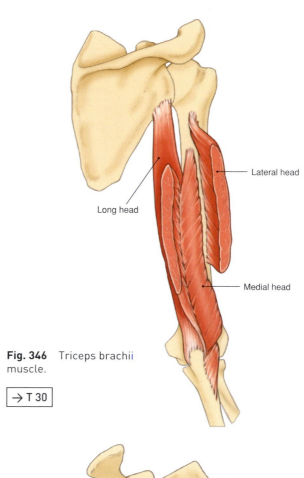

Fig. 346 Triceps brachii muscle.

→ T 30

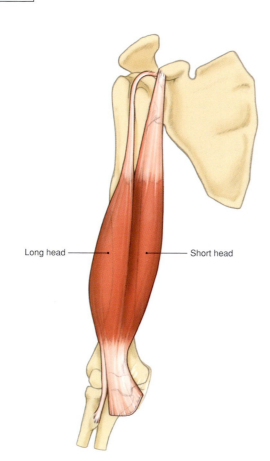

Fig. 347 Biceps brachii muscle.

→ T 29

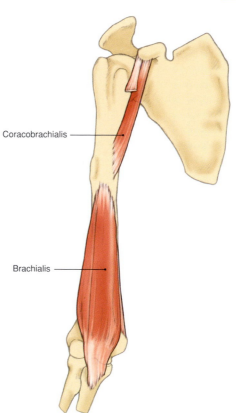

Fig. 348 Brachial and coracobrachial muscles.

→ T 29

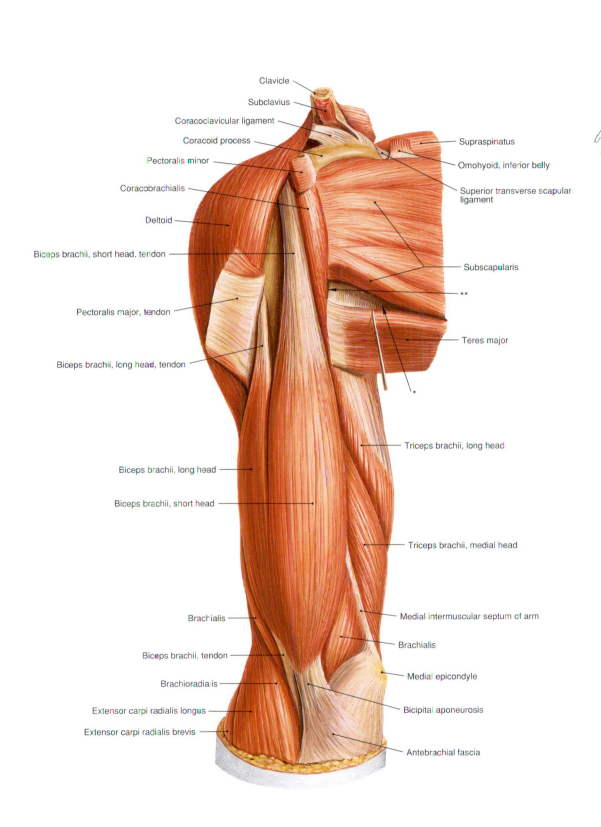

Clavicle

Subclavius

Coracoclavicular ligament

Coracoid process

Pectoralis minor

Coracobrachialis

Deltoid

Biceps brachii, short head, tendon

Pectoralis major, tendon

Biceps brachii, long head, tendon

Biceps brachii, long head

Biceps brachii, short head

Brachialis

Biceps brachii, tendon

Brachioradialis

Extensor carpi radialis longus

Extensor carpi radialis brevis

Supraspinatus

Omohyoid, inferior belly

Superior transverse scapular ligament

Subscapularis

**

Teres major

*

Triceps brachii, long head

Triceps brachii, medial head

Medial intermuscular septum of arm

Brachialis

Medial epicondyle

Bicipital aponeurosis

Antebrachial fascia

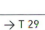

Fig. 349   Muscles of the arm;
flexor aspect, superficial layer.

*   Triangular space
** Quadrangular space

→ T 29

Muscles of the arm

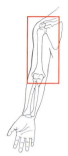

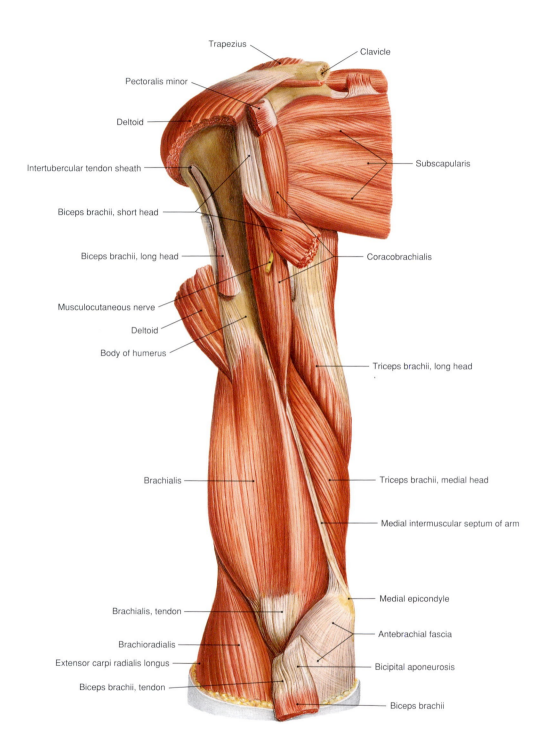

Trapezius

Clavicle

Pectoralis minor

Deltoid

Intertubercular tendon sheath

Subscapularis

Biceps brachii, short head

Biceps brachii, long head

Coracobrachialis

Musculocutaneous nerve

Deltoid

Body of humerus

Triceps brachii, long head

Brachialis

Triceps brachii, medial head

Medial intermuscular septum of arm

Medial epicondyle

Brachialis, tendon

Antebrachial fascia

Brachioradialis

Extensor carpi radialis longus

Bicipital aponeurosis

Biceps brachii, tendon

Biceps brachii

→ T 29

Fig. 350 Muscles of the arm;
flexor aspect, deep layer.

Muscles of the arm

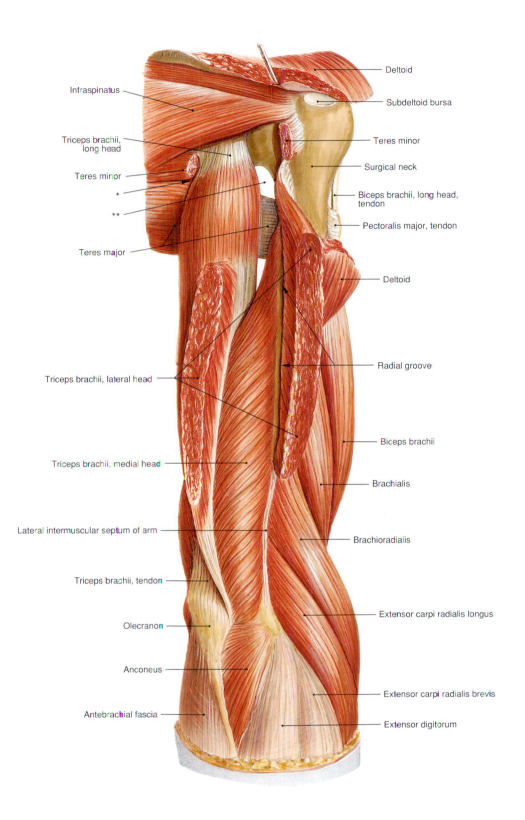

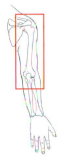

Deltoid

Subdeltoid bursa

Teres minor

Surgical neck

Biceps brachii, long head, tendon

Pectoralis major, tendon

Deltoid

Radial groove

Biceps brachii

Brachialis

Brachioradialis

Extensor carpi radialis longus

Extensor carpi radialis brevis

Extensor digitorum

Infraspinatus

Triceps brachii, long head

Teres minor

*

**

Teres major

Triceps brachii, lateral head

Triceps brachii, medial head

Lateral intermuscular septum of arm

Triceps brachii, tendon

Olecranon

Anconeus

Antebrachial fascia

Fig. 351   Muscles of the arm;
extensor aspect, deep layer.

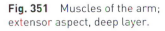

* Triangular space
** Quadrangular space

Origins and insertions of the ventral muscles of the forearm

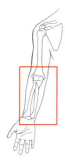

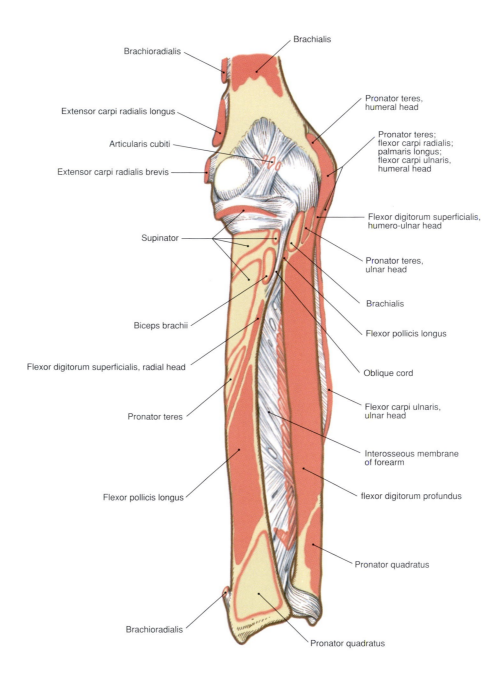

Brachialis

Brachioradialis

Extensor carpi radialis longus

Articularis cubiti

Extensor carpi radialis brevis

Supinator

Biceps brachii

Flexor digitorum superficialis, radial head

Pronator teres

Flexor pollicis longus

Brachioradialis

Pronator teres, humeral head

Pronator teres; flexor carpi radialis; palmaris longus; flexor carpi ulnaris, humeral head

Flexor digitorum superficialis, humero-ulnar head

Pronator teres, ulnar head

Brachialis

Flexor pollicis longus

Oblique cord

Flexor carpi ulnaris, ulnar head

Interosseous membrane of forearm

flexor digitorum profundus

Pronator quadratus

Pronator quadratus

→ T 31–T 33

Fig. 352   Origins and insertions of the muscles
at the radius, the ulna and the distal part of the humerus.

Muscles of the forearm

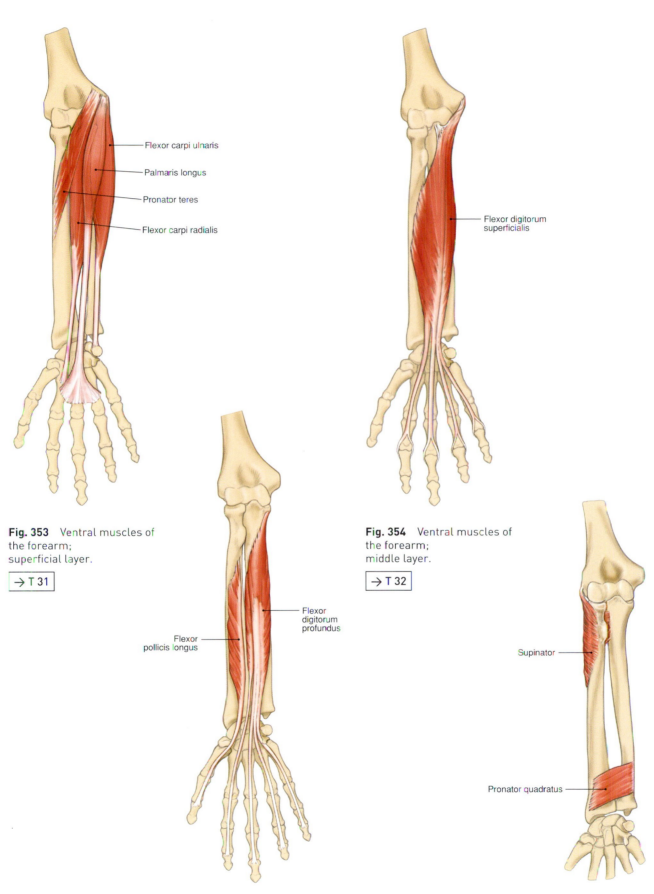

Flexor carpi ulnaris
Palmaris longus
Pronator teres
Flexor carpi radialis

Fig. 353 Ventral muscles of the forearm; superficial layer.

→ T 31

Flexor digitorum superficialis

Fig. 354 Ventral muscles of the forearm; middle layer.

→ T 32

Flexor digitorum profundus
Flexor pollicis longus

Fig. 355 Ventral muscles of the forearm; deep layer.

→ T 31, T32

Supinator

Pronator quadratus

Fig. 356 Ventral muscles of the forearm; deepest layer.

→ T 31, T 35

Muscles of the forearm

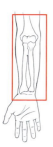

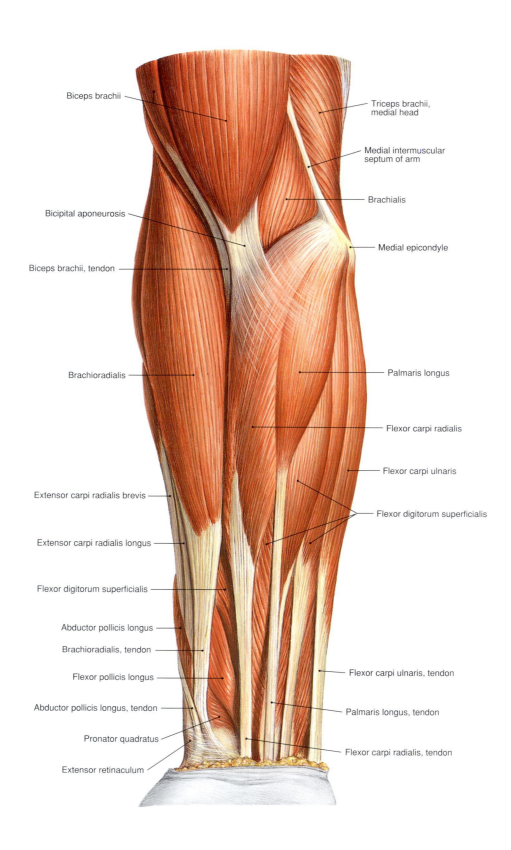

Biceps brachii

Bicipital aponeurosis

Biceps brachii, tendon

Brachioradialis

Extensor carpi radialis brevis

Extensor carpi radialis longus

Flexor digitorum superficialis

Abductor pollicis longus

Brachioradialis, tendon

Flexor pollicis longus

Abductor pollicis longus, tendon

Pronator quadratus

Extensor retinaculum

Triceps brachii, medial head

Medial intermuscular septum of arm

Brachialis

Medial epicondyle

Palmaris longus

Flexor carpi radialis

Flexor carpi ulnaris

Flexor digitorum superficialis

Flexor carpi ulnaris, tendon

Palmaris longus, tendon

Flexor carpi radialis, tendon

→ T 31

Fig. 357 Muscles of the forearm; flexor aspect, superficial layer.

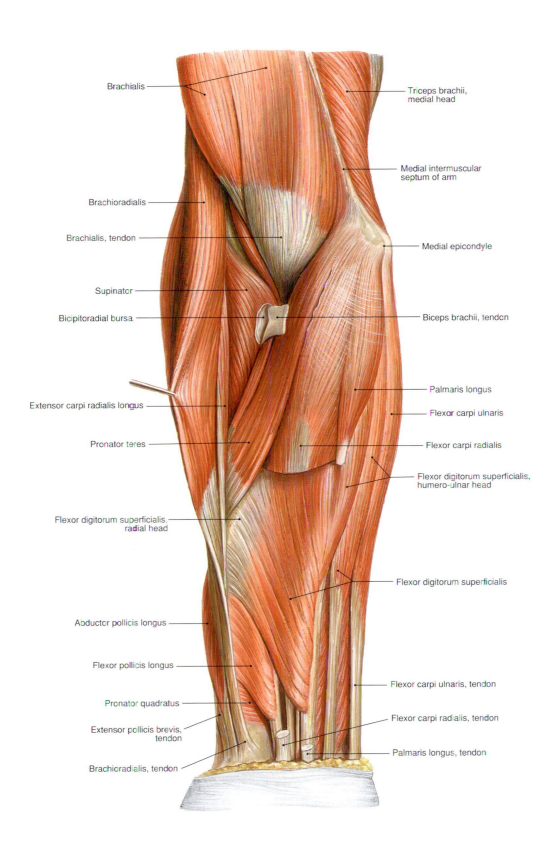

Brachialis

Triceps brachii, medial head

Medial intermuscular septum of arm

Brachioradialis

Brachialis, tendon

Medial epicondyle

Supinator

Bicipitoradial bursa

Biceps brachii, tendon

Palmaris longus

Extensor carpi radialis longus

Flexor carpi ulnaris

Pronator teres

Flexor carpi radialis

Flexor digitorum superficialis, humero-ulnar head

Flexor digitorum superficialis, radial head

Flexor digitorum superficialis

Abductor pollicis longus

Flexor pollicis longus

Pronator quadratus

Flexor carpi ulnaris, tendon

Flexor carpi radialis, tendon

Extensor pollicis brevis, tendon

Palmaris longus, tendon

Brachioradialis, tendon

Fig. 358 Muscles of the forearm; flexor aspect, middle layer.

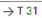 → T 31

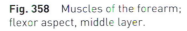

Muscles of the forearm

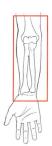

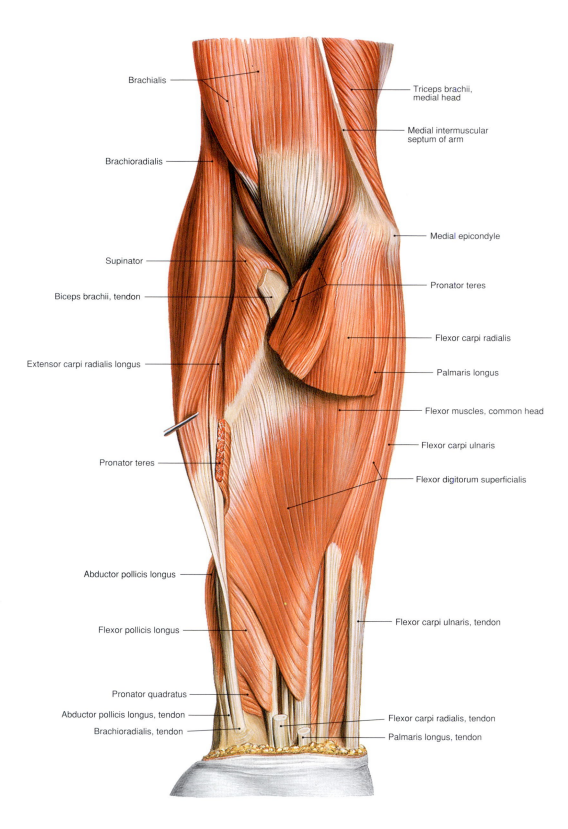

Brachialis

Triceps brachii, medial head

Medial intermuscular septum of arm

Brachioradialis

Medial epicondyle

Supinator

Pronator teres

Biceps brachii, tendon

Flexor carpi radialis

Extensor carpi radialis longus

Palmaris longus

Flexor muscles, common head

Flexor carpi ulnaris

Pronator teres

Flexor digitorum superficialis

Abductor pollicis longus

Flexor carpi ulnaris, tendon

Flexor pollicis longus

Pronator quadratus

Abductor pollicis longus, tendon

Flexor carpi radialis, tendon

Brachioradialis, tendon

Palmaris longus, tendon

→ T 31, T 32

Fig. 359 Muscles of the forearm; flexor aspect, middle layer after section of the pronator teres muscle.

Muscles of the forearm

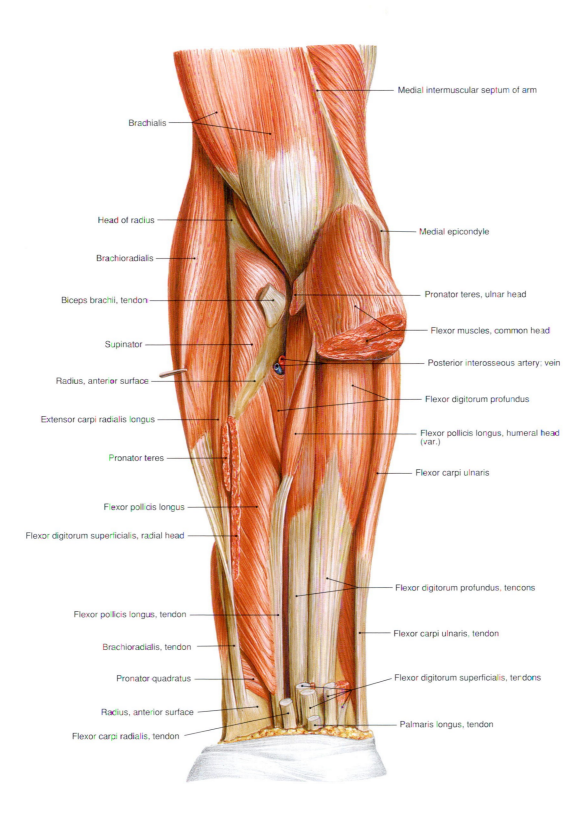

Medial intermuscular septum of arm

Brachialis

Head of radius

Medial epicondyle

Brachioradialis

Biceps brachii, tendon

Pronator teres, ulnar head

Supinator

Flexor muscles, common head

Radius, anterior surface

Posterior interosseous artery; vein

Extensor carpi radialis longus

Flexor digitorum profundus

Pronator teres

Flexor pollicis longus, humeral head (var.)

Flexor pollicis longus

Flexor carpi ulnaris

Flexor digitorum superficialis, radial head

Flexor digitorum profundus, tencons

Flexor pollicis longus, tendon

Flexor carpi ulnaris, tendon

Brachioradialis, tendon

Pronator quadratus

Flexor digitorum superficialis, terdons

Radius, anterior surface

Flexor carpi radialis, tendon

Palmaris longus, tendon

Fig. 360 Muscles of the forearm; flexor aspect, deep layer.

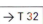 → T 32

Origins and insertions of the dorsal muscles of the forearm

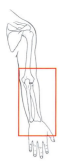

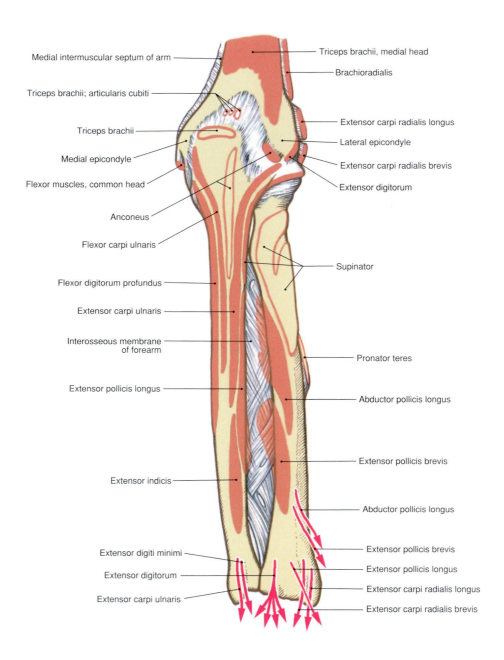

Medial intermuscular septum of arm

Triceps brachii, medial head

Brachioradialis

Triceps brachii; articularis cubiti

Triceps brachii

Extensor carpi radialis longus

Lateral epicondyle

Medial epicondyle

Extensor carpi radialis brevis

Flexor muscles, common head

Extensor digitorum

Anconeus

Flexor carpi ulnaris

Supinator

Flexor digitorum profundus

Extensor carpi ulnaris

Interosseous membrane of forearm

Pronator teres

Extensor pollicis longus

Abductor pollicis longus

Extensor pollicis brevis

Extensor indicis

Abductor pollicis longus

Extensor digiti minimi

Extensor pollicis brevis

Extensor digitorum

Extensor pollicis longus

Extensor carpi ulnaris

Extensor carpi radialis longus

Extensor carpi radialis brevis

→ T 34, T 35

Fig. 361 Origins and insertions of the muscles at the radius, the ulna and the distal part of the humerus.

Muscles of the forearm

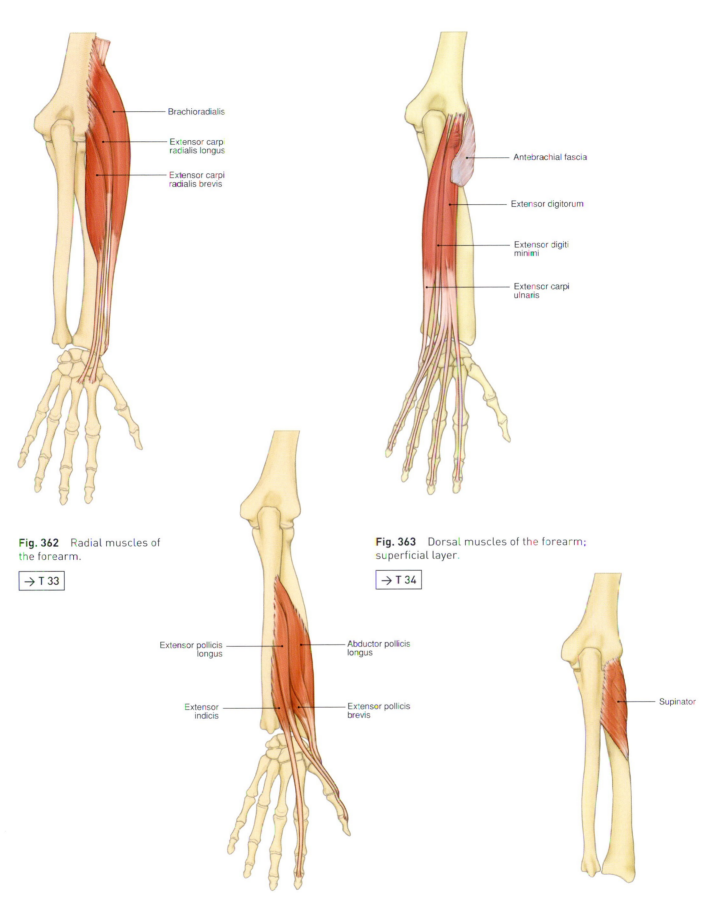

Brachioradialis

Extensor carpi radialis longus

Extensor carpi radialis brevis

Fig. 362 Radial muscles of the forearm.

→ T 33

Antebrachial fascia

Extensor digitorum

Extensor digiti minimi

Extensor carpi ulnaris

Fig. 363 Dorsal muscles of the forearm; superficial layer.

→ T 34

Extensor pollicis longus

Abductor pollicis longus

Extensor indicis

Extensor pollicis brevis

Fig. 364 Dorsal muscles of the forearm; middle layer.

→ T 35

Supinator

Fig. 365 Dorsal muscles of the forearm; deep layer.

→ T35

Muscles of the forearm

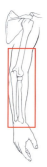

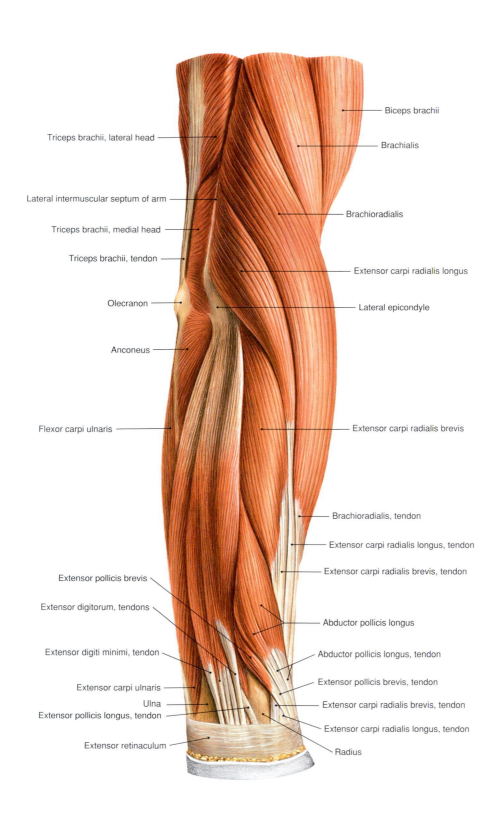

Triceps brachii, lateral head

Lateral intermuscular septum of arm

Triceps brachii, medial head

Triceps brachii, tendon

Olecranon

Anconeus

Flexor carpi ulnaris

Extensor pollicis brevis

Extensor digitorum, tendons

Extensor digiti minimi, tendon

Extensor carpi ulnaris

Ulna

Extensor pollicis longus, tendon

Extensor retinaculum

Biceps brachii

Brachialis

Brachioradialis

Extensor carpi radialis longus

Lateral epicondyle

Extensor carpi radialis brevis

Brachioradialis, tendon

Extensor carpi radialis longus, tendon

Extensor carpi radialis brevis, tendon

Abductor pollicis longus

Abductor pollicis longus, tendon

Extensor pollicis brevis, tendon

Extensor carpi radialis brevis, tendon

Extensor carpi radialis longus, tendon

Radius

→ T 33

Fig. 366 Muscles of the forearm and
the distal part of the arm;
lateral view;
intermediate position of the forearm between supination and pronation.

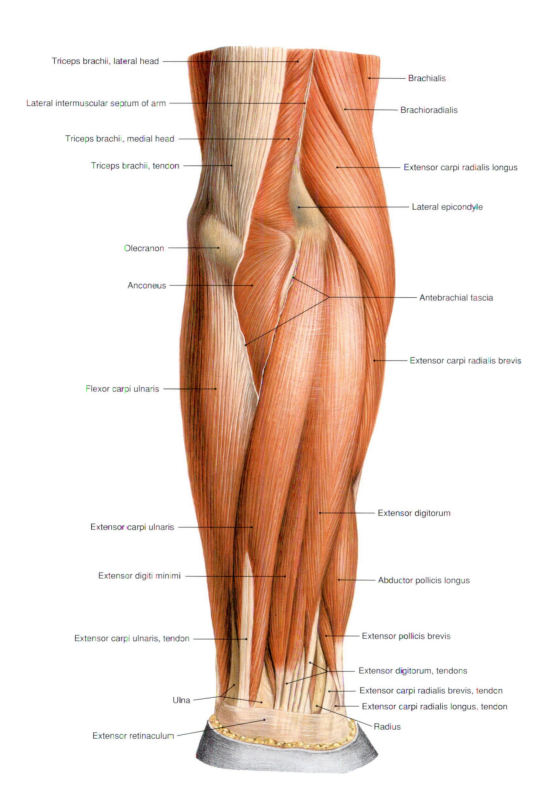

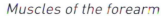

Triceps brachii, lateral head

Brachialis

Lateral intermuscular septum of arm

Brachioradialis

Triceps brachii, medial head

Triceps brachii, tendon

Extensor carpi radialis longus

Lateral epicondyle

Olecranon

Anconeus

Antebrachial fascia

Extensor carpi radialis brevis

Flexor carpi ulnaris

Extensor digitorum

Extensor carpi ulnaris

Extensor digiti minimi

Abductor pollicis longus

Extensor pollicis brevis

Extensor carpi ulnaris, tendon

Extensor digitorum, tendons

Extensor carpi radialis brevis, tendon

Ulna

Extensor carpi radialis longus, tendon

Radius

Extensor retinaculum

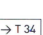

Fig. 367   Muscles of the forearm and
the distal part of the arm;
extensor aspect, superficial layer;
intermediate position of the forearm between
supination and pronation.

→ T 34

Muscles of the forearm

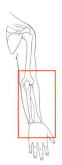

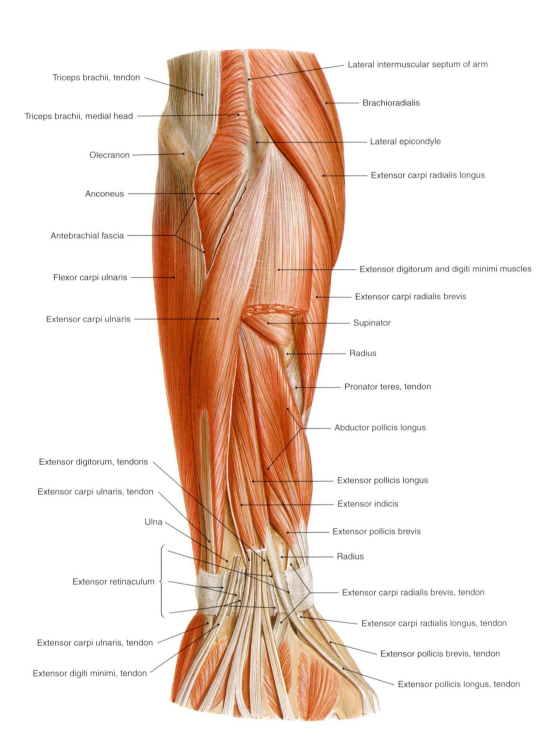

Triceps brachii, tendon

Triceps brachii, medial head

Olecranon

Anconeus

Antebrachial fascia

Flexor carpi ulnaris

Extensor carpi ulnaris

Extensor digitorum, tendons

Extensor carpi ulnaris, tendon

Ulna

Extensor retinaculum

Extensor carpi ulnaris, tendon

Extensor digiti minimi, tendon

Lateral intermuscular septum of arm

Brachioradialis

Lateral epicondyle

Extensor carpi radialis longus

Extensor digitorum and digiti minimi muscles

Extensor carpi radialis brevis

Supinator

Radius

Pronator teres, tendon

Abductor pollicis longus

Extensor pollicis longus

Extensor indicis

Extensor pollicis brevis

Radius

Extensor carpi radialis brevis, tendon

Extensor carpi radialis longus, tendon

Extensor pollicis brevis, tendon

Extensor pollicis longus, tendon

→ T 34, T 35

Fig. 368   Muscles of the forearm; extensor aspect, middle layer; intermediate position of the forearm between supination and pronation.

Muscles of the forearm

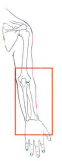

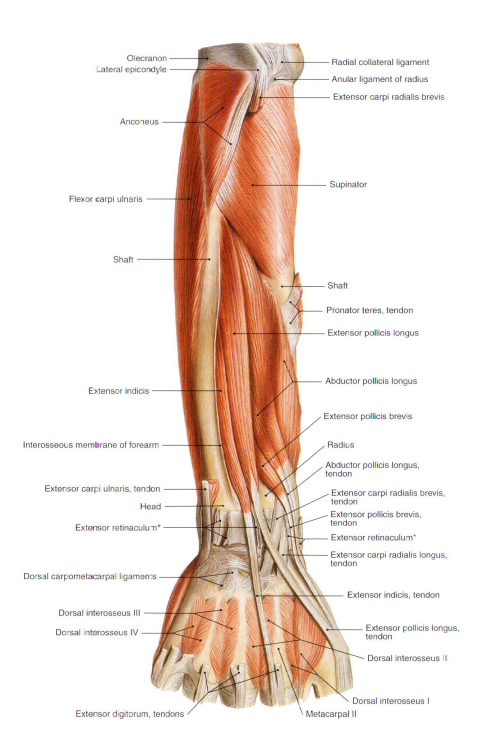

Olecranon — Radial collateral ligament
Lateral epicondyle — Anular ligament of radius
— Extensor carpi radialis brevis
Anconeus —
Supinator
Flexor carpi ulnaris —
Shaft —
— Shaft
— Pronator teres, tendon
— Extensor pollicis longus
Extensor indicis — — Abductor pollicis longus
— Extensor pollicis brevis
Interosseous membrane of forearm — — Radius
Abductor pollicis longus, tendon
Extensor carpi ulnaris, tendon — Extensor carpi radialis brevis, tendon
Head — Extensor pollicis brevis, tendon
Extensor retinaculum* — — Extensor retinaculum*
Extensor carpi radialis longus, tendon
Dorsal carpometacarpal ligaments — — Extensor indicis, tendon
Dorsal interosseus III — Extensor pollicis longus, tendon
Dorsal interosseus IV — — Dorsal interosseus II
— Dorsal interosseus I
Extensor digitorum, tendons — Metacarpal II

Fig. 369 Muscles of the forearm and the hand;
extensor aspect, deep layer;
intermediate position of the forearm between
supination and pronation.

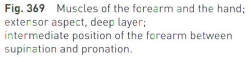 → T 35

* The tendon compartments formed by the extensor retinaculum have been opened
longitudinally.

Muscles of the forearm

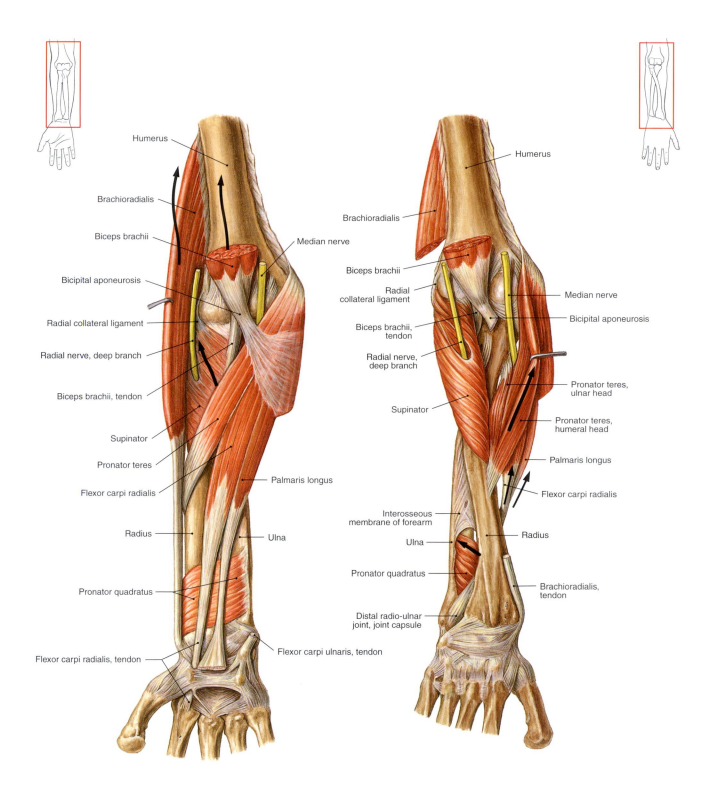

Humerus
Brachioradialis
Biceps brachii
Bicipital aponeurosis
Radial collateral ligament
Radial nerve, deep branch
Biceps brachii, tendon
Supinator
Pronator teres
Flexor carpi radialis
Radius
Pronator quadratus
Flexor carpi radialis, tendon
Median nerve
Palmaris longus
Ulna
Flexor carpi ulnaris, tendon

Humerus
Brachioradialis
Biceps brachii
Radial collateral ligament
Biceps brachii, tendon
Radial nerve, deep branch
Supinator
Interosseous membrane of forearm
Ulna
Pronator quadratus
Distal radio-ulnar joint, joint capsule
Median nerve
Bicipital aponeurosis
Pronator teres, ulnar head
Pronator teres, humeral head
Palmaris longus
Flexor carpi radialis
Radius
Brachioradialis, tendon

Fig. 370 Forearm in supination; ventropalmar view.
Arrows indicate the direction of force generated by the main supinator muscles.

→ T 32, T 33, T 35

Fig. 371 Forearm in pronation; ventral view of the elbow region, dorsal view of the dorsum of the hand.
Arrows indicate the direction of force generated by the main pronator muscles.

→ T 32, T 33, T 35

Origins and insertions of the muscles of the hand

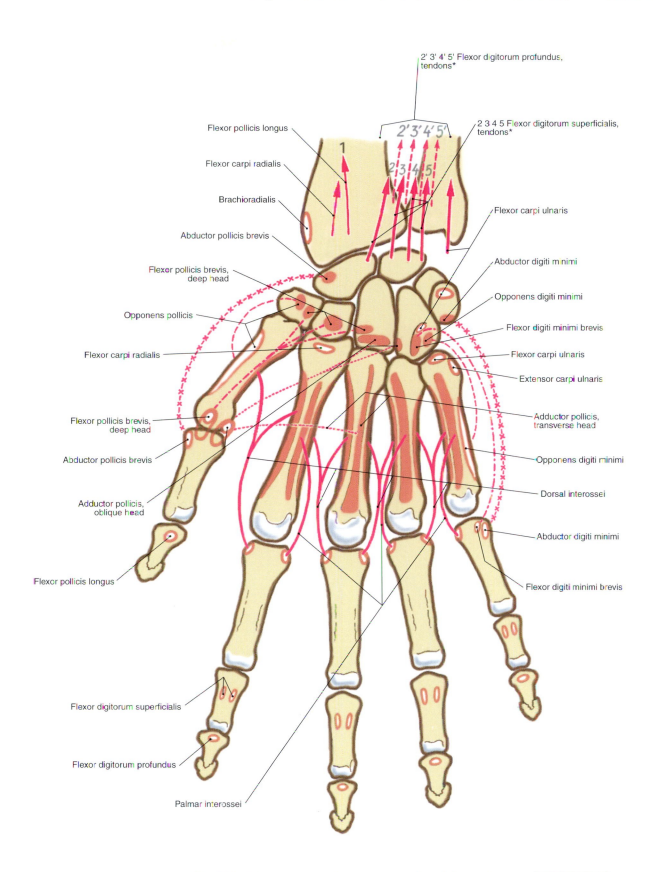

2' 3' 4' 5' Flexor digitorum profundus, tendons*

Flexor pollicis longus

Flexor carpi radialis

Brachioradialis

Abductor pollicis brevis

Flexor pollicis brevis, deep head

Opponens pollicis

Flexor carpi radialis

Flexor pollicis brevis, deep head

Abductor pollicis brevis

Adductor pollicis, oblique head

Flexor pollicis longus

Flexor digitorum superficialis

Flexor digitorum profundus

Palmar interossei

2 3 4 5 Flexor digitorum superficialis, tendons*

Flexor carpi ulnaris

Abductor digiti minimi

Opponens digiti minimi

Flexor digiti minimi brevis

Flexor carpi ulnaris

Extensor carpi ulnaris

Adductor pollicis, transverse head

Opponens digiti minimi

Dorsal interossei

Abductor digiti minimi

Flexor digiti minimi brevis

Fig. 372   Origins and insertions of the muscles of the hand at the bones of the hand.

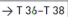 → T 36–T 38

* The flexors insert at the second to fifth digit.

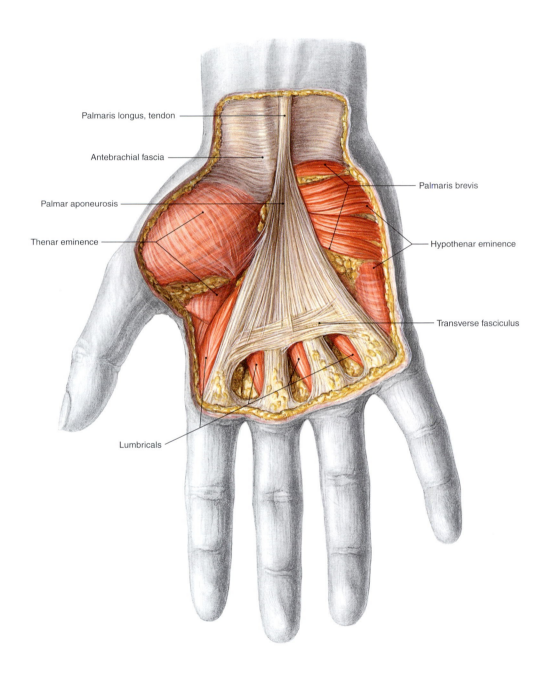

Palmaris longus, tendon

Antebrachial fascia

Palmar aponeurosis

Thenar eminence

Palmaris brevis

Hypothenar eminence

Transverse fasciculus

Lumbricals

→ T 31, T 36–T 38

Fig. 373 Muscles of the palm; superficial layer.

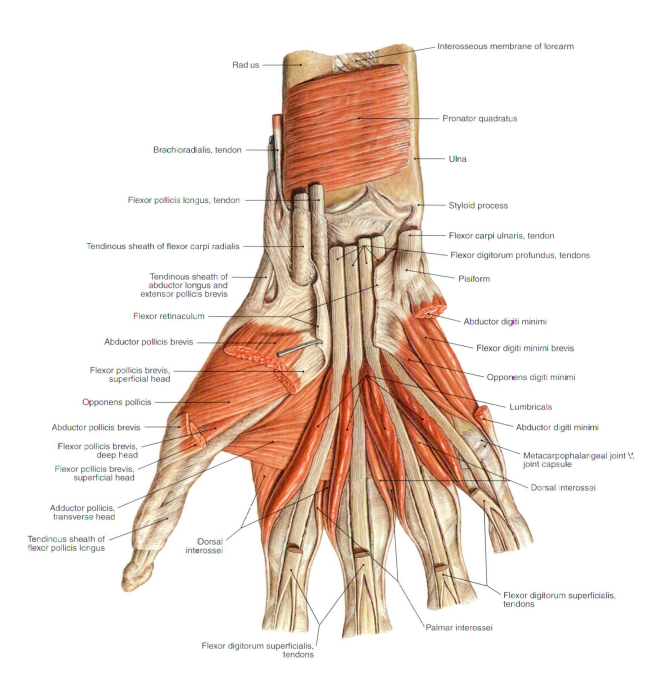

Interosseous membrane of forearm

Rad us

Pronator quadratus

Brachioradialis, tendon

Ulna

Flexor pollicis longus, tendon

Styloid process

Flexor carpi ulnaris, tendon

Tendinous sheath of flexor carpi radialis

Flexor digitorum profundus, tendons

Tendinous sheath of abductor longus and extensor pollicis brevis

Pisiform

Flexor retinaculum

Abductor digiti minimi

Abductor pollicis brevis

Flexor digiti minimi brevis

Flexor pollicis brevis, superficial head

Opponens digiti minimi

Opponens pollicis

Lumbricals

Abductor pollicis brevis

Abductor digiti minimi

Flexor pollicis brevis, deep head

Metacarpophalangeal joint V, joint capsule

Flexor pollicis brevis, superficial head

Adductor pollicis, transverse head

Dorsal interossei

Tendinous sheath of flexor pollicis longus

Dorsal interossei

Flexor digitorum superficialis, tendons

Palmar interossei

Flexor digitorum superficialis, tendons

Fig. 374 Muscles of the palm; middle layer.

→ T 32, T 36–T 38

Tendon sheaths of the hand

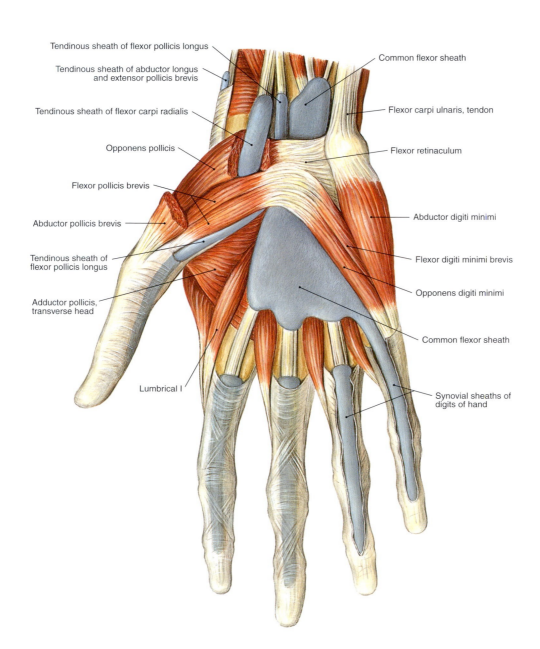

Tendinous sheath of flexor pollicis longus

Tendinous sheath of abductor longus and extensor pollicis brevis

Tendinous sheath of flexor carpi radialis

Opponens pollicis

Flexor pollicis brevis

Abductor pollicis brevis

Tendinous sheath of flexor pollicis longus

Adductor pollicis, transverse head

Lumbrical I

Common flexor sheath

Flexor carpi ulnaris, tendon

Flexor retinaculum

Abductor digiti minimi

Flexor digiti minimi brevis

Opponens digiti minimi

Common flexor sheath

Synovial sheaths of digits of hand

Fig. 375   Tendon sheaths of the hand.

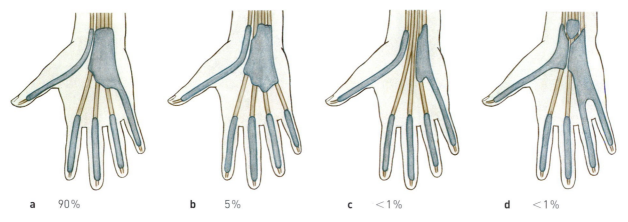

a   90 %   **b**   5 %   **c**   < 1 %   **d**   < 1 %

Fig. 376 a–d   Frequent variations of the palmar tendon sheaths.

Muscles of the hand

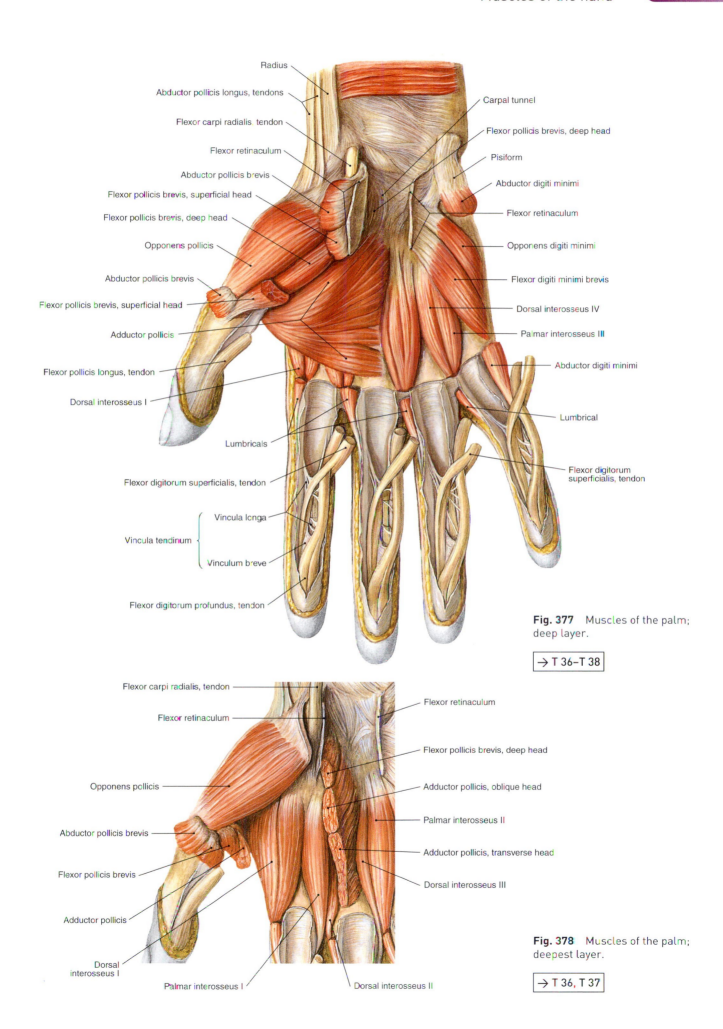

Radius

Abductor pollicis longus, tendons

Flexor carpi radialis, tendon

Flexor retinaculum

Abductor pollicis brevis

Flexor pollicis brevis, superficial head

Flexor pollicis brevis, deep head

Opponens pollicis

Abductor pollicis brevis

Flexor pollicis brevis, superficial head

Adductor pollicis

Flexor pollicis longus, tendon

Dorsal interosseus I

Lumbricals

Flexor digitorum superficialis, tendon

Vincula longa

Vincula tendinum

Vinculum breve

Flexor digitorum profundus, tendon

Carpal tunnel

Flexor pollicis brevis, deep head

Pisiform

Abductor digiti minimi

Flexor retinaculum

Opponens digiti minimi

Flexor digiti minimi brevis

Dorsal interosseus IV

Palmar interosseus III

Abductor digiti minimi

Lumbrical

Flexor digitorum superficialis, tendon

Fig. 377 Muscles of the palm; deep layer.

→ T 36–T 38

Flexor carpi radialis, tendon

Flexor retinaculum

Opponens pollicis

Abductor pollicis brevis

Flexor pollicis brevis

Adductor pollicis

Dorsal interosseus I

Palmar interosseus I

Flexor retinaculum

Flexor pollicis brevis, deep head

Adductor pollicis, oblique head

Palmar interosseus II

Adductor pollicis, transverse head

Dorsal interosseus III

Dorsal interosseus II

Fig. 378 Muscles of the palm; deepest layer.

→ T 36, T 37

Muscles of the hand

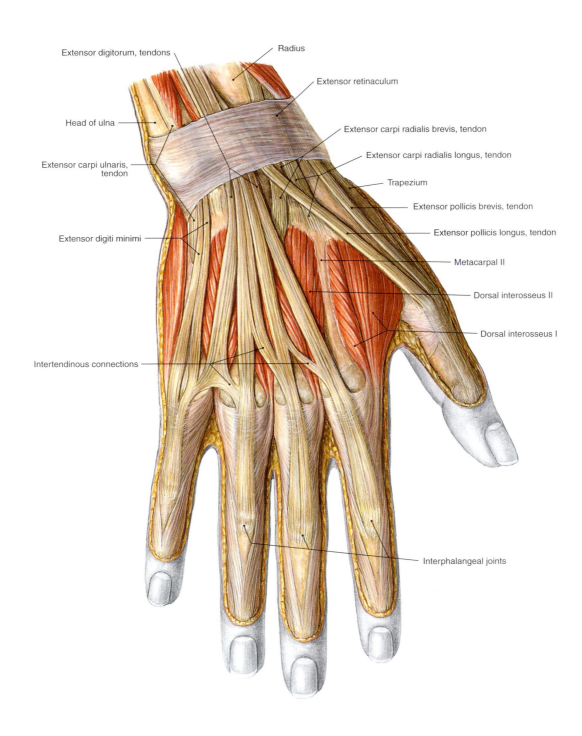

Extensor digitorum, tendons

Radius

Extensor retinaculum

Head of ulna

Extensor carpi radialis brevis, tendon

Extensor carpi radialis longus, tendon

Extensor carpi ulnaris, tendon

Trapezium

Extensor pollicis brevis, tendon

Extensor digiti minimi

Extensor pollicis longus, tendon

Metacarpal II

Dorsal interosseus II

Dorsal interosseus I

Intertendinous connections

Interphalangeal joints

→ T 34, T 35, T 37

Fig. 379   Muscles of the dorsum of the hand.

Tendon sheaths of the hand

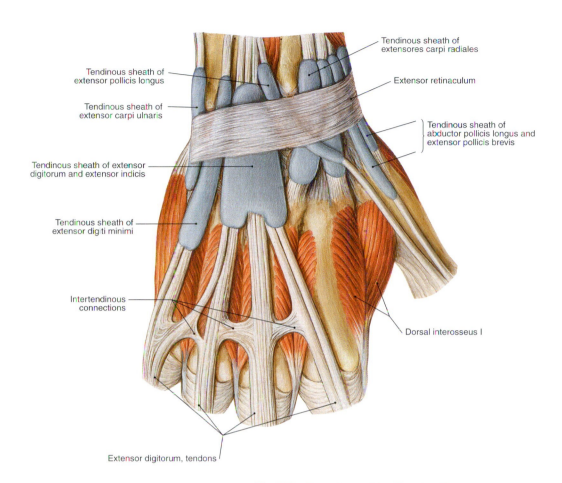

Tendinous sheath of
extensores carpi radiales

Tendinous sheath of
extensor pollicis longus

Extensor retinaculum

Tendinous sheath of
extensor carpi ulnaris

Tendinous sheath of
abductor pollicis longus and
extensor pollicis brevis

Tendincus sheath of extensor
digitorum and extensor indicis

Tendinous sheath of
extensor digiti minimi

Intertendinous
connections

Dorsal interosseus I

Extensor digitorum, tendons

Fig. 380 Dorsal carpal tendon sheath.

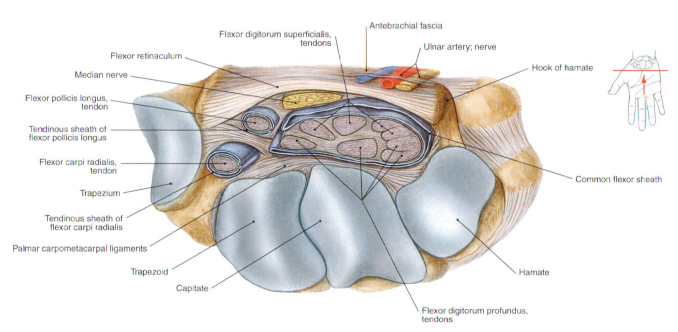

Flexor digitorum superficialis,
tendons

Antebrachial fascia

Ulnar artery; nerve

Flexor retinaculum

Median nerve

Hook of hamate

Flexor pollicis longus,
tendon

Tendinous sheath of
flexor pollicis longus

Flexor carpi radialis,
tendon

Common flexor sheath

Trapezium

Tendinous sheath of
flexor carpi radialis

Palmar carpometacarpal ligaments

Trapezoid

Hamate

Capitate

Flexor digitorum profundus,
tendons

Fig. 381 Palmar carpal tendon sheaths;
transverse section.

The compression of the median nerve
in the carpal tunnel is known as
"carpal tunnel syndrome".

Muscles of the hand

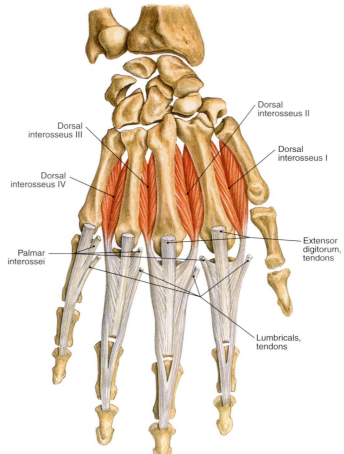

Fig. 382 Dorsal interosseous muscles; dorsal view.

→ T 37

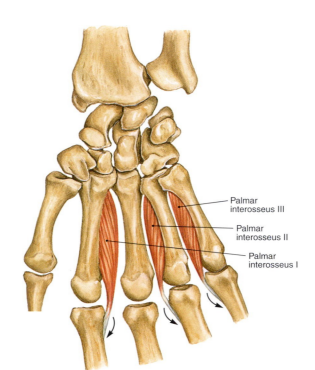

Fig. 383 Palmar interosseous muscles; palmar view.
The tendons of the interosseous and the lumbrical muscles radiate into the so-called dorsal aponeurosis of the fingers (arrows).

→ T 37

Muscles of the hand

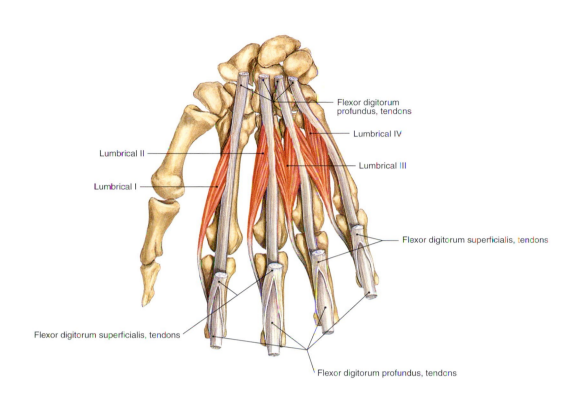

Flexor digitorum profundus, tendons

Lumbrical IV

Lumbrical II

Lumbrical III

Lumbrical I

Flexor digitorum superficialis, tendons

Flexor digitorum superficialis, tendons

Flexor digitorum profundus, tendons

Fig. 384 Lumbrical muscles; palmar view.

$\rightarrow$ T 37

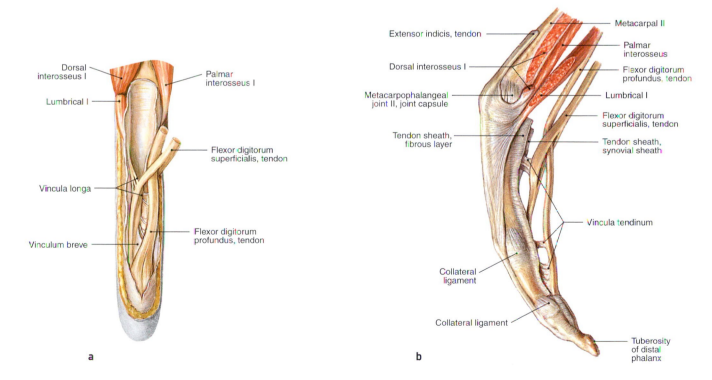

Dorsal interosseus I

Palmar interosseus I

Lumbrical I

Flexor digitorum superficialis, tendon

Vincula longa

Vinculum breve

Flexor digitorum profundus, tendon

a

Extensor indicis, tendon

Metacarpal II

Palmar interosseus

Dorsal interosseus I

Flexor digitorum profundus, tendon

Metacarpophalangeal joint II, joint capsule

Lumbrical I

Flexor digitorum superficialis, tendon

Tendon sheath, fibrous layer

Tendon sheath, synovial sheath

Vincula tendinum

Collateral ligament

Collateral ligament

Tuberosity of distal phalanx

b

Fig. 385 a, b Tendon insertions at the index; the tendons of both flexors have been dissected from the tendon sheath.
a Palmar view
b Lateral view

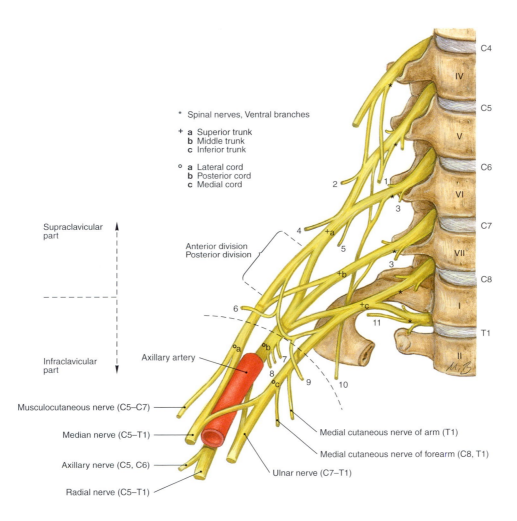

* Spinal nerves, Ventral branches

\+ **a** Superior trunk
b Middle trunk
c Inferior trunk

° **a** Lateral cord
b Posterior cord
c Medial cord

Supraclavicular part

Anterior division
Posterior division

Infraclavicular part

Axillary artery

Musculocutaneous nerve (C5–C7)

Median nerve (C5–T1)

Axillary nerve (C5, C6)

Radial nerve (C5–T1)

Medial cutaneous nerve of arm (T1)

Medial cutaneous nerve of forearm (C8, T1)

Ulnar nerve (C7–T1)

1 Phrenic nerve (Cervical plexus)
2 Dorsal scapular nerve (C5)
3 Muscular branches
4 Suprascapular nerve (C5, C6)
5 Subclavian nerve (C5, C6)
6 Lateral pectoral nerve (C5–C7)
7 Subscapular nerve (C5–C7)
8 Thoracodorsal nerve (C6–C8)
9 Medial pectoral nerve (C8, T1)
10 Long thoracic nerve (C5–C7)
11 Intercostal nerve (T1)

→ T 24, T 25

Fig. 386   Brachial plexus.

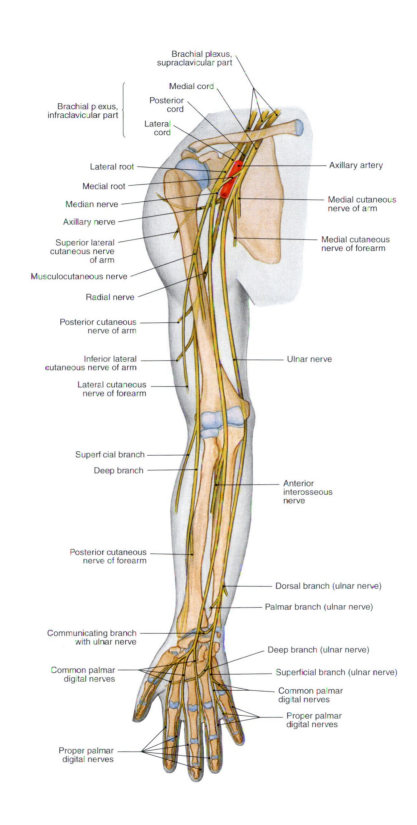

Brachial plexus,
supraclavicular part

Medial cord

Posterior
cord

Brachial plexus,
infraclavicular part

Lateral
cord

Lateral root

Medial root

Median nerve

Axillary nerve

Superior lateral
cutaneous nerve
of arm

Musculocutaneous nerve

Radial nerve

Posterior cutaneous
nerve of arm

Inferior lateral
cutaneous nerve of arm

Lateral cutaneous
nerve of forearm

Superficial branch

Deep branch

Posterior cutaneous
nerve of forearm

Communicating branch
with ulnar nerve

Common palmar
digital nerves

Proper palmar
digital nerves

Axillary artery

Medial cutaneous
nerve of arm

Medial cutaneous
nerve of forearm

Ulnar nerve

Anterior
interosseous
nerve

Dorsal branch (ulnar nerve)

Palmar branch (ulnar nerve)

Deep branch (ulnar nerve)

Superficial branch (ulnar nerve)

Common palmar
digital nerves

Proper palmar
digital nerves

Fig. 387   Nerves of the upper limb;
overview.

→ T 24, T 25

Cutaneous innervation

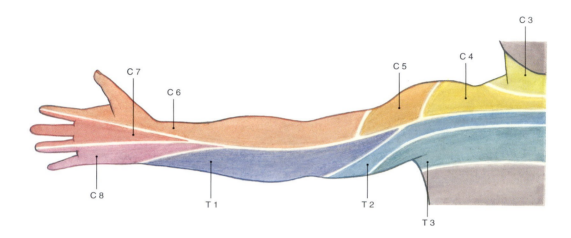

→ T 24   **Fig. 388**   Segmental cutaneous innervation (dermatomes) of the upper limb.

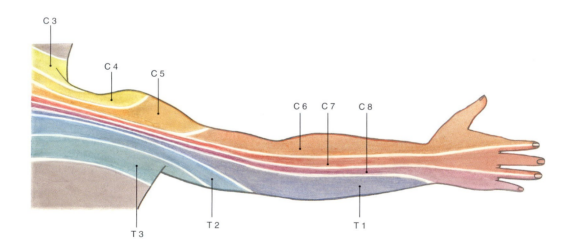

→ T 24   **Fig. 389**   Segmental cutaneous innervation (dermatomes) of the upper limb.

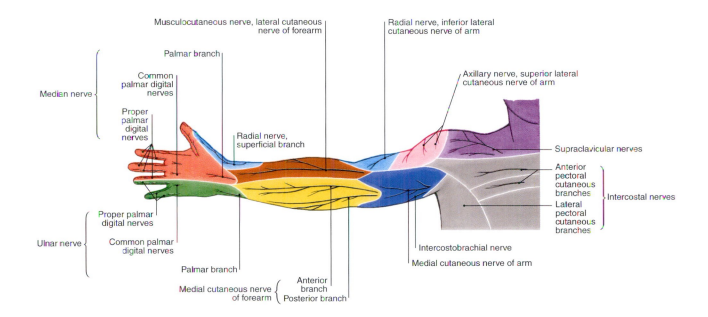

Musculocutaneous nerve, lateral cutaneous nerve of forearm

Radial nerve, inferior lateral cutaneous nerve of arm

Palmar branch

Common palmar digital nerves

Axillary nerve, superior lateral cutaneous nerve of arm

Median nerve

Proper palmar digital nerves

Radial nerve, superficial branch

Supraclavicular nerves

Anterior pectoral cutaneous branches

Intercostal nerves

Lateral pectoral cutaneous branches

Proper palmar digital nerves

Ulnar nerve

Common palmar digital nerves

Palmar branch

Medial cutaneous nerve of forearm { Anterior branch / Posterior branch }

Intercostobrachial nerve

Medial cutaneous nerve of arm

Fig. 390   Cutaneous nerves of the upper limb.   → T 24

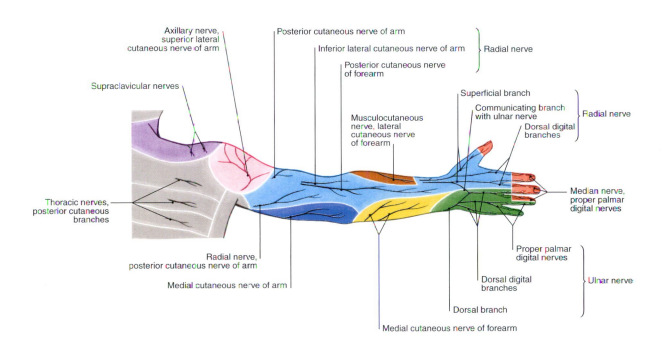

Axillary nerve, superior lateral cutaneous nerve of arm

Posterior cutaneous nerve of arm

Inferior lateral cutaneous nerve of arm

Radial nerve

Posterior cutaneous nerve of forearm

Supraclavicular nerves

Superficial branch

Communicating branch with ulnar nerve

Radial nerve

Dorsal digital branches

Musculocutaneous nerve, lateral cutaneous nerve of forearm

Thoracic nerves, posterior cutaneous branches

Median nerve, proper palmar digital nerves

Radial nerve, posterior cutaneous nerve of arm

Proper palmar digital nerves

Medial cutaneous nerve of arm

Dorsal digital branches

Ulnar nerve

Dorsal branch

Medial cutaneous nerve of forearm

Fig. 391   Cutaneous nerves of the upper limb.   → T 24

Musculocutaneous nerve

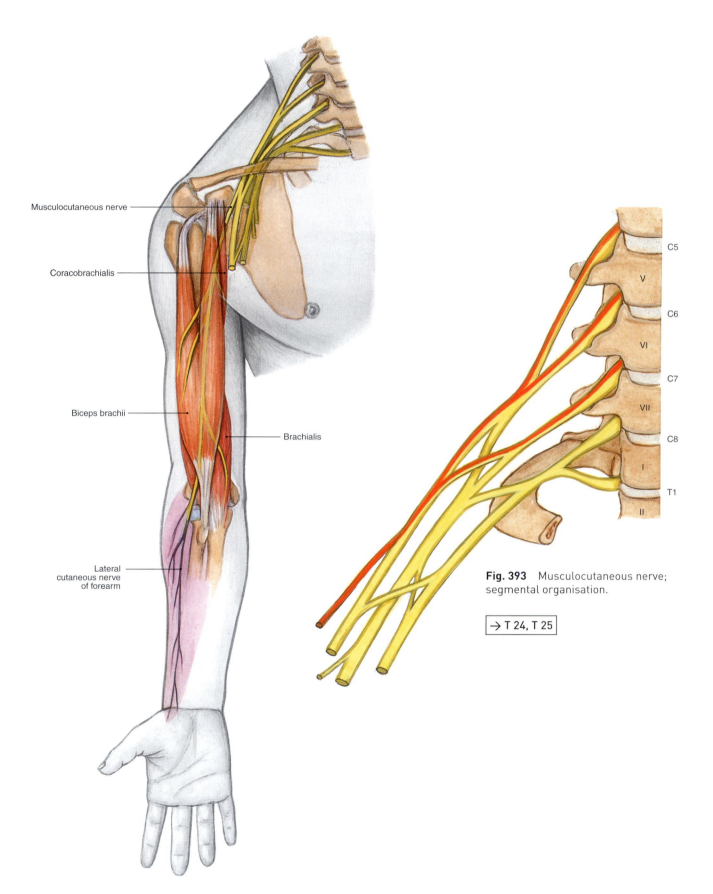

Musculocutaneous nerve

Coracobrachialis

Biceps brachii

Brachialis

Lateral
cutaneous nerve
of forearm

C5
V
C6
VI
C7
VII
C8
I
T1
II

Fig. 393 Musculocutaneous nerve;
segmental organisation.

→ T 24, T 25

Fig. 392 Musculocutaneous nerve;
supplying areas.
The skin branches and the
cutaneous innervation are
illustrated in blue.

→ 46, 386, T 24, T 25

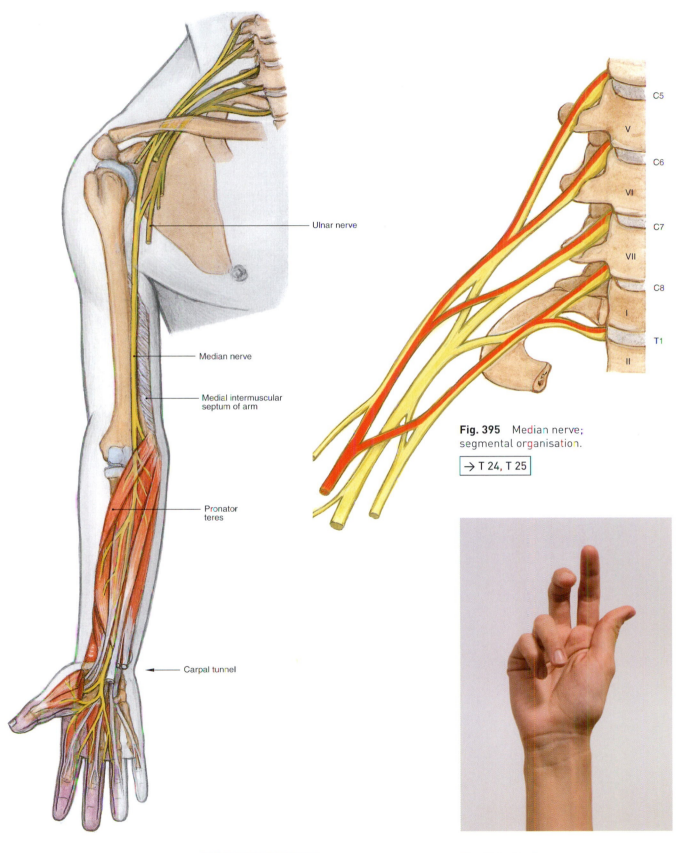

Ulnar nerve

Median nerve

Medial intermuscular
septum of arm

Pronator
teres

Carpal tunnel

C5

V

C6

VI

C7

VII

C8

I

T1

II

Fig. 395   Median nerve;
segmental organisation.

→ T 24, T 25

Fig. 394   Median nerve;
supplying areas.

→ 46, 386, T 24, T 25

Fig. 396   Median nerve;
proximal palsy: typical
posture.

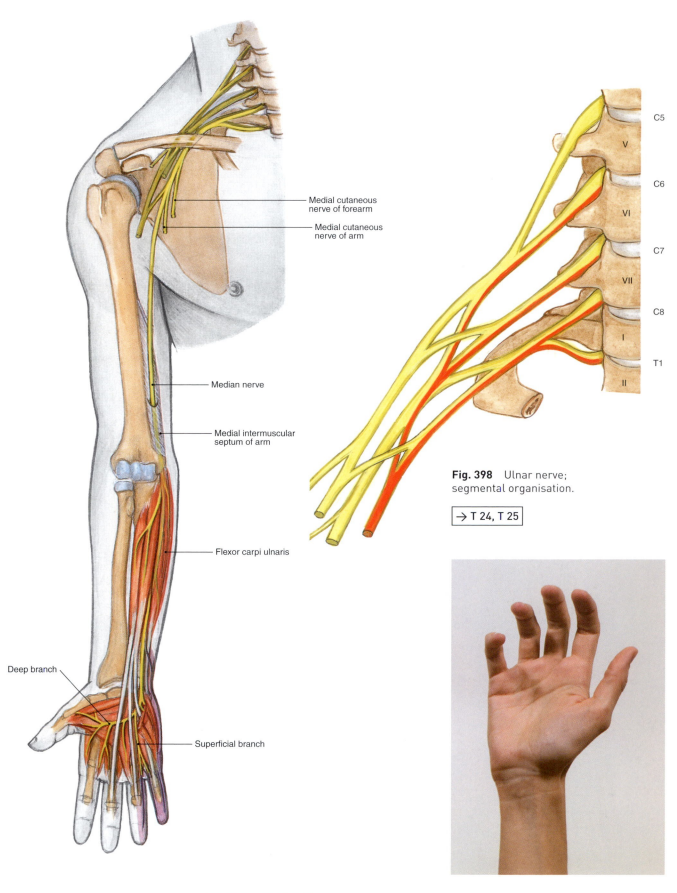

Medial cutaneous
nerve of forearm

Medial cutaneous
nerve of arm

Median nerve

Medial intermuscular
septum of arm

Flexor carpi ulnaris

Deep branch

Superficial branch

C5
V
C6
VI
C7
VII
C8
I
T1
II

Fig. 398 Ulnar nerve;
segmental organisation.

→ T 24, T 25

Fig. 397 Ulnar nerve;
supplying areas.

→ 46, 386, T 24, T 25

Fig. 399 Ulnar nerve;
proximal palsy.

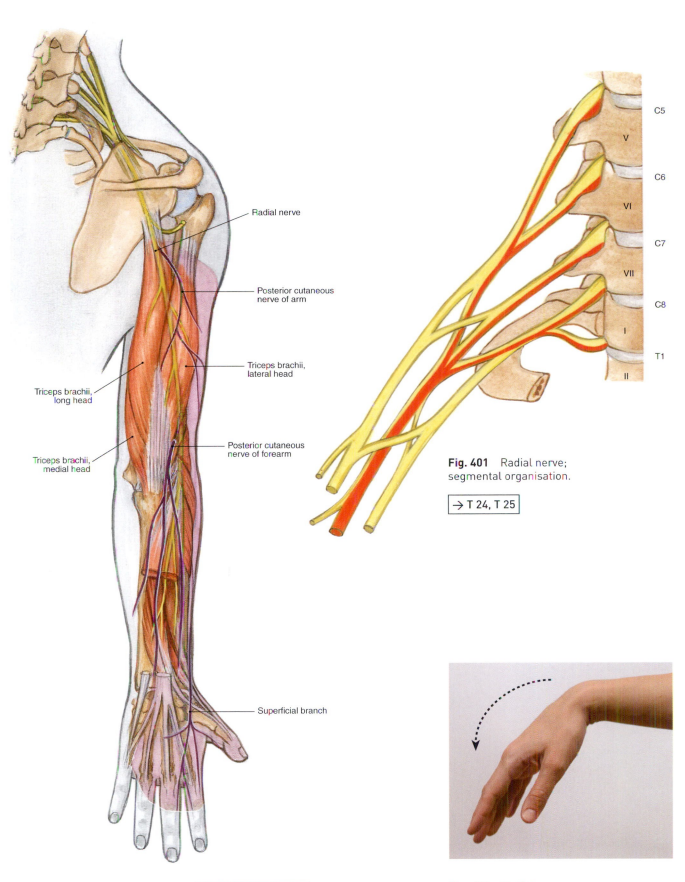

Radial nerve

Posterior cutaneous
nerve of arm

Triceps brachii,
lateral head

Triceps brachii,
long head

Posterior cutaneous
nerve of forearm

Triceps brachii,
medial head

Superficial branch

Fig. 400 Radial nerve;
supplying areas.

→ 46, 386, T 24, T 25

C5

V

C6

VI

C7

VII

C8

I

T1

II

Fig. 401 Radial nerve;
segmental organisation.

→ T 24, T 25

Fig. 402 Radial nerve;
proximal palsy.

Axillary nerve

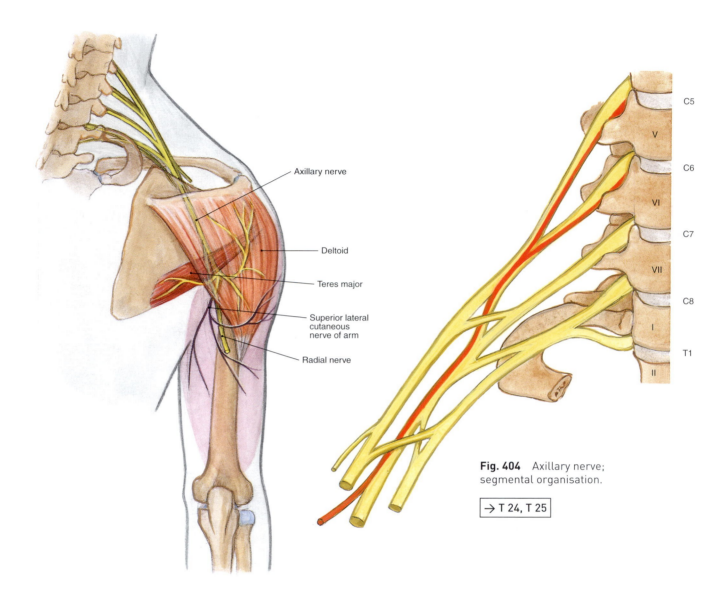

Axillary nerve

Deltoid

Teres major

Superior lateral
cutaneous
nerve of arm

Radial nerve

C5

V

C6

VI

C7

VII

C8

I

T1

II

Fig. 404 Axillary nerve;
segmental organisation.

→ T 24, T 25

Fig. 403 Axillary nerve;
supplying areas.
The axillary nerve passes to the
dorsal side of the arm through the
quadrangular space along with the
posterior circumflex humeral artery.

→ 44, 386, T 24, T 25

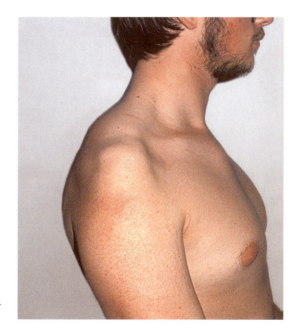

Fig. 405 Axillary nerve;
palsy: deltoid muscle atrophy.

Arteries of the upper limb

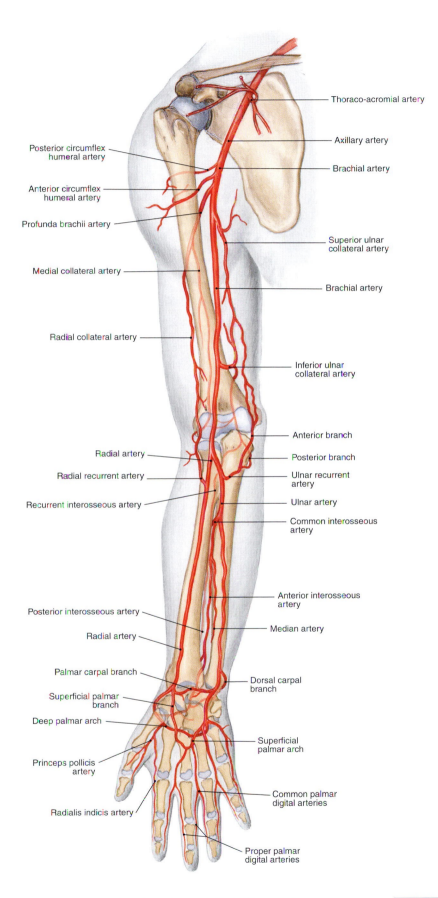

Thoraco-acromial artery

Axillary artery

Brachial artery

Posterior circumflex humeral artery

Anterior circumflex humeral artery

Profunda brachii artery

Superior ulnar collateral artery

Medial collateral artery

Brachial artery

Radial collateral artery

Inferior ulnar collateral artery

Anterior branch

Radial artery

Posterior branch

Radial recurrent artery

Ulnar recurrent artery

Recurrent interosseous artery

Ulnar artery

Common interosseous artery

Anterior interosseous artery

Posterior interosseous artery

Median artery

Radial artery

Palmar carpal branch

Dorsal carpal branch

Superficial palmar branch

Deep palmar arch

Superficial palmar arch

Princeps pollicis artery

Radialis indicis artery

Common palmar digital arteries

Proper palmar digital arteries

Fig. 406 Arteries of the upper limb; overview.
Arteries adjacent to the elbow joint form the cubital anastomosis.

→ 264

Lymphatics of the axilla

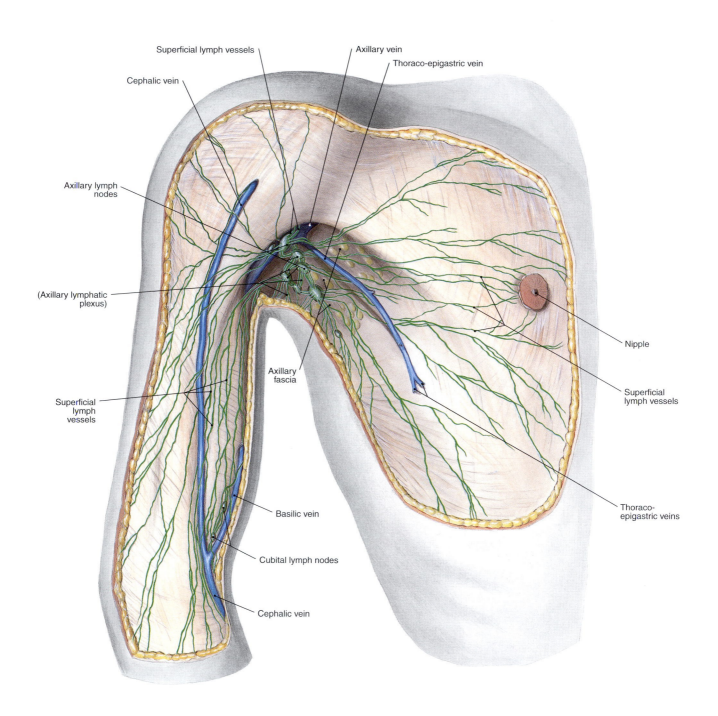

Superficial lymph vessels

Axillary vein

Thoraco-epigastric vein

Cephalic vein

Axillary lymph nodes

(Axillary lymphatic plexus)

Axillary fascia

Nipple

Superficial lymph vessels

Superficial lymph vessels

Basilic vein

Cubital lymph nodes

Cephalic vein

Thoraco-epigastric veins

→ 42

408

Fig. 407 Superficial lymphatics, lymph nodes and vein trunks in the regions of the arm, the lateral thoracic wall and the axilla.

Fascia of the chest, the shoulder and the axilla

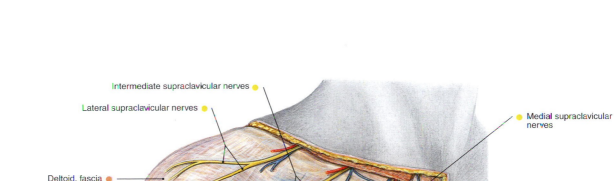

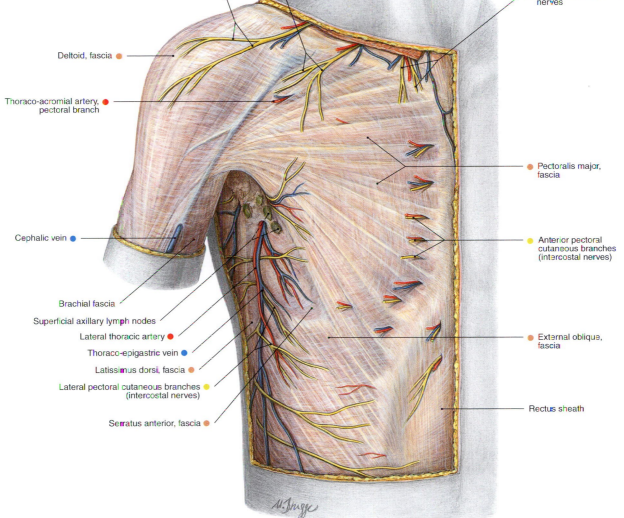

Intermediate supraclavicular nerves ●

Lateral supraclavicular nerves ●

Medial supraclavicular nerves ●

Deltoid, fascia ●

Thoraco-acromial artery, ● pectoral branch

Pectoralis major, fascia ●

Anterior pectoral cutaneous branches (intercostal nerves) ●

Cephalic vein ●

Brachial fascia

Superficial axillary lymph nodes

Lateral thoracic artery ●

Thoraco-epigastric vein ●

Latissimus dorsi, fascia ●

Lateral pectoral cutaneous branches ● (intercostal nerves)

Serratus anterior, fascia ●

External oblique, fascia ●

Rectus sheath

Fig. 408 Vessels and nerves in the regions of the upper arm as well as the shoulder, and the clavipectoral triangle.

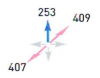

253   409

407

Clavipectoral triangle

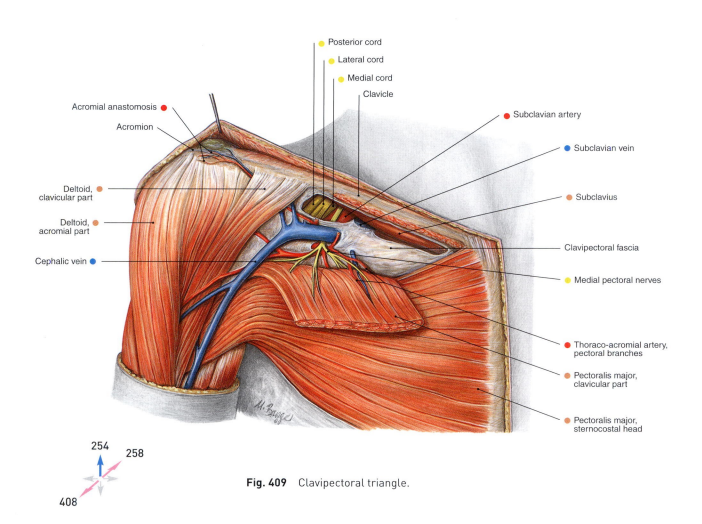

Posterior cord
Lateral cord
Medial cord
Clavicle
Acromial anastomosis
Acromion
Subclavian artery
Subclavian vein
Deltoid, clavicular part
Subclavius
Deltoid, acromial part
Clavipectoral fascia
Cephalic vein
Medial pectoral nerves
Thoraco-acromial artery, pectoral branches
Pectoralis major, clavicular part
Pectoralis major, sternocostal head

254
258
408

Fig. 409 Clavipectoral triangle.

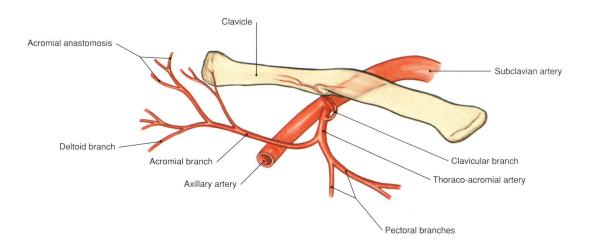

Clavicle
Acromial anastomosis
Subclavian artery
Deltoid branch
Acromial branch
Axillary artery
Clavicular branch
Thoraco-acromial artery
Pectoral branches

Fig. 410 Branching pattern of the thoraco-acromial artery.

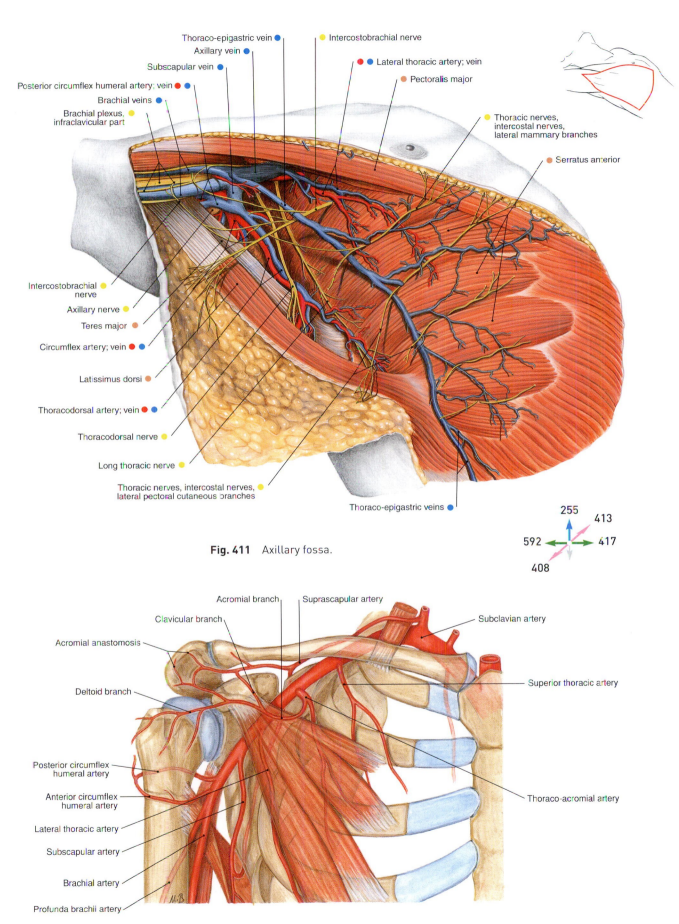

Thoraco-epigastric vein ●
Axillary vein ●
Subscapular vein ●
Posterior circumflex humeral artery; vein ● ●
Brachial veins ●
Brachial plexus, infraclavicular part ●

Intercostobrachial nerve ●
Lateral thoracic artery; vein ● ●
Pectoralis major ●
Thoracic nerves, intercostal nerves, lateral mammary branches ●
Serratus anterior ●

Intercostobrachial nerve ●
Axillary nerve ●
Teres major ●
Circumflex artery; vein ● ●
Latissimus dorsi ●
Thoracodorsal artery; vein ● ●
Thoracodorsal nerve ●
Long thoracic nerve
Thoracic nerves, intercostal nerves, lateral pectoral cutaneous branches ●
Thoraco-epigastric veins ●

255
413
592   417
408

Fig. 411   Axillary fossa.

Acromial branch
Suprascapular artery
Clavicular branch
Acromial anastomosis
Subclavian artery

Deltoid branch
Superior thoracic artery

Posterior circumflex humeral artery
Anterior circumflex humeral artery
Lateral thoracic artery
Subscapular artery
Brachial artery
Profunda brachii artery
Thoraco-acromial artery

Fig. 412   Arteries of the shoulder region.

Neck and axillary fossa

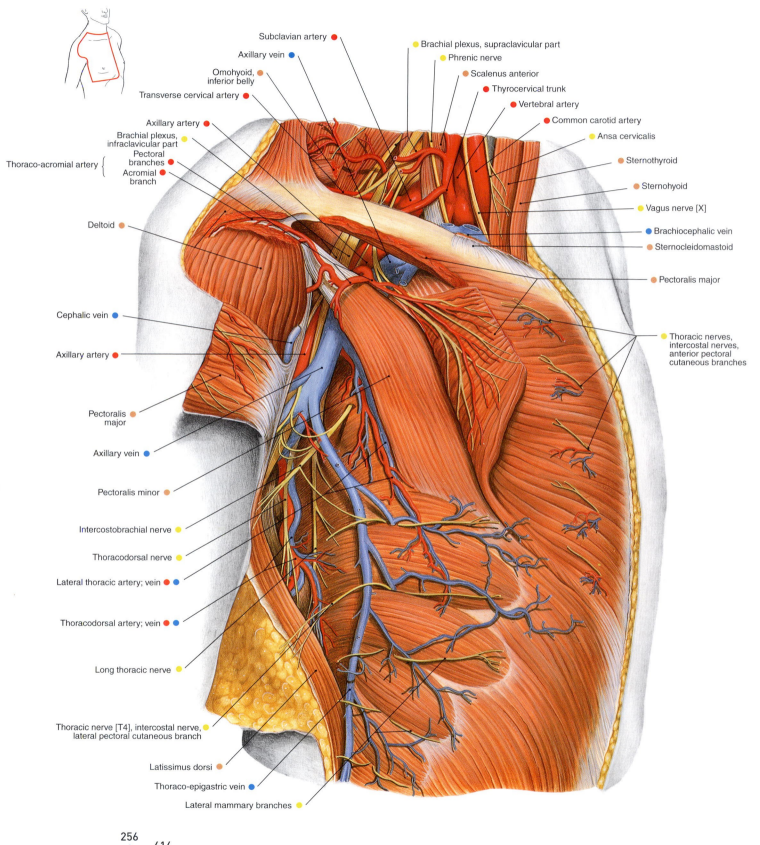

Subclavian artery
Axillary vein
Omohyoid, inferior belly
Transverse cervical artery
Axillary artery
Brachial plexus, infraclavicular part
Pectoral branches
Thoraco-acromial artery
Acromial branch
Deltoid
Cephalic vein
Axillary artery
Pectoralis major
Axillary vein
Pectoralis minor
Intercostobrachial nerve
Thoracodorsal nerve
Lateral thoracic artery; vein
Thoracodorsal artery; vein
Long thoracic nerve
Thoracic nerve [T4], intercostal nerve, lateral pectoral cutaneous branch
Latissimus dorsi
Thoraco-epigastric vein
Lateral mammary branches

Brachial plexus, supraclavicular part
Phrenic nerve
Scalenus anterior
Thyrocervical trunk
Vertebral artery
Common carotid artery
Ansa cervicalis
Sternothyroid
Sternohyoid
Vagus nerve [X]
Brachiocephalic vein
Sternocleidomastoid
Pectoralis major
Thoracic nerves, intercostal nerves, anterior pectoral cutaneous branches

256
414
411
417

Fig. 413 Lateral thoracic wall; infraclavicular fossa and axillary fossa.

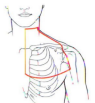

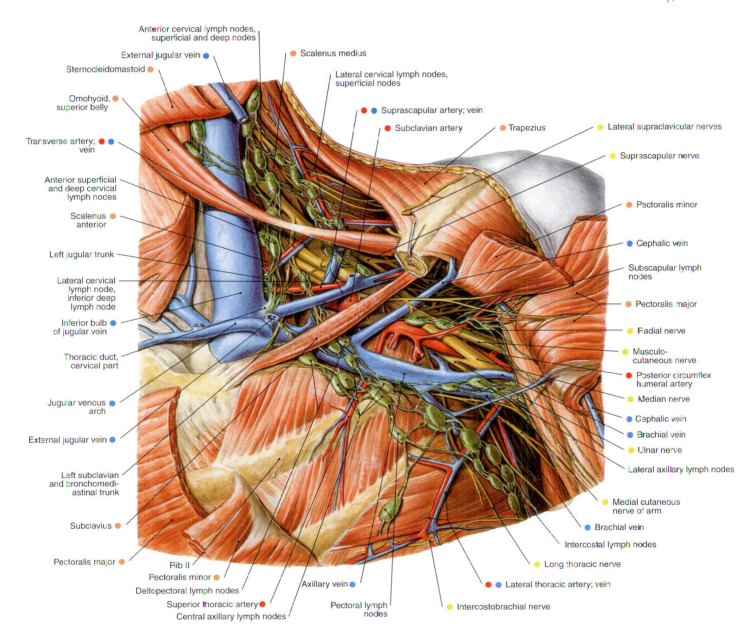

Anterior cervical lymph nodes, superficial and deep nodes

External jugular vein ●

Sternocleidomastoid ●

Omohyoid, ● superior belly

Transverse artery; ● ● vein

Anterior superficial and deep cervical lymph nodes

Scalenus anterior ●

Left jugular trunk

Lateral cervical lymph node, inferior deep lymph node

Inferior bulb ● of jugular vein

Thoracic duct, cervical part

Jugular venous ● arch

External jugular vein ●

Left subclavian and bronchomedi-astinal trunk

Subclavius ●

Pectoralis major ●

Rib II

Pectoralis minor ●

Deltopectoral lymph nodes

Superior thoracic artery ●

Central axillary lymph nodes

Axillary vein ●

Pectoral lymph nodes

Intercostobrachial nerve ●

Scalenus medius ●

Lateral cervical lymph nodes, superficial nodes

Suprascapular artery; vein ● ●

Subclavian artery ●

Trapezius ●

Lateral supraclavicular nerves ●

Suprascapular nerve ●

Pectoralis minor ●

Cephalic vein ●

Subscapular lymph nodes

Pectoralis major ●

Radial nerve ●

Musculo-cutaneous nerve ●

Posterior circumflex humeral artery ●

Median nerve ●

Cephalic vein ●

Brachial vein ●

Ulnar nerve ●

Lateral axillary lymph nodes

Medial cutaneous nerve of arm ●

Brachial vein ●

Intercostal lymph nodes

Long thoracic nerve ●

Lateral thoracic artery; vein ● ●

Fig. 414 Axillary fossa and deep cervical region; exemplary illustration of lymphatics and lymph nodes.

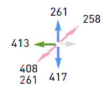

261
258
413
408
261 417

Vessels and nerves of the arm

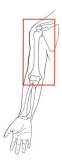

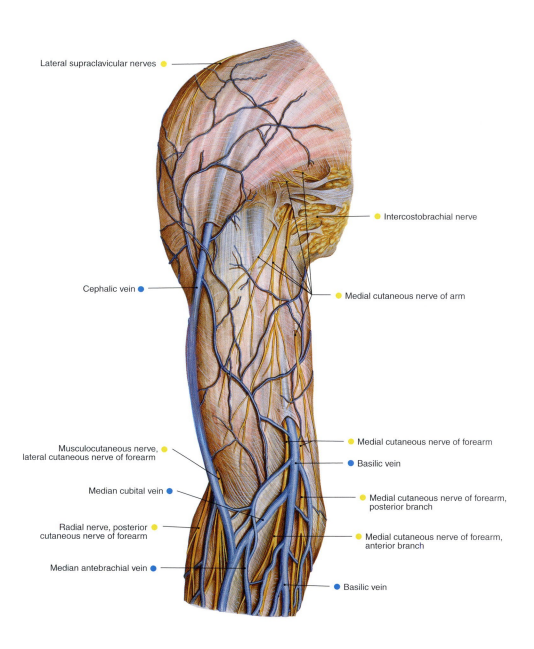

Lateral supraclavicular nerves ●

Intercostobrachial nerve ●

Cephalic vein ●

Medial cutaneous nerve of arm ●

Medial cutaneous nerve of forearm ●

Musculocutaneous nerve, lateral cutaneous nerve of forearm ●

Basilic vein ●

Median cubital vein ●

Medial cutaneous nerve of forearm, posterior branch ●

Radial nerve, posterior cutaneous nerve of forearm ●

Medial cutaneous nerve of forearm, anterior branch ●

Median antebrachial vein ●

Basilic vein ●

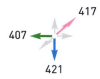

417

407

421

Fig. 415 Epifascial vessels and nerves of the shoulder, the anterior region of the arm and the anterior region of the elbow.

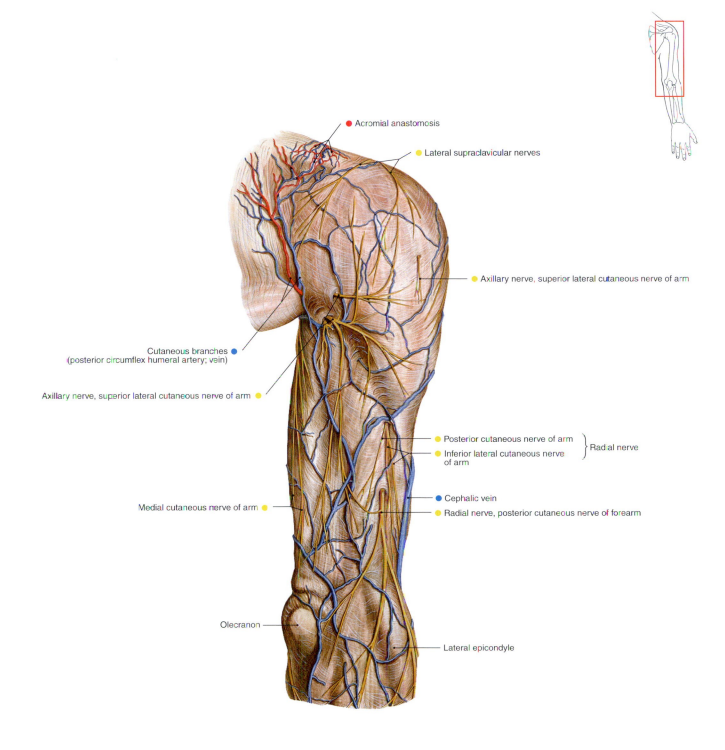

● Acromial anastomosis

● Lateral supraclavicular nerves

● Axillary nerve, superior lateral cutaneous nerve of arm

Cutaneous branches ●
(posterior circumflex humeral artery; vein)

Axillary nerve, superior lateral cutaneous nerve of arm ●

● Posterior cutaneous nerve of arm } Radial nerve
● Inferior lateral cutaneous nerve
of arm

Medial cutaneous nerve of arm ●

● Cephalic vein

● Radial nerve, posterior cutaneous nerve of forearm

Olecranon

Lateral epicondyle

Fig. 416   Epifascial vessels and nerves of the shoulder,
the posterior region of the arm and the posterior region
of the elbow.

419

422

Vessels and nerves of the arm

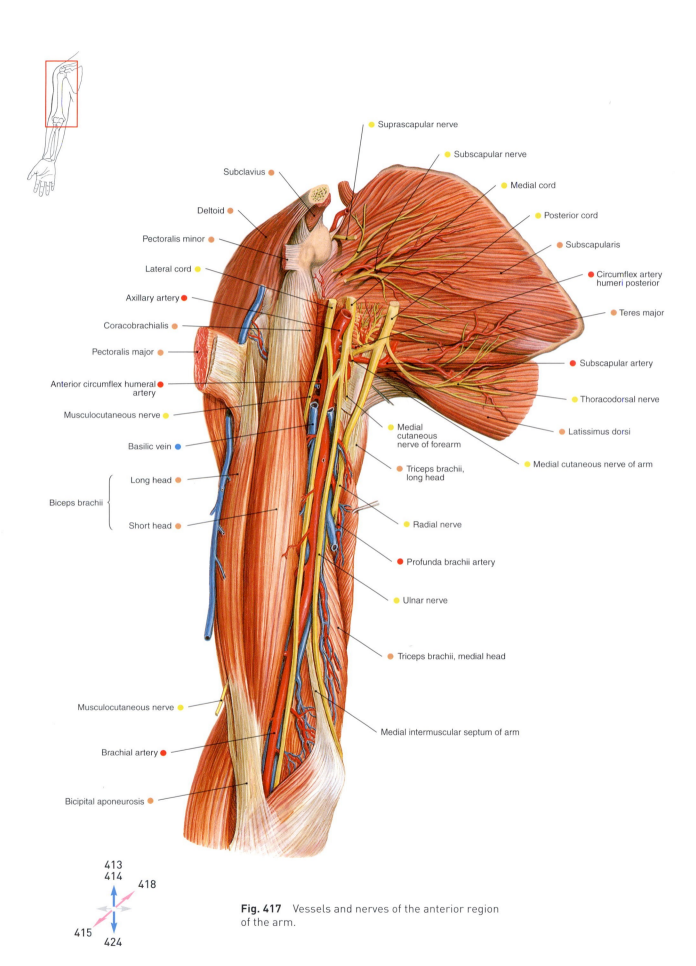

Suprascapular nerve

Subscapular nerve

Medial cord

Posterior cord

Subclavius

Deltoid

Subscapularis

Pectoralis minor

Circumflex artery humeri posterior

Lateral cord

Teres major

Axillary artery

Coracobrachialis

Subscapular artery

Pectoralis major

Anterior circumflex humeral artery

Thoracodorsal nerve

Musculocutaneous nerve

Latissimus dorsi

Basilic vein

Medial cutaneous nerve of forearm

Medial cutaneous nerve of arm

Long head

Triceps brachii, long head

Biceps brachii

Radial nerve

Short head

Profunda brachii artery

Ulnar nerve

Triceps brachii, medial head

Musculocutaneous nerve

Medial intermuscular septum of arm

Brachial artery

Bicipital aponeurosis

413
414
418

415
424

Fig. 417   Vessels and nerves of the anterior region of the arm.

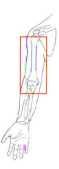

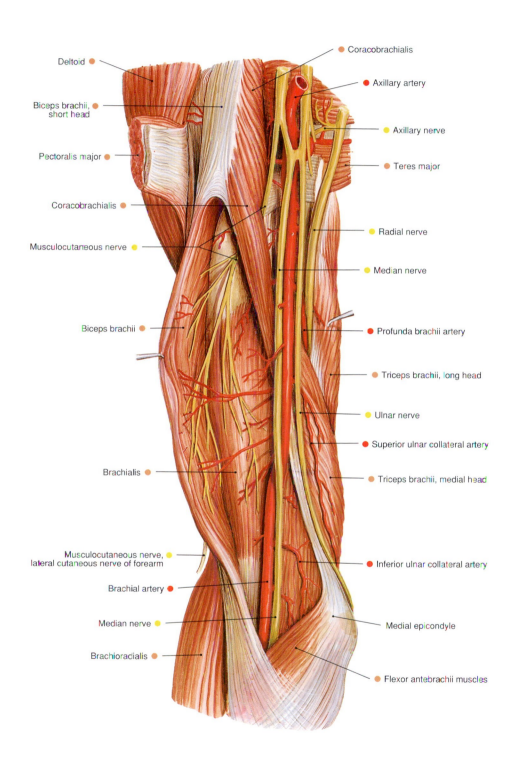

Deltoid ●

Biceps brachii, ●
short head

Pectoralis major ●

Coracobrachialis ●

Musculocutaneous nerve ●

Biceps brachii ●

Brachialis ●

Musculocutaneous nerve, ●
lateral cutaneous nerve of forearm

Brachial artery ●

Median nerve ●

Brachioradialis ●

● Coracobrachialis

● Axillary artery

● Axillary nerve

● Teres major

● Radial nerve

● Median nerve

● Profunda brachii artery

● Triceps brachii, long head

● Ulnar nerve

● Superior ulnar collateral artery

● Triceps brachii, medial head

● Inferior ulnar collateral artery

Medial epicondyle

● Flexor antebrachii muscles

Fig. 418   Arteries and nerves of the anterior region
of the arm.

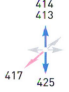

414
413

417   425

Arteries and nerves of the arm

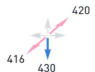

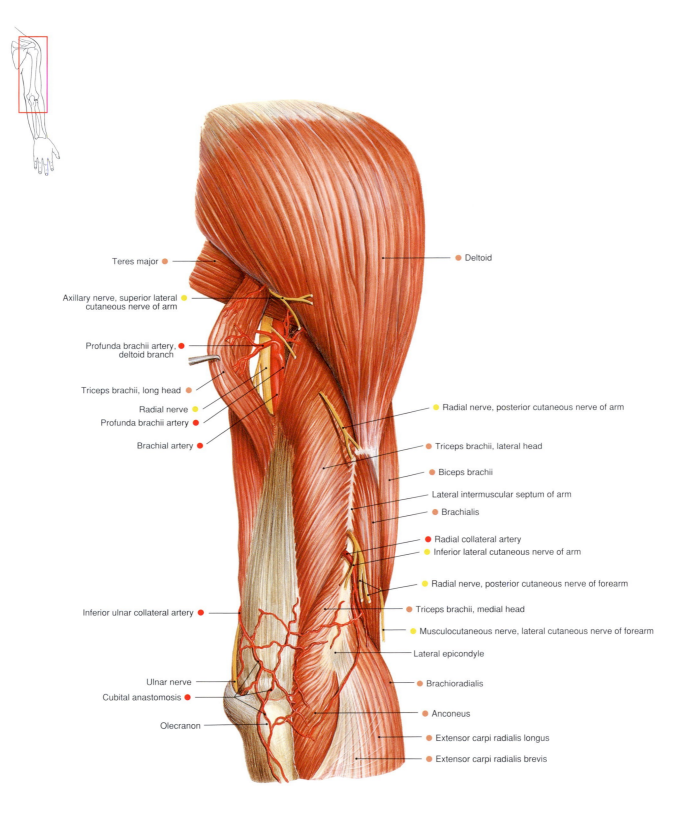

Teres major ●

Axillary nerve, superior lateral
cutaneous nerve of arm ●

Profunda brachii artery,
deltoid branch ●

Triceps brachii, long head ●

Radial nerve ●
Profunda brachii artery ●

Brachial artery ●

Inferior ulnar collateral artery ●

Ulnar nerve
Cubital anastomosis ●

Olecranon

● Deltoid

● Radial nerve, posterior cutaneous nerve of arm

● Triceps brachii, lateral head

● Biceps brachii

Lateral intermuscular septum of arm

● Brachialis

● Radial collateral artery
● Inferior lateral cutaneous nerve of arm

● Radial nerve, posterior cutaneous nerve of forearm

● Triceps brachii, medial head

● Musculocutaneous nerve, lateral cutaneous nerve of forearm

Lateral epicondyle

● Brachioradialis

● Anconeus

● Extensor carpi radialis longus
● Extensor carpi radialis brevis

420

416
430

Fig. 419 Arteries and nerves of the posterior region
of the arm.

Arteries and nerves of the arm

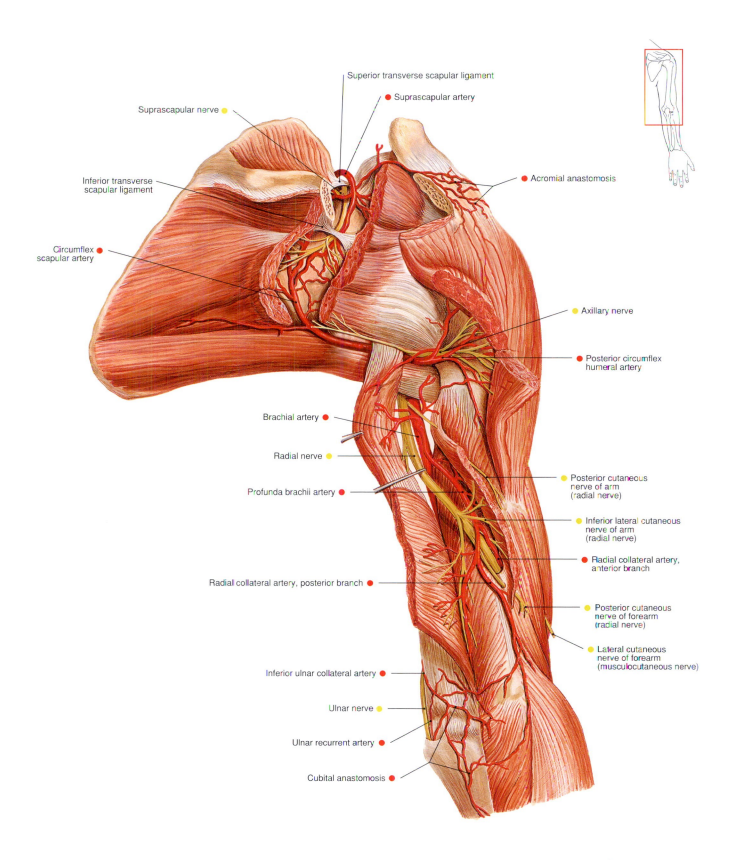

Superior transverse scapular ligament

Suprascapular nerve ●

● Suprascapular artery

Inferior transverse
scapular ligament

● Acromial anastomosis

Circumflex ●
scapular artery

● Axillary nerve

● Posterior circumflex
humeral artery

Brachial artery ●

Radial nerve ●

● Posterior cutaneous
nerve of arm
(radial nerve)

Profunda brachii artery ●

● Inferior lateral cutaneous
nerve of arm
(radial nerve)

● Radial collateral artery,
anterior branch

Radial collateral artery, posterior branch ●

● Posterior cutaneous
nerve of forearm
(radial nerve)

● Lateral cutaneous
nerve of forearm
(musculocutaneous nerve)

Inferior ulnar collateral artery ●

Ulnar nerve ●

Ulnar recurrent artery ●

Cubital anastomosis ●

Fig. 420   Arteries and nerves of the scapular region
and the posterior region of the arm.

419

430
431

Veins and nerves of the forearm

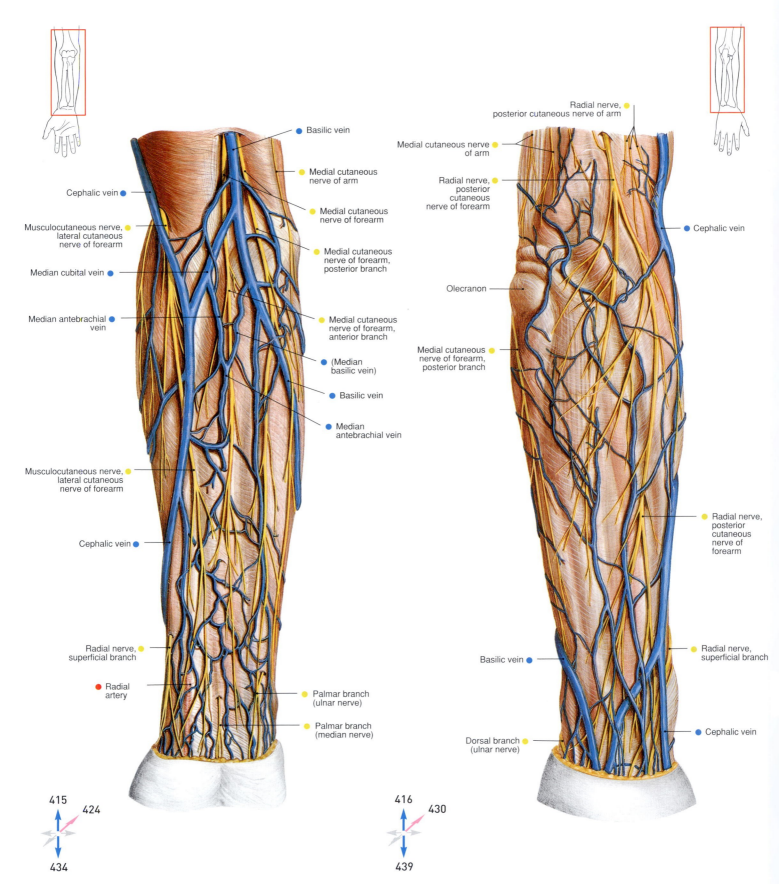

Basilic vein

Medial cutaneous nerve of arm

Cephalic vein

Medial cutaneous nerve of forearm

Musculocutaneous nerve, lateral cutaneous nerve of forearm

Medial cutaneous nerve of forearm, posterior branch

Median cubital vein

Median antebrachial vein

Medial cutaneous nerve of forearm, anterior branch

(Median basilic vein)

Basilic vein

Median antebrachial vein

Musculocutaneous nerve, lateral cutaneous nerve of forearm

Cephalic vein

Radial nerve, superficial branch

Radial artery

Palmar branch (ulnar nerve)

Palmar branch (median nerve)

Radial nerve, posterior cutaneous nerve of arm

Medial cutaneous nerve of arm

Radial nerve, posterior cutaneous nerve of forearm

Cephalic vein

Olecranon

Medial cutaneous nerve of forearm, posterior branch

Radial nerve, posterior cutaneous nerve of forearm

Basilic vein

Radial nerve, superficial branch

Cephalic vein

Dorsal branch (ulnar nerve)

415
424
434

416
430
439

Fig. 421 Veins and nerves of the anterior region of the forearm; epifascial layer.

Fig. 422 Veins and nerves of the posterior region of the forearm; epifascial layer.

Veins of the cubital fossa

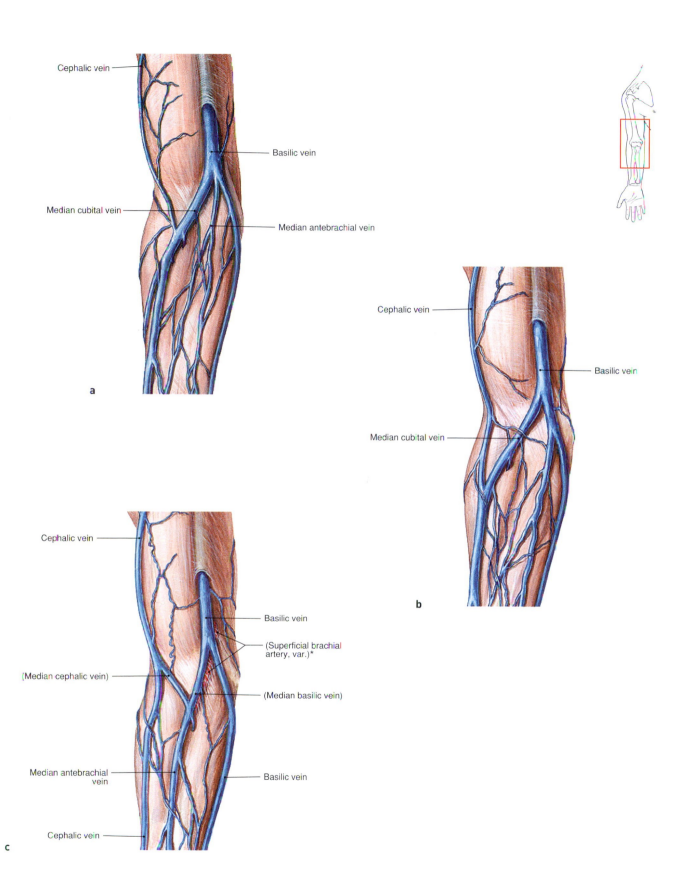

Cephalic vein

Basilic vein

Median cubital vein

Median antebrachial vein

a

Cephalic vein

Basilic vein

Median cubital vein

b

Cephalic vein

Basilic vein

(Superficial brachial artery, var.)*

(Median cephalic vein)

(Median basilic vein)

Median antebrachial vein

Basilic vein

Cephalic vein

c

Fig. 423 a–c   Variations in the epifascial veins of the cubital fossa.

* With regard to intravenous injections, this rare variation is particularly important, as a supposedly intravenous injection can mistakenly become intra-arterial.

Arteries and nerves of the arm

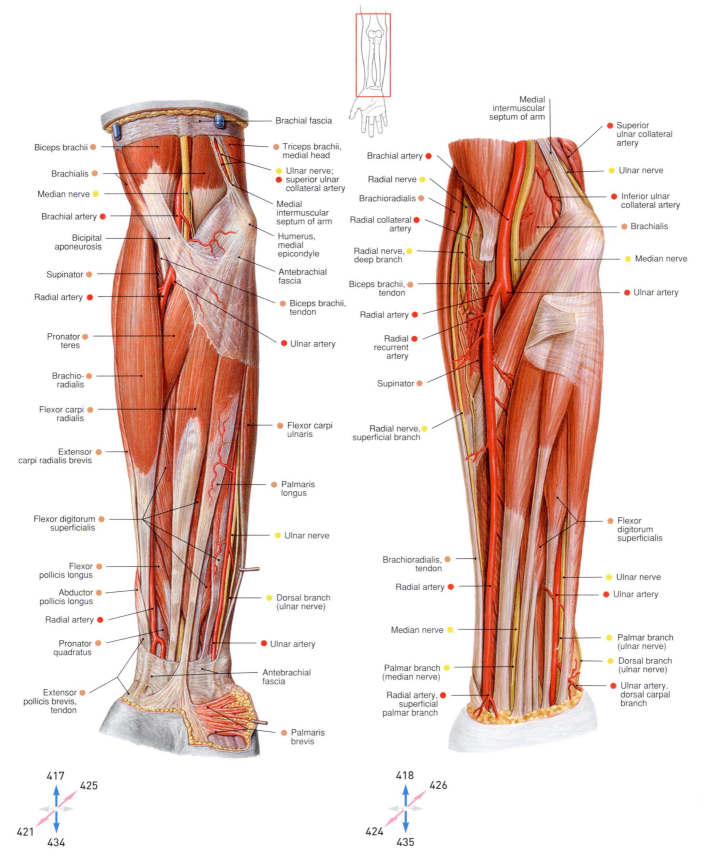

Brachial fascia

Biceps brachii ●

Brachialis ●

Median nerve ●

Brachial artery ●

Bicipital aponeurosis

Supinator ●

Radial artery ●

Pronator teres ●

Brachio-radialis ●

Flexor carpi radialis

Extensor carpi radialis brevis ●

Flexor digitorum superficialis ●

Flexor pollicis longus ●

Abductor pollicis longus ●

Radial artery ●

Pronator quadratus ●

Extensor pollicis brevis, tendon ●

● Triceps brachii, medial head

● Ulnar nerve;
● superior ulnar collateral artery

Medial intermuscular septum of arm

Humerus, medial epicondyle

Antebrachial fascia

● Biceps brachii, tendon

● Ulnar artery

● Flexor carpi ulnaris

● Palmaris longus

● Ulnar nerve

● Dorsal branch (ulnar nerve)

● Ulnar artery

Antebrachial fascia

● Palmaris brevis

417
425
421
434

Fig. 424 Arteries and nerves of the anterior region of the forearm; subfascial layer.

Medial intermuscular septum of arm

Brachial artery ●

Radial nerve ●

Brachioradialis ●

Radial collateral artery ●

Radial nerve, deep branch ●

Biceps brachii, tendon ●

Radial artery ●

Radial recurrent artery ●

Supinator ●

Radial nerve, superficial branch ●

Brachioradialis, tendon ●

Radial artery ●

Median nerve ●

Palmar branch (median nerve) ●

Radial artery, superficial palmar branch ●

● Superior ulnar collateral artery

● Ulnar nerve

● Inferior ulnar collateral artery

● Brachialis

● Median nerve

● Ulnar artery

● Flexor digitorum superficialis

● Ulnar nerve

● Ulnar artery

● Palmar branch (ulnar nerve)

● Dorsal branch (ulnar nerve)

● Ulnar artery, dorsal carpal branch

418
426
424
435

Fig. 425 Arteries and nerves of the anterior region of the forearm; course of the radial artery.

Arteries and nerves of the arm

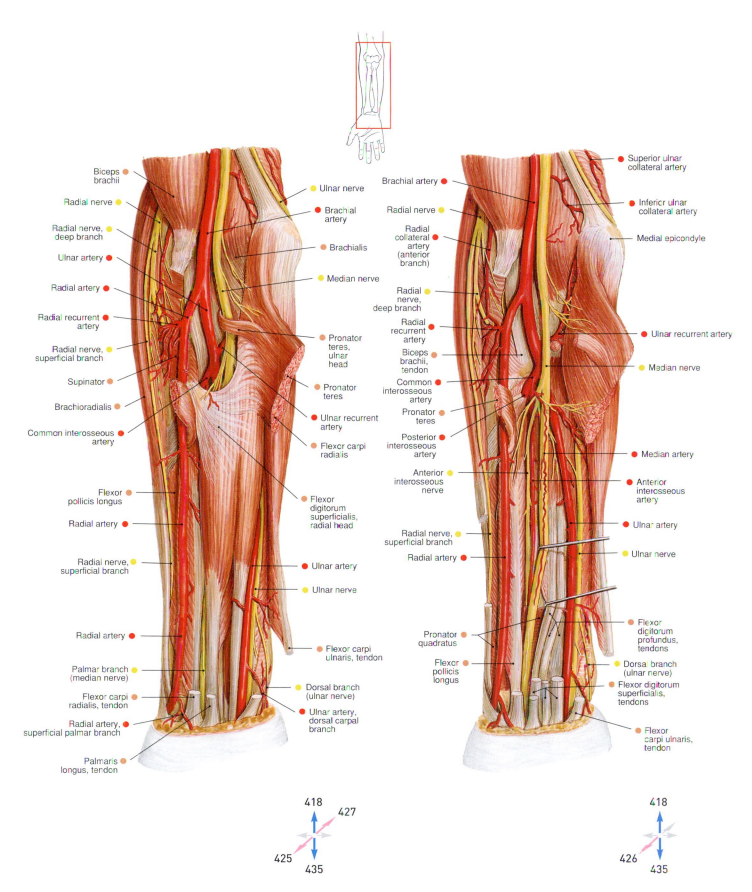

Biceps brachii

Radial nerve

Radial nerve, deep branch

Ulnar artery

Radial artery

Radial recurrent artery

Radial nerve, superficial branch

Supinator

Brachioradialis

Common interosseous artery

Flexor pollicis longus

Radial artery

Radial nerve, superficial branch

Radial artery

Palmar branch (median nerve)

Flexor carpi radialis, tendon

Radial artery, superficial palmar branch

Palmaris longus, tendon

Ulnar nerve

Brachial artery

Brachialis

Median nerve

Pronator teres, ulnar head

Pronator teres

Ulnar recurrent artery

Flexor carpi radialis

Flexor digitorum superficialis, radial head

Ulnar artery

Ulnar nerve

Flexor carpi ulnaris, tendon

Dorsal branch (ulnar nerve)

Ulnar artery, dorsal carpal branch

Brachial artery

Radial nerve

Radial collateral artery (anterior branch)

Radial nerve, deep branch

Radial recurrent artery

Biceps brachii, tendon

Common interosseous artery

Pronator teres

Posterior interosseous artery

Anterior interosseous nerve

Radial nerve, superficial branch

Radial artery

Pronator quadratus

Flexor pollicis longus

Superior ulnar collateral artery

Inferior ulnar collateral artery

Medial epicondyle

Ulnar recurrent artery

Median nerve

Median artery

Anterior interosseous artery

Ulnar artery

Ulnar nerve

Flexor digitorum profundus, tendons

Dorsal branch (ulnar nerve)

Flexor digitorum superficialis, tendons

Flexor carpi ulnaris, tendon

418
427
425
435

418
426
435

Fig. 426 Arteries and nerves of the anterior region of the forearm; deep layer.

Fig. 427 Arteries and nerves of the anterior region of the forearm; deep layer after partial removal of the flexor digitorum superficialis muscle.

Arteries and nerves of the cubital fossa

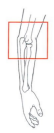

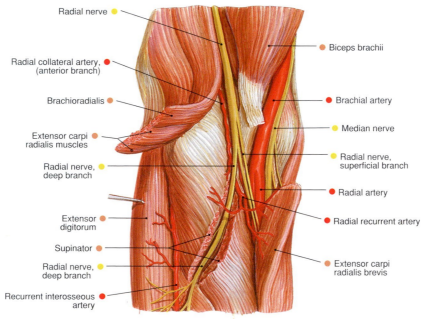

Radial nerve ●

Radial collateral artery, ● (anterior branch)

Brachioradialis ●

Extensor carpi ● radialis muscles

Radial nerve, ● deep branch

Extensor ● digitorum

Supinator ●

Radial nerve, ● deep branch

Recurrent interosseous ● artery

● Biceps brachii

● Brachial artery

● Median nerve

● Radial nerve, superficial branch

● Radial artery

● Radial recurrent artery

● Extensor carpi radialis brevis

418

427 ⤡ 427

Fig. 428 Arteries and nerves of the anterior region of the elbow; after removal of the radial muscles of the forearm; lateral (radial) view.

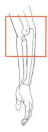

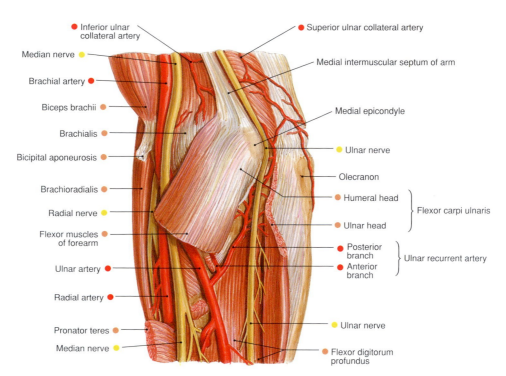

● Inferior ulnar collateral artery

Median nerve ●

Brachial artery ●

Biceps brachii ●

Brachialis ●

Bicipital aponeurosis ●

Brachioradialis ●

Radial nerve ●

Flexor muscles ● of forearm

Ulnar artery ●

Radial artery ●

Pronator teres ●

Median nerve ●

● Superior ulnar collateral artery

Medial intermuscular septum of arm

Medial epicondyle

● Ulnar nerve

Olecranon

● Humeral head ⎫
 ⎬ Flexor carpi ulnaris
● Ulnar head ⎭

● Posterior branch ⎫
 ⎬ Ulnar recurrent artery
● Anterior branch ⎭

● Ulnar nerve

● Flexor digitorum profundus

418

425 ⤡ 427

Fig. 429 Arteries and nerves of the anterior region of the elbow; after partial removal of the flexor muscles of the forearm; medial (ulnar) view.

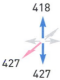

Arteries and nerves of the forearm

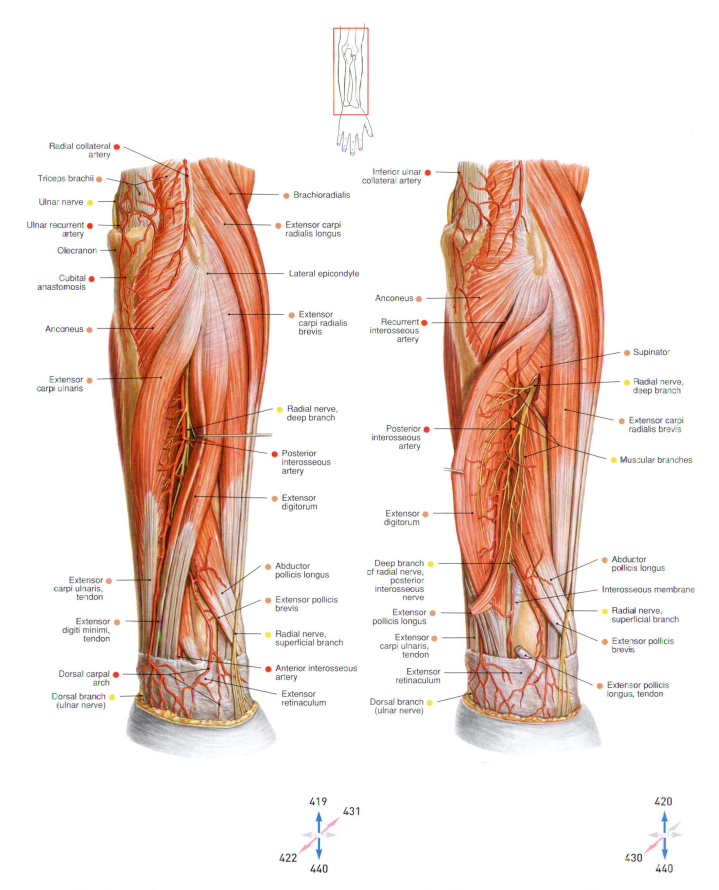

Radial collateral artery

Triceps brachii

Ulnar nerve

Ulnar recurrent artery

Olecranon

Cubital anastomosis

Anconeus

Extensor carpi ulnaris

Brachioradialis

Extensor carpi radialis longus

Lateral epicondyle

Extensor carpi radialis brevis

Radial nerve, deep branch

Posterior interosseous artery

Extensor digitorum

Abductor pollicis longus

Extensor pollicis brevis

Radial nerve, superficial branch

Extensor carpi ulnaris, tendon

Extensor digiti minimi, tendon

Dorsal carpal arch

Dorsal branch (ulnar nerve)

Anterior interosseous artery

Extensor retinaculum

419
431
422
440

Inferior ulnar collateral artery

Anconeus

Recurrent interosseous artery

Posterior interosseous artery

Extensor digitorum

Deep branch of radial nerve, posterior interosseous nerve

Extensor pollicis longus

Extensor carpi ulnaris, tendon

Extensor retinaculum

Dorsal branch (ulnar nerve)

Supinator

Radial nerve, deep branch

Extensor carpi radialis brevis

Muscular branches

Abductor pollicis longus

Interosseous membrane

Radial nerve, superficial branch

Extensor pollicis brevis

Extensor pollicis longus, tendon

420
430
440

Fig. 430 Arteries and nerves of the posterior region of the forearm; superficial layer.

Fig. 431 Arteries and nerves of the posterior region of the forearm; deep layer.

Arteries of the hand

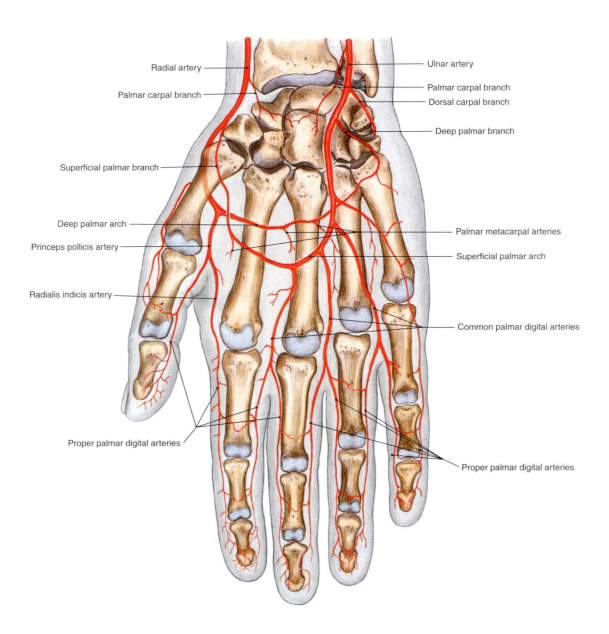

Radial artery

Palmar carpal branch

Superficial palmar branch

Deep palmar arch

Princeps pollicis artery

Radialis indicis artery

Proper palmar digital arteries

Ulnar artery

Palmar carpal branch

Dorsal carpal branch

Deep palmar branch

Palmar metacarpal arteries

Superficial palmar arch

Common palmar digital arteries

Proper palmar digital arteries

Fig. 432   Arteries of the palm; overview.

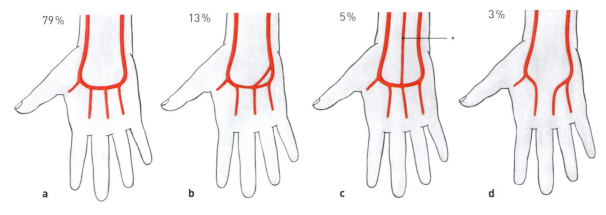

79 %   13 %   5 %   3 %

a   b   c   *   d

Fig. 433 a–d   Variations of the deep palmar arch.
a   "Textbook case", simple, closed arch
b   Doubling of the ulnar part

c   Anastomosis with the anterior interosseous artery (*)
d   The radial artery supplies both radial fingers, whereas the ulnar artery supplies the three ulnar fingers.

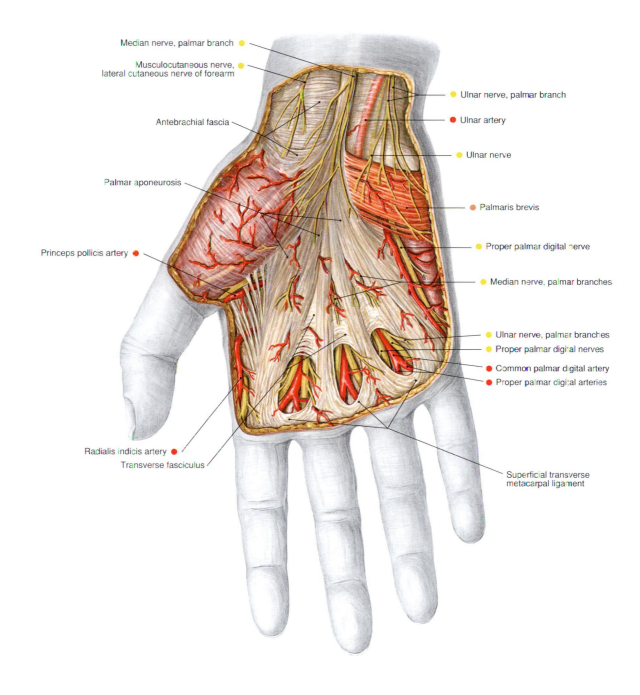

Median nerve, palmar branch ●

Musculocutaneous nerve, ●
lateral cutaneous nerve of forearm

Antebrachial fascia

Palmar aponeurosis

Princeps pollicis artery ●

Radialis indicis artery ●
Transverse fasciculus

● Ulnar nerve, palmar branch

● Ulnar artery

Ulnar nerve

● Palmaris brevis

● Proper palmar digital nerve

● Median nerve, palmar branches

● Ulnar nerve, palmar branches
● Proper palmar digital nerves
● Common palmar digital artery
● Proper palmar digital arteries

Superficial transverse
metacarpal ligament

Fig. 434   Arteries and nerves of the palm;
superficial layer.

Arteries and nerves of the hand

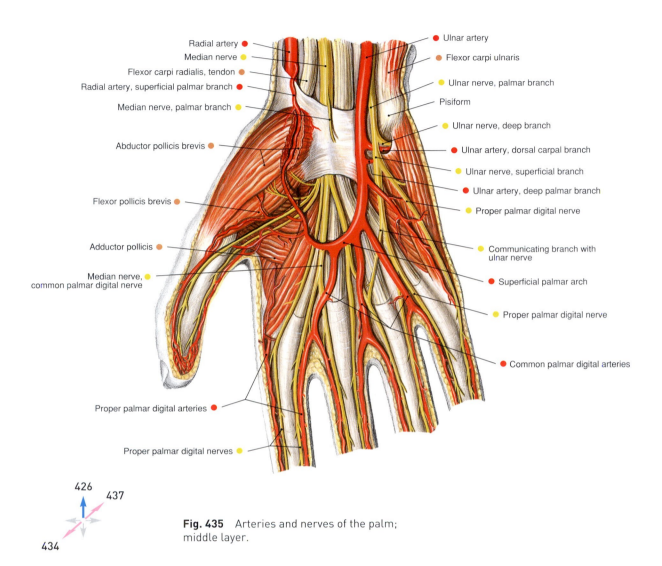

Radial artery ●
Median nerve ●
Flexor carpi radialis, tendon ●
Radial artery, superficial palmar branch ●
Median nerve, palmar branch ●
Abductor pollicis brevis ●
Flexor pollicis brevis ●
Adductor pollicis ●
Median nerve, common palmar digital nerve ●
Proper palmar digital arteries ●
Proper palmar digital nerves ●

● Ulnar artery
● Flexor carpi ulnaris
● Ulnar nerve, palmar branch
Pisiform
● Ulnar nerve, deep branch
● Ulnar artery, dorsal carpal branch
● Ulnar nerve, superficial branch
● Ulnar artery, deep palmar branch
● Proper palmar digital nerve
● Communicating branch with ulnar nerve
● Superficial palmar arch
● Proper palmar digital nerve
● Common palmar digital arteries

426
437
434

Fig. 435 Arteries and nerves of the palm; middle layer.

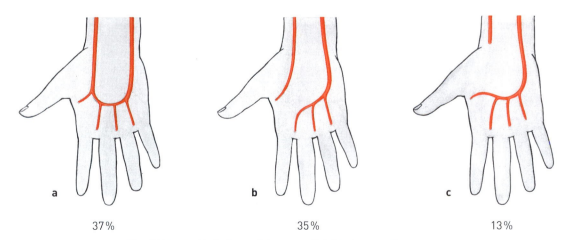

37%   35%   13%

a   b   c

Fig. 436 a–c Variations of the superficial palmar arch.
a "Textbook case", closed arch
b The ulnar artery supplies the three ulnar fingers.
c All fingers are supplied by the ulnar artery.

Arteries and nerves of the hand

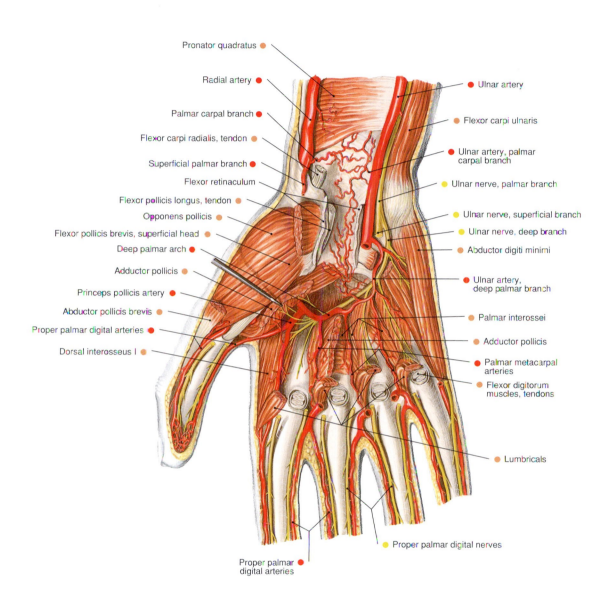

Pronator quadratus ●

Radial artery ●

Palmar carpal branch ●

Flexor carpi radialis, tendon ●

Superficial palmar branch ●

Flexor retinaculum

Flexor pollicis longus, tendon ●

Opponens pollicis ●

Flexor pollicis brevis, superficial head ●

Deep palmar arch ●

Adductor pollicis ●

Princeps pollicis artery ●

Abductor pollicis brevis ●

Proper palmar digital arteries ●

Dorsal interosseus I ●

● Ulnar artery

● Flexor carpi ulnaris

● Ulnar artery, palmar carpal branch

● Ulnar nerve, palmar branch

● Ulnar nerve, superficial branch

● Ulnar nerve, deep branch

● Abductor digiti minimi

● Ulnar artery, deep palmar branch

● Palmar interossei

● Adductor pollicis

● Palmar metacarpal arteries

● Flexor digitorum muscles, tendons

● Lumbricals

● Proper palmar digital nerves

Proper palmar ●
digital arteries

Fig. 437 Arteries and nerves of the palm; deep layer.

427

435

Arteries and nerves of the hand

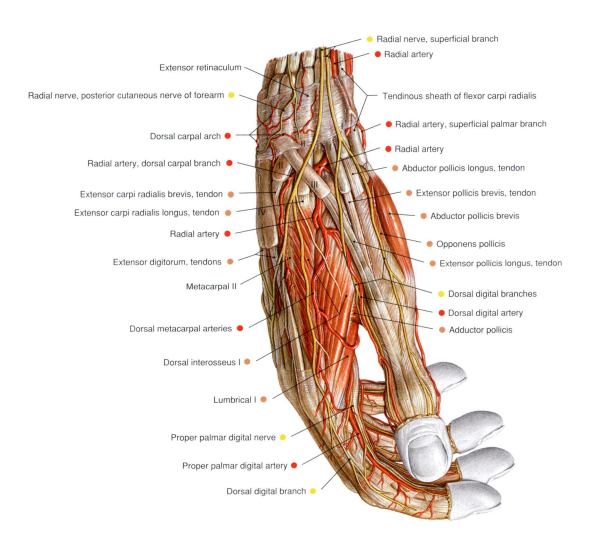

Radial nerve, superficial branch ●

Radial artery ●

Extensor retinaculum

Radial nerve, posterior cutaneous nerve of forearm ●

Tendinous sheath of flexor carpi radialis

Dorsal carpal arch ●

Radial artery, superficial palmar branch ●

Radial artery, dorsal carpal branch ●

Radial artery ●

Abductor pollicis longus, tendon ●

Extensor carpi radialis brevis, tendon ●

Extensor pollicis brevis, tendon ●

Extensor carpi radialis longus, tendon ●

Abductor pollicis brevis ●

Radial artery ●

Opponens pollicis ●

Extensor digitorum, tendons ●

Extensor pollicis longus, tendon ●

Metacarpal II

Dorsal digital branches ●

Dorsal digital artery ●

Dorsal metacarpal arteries ●

Adductor pollicis ●

Dorsal interosseus I ●

Lumbrical I ●

Proper palmar digital nerve ●

Proper palmar digital artery ●

Dorsal digital branch ●

I–IV Tendinous sheath of extensores:
I   Tendinous sheath of abductor longus
     and extensor pollicis brevis
II   Tendinous sheath of extensores carpi radiales
III Tendinous sheath of extensor pollicis longus
IV   Tendinous sheath of extensor digitorum
     and extensor indicis

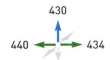

430

440 ← → 434

Fig. 438   Arteries and nerves of the hand.

Vessels and nerves of the hand

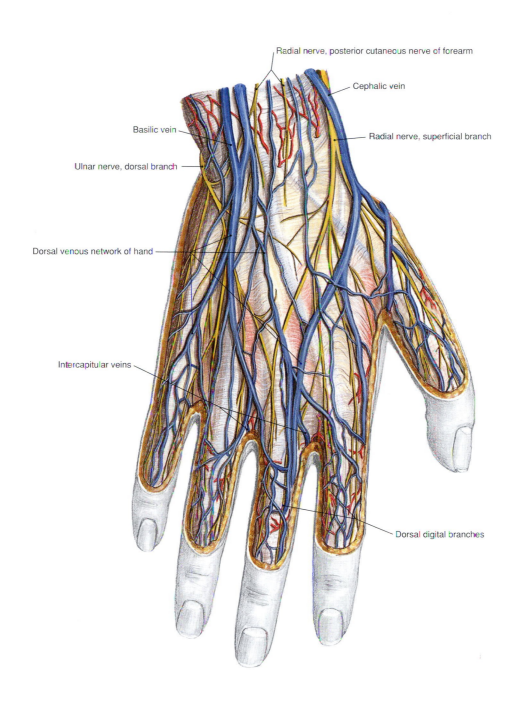

Radial nerve, posterior cutaneous nerve of forearm

Cephalic vein

Basilic vein

Radial nerve, superficial branch

Ulnar nerve, dorsal branch

Dorsal venous network of hand

Intercapitular veins

Dorsal digital branches

Fig. 439 Vessels and nerves of the dorsum of
the hand; superficial layer.

422

440

Arteries and nerves of the hand

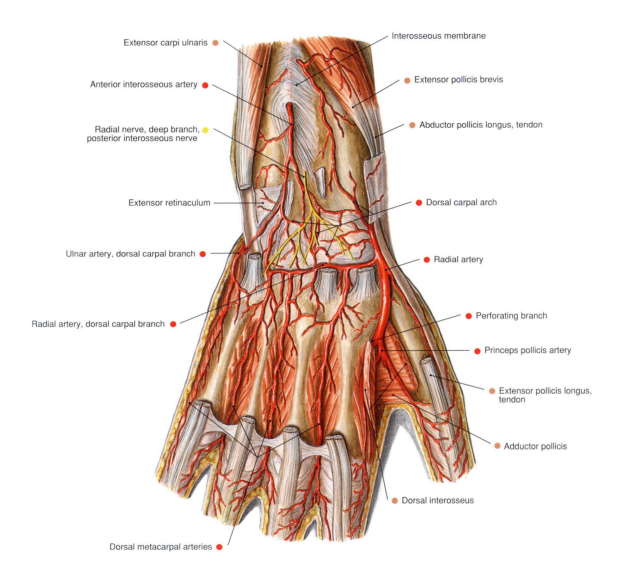

Extensor carpi ulnaris ●

Anterior interosseous artery ●

Radial nerve, deep branch,
posterior interosseous nerve ●

Extensor retinaculum —

Ulnar artery, dorsal carpal branch ●

Radial artery, dorsal carpal branch ●

Dorsal metacarpal arteries ●

Interosseous membrane

● Extensor pollicis brevis

● Abductor pollicis longus, tendon

● Dorsal carpal arch

● Radial artery

● Perforating branch

● Princeps pollicis artery

● Extensor pollicis longus,
tendon

● Adductor pollicis

● Dorsal interosseus

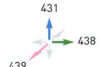

431
438
439

Fig. 440 Arteries and nerves of the dorsum of
the hand; deep layer.

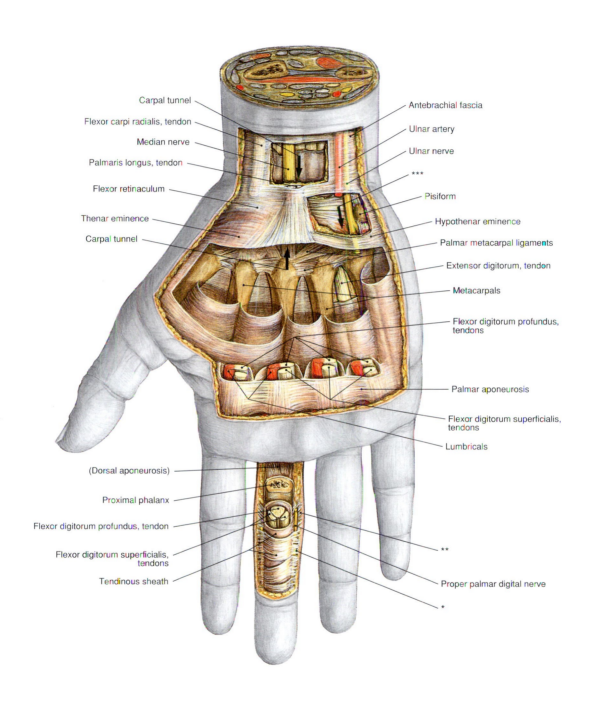

Carpal tunnel

Flexor carpi radialis, tendon

Median nerve

Palmaris longus, tendon

Flexor retinaculum

Thenar eminence

Carpal tunnel

Antebrachial fascia

Ulnar artery

Ulnar nerve

***

Pisiform

Hypothenar eminence

Palmar metacarpal ligaments

Extensor digitorum, tendon

Metacarpals

Flexor digitorum profundus, tendons

Palmar aponeurosis

Flexor digitorum superficialis, tendons

Lumbricals

(Dorsal aponeurosis)

Proximal phalanx

Flexor digitorum profundus, tendon

Flexor digitorum superficialis, tendons

Tendinous sheath

**

Proper palmar digital nerve

*

Fig. 441   Fascial compartments of the hand.

*   Clinical term: ligament of GRAYSON
**   Clinical term: ligament of CLELAND
*** Clinical term: ulnar canal (loge de GUYON)

Hand, sagittal section

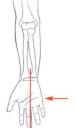

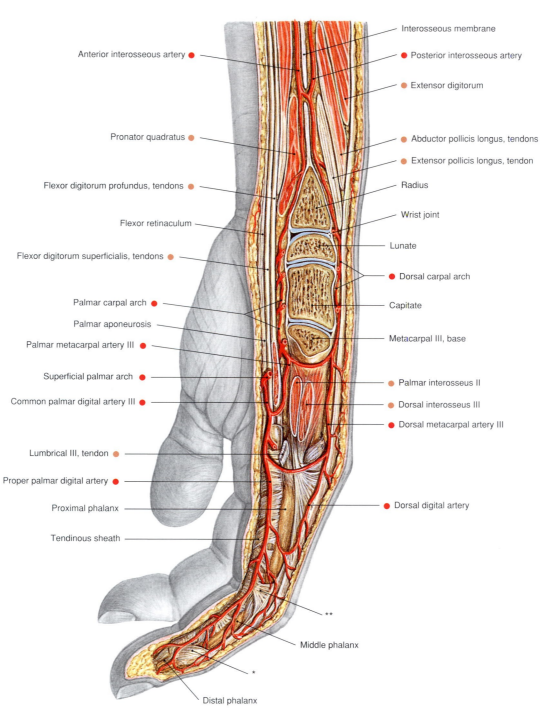

Anterior interosseous artery ●

Pronator quadratus ●

Flexor digitorum profundus, tendons ●

Flexor retinaculum

Flexor digitorum superficialis, tendons ●

Palmar carpal arch ●

Palmar aponeurosis

Palmar metacarpal artery III ●

Superficial palmar arch ●

Common palmar digital artery III ●

Lumbrical III, tendon ●

Proper palmar digital artery ●

Proximal phalanx

Tendinous sheath

Distal phalanx

Interosseous membrane

● Posterior interosseous artery

● Extensor digitorum

● Abductor pollicis longus, tendons

● Extensor pollicis longus, tendon

Radius

Wrist joint

Lunate

● Dorsal carpal arch

Capitate

Metacarpal III, base

● Palmar interosseus II

● Dorsal interosseus III

● Dorsal metacarpal artery III

● Dorsal digital artery

**

Middle phalanx

*

Fig. 442   Hand;
sagittal section at the level of the ulnar plane of the middle finger.

*   Clinical term: ligament of CLELAND
** Clinical term: ligament of GRAYSON

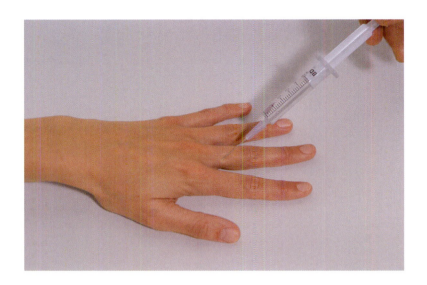

Fig. 443   Points of injection for regional
conduction anaesthesia at the middle finger.

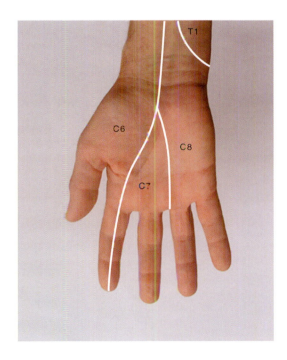

Fig. 444   Palm;
segmental cutaneous innervation.

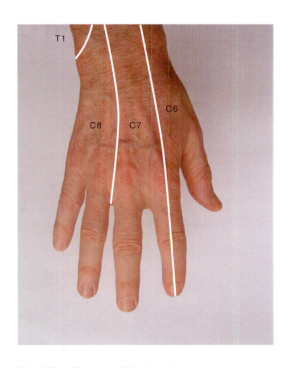

Fig. 445   Dorsum of the hand;
segmental cutaneous innervation.

Arm, transverse sections

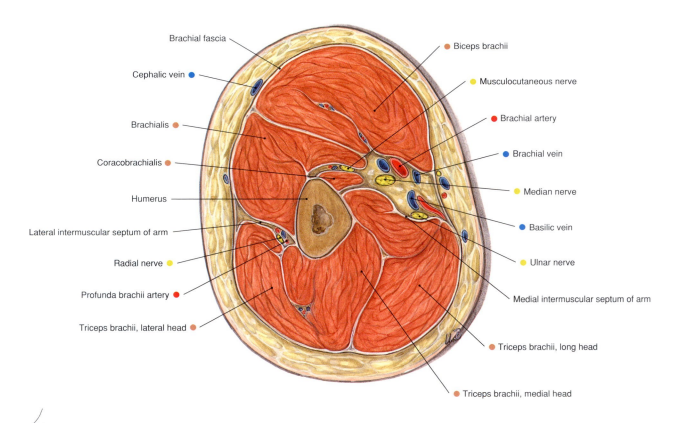

Brachial fascia

Cephalic vein ●

Brachialis ●

Coracobrachialis ●

Humerus

Lateral intermuscular septum of arm

Radial nerve ●

Profunda brachii artery ●

Triceps brachii, lateral head ●

Biceps brachii ●

Musculocutaneous nerve ●

Brachial artery ●

Brachial vein ●

Median nerve ●

Basilic vein ●

Ulnar nerve ●

Medial intermuscular septum of arm

Triceps brachii, long head ●

Triceps brachii, medial head ●

Fig. 446 Arm;
transverse section.

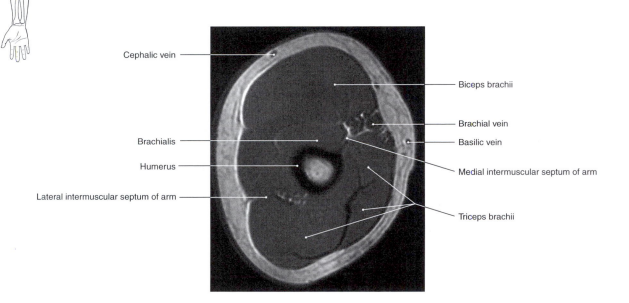

Cephalic vein

Brachialis

Humerus

Lateral intermuscular septum of arm

Biceps brachii

Brachial vein

Basilic vein

Medial intermuscular septum of arm

Triceps brachii

Fig. 447 Arm;
magnetic resonance tomographic image (MRI);
cross-section at the level of the middle of the arm;
distal view.

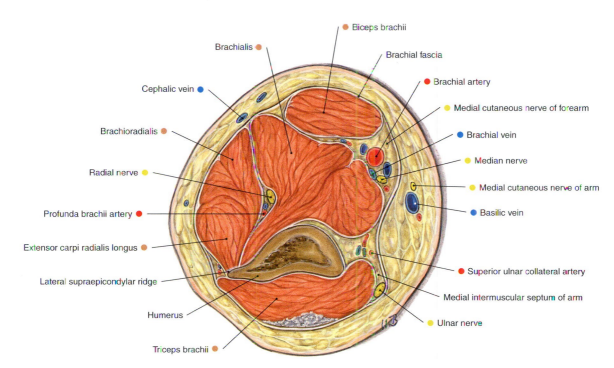

Biceps brachii

Brachialis

Brachial fascia

Cephalic vein

Brachial artery

Brachioradialis

Medial cutaneous nerve of forearm

Brachial vein

Radial nerve

Median nerve

Medial cutaneous nerve of arm

Profunda brachii artery

Basilic vein

Extensor carpi radialis longus

Lateral supraepicondylar ridge

Superior ulnar collateral artery

Medial intermuscular septum of arm

Humerus

Ulnar nerve

Triceps brachii

Fig. 448   Arm;
transverse section through the lower third of the arm.

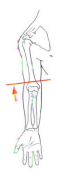

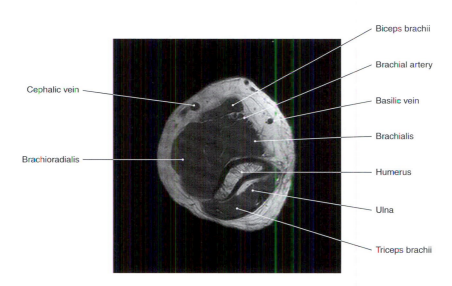

Cephalic vein

Biceps brachii

Brachial artery

Basilic vein

Brachialis

Brachioradialis

Humerus

Ulna

Triceps brachii

Fig. 449   Arm;
magnetic resonance tomographic image (MRI);
cross-section at the level of the lower third of the arm;
distal view.

Forearm, transverse sections

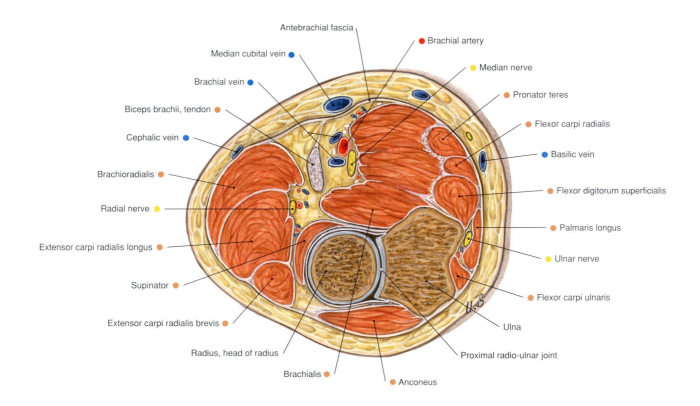

Antebrachial fascia

Median cubital vein ●

Brachial vein ●

Biceps brachii, tendon ●

Cephalic vein ●

Brachioradialis ●

Radial nerve ●

Extensor carpi radialis longus ●

Supinator ●

Extensor carpi radialis brevis ●

Radius, head of radius

Brachialis ●

Anconeus ●

● Brachial artery

● Median nerve

● Pronator teres

● Flexor carpi radialis

● Basilic vein

● Flexor digitorum superficialis

● Palmaris longus

● Ulnar nerve

● Flexor carpi ulnaris

Ulna

Proximal radio-ulnar joint

Fig. 450   Forearm;
transverse section at the level of the
proximal radio-ulnar joint.

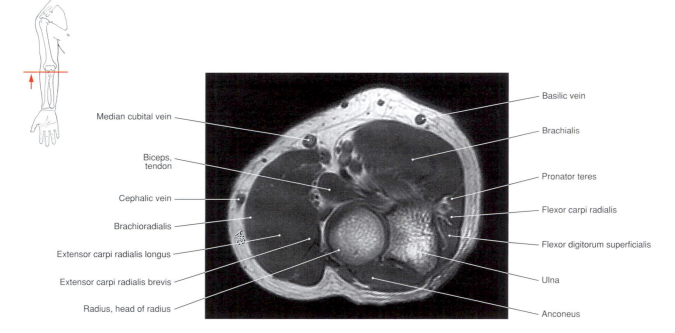

Median cubital vein

Biceps, tendon

Cephalic vein

Brachioradialis

Extensor carpi radialis longus

Extensor carpi radialis brevis

Radius, head of radius

Basilic vein

Brachialis

Pronator teres

Flexor carpi radialis

Flexor digitorum superficialis

Ulna

Anconeus

Fig. 451   Forearm;
magnetic resonance tomographic image (MRI);
cross-section at the level of the elbow joint;
distal view.

Forearm, transverse sections

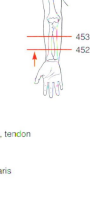

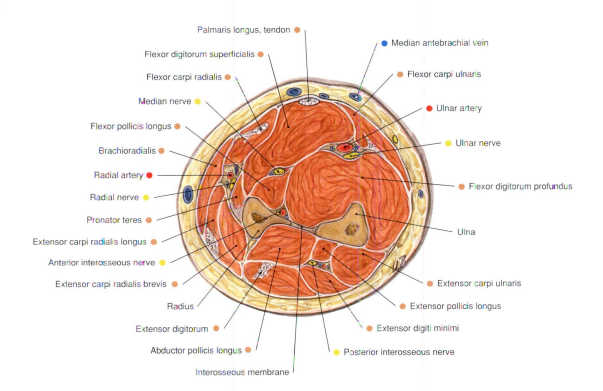

Palmaris longus, tendon ●
Flexor digitorum superficialis ●
Flexor carpi radialis ●
Median nerve ●
Flexor pollicis longus ●
Brachioradialis ●
Radial artery ●
Radial nerve ●
Pronator teres ●
Extensor carpi radialis longus ●
Anterior interosseous nerve ●
Extensor carpi radialis brevis ●
Radius
Extensor digitorum ●
Abductor pollicis longus ●
Interosseous membrane

● Median antebrachial vein
● Flexor carpi ulnaris
● Ulnar artery
● Ulnar nerve
● Flexor digitorum profundus
Ulna
● Extensor carpi ulnaris
● Extensor pollicis longus
● Extensor digiti minimi
● Posterior interosseous nerve

Fig. 452 Forearm;
transverse section through the lower third of
the forearm.

453
452

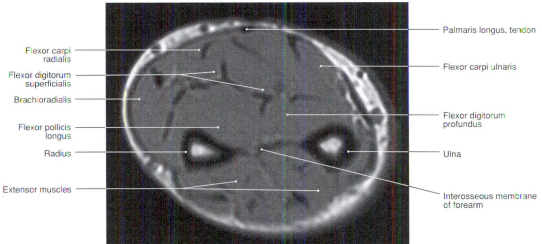

Flexor carpi
radialis
Flexor digitorum
superficialis
Brachioradialis
Flexor pollicis
longus
Radius
Extensor muscles

Palmaris longus, tendon
Flexor carpi ulnaris
Flexor digitorum
profundus
Ulna
Interosseous membrane
of forearm

Fig. 453 Forearm;
magnetic resonance tomographic image (MRI);
cross-section at the level of the middle of the forearm;
distal view.

Forearm, transverse sections

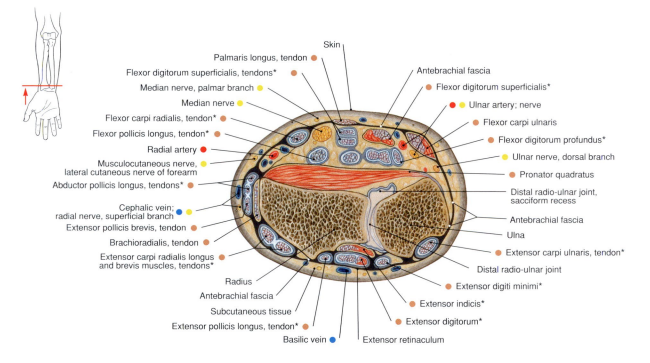

Skin
Palmaris longus, tendon ●
Flexor digitorum superficialis, tendons* ●
Median nerve, palmar branch ●
Median nerve ●
Flexor carpi radialis, tendon* ●
Flexor pollicis longus, tendon* ●
Radial artery ●
Musculocutaneous nerve, lateral cutaneous nerve of forearm ●
Abductor pollicis longus, tendons* ●
Cephalic vein; radial nerve, superficial branch ● ●
Extensor pollicis brevis, tendon ●
Brachioradialis, tendon ●
Extensor carpi radialis longus and brevis muscles, tendons* ●
Radius
Antebrachial fascia
Subcutaneous tissue
Extensor pollicis longus, tendon* ●
Basilic vein ●
Extensor retinaculum

Antebrachial fascia
Flexor digitorum superficialis* ●
Ulnar artery; nerve ● ●
Flexor carpi ulnaris ●
Flexor digitorum profundus* ●
Ulnar nerve, dorsal branch ●
Pronator quadratus ●
Distal radio-ulnar joint, sacciform recess
Antebrachial fascia
Ulna
Extensor carpi ulnaris, tendon* ●
Distal radio-ulnar joint
Extensor digiti minimi* ●
Extensor indicis* ●
Extensor digitorum* ●

Fig. 454 Forearm; transverse section at the level of the distal radio-ulnar joint. At this level, the muscle tendons marked with * run within tendon sheaths.

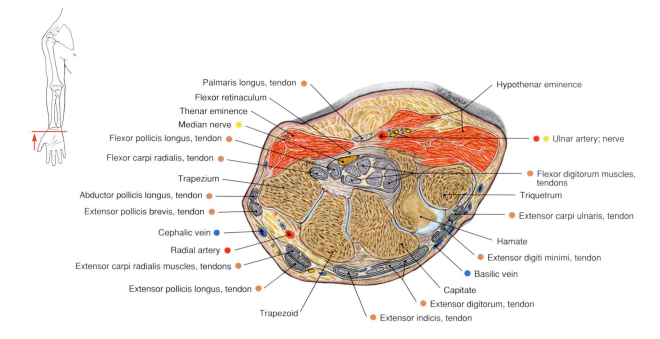

Palmaris longus, tendon ●
Flexor retinaculum
Thenar eminence
Median nerve ●
Flexor pollicis longus, tendon ●
Flexor carpi radialis, tendon ●
Trapezium
Abductor pollicis longus, tendon ●
Extensor pollicis brevis, tendon ●
Cephalic vein ●
Radial artery ●
Extensor carpi radialis muscles, tendons ●
Extensor pollicis longus, tendon ●
Trapezoid

Hypothenar eminence
Ulnar artery; nerve ● ●
Flexor digitorum muscles, tendons ●
Triquetrum
Extensor carpi ulnaris, tendon ●
Hamate
Extensor digiti minimi, tendon ●
Basilic vein ●
Capitate
Extensor digitorum, tendon ●
Extensor indicis, tendon ●

Fig. 455 Wrist; transverse section at the level of the hook of the hamate bone.

* Carpal tunnel
** ulnar canal (loge de GUYON)

Hand, transverse sections

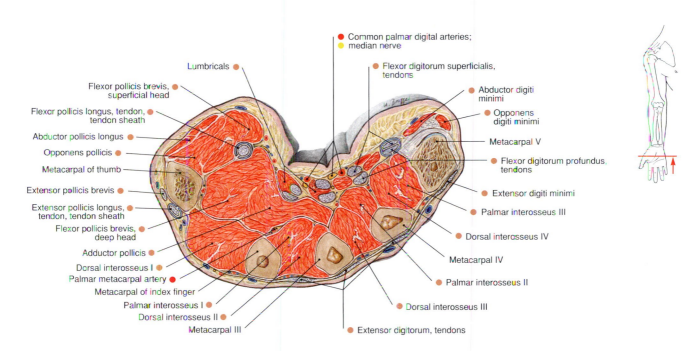

Lumbricals

Flexor pollicis brevis,
superficial head

Flexor pollicis longus, tendon,
tendon sheath

Abductor pollicis longus

Opponens pollicis

Metacarpal of thumb

Extensor pollicis brevis

Extensor pollicis longus,
tendon, tendon sheath

Flexor pollicis brevis,
deep head

Adductor pollicis

Dorsal interosseus I

Palmar metacarpal artery

Metacarpal of index finger

Palmar interosseus I

Dorsal interosseus II

Metacarpal III

Common palmar digital arteries;
median nerve

Flexor digitorum superficialis,
tendons

Abductor digiti
minimi

Opponens
digiti minimi

Metacarpal V

Flexor digitorum profundus,
tendons

Extensor digiti minimi

Palmar interosseus III

Dorsal interosseus IV

Metacarpal IV

Palmar interosseus II

Dorsal interosseus III

Extensor digitorum, tendons

Fig. 456   Metacarpus; transverse section at the level of the third metacarpal bone.

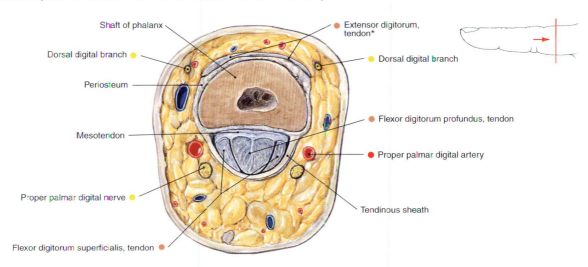

Shaft of phalanx

Dorsal digital branch

Periosteum

Mesotendon

Proper palmar digital nerve

Flexor digitorum superficialis, tendon

Extensor digitorum,
tendon*

Dorsal digital branch

Flexor digitorum profundus, tendon

Proper palmar digital artery

Tendinous sheath

Fig. 457   Middle finger;
transverse section through the shaft of the proximal phalanx.

*   So-called dorsal aponeurosis into which the branching tendon
of the extensor digitorum muscle, as well as the tendons of the
interosseous and lumbrical muscles radiate

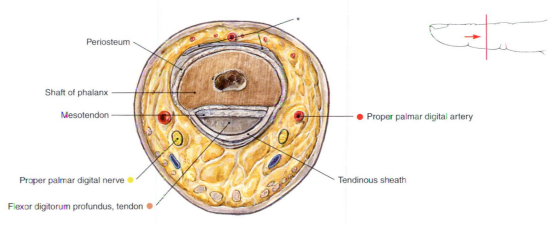

Periosteum

Shaft of phalanx

Mesotendon

Proper palmar digital nerve

Flexor digitorum profundus, tendon

Proper palmar digital artery

Tendinous sheath

Fig. 458   Middle finger;
transverse section through the shaft of the middle phalanx.

*   So-called dorsal aponeurosis

Regions

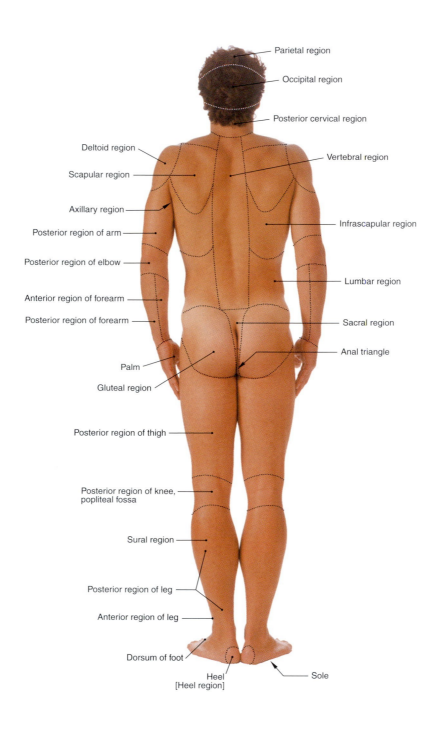

Parietal region

Occipital region

Posterior cervical region

Deltoid region

Vertebral region

Scapular region

Axillary region

Infrascapular region

Posterior region of arm

Posterior region of elbow

Lumbar region

Anterior region of forearm

Posterior region of forearm

Sacral region

Anal triangle

Palm

Gluteal region

Posterior region of thigh

Posterior region of knee, popliteal fossa

Sural region

Posterior region of leg

Anterior region of leg

Dorsum of foot

Heel
[Heel region]

Sole

Fig. 459   Regions of the human body.

Skeleton of the trunk

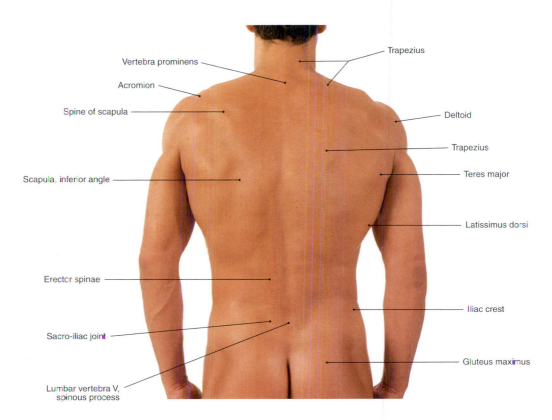

Vertebra prominens

Acromion

Spine of scapula

Scapula, inferior angle

Erector spinae

Sacro-iliac joint

Lumbar vertebra V,
spinous process

Trapezius

Deltoid

Trapezius

Teres major

Latissimus dorsi

Iliac crest

Gluteus maximus

Fig. 460 Back;
surface anatomy.

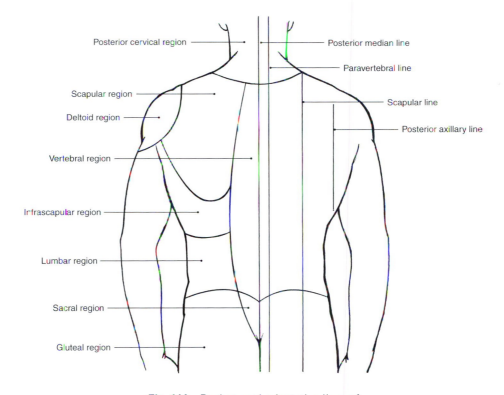

Posterior cervical region

Scapular region

Deltoid region

Vertebral region

Infrascapular region

Lumbar region

Sacral region

Gluteal region

Posterior median line

Paravertebral line

Scapular line

Posterior axillary line

Fig. 461 Regions and orientation lines of
the back.

Skeleton of the trunk

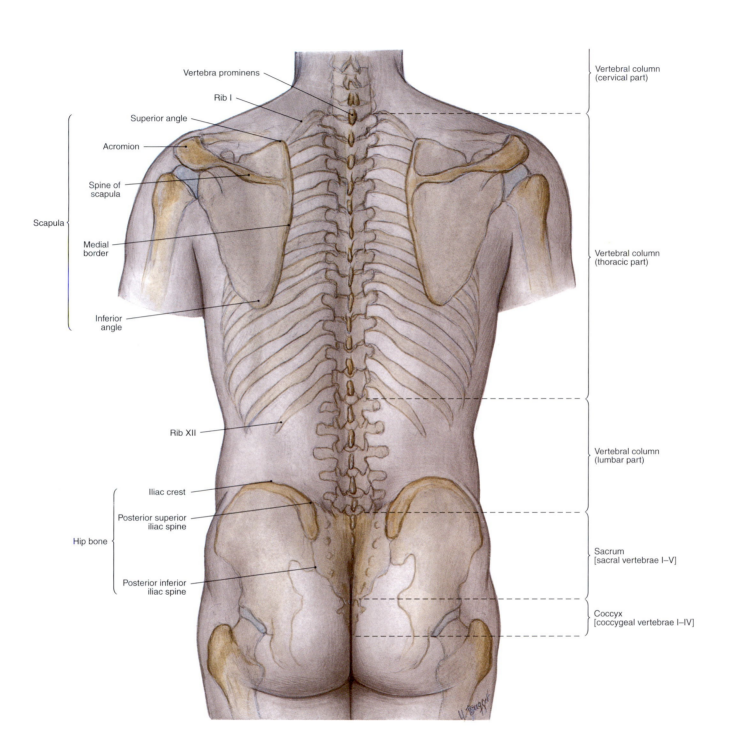

Vertebra prominens

Rib I

Superior angle

Acromion

Spine of scapula

Scapula

Medial border

Inferior angle

Rib XII

Iliac crest

Posterior superior iliac spine

Hip bone

Posterior inferior iliac spine

Vertebral column (cervical part)

Vertebral column (thoracic part)

Vertebral column (lumbar part)

Sacrum [sacral vertebrae I–V]

Coccyx [coccygeal vertebrae I–IV]

Fig. 462 Skeletal system of the trunk.

Skeleton of the trunk

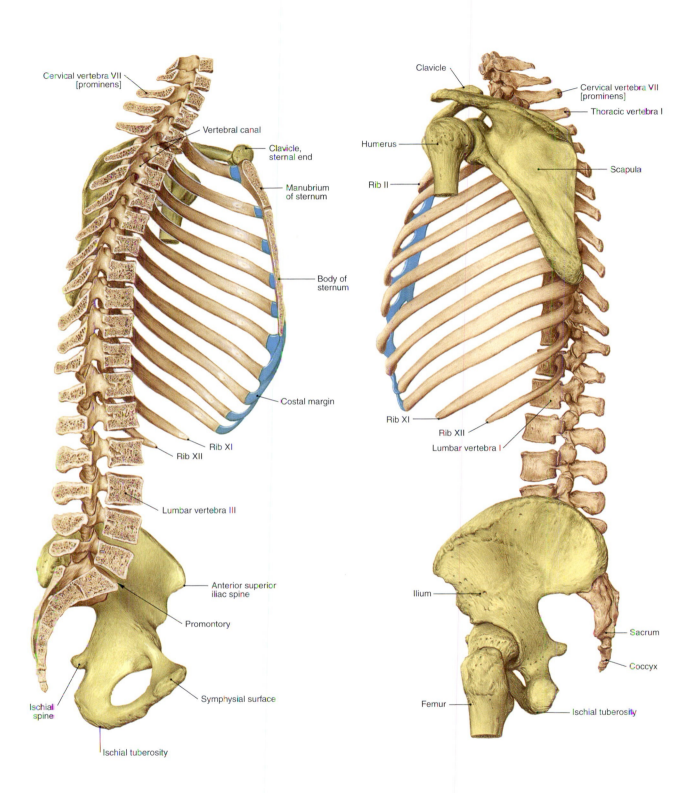

Cervical vertebra VII [prominens]

Vertebral canal

Clavicle, sternal end

Manubrium of sternum

Body of sternum

Costal margin

Rib XI

Rib XII

Lumbar vertebra III

Anterior superior iliac spine

Promontory

Symphysial surface

Ischial spine

Ischial tuberosity

Clavicle

Cervical vertebra VII [prominens]

Thoracic vertebra I

Humerus

Scapula

Rib II

Rib XI

Rib XII

Lumbar vertebra I

Ilium

Sacrum

Coccyx

Femur

Ischial tuberosity

Fig. 463 Vertebral column; pectoral girdle and pelvic girdle; median section through the vertebral column; medial view.

Fig. 464 Vertebral column; pectoral girdle and pelvic girdle; median section through the vertebral column; viewed from the left.

Vertebral column

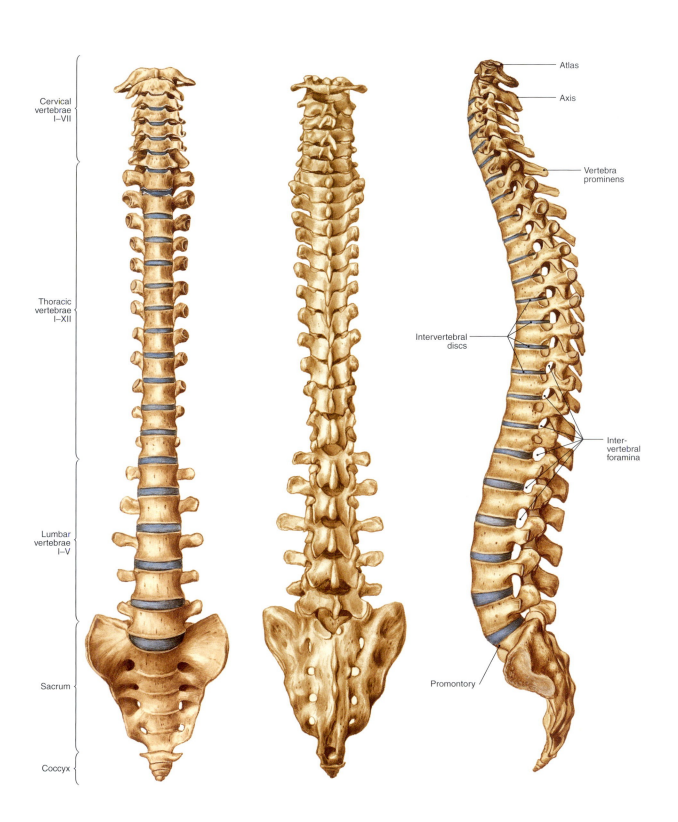

Cervical
vertebrae
I–VII

Thoracic
vertebrae
I–XII

Lumbar
vertebrae
I–V

Sacrum

Coccyx

Atlas

Axis

Vertebra
prominens

Intervertebral
discs

Inter-
vertebral
foramina

Promontory

Fig. 465 Vertebral column;
ventral view.

Fig. 466 Vertebral column;
dorsal view.

Fig. 467 Vertebral column;
viewed from the left.

Vertebral column, development

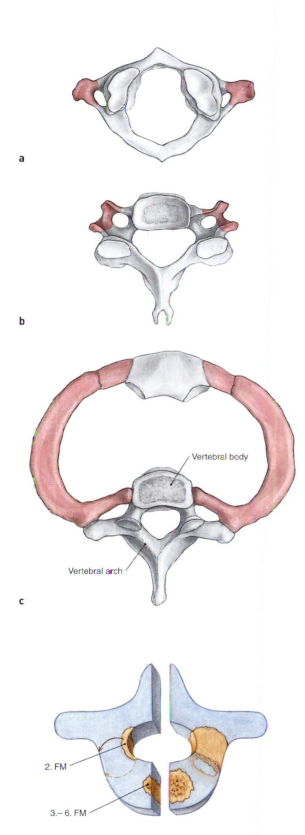

Vertebral body

Vertebral arch

a

b

c

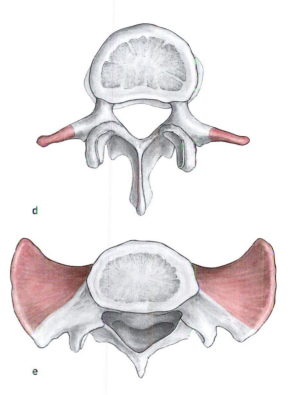

d

e

Fig. 468 a–e Regional characteristics of the vertebrae. Only in the thoracic region of the vertebral column do the lateral parts (labelled in red) remain separated and form ribs.

a First cervical vertebra, atlas
b Fourth cervical vertebra
c First thoracic vertebra with corresponding ribs and sternum
d Third lumbar vertebra
e Sacrum

2. FM

3.– 6. FM

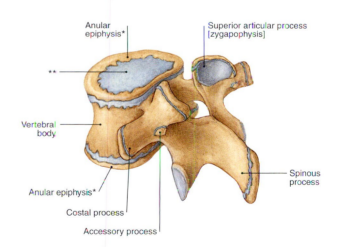

Anular epiphysis*

Superior articular process [zygapophysis]

**

Vertebral body

Spinous process

Anular epiphysis*

Costal process

Accessory process

Fig. 469 Vertebral development.
Demonstration of the appearance of primary ossification centres in a lumbar vertebra (pedicle: second foetal month; corpus: third to sixth foetal month).
Synostosis of the ossification centres of the vertebral arch with those of the corpus occurs between the third and the sixth year of life.

Fig. 470 Vertebral development.
Circular ossification centres (= rims*) appear in the epiphyses of the vertebrae during the eighth year of life and fuse with the vertebral bodies until the eighteenth year of life.
The central portions of the epiphyses remain as hyaline cartilaginous laminae ** throughout life.
Secondary ossification centres (apophyses) develop at the processes.

Atlas and axis

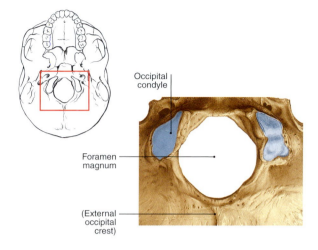

Fig. 471 Occipital bone;
section illustrating the foramen magnum and the
articular surfaces of the atlanto-occipital joint;
inferior view.

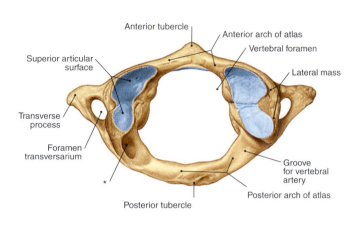

Fig. 472 First cervical vertebra, atlas;
superior view.
The superior articular surfaces of the atlas are
frequently divided.

* Canal for vertebral artery as a variation

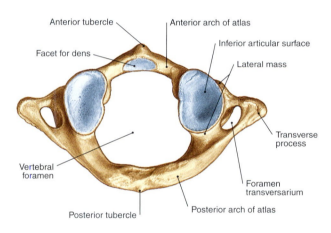

Fig. 473 First cervical vertebra, atlas;
inferior view.

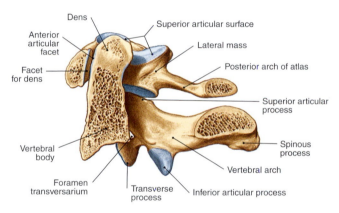

Fig. 474 First and second cervical vertebrae,
atlas and axis;
median section.

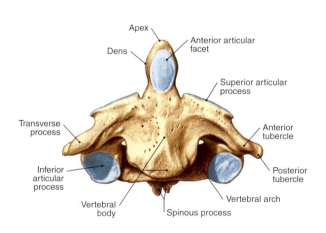

Fig. 475 Second cervical vertebra, axis;
ventral view.

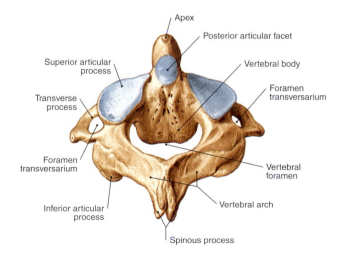

Fig. 476 Second cervical vertebra, axis;
dorsosuperior view.

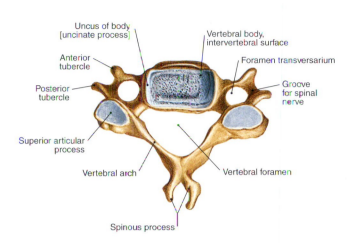

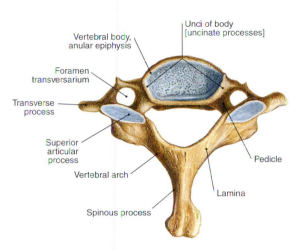

Fig. 477 Fifth cervical vertebra; superior view.
The tips of the spinous processes of the cervical vertebrae II–VI are frequently divided.

Fig. 478 Seventh cervical vertebra; superior view.
In general the seventh cervical vertebra can be easily iden-tified by its protruding spinous process and is referred to as vertebra prominens. In fact, the spinous process of the first thoracic vertebra often protrudes even further.

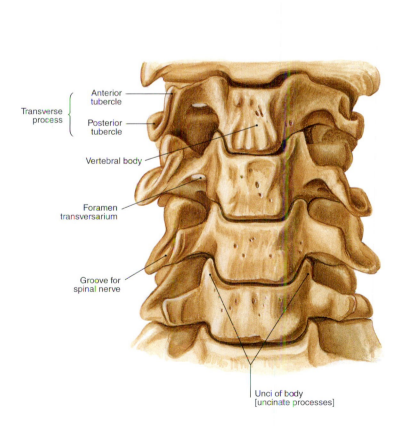

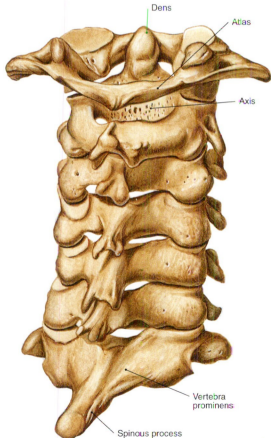

Fig. 479 Second to seventh cervical vertebrae; ventral view.

Fig. 480 First to seventh cervical vertebrae; dorsolateral view.

Thoracic and lumbar vertebrae

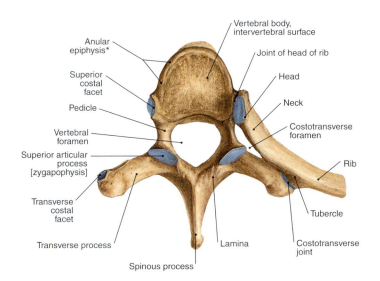

Fig. 481 Vertebra;
typical structural features exemplified by the
fifth thoracic vertebra;
superior view.

* Also: rim of vertebral body

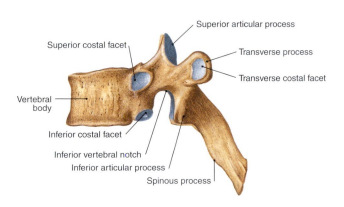

Fig. 482 Sixth thoracic vertebra;
viewed from the left.

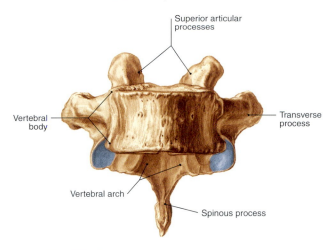

Fig. 483 Tenth thoracic vertebra;
ventral view.

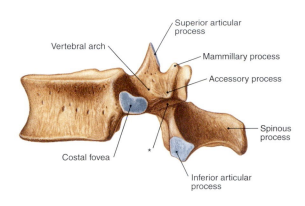

Fig. 484 Twelfth thoracic vertebra;
viewed from the left.

* Region of the vertebral arch between the superior and
inferior articular processes
(„isthmus" = interarticular portion)

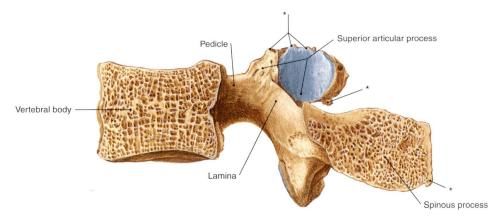

Fig. 485 Third lumbar vertebra;
median section; specimen of an older individual.

* Ossification of the ligamentous insertions

Thoracic and lumbar vertebrae

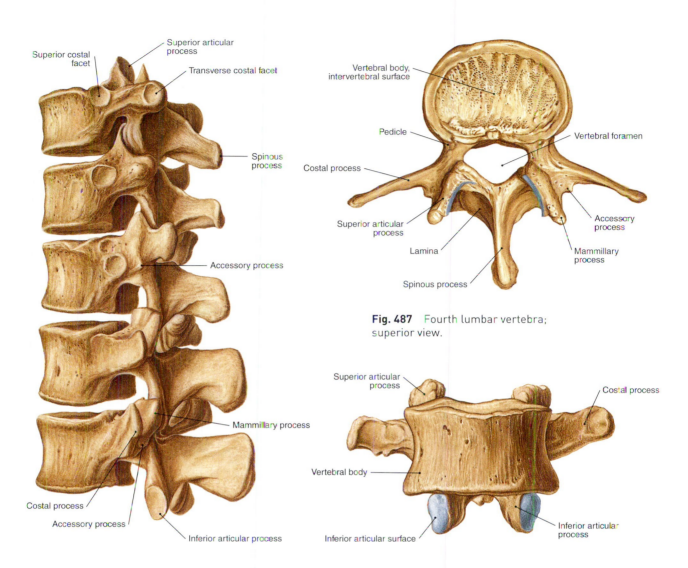

Superior costal facet

Superior articular process

Transverse costal facet

Spinous process

Accessory process

Mammillary process

Costal process

Accessory process

Inferior articular process

Fig. 486 Tenth to twelfth thoracic vertebrae and first to second lumbar vertebrae; dorsal view from the left.

Vertebral body, intervertebral surface

Pedicle

Costal process

Superior articular process

Lamina

Spinous process

Vertebral foramen

Accessory process

Mammillary process

Fig. 487 Fourth lumbar vertebra; superior view.

Superior articular process

Costal process

Vertebral body

Inferior articular surface

Inferior articular process

Fig. 488 Fourth lumbar vertebra; ventral view.

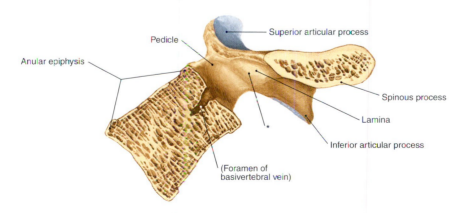

Anular epiphysis

Pedicle

Superior articular process

Spinous process

Lamina

Inferior articular process

*

(Foramen of basivertebral vein)

Fig. 489 Fifth lumbar vertebra; median section.
Note the characteristic wedge-shape of the body of the fifth lumbar vertebra.

* Region of the vertebral arch between the superior and inferior articular process. Here in the fifth and less frequently in the fourth lumbar vertebra a cleft, bridged by connective tissue (spondylolysis) can be formed. This is probably caused by local bending stress. As a consequence, the superior vertebra may slip (olisthesis) onto the inferior vertebra (spondylolisthesis).

Sacrum

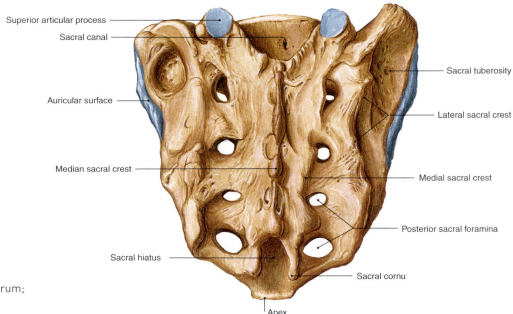

Superior articular process
Sacral canal
Sacral tuberosity
Auricular surface
Lateral sacral crest
Median sacral crest
Medial sacral crest
Posterior sacral foramina
Sacral hiatus
Sacral cornu
Apex

Fig. 490 Sacrum;
dorsal view.

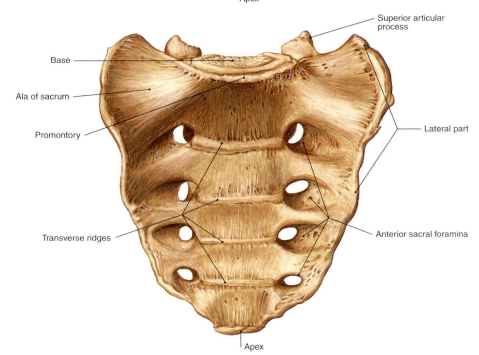

Superior articular process
Base
Ala of sacrum
Promontory
Lateral part
Transverse ridges
Anterior sacral foramina
Apex

Fig. 491 Sacrum;
ventroinferior view.

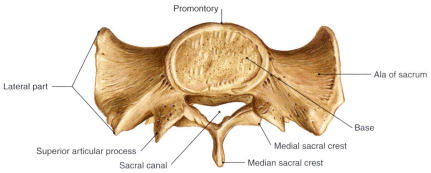

Promontory
Lateral part
Ala of sacrum
Base
Superior articular process
Medial sacral crest
Sacral canal
Median sacral crest

Fig. 492 Sacrum;
the bone has been sectioned at the
level of the second sacral vertebra;
superior view.

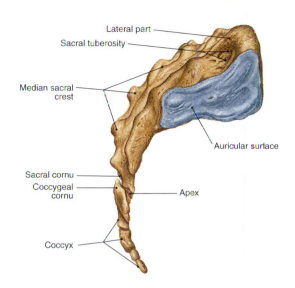

Fig. 493 Sacrum; viewed from the right.

Lateral part
Sacral tuberosity
Median sacral crest
Auricular surface
Sacral cornu
Coccygeal cornu
Apex
Coccyx

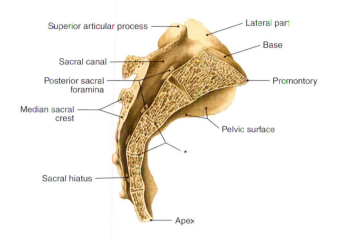

Fig. 494 Sacrum; median section.

* Remnants of intervertebral disc tissue persist even in the adult.

Superior articular process
Sacral canal
Posterior sacral foramina
Median sacral crest
Sacral hiatus
Lateral part
Base
Promontory
Pelvic surface
*
Apex

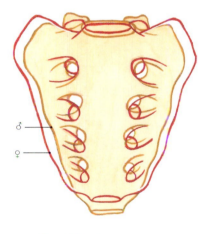

Fig. 495 Sacrum; gender differences.

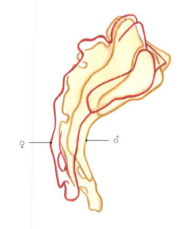

Fig. 496 Sacrum; gender differences.

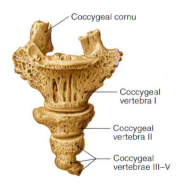

Fig. 497 Coccyx; ventrosuperior view.

Coccygeal cornu
Coccygeal vertebra I
Coccygeal vertebra II
Coccygeal vertebrae III–V

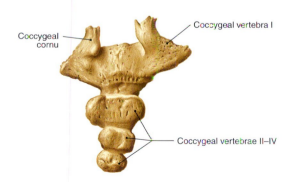

Fig. 498 Coccyx; dorsoinferior view.

Coccygeal cornu
Coccygeal vertebra I
Coccygeal vertebrae II–IV

Cervical part of the vertebral column, radiography

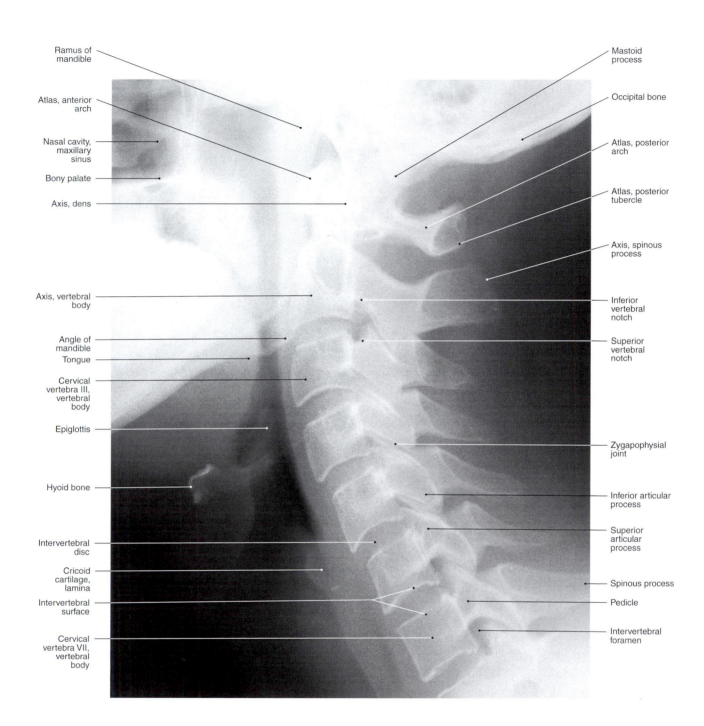

Ramus of mandible

Atlas, anterior arch

Nasal cavity, maxillary sinus

Bony palate

Axis, dens

Axis, vertebral body

Angle of mandible

Tongue

Cervical vertebra III, vertebral body

Epiglottis

Hyoid bone

Intervertebral disc

Cricoid cartilage, lamina

Intervertebral surface

Cervical vertebra VII, vertebral body

Mastoid process

Occipital bone

Atlas, posterior arch

Atlas, posterior tubercle

Axis, spinous process

Inferior vertebral notch

Superior vertebral notch

Zygapophysial joint

Inferior articular process

Superior articular process

Spinous process

Pedicle

Intervertebral foramen

Fig. 499 Cervical vertebrae;
lateral radiograph of the cervical part of the vertebral column;
upright position; the central beam is directed
onto the third cervical vertebra;
shoulders are pulled downwards.

Cervical part of the vertebral column, radiography

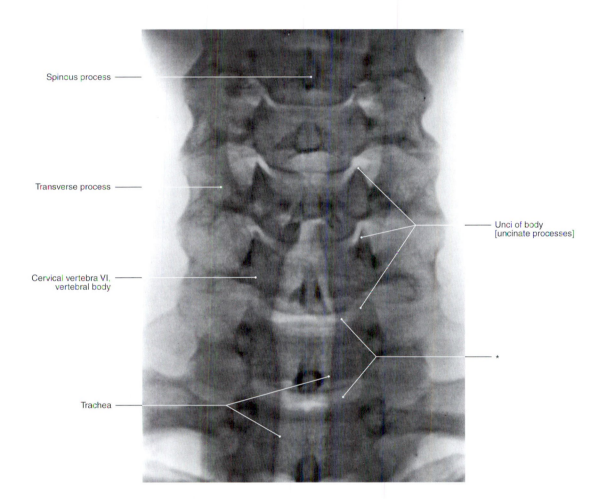

Spinous process

Transverse process

Cervical vertebra VI, vertebral body

Trachea

Unci of body [uncinate processes]

*

Fig. 500   Cervical vertebrae;
AP-radiograph of the cervical part of the vertebral column;
upright position; the central beam is directed
onto the third cervical vertebra.

*   Intervertebral disc spaces

Thoracic part of the vertebral column, radiography

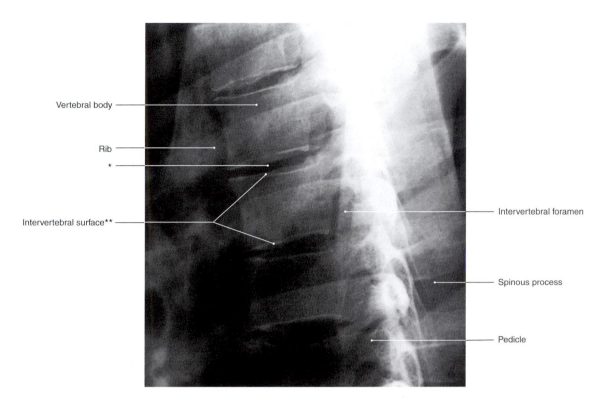

Vertebral body

Rib

*

Intervertebral surface**

Intervertebral foramen

Spinous process

Pedicle

Fig. 501 Thoracic vertebrae;
lateral radiograph of the thoracic part of the vertebral column;
upright position with the thorax in inspiration;
the central beam is directed onto the sixth thoracic vertebra.

* Intervertebral disc space
** Clinical term: end-plates

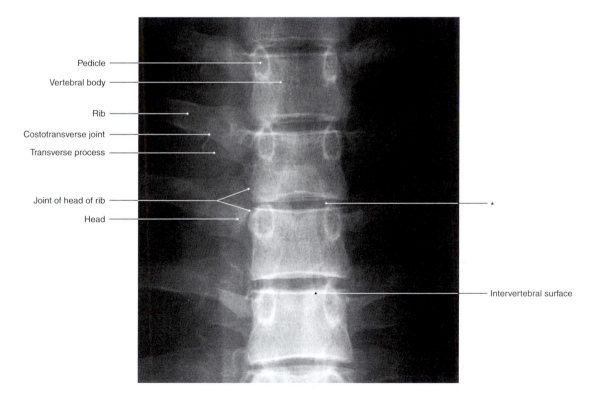

Pedicle

Vertebral body

Rib

Costotransverse joint

Transverse process

Joint of head of rib

Head

*

Intervertebral surface

Fig. 502 Thoracic vertebrae;
AP-radiograph of the thoracic part of the vertebral column;
upright position with the thorax in inspiration;
the central beam is directed onto the sixth thoracic vertebra.

* Intervertebral disc space

Lumbar part of the vertebral column, radiography

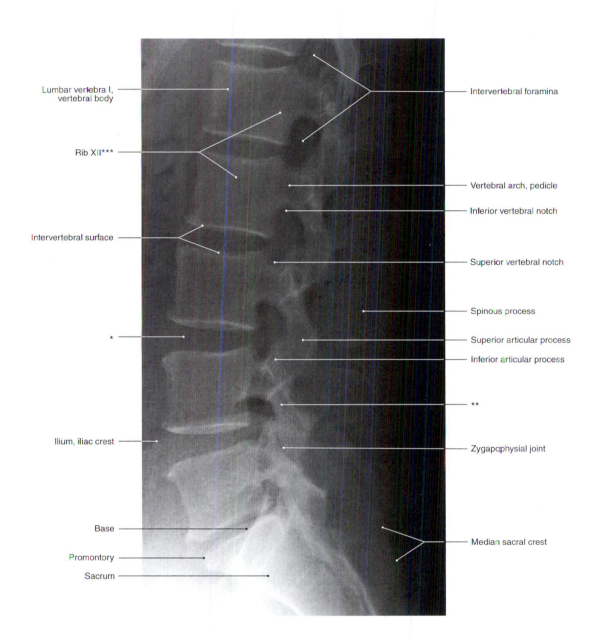

Lumbar vertebra I,
vertebral body

Rib XII***

Intervertebral surface

*

Ilium, iliac crest

Base

Promontory

Sacrum

Intervertebral foramina

Vertebral arch, pedicle

Inferior vertebral notch

Superior vertebral notch

Spinous process

Superior articular process

Inferior articular process

**

Zygapophysial joint

Median sacral crest

Fig. 503 Lumbar vertebrae;
lateral radiograph of the lumbar part of the vertebral column;
upright position;
the central beam is directed onto the second lumbar vertebra.
In this case, the anterior edges of the lower lumbar vertebrae
are oblique due to pathological alterations.

* Intervertebral disc space

** Region of the vertebral arch between the superior and inferior
articular processes ("isthmus" = interarticular portion)

*** The marks indicate the position of the twelfth rib, which is poorly
visible in this copy of the radiograph.

Lumbar part of the vertebral column, radiography

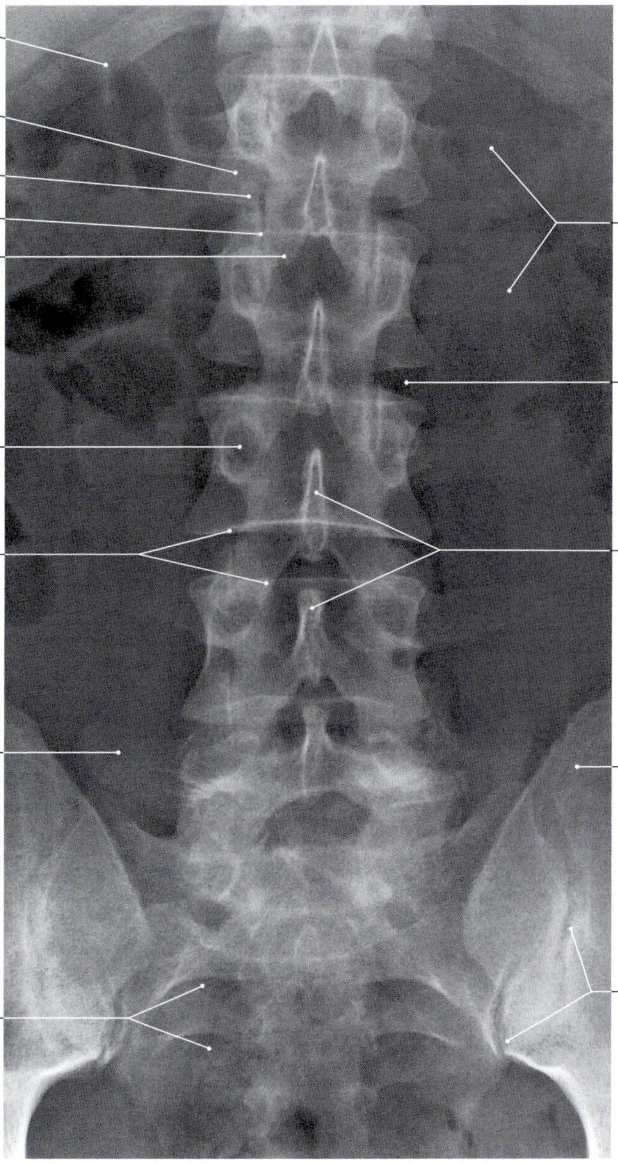

Rib XII

Lumbar vertebra I, vertebral body

Superior articular process

Zygapophysial joint

Inferior articular process

Pedicle

Intervertebral surface

Costal process

Anterior sacral foramina

Costal processes

*

Spinous processes

Hip bone; ilium

Sacro-iliac joint

Fig. 504 Lumbar vertebrae;
AP-radiograph of the lumbar part of the vertebral column
and the sacrum;
upright position; the central beam is directed onto the second
lumbar vertebra.

* Intervertebral disc space

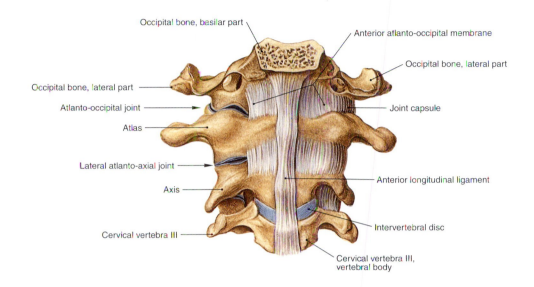

Occipital bone, basilar part

Anterior atlanto-occipital membrane

Occipital bone, lateral part

Occipital bone, lateral part

Atlanto-occipital joint

Joint capsule

Atlas

Lateral atlanto-axial joint

Anterior longitudinal ligament

Axis

Cervical vertebra III

Intervertebral disc

Cervical vertebra III, vertebral body

Fig. 505   Craniocervical junctions and the upper cervical part of the vertebral column; ventral view.

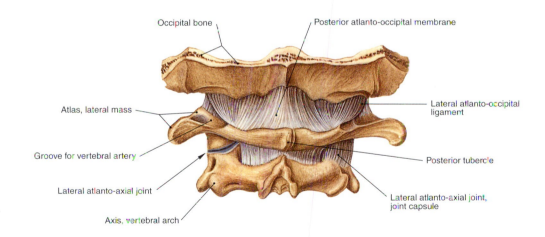

Occipital bone

Posterior atlanto-occipital membrane

Atlas, lateral mass

Lateral atlanto-occipital ligament

Groove for vertebral artery

Posterior tubercle

Lateral atlanto-axial joint

Lateral atlanto-axial joint, joint capsule

Axis, vertebral arch

Fig. 506   Craniocervical junctions; dorsal view.

Craniocervical junctions

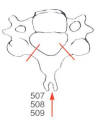

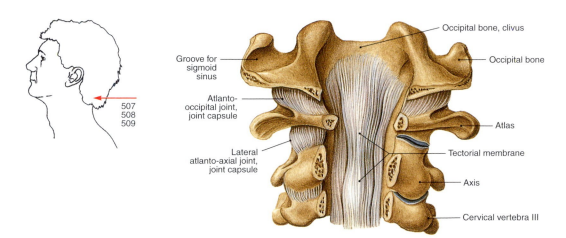

507
508
509

Occipital bone, clivus

Groove for sigmoid sinus

Occipital bone

Atlanto-occipital joint, joint capsule

Atlas

Tectorial membrane

Lateral atlanto-axial joint, joint capsule

Axis

Cervical vertebra III

Fig. 507 Craniocervical junctions, deep ligaments; dorsal view.

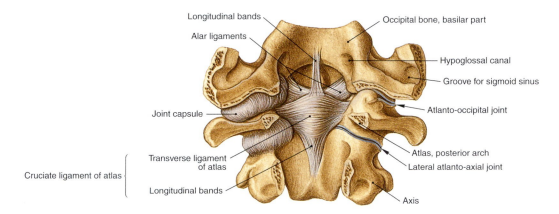

Longitudinal bands

Occipital bone, basilar part

Alar ligaments

Hypoglossal canal

Groove for sigmoid sinus

Joint capsule

Atlanto-occipital joint

Cruciate ligament of atlas

Transverse ligament of atlas

Atlas, posterior arch

Lateral atlanto-axial joint

Longitudinal bands

Axis

Fig. 508 Craniocervical junctions, deep ligaments; dorsal view.

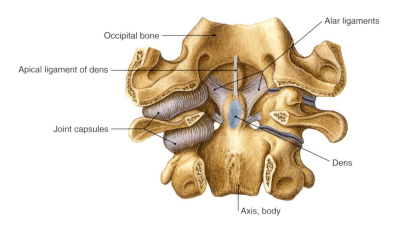

Alar ligaments

Occipital bone

Apical ligament of dens

Joint capsules

Dens

Axis, body

Fig. 509 Craniocervical junctions, deep ligaments; dorsal view.
The alar ligaments frequently extend to the lateral masses of the atlas.

Craniocervical junctions

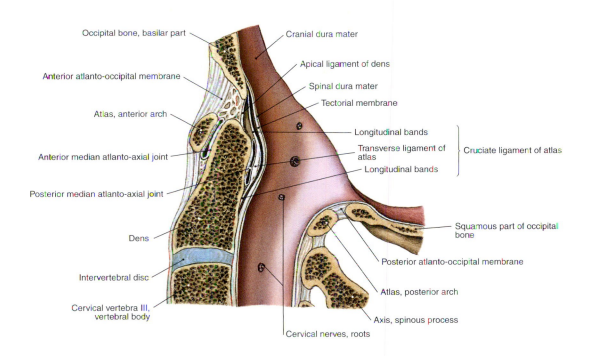

Occipital bone, basilar part
Cranial dura mater
Apical ligament of dens
Anterior atlanto-occipital membrane
Spinal dura mater
Atlas, anterior arch
Tectorial membrane
Longitudinal bands
Anterior median atlanto-axial joint
Transverse ligament of atlas
Cruciate ligament of atlas
Longitudinal bands
Posterior median atlanto-axial joint
Dens
Squamous part of occipital bone
Posterior atlanto-occipital membrane
Intervertebral disc
Atlas, posterior arch
Axis, spinous process
Cervical vertebra III, vertebral body
Cervical nerves, roots

Fig. 510 Craniocervical junctions; median section.

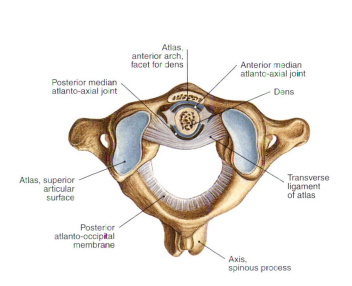

Atlas, anterior arch, facet for dens
Posterior median atlanto-axial joint
Anterior median atlanto-axial joint
Dens
Atlas, superior articular surface
Transverse ligament of atlas
Posterior atlanto-occipital membrane
Axis, spinous process

Fig. 511 Craniocervical junctions; superior view.

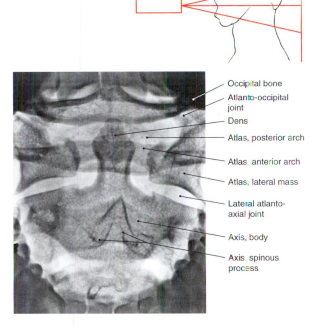

Occipital bone
Atlanto-occipital joint
Dens
Atlas, posterior arch
Atlas, anterior arch
Atlas, lateral mass
Lateral atlanto-axial joint
Axis, body
Axis, spinous process

Fig. 512 Craniocervical junctions; AP-radiograph.

Ligaments of the vertebral column

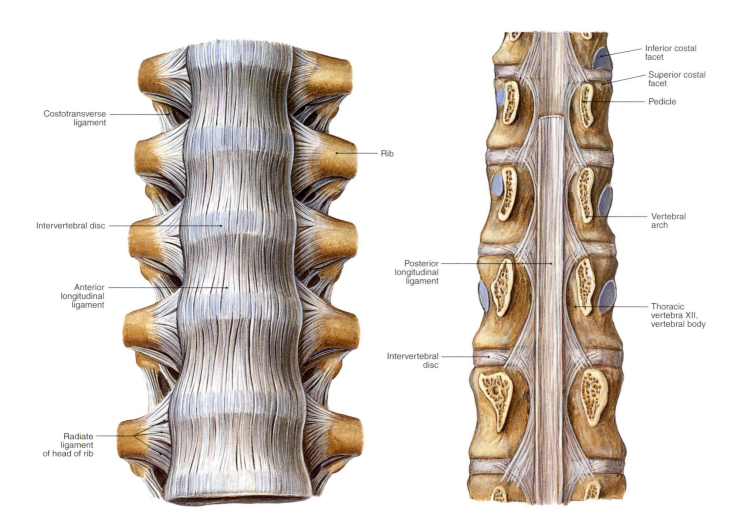

Costotransverse ligament

Rib

Intervertebral disc

Anterior longitudinal ligament

Radiate ligament of head of rib

Inferior costal facet

Superior costal facet

Pedicle

Vertebral arch

Posterior longitudinal ligament

Thoracic vertebra XII, vertebral body

Intervertebral disc

Fig. 513 Ligaments of the vertebral column; exemplified by the lower thoracic part of the vertebral column; ventral view.

Fig. 514 Ligaments of the vertebral column; exemplified by the lower thoracic and the upper lumbar part of the vertebral column; dorsal view.

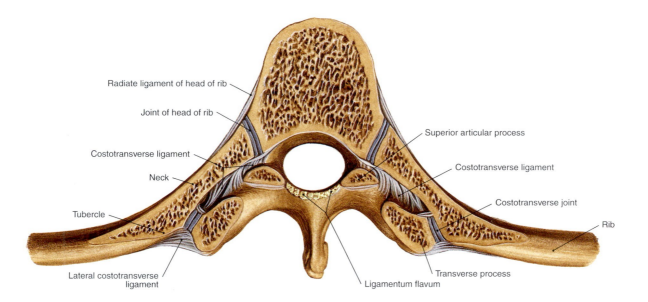

Radiate ligament of head of rib

Joint of head of rib

Costotransverse ligament

Neck

Tubercle

Lateral costotransverse ligament

Superior articular process

Costotransverse ligament

Costotransverse joint

Rib

Transverse process

Ligamentum flavum

Fig. 515 Costovertebral joints; cross-section at the level of the lower part of the joint at a head of a rib; superior view.

Ligaments of the vertebral column

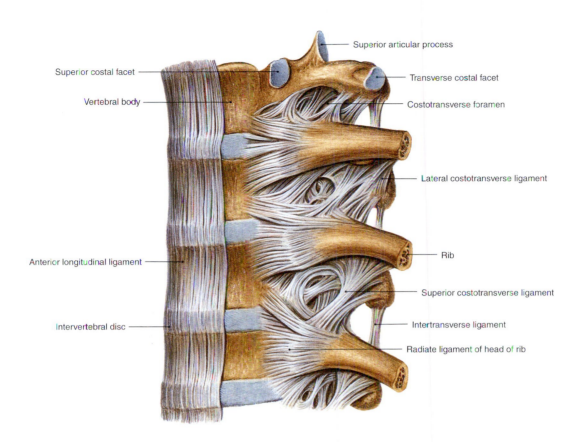

Superior articular process

Superior costal facet

Vertebral body

Transverse costal facet

Costotransverse foramen

Lateral costotransverse ligament

Anterior longitudinal ligament

Rib

Superior costotransverse ligament

Intervertebral disc

Intertransverse ligament

Radiate ligament of head of rib

Fig. 516 Ligaments of the vertebral column and the costovertebral joints;
lateral parts of the anterior longitudinal ligament have been removed;
viewed from the left.

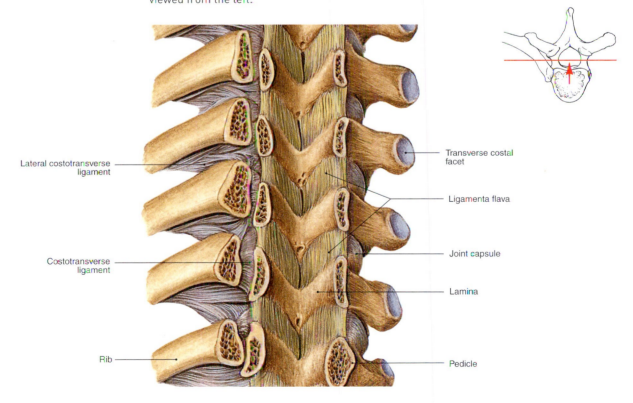

Lateral costotransverse ligament

Transverse costal facet

Ligamenta flava

Costotransverse ligament

Joint capsule

Lamina

Rib

Pedicle

Fig. 517 Junctions between the vertebral arches;
ventral view.

Costovertebral joints

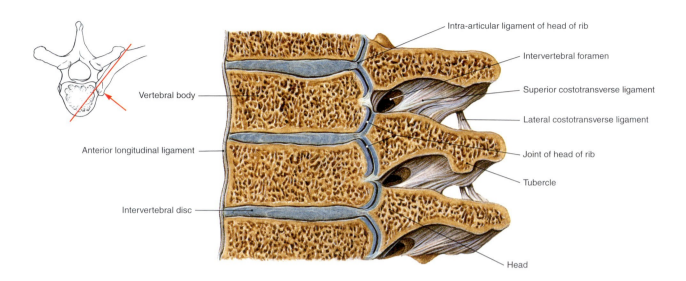

Intra-articular ligament of head of rib

Intervertebral foramen

Vertebral body

Superior costotransverse ligament

Lateral costotransverse ligament

Anterior longitudinal ligament

Joint of head of rib

Tubercle

Intervertebral disc

Head

Fig. 518 Costovertebral joints;
ventral view from the left.

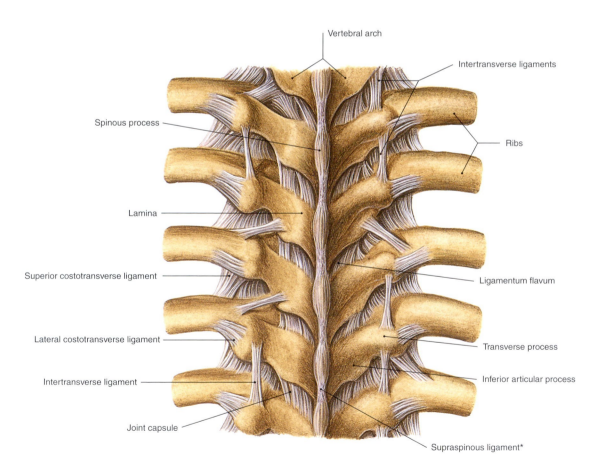

Vertebral arch

Intertransverse ligaments

Spinous process

Ribs

Lamina

Superior costotransverse ligament

Ligamentum flavum

Lateral costotransverse ligament

Transverse process

Intertransverse ligament

Inferior articular process

Joint capsule

Supraspinous ligament*

Fig. 519 Ligaments of the vertebral arches and the
costovertebral joints;
dorsal view.

* The median portion of the thoracolumbar fascia is referred to as
supraspinous ligament.

Ligaments of the lumbar part of the vertebral column

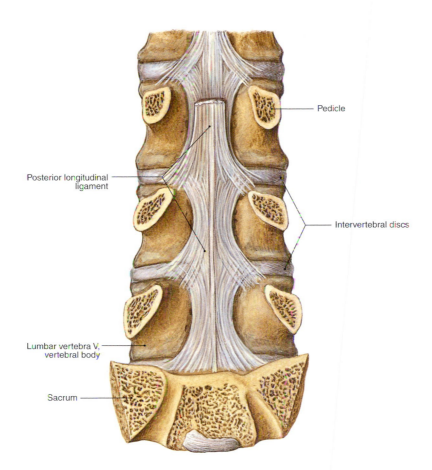

Pedicle

Posterior longitudinal ligament

Intervertebral discs

Lumbar vertebra V, vertebral body

Sacrum

Fig. 520   Ligaments of the lumbar part of the vertebral column.

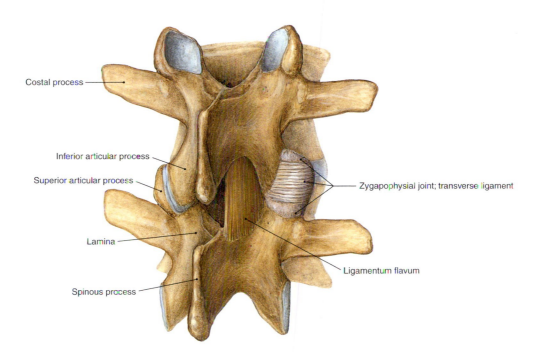

Costal process

Inferior articular process

Superior articular process

Zygapophysial joint; transverse ligament

Lamina

Ligamentum flavum

Spinous process

Fig. 521   Vertebral joints of the lumbar part of the vertebral column;
dorsal view from the right.

Reinforcement of the interarticular joints by strong and transverse fibres (transverse ligaments) is restricted to the lumbar part of the vertebral column.

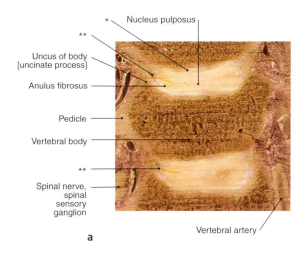

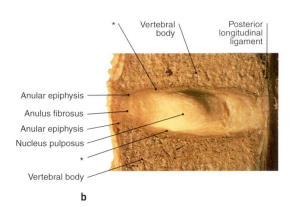

Nucleus pulposus
Uncus of body [uncinate process]
Anulus fibrosus
Pedicle
Vertebral body
Spinal nerve, spinal sensory ganglion
Vertebral artery

a

Vertebral body
Posterior longitudinal ligament
Anular epiphysis
Anulus fibrosus
Anular epiphysis
Nucleus pulposus
Vertebral body

b

Fig. 522 a, b Intervertebral discs
a Cervical intervertebral discs; frontal section
b Lumbar intervertebral disc; median section

* Hyaline cartilaginous covering of the end-plates of the vertebral bodies reflecting the non-ossified portion of the epiphyses

** In the first decade of life, so-called uncovertebral clefts develop in the lateral zones of the cervical intervertebral discs, which can progress further towards the middle in the following decades.

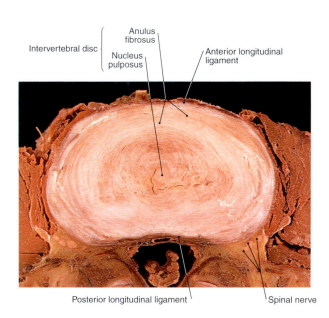

Intervertebral disc
Anulus fibrosus
Nucleus pulposus
Anterior longitudinal ligament
Posterior longitudinal ligament
Spinal nerve

Fig. 523 Lumbar intervertebral disc; superior view.

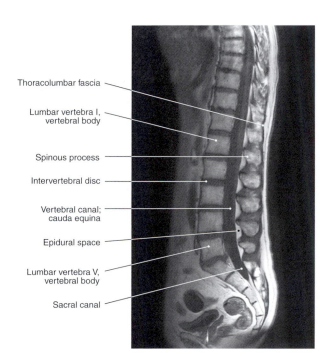

Thoracolumbar fascia
Lumbar vertebra I, vertebral body
Spinous process
Intervertebral disc
Vertebral canal; cauda equina
Epidural space
Lumbar vertebra V, vertebral body
Sacral canal

Fig. 524 Lumbar parts of the vertebral column; magnetic resonance tomographic image (MRI); median section.

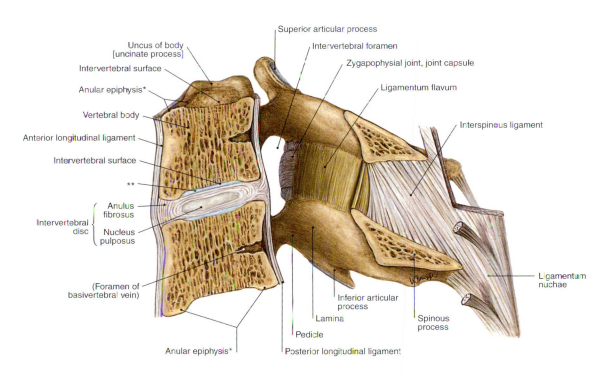

Uncus of body [uncinate process]
Intervertebral surface
Anular epiphysis*
Vertebral body
Anterior longitudinal ligament
Intervertebral surface
**
Anulus fibrosus
Intervertebral disc
Nucleus pulposus
(Foramen of basivertebral vein)
Anular epiphysis*

Superior articular process
Intervertebral foramen
Zygapophysial joint, joint capsule
Ligamentum flavum
Interspinous ligament
Ligamentum nuchae
Inferior articular process
Lamina
Spinous process
Pedicle
Posterior longitudinal ligament

Fig. 525   Cervical motion segment;
schematic median section.

* Also: rim of vertebral body
** Hyaline cartilaginous covering of the end-plate of the vertebral body
reflecting the non-ossified portion of the epiphysis

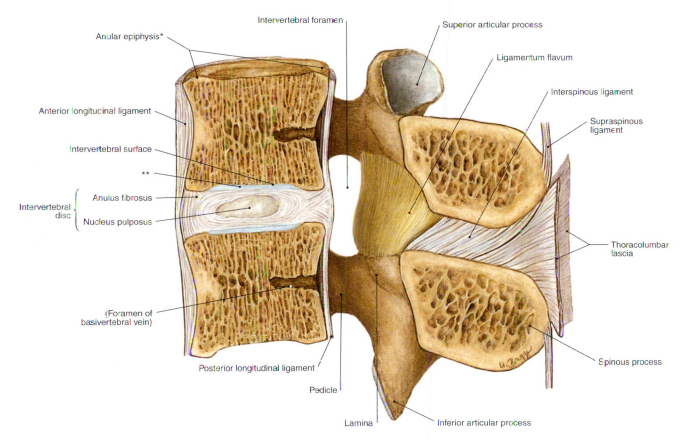

Anular epiphysis*
Anterior longitudinal ligament
Intervertebral surface
**
Anulus fibrosus
Intervertebral disc
Nucleus pulposus
(Foramen of basivertebral vein)
Posterior longitudinal ligament
Pedicle
Lamina

Intervertebral foramen
Superior articular process
Ligamentum flavum
Interspinous ligament
Supraspinous ligament
Thoracolumbar fascia
Spinous process
Inferior articular process

Fig. 526   Lumbar motion segment;
schematic median section.

* Also: rim of vertebral body
** Hyaline cartilaginous covering of the end-plate of the vertebral
body reflecting the non-ossified portion of the epiphysis

Superficial muscles of the back

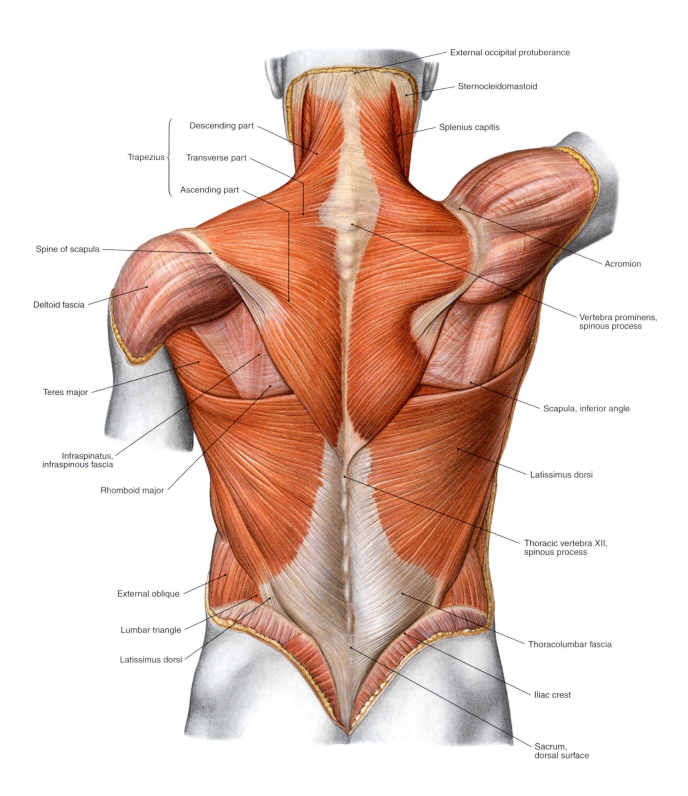

External occipital protuberance

Sternocleidomastoid

Splenius capitis

Descending part

Transverse part

Trapezius {

Ascending part

Spine of scapula

Deltoid fascia

Acromion

Vertebra prominens, spinous process

Teres major

Scapula, inferior angle

Infraspinatus, infraspinous fascia

Rhomboid major

Latissimus dorsi

Thoracic vertebra XII, spinous process

External oblique

Lumbar triangle

Latissimus dorsi

Thoracolumbar fascia

Iliac crest

Sacrum, dorsal surface

→ T 17, T 18

Fig. 527   Muscles of the back;
superficial layer of the trunk-arm and trunk-shoulder
girdle muscles.

Superficial muscles of the back

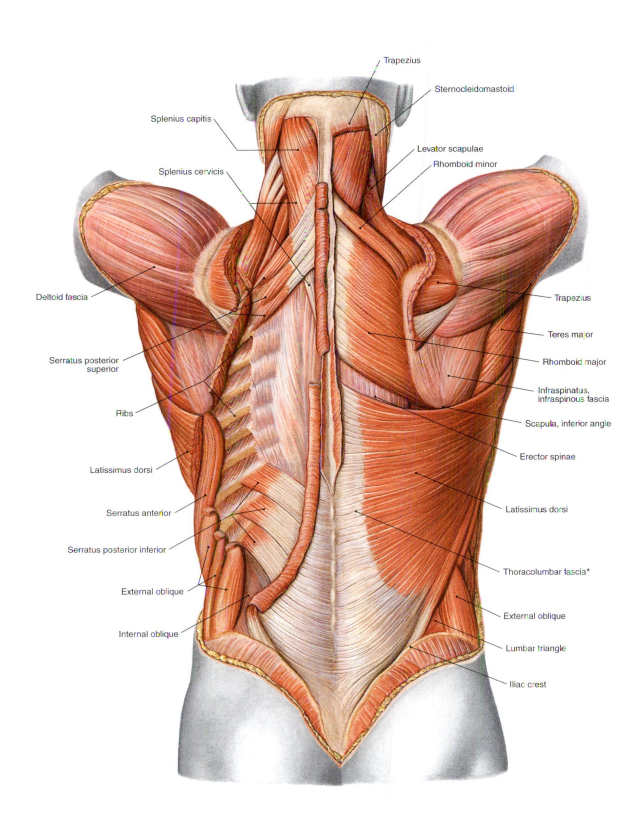

Trapezius
Sternocleidomastoid
Splenius capitis
Levator scapulae
Rhomboid minor
Splenius cervicis
Deltoid fascia
Trapezius
Teres major
Serratus posterior superior
Rhomboid major
Ribs
Infraspinatus, infraspinous fascia
Scapula, inferior angle
Erector spinae
Latissimus dorsi
Serratus anterior
Latissimus dorsi
Serratus posterior inferior
Thoracolumbar fascia*
External oblique
External oblique
Internal oblique
Lumbar triangle
Iliac crest

Fig. 528 Muscles of the back;
deep layer of the trunk-arm and trunk-shoulder
girdle muscles.

→ T 17–T 19

* The so-called thoracolumbar fascia forms a dense
aponeurosis.

Deep muscles of the back

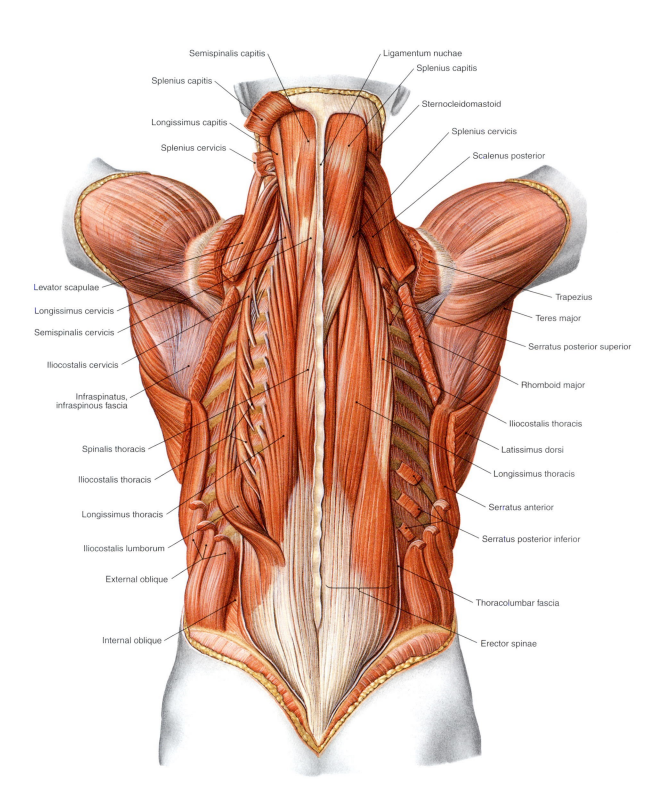

Semispinalis capitis

Splenius capitis

Longissimus capitis

Splenius cervicis

Ligamentum nuchae

Splenius capitis

Sternocleidomastoid

Splenius cervicis

Scalenus posterior

Levator scapulae

Longissimus cervicis

Semispinalis cervicis

Iliocostalis cervicis

Infraspinatus, infraspinous fascia

Spinalis thoracis

Iliocostalis thoracis

Longissimus thoracis

Iliocostalis lumborum

External oblique

Internal oblique

Trapezius

Teres major

Serratus posterior superior

Rhomboid major

Iliocostalis thoracis

Latissimus dorsi

Longissimus thoracis

Serratus anterior

Serratus posterior inferior

Thoracolumbar fascia

Erector spinae

→ T 20 a, b

Fig. 529 Muscles of the back; superficial layer of the deep (autochthonous) muscles.

Muscles of the back, sections

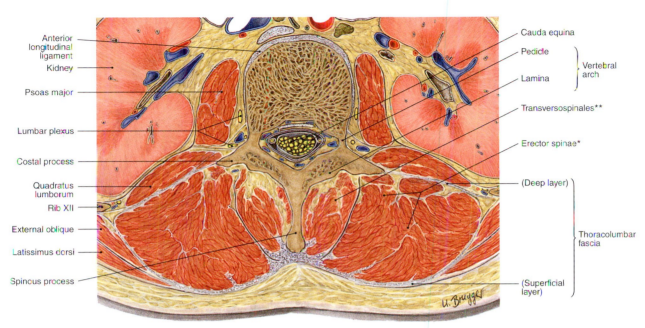

Anterior longitudinal ligament
Kidney
Psoas major
Lumbar plexus
Costal process
Quadratus lumborum
Rib XII
External oblique
Latissimus dorsi
Spinous process

Cauda equina
Pedicle ⎫ Vertebral
Lamina ⎭ arch
Transversospinales**
Erector spinae*
(Deep layer) ⎫
Thoracolumbar fascia
(Superficial layer) ⎭

U. Brugger

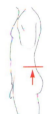

Fig. 530 Muscles of the back;
cross-section at the level of the second lumbar vertebra;
inferior view.

The deep (autochthonous) muscles of the back lie within an osteofibrous tube formed by dorsal parts of the vertebrae and the surrounding aponeurotic thoracolumbar fascia. The muscles are divided into a lateral * and a medial ** tract.

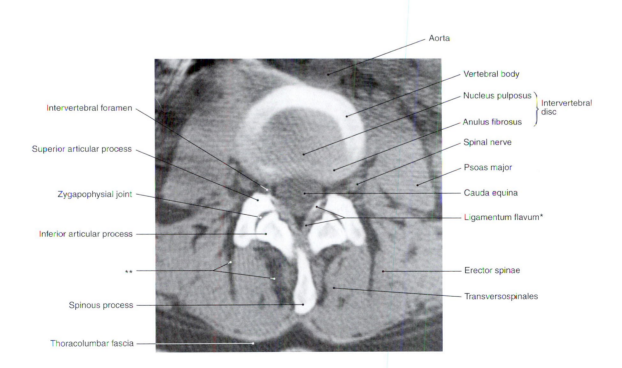

Intervertebral foramen
Superior articular process
Zygapophysial joint
Inferior articular process
**
Spinous process
Thoracolumbar fascia

Aorta
Vertebral body
Nucleus pulposus ⎫ Intervertebral
Anulus fibrosus ⎭ disc
Spinal nerve
Psoas major
Cauda equina
Ligamentum flavum*
Erector spinae
Transversospinales

Fig. 531 Muscles of the back;
computed tomographic cross-section (CT) at the level of the intervertebral disc between the third and the fourth lumbar vertebra;
inferior view.

* Calcification or ossification frequently occurs at the sites of insertion of the ligamenta flava, even in younger individuals.
** Adipose tissue deposits

Deep muscles of the back

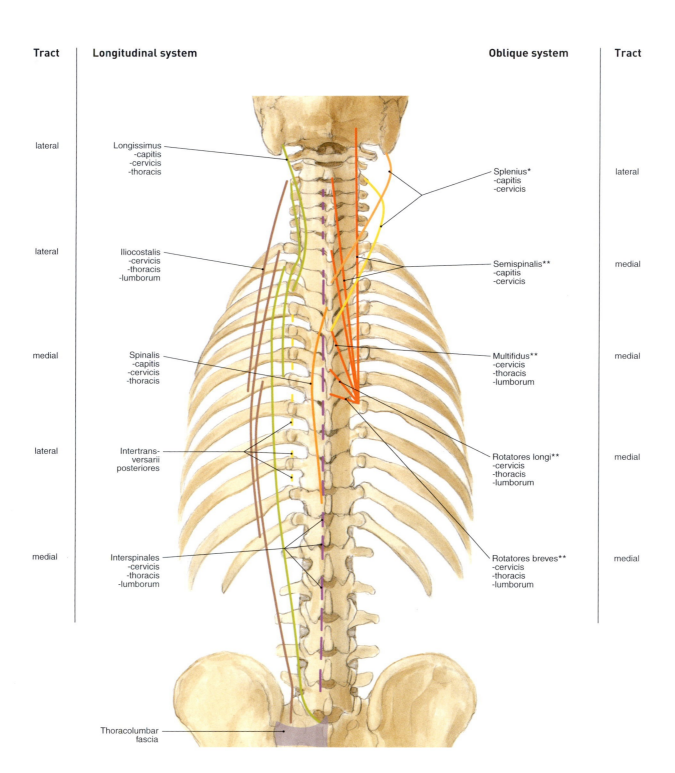

Tract	Longitudinal system		Oblique system	Tract
lateral	Longissimus -capitis -cervicis -thoracis		Splenius* -capitis -cervicis	lateral
lateral	Iliocostalis -cervicis -thoracis -lumborum		Semispinalis** -capitis -cervicis	medial
medial	Spinalis -capitis -cervicis -thoracis		Multifidus** -cervicis -thoracis -lumborum	medial
lateral	Intertrans- versarii posteriores		Rotatores longi** -cervicis -thoracis -lumborum	medial
medial	Interspinales -cervicis -thoracis -lumborum		Rotatores breves** -cervicis -thoracis -lumborum	medial
	Thoracolumbar fascia			

Fig. 532 Deep (autochthonous) muscles of the back;
diagram of the different groups of muscles.
The deep (autochthonous) muscles of the back can be
divided into a longitudinal and an oblique system, as
well as into a medial and a lateral tract.

* Spinotransverse
** Transversospinal

Deep muscles of the back

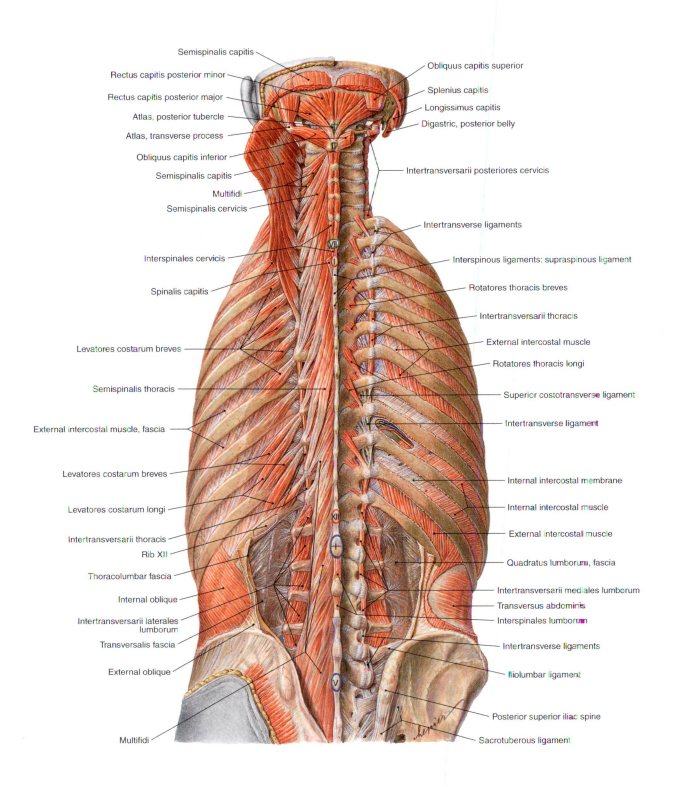

Semispinalis capitis

Rectus capitis posterior minor

Rectus capitis posterior major

Atlas, posterior tubercle

Atlas, transverse process

Obliquus capitis inferior

Semispinalis capitis

Multifidi

Semispinalis cervicis

Interspinales cervicis

Spinalis capitis

Levatores costarum breves

Semispinalis thoracis

External intercostal muscle, fascia

Levatores costarum breves

Levatores costarum longi

Intertransversarii thoracis

Rib XII

Thoracolumbar fascia

Internal oblique

Intertransversarii laterales lumborum

Transversalis fascia

External oblique

Multifidi

Obliquus capitis superior

Splenius capitis

Longissimus capitis

Digastric, posterior belly

Intertransversarii posteriores cervicis

Intertransverse ligaments

Interspinous ligaments; supraspinous ligament

Rotatores thoracis breves

Intertransversarii thoracis

External intercostal muscle

Rotatores thoracis longi

Superior costotransverse ligament

Intertransverse ligament

Internal intercostal membrane

Internal intercostal muscle

External intercostal muscle

Quadratus lumborum, fascia

Intertransversarii mediales lumborum

Transversus abdominis

Interspinales lumborum

Intertransverse ligaments

Iliolumbar ligament

Posterior superior iliac spine

Sacrotuberous ligament

Fig. 533 Muscles of the back and suboccipital muscles.

→ T 20 b, c

Deep muscles of the back

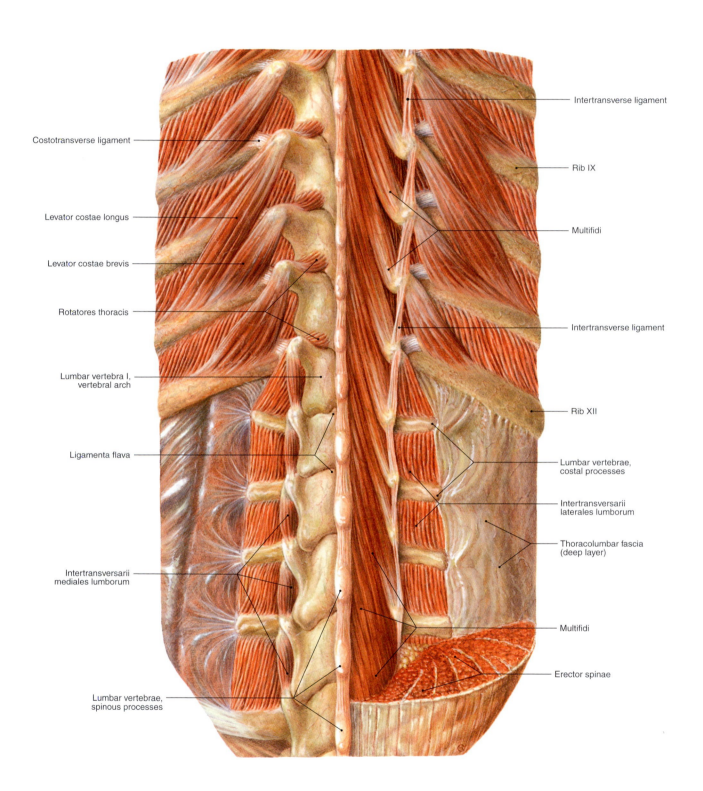

Intertransverse ligament

Costotransverse ligament

Rib IX

Levator costae longus

Multifidi

Levator costae brevis

Rotatores thoracis

Intertransverse ligament

Lumbar vertebra I,
vertebral arch

Rib XII

Ligamenta flava

Lumbar vertebrae,
costal processes

Intertransversarii
laterales lumborum

Thoracolumbar fascia
(deep layer)

Intertransversarii
mediales lumborum

Multifidi

Erector spinae

Lumbar vertebrae,
spinous processes

→ T 20 a, b

Fig. 534 Muscles of the back;
deepest layer in the region of the lower thoracic and the lumbar
part of the vertebral column.

Suboccipital muscles

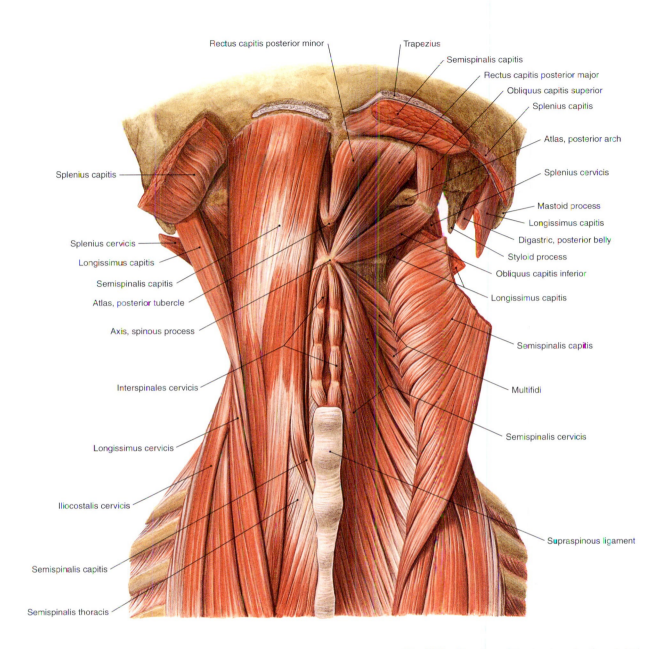

Rectus capitis posterior minor

Trapezius

Semispinalis capitis

Rectus capitis posterior major

Obliquus capitis superior

Splenius capitis

Atlas, posterior arch

Splenius cervicis

Mastoid process

Longissimus capitis

Digastric, posterior belly

Styloid process

Obliquus capitis inferior

Longissimus capitis

Semispinalis capitis

Multifidi

Semispinalis cervicis

Supraspinous ligament

Splenius capitis

Splenius cervicis

Longissimus capitis

Semispinalis capitis

Atlas, posterior tubercle

Axis, spinous process

Interspinales cervicis

Longissimus cervicis

Iliocostalis cervicis

Semispinalis capitis

Semispinalis thoracis

Fig. 535 Muscles of the back and suboccipital muscles.

→ T 20 b, c

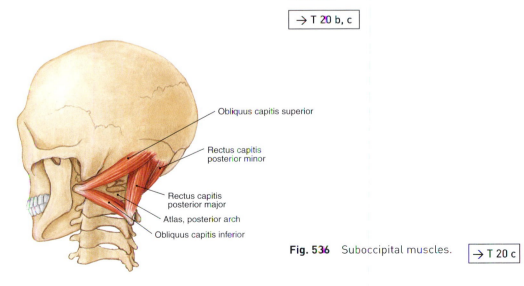

Obliquus capitis superior

Rectus capitis posterior minor

Rectus capitis posterior major

Atlas, posterior arch

Obliquus capitis inferior

Fig. 536 Suboccipital muscles. → T 20 c

Suboccipital muscles

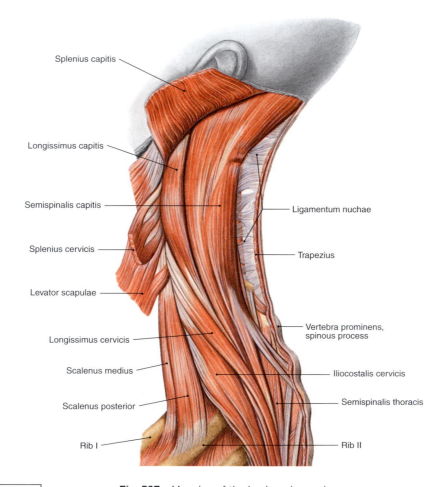

Splenius capitis

Longissimus capitis

Semispinalis capitis

Splenius cervicis

Levator scapulae

Longissimus cervicis

Scalenus medius

Scalenus posterior

Rib I

Ligamentum nuchae

Trapezius

Vertebra prominens, spinous process

Iliocostalis cervicis

Semispinalis thoracis

Rib II

→ T 20 a, b

Fig. 537 Muscles of the back and muscles of the neck.

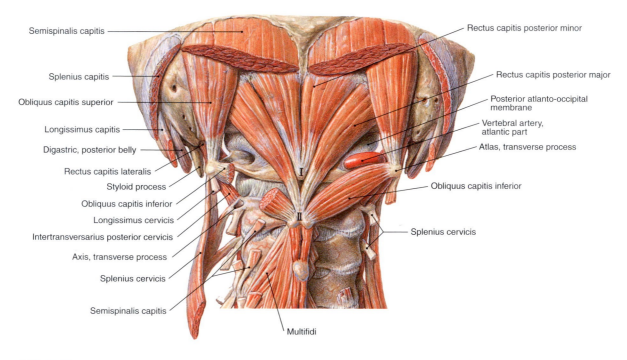

Semispinalis capitis

Splenius capitis

Obliquus capitis superior

Longissimus capitis

Digastric, posterior belly

Rectus capitis lateralis

Styloid process

Obliquus capitis inferior

Longissimus cervicis

Intertransversarius posterior cervicis

Axis, transverse process

Splenius cervicis

Semispinalis capitis

Multifidi

Rectus capitis posterior minor

Rectus capitis posterior major

Posterior atlanto-occipital membrane

Vertebral artery, atlantic part

Atlas, transverse process

Obliquus capitis inferior

Splenius cervicis

→ T 20 c

Fig. 538 Suboccipital muscles.

I = Posterior tubercle of the atlas
II = Spinous process of the axis

Vertebral column, sections

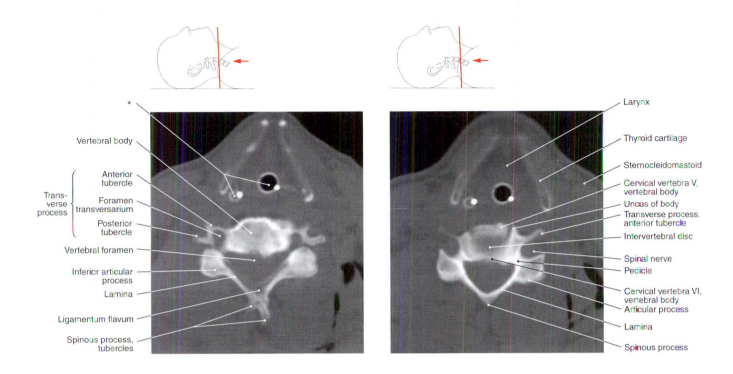

*
Vertebral body
Anterior tubercle
Transverse process { Foramen transversarium
Posterior tubercle
Vertebral foramen
Inferior articular process
Lamina
Ligamentum flavum
Spinous process, tubercles

Larynx
Thyroid cartilage
Sternocleidomastoid
Cervical vertebra V, vertebral body
Uncus of body
Transverse process, anterior tubercle
Intervertebral disc
Spinal nerve
Pedicle
Cervical vertebra VI, vertebral body
Articular process
Lamina
Spinous process

Fig. 539 Cervical part of the vertebral column; computed tomographic cross-section (CT) at the level of the intervertebral disc between the fourth and the fifth cervical vertebra.

* Endotracheal tube and endoscope

Fig. 540 Cervical part of the vertebral column; computed tomographic cross-section (CT) at the level of the fifth and the sixth cervical vertebra.

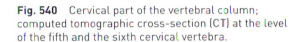

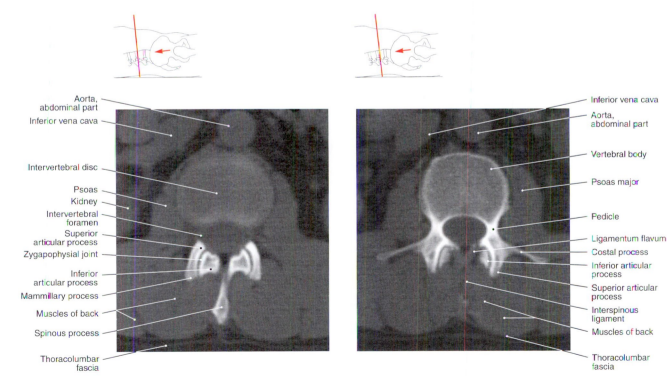

Aorta, abdominal part
Inferior vena cava
Intervertebral disc
Psoas
Kidney
Intervertebral foramen
Superior articular process
Zygapophysial joint
Inferior articular process
Mammillary process
Muscles of back
Spinous process
Thoracolumbar fascia

Inferior vena cava
Aorta, abdominal part
Vertebral body
Psoas major
Pedicle
Ligamentum flavum
Costal process
Inferior articular process
Superior articular process
Interspinous ligament
Muscles of back
Thoracolumbar fascia

Fig. 541 Lumbar part of the vertebral column; computed tomographic cross-section (CT) at the level of the intervertebral disc between the second and the third lumbar vertebra.

Fig. 542 Lumbar part of the vertebral column; computed tomographic cross-section (CT) at the level of the pedicles of the third lumbar vertebra.

Cutaneous innervation

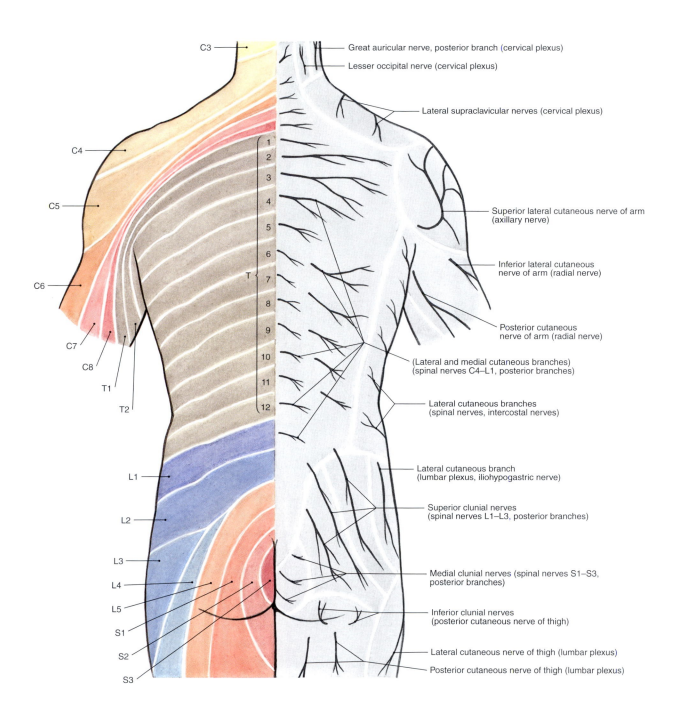

C3 — Great auricular nerve, posterior branch (cervical plexus)

Lesser occipital nerve (cervical plexus)

Lateral supraclavicular nerves (cervical plexus)

C4

C5

Superior lateral cutaneous nerve of arm
(axillary nerve)

Inferior lateral cutaneous
nerve of arm (radial nerve)

C6

Posterior cutaneous
nerve of arm (radial nerve)

C7

C8

(Lateral and medial cutaneous branches)
(spinal nerves C4–L1, posterior branches)

T1

T2

Lateral cutaneous branches
(spinal nerves, intercostal nerves)

Lateral cutaneous branch
(lumbar plexus, iliohypogastric nerve)

L1

L2

Superior clunial nerves
(spinal nerves L1–L3, posterior branches)

L3

L4

L5

Medial clunial nerves (spinal nerves S1–S3,
posterior branches)

S1

Inferior clunial nerves
(posterior cutaneous nerve of thigh)

S2

Lateral cutaneous nerve of thigh (lumbar plexus)

Posterior cutaneous nerve of thigh (lumbar plexus)

S3

Fig. 543 Segmental cutaneous innervation (dermatomes)
and cutaneous nerves of the back.

Vessels and nerves of the back

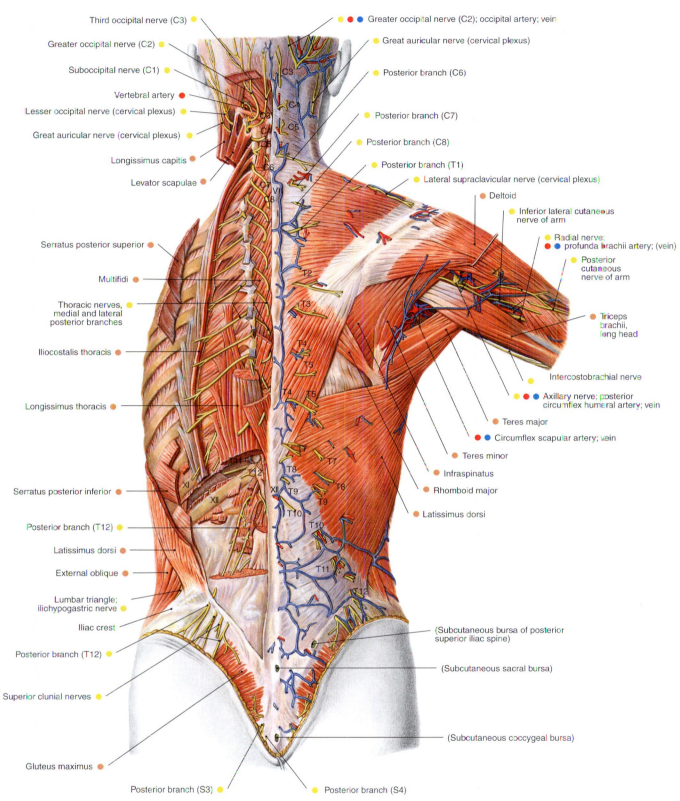

Third occipital nerve (C3)

Greater occipital nerve (C2)

Suboccipital nerve (C1)

Vertebral artery ●

Lesser occipital nerve (cervical plexus)

Great auricular nerve (cervical plexus)

Longissimus capitis

Levator scapulae

Serratus posterior superior

Multifidi

Thoracic nerves,
medial and lateral
posterior branches

Iliocostalis thoracis

Longissimus thoracis

Serratus posterior inferior

Posterior branch (T12)

Latissimus dorsi

External oblique

Lumbar triangle;
iliohypogastric nerve

Iliac crest

Posterior branch (T12)

Superior clunial nerves

Gluteus maximus

Posterior branch (S3)

●● ● Greater occipital nerve (C2); occipital artery; vein

Great auricular nerve (cervical plexus)

Posterior branch (C6)

Posterior branch (C7)

Posterior branch (C8)

Posterior branch (T1)

Lateral supraclavicular nerve (cervical plexus)

Deltoid

Inferior lateral cutaneous
nerve of arm

Radial nerve;
●● ● profunda brachii artery; (vein)

Posterior
cutaneous
nerve of arm

Triceps
brachii,
long head

Intercostobrachial nerve

●● ● Axillary nerve; posterior
circumflex humeral artery; vein

Teres major

●● Circumflex scapular artery; vein

Teres minor

Infraspinatus

Rhomboid major

Latissimus dorsi

(Subcutaneous bursa of posterior
superior iliac spine)

(Subcutaneous sacral bursa)

(Subcutaneous coccygeal bursa)

Posterior branch (S4)

545
546

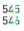

Fig. 544 Vessels and nerves of the back.

* Vessels and nerves of the triangular space
** Vessels and nerves of the quadrangular space

Vessels and nerves of the posterior cervical region

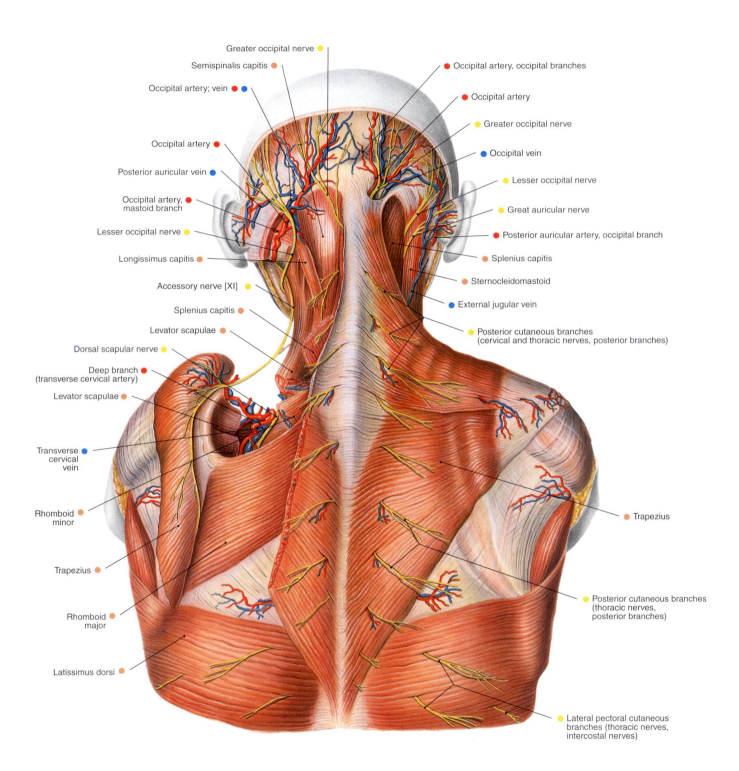

Greater occipital nerve ●
Semispinalis capitis ●
Occipital artery; vein ● ●
Occipital artery ●
Posterior auricular vein ●
Occipital artery, mastoid branch ●
Lesser occipital nerve ●
Longissimus capitis ●
Accessory nerve [XI] ●
Splenius capitis ●
Levator scapulae ●
Dorsal scapular nerve ●
Deep branch (transverse cervical artery) ●
Levator scapulae ●
Transverse cervical vein ●
Rhomboid minor ●
Trapezius ●
Rhomboid major ●
Latissimus dorsi ●

● Occipital artery, occipital branches
● Occipital artery
● Greater occipital nerve
● Occipital vein
● Lesser occipital nerve
● Great auricular nerve
● Posterior auricular artery, occipital branch
● Splenius capitis
● Sternocleidomastoid
● External jugular vein
● Posterior cutaneous branches (cervical and thoracic nerves, posterior branches)
● Trapezius
● Posterior cutaneous branches (thoracic nerves, posterior branches)
● Lateral pectoral cutaneous branches (thoracic nerves, intercostal nerves)

546
544

Fig. 545 Vessels and nerves of the occipital region, the posterior cervical region and the upper back.

Vessels and nerves of the posterior cervical region

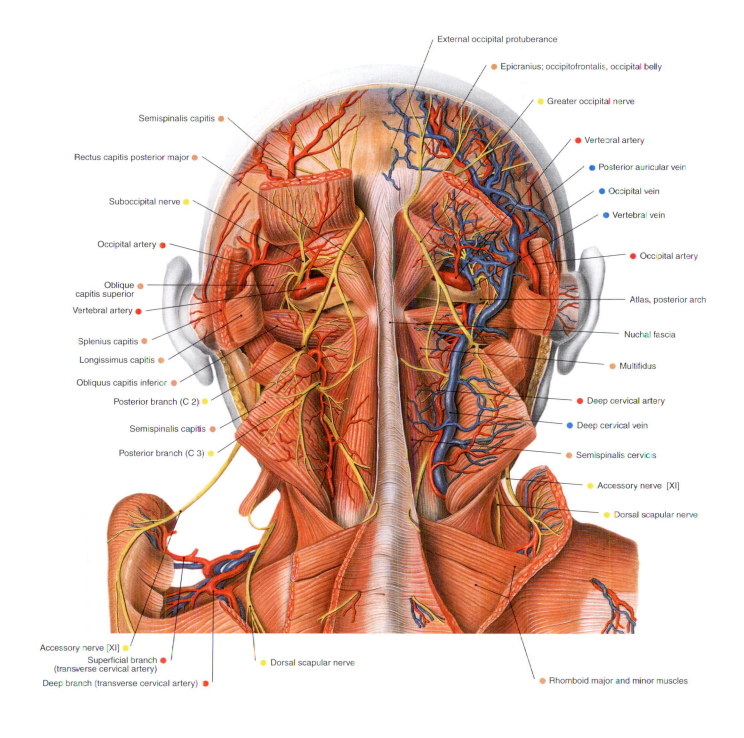

External occipital protuberance

● Epicranius; occipitofrontalis, occipital belly

● Greater occipital nerve

● Vertebral artery

● Posterior auricular vein

● Occipital vein

● Vertebral vein

● Occipital artery

Atlas, posterior arch

Nuchal fascia

● Multifidus

● Deep cervical artery

● Deep cervical vein

● Semispinalis cervicis

● Accessory nerve [XI]

● Dorsal scapular nerve

● Rhomboid major and minor muscles

Semispinalis capitis ●

Rectus capitis posterior major ●

Suboccipital nerve ●

Occipital artery ●

Oblique ● capitis superior

Vertebral artery ●

Splenius capitis ●

Longissimus capitis ●

Obliquus capitis inferior ●

Posterior branch (C 2) ●

Semispinalis capitis ●

Posterior branch (C 3) ●

Accessory nerve [XI] ●
Superficial branch ● (transverse cervical artery)
Deep branch (transverse cervical artery) ●

● Dorsal scapular nerve

Fig. 546   Vessels and nerves of the occipital region
and the posterior cervical region.

547

545

Cervical part of the vertebral canal

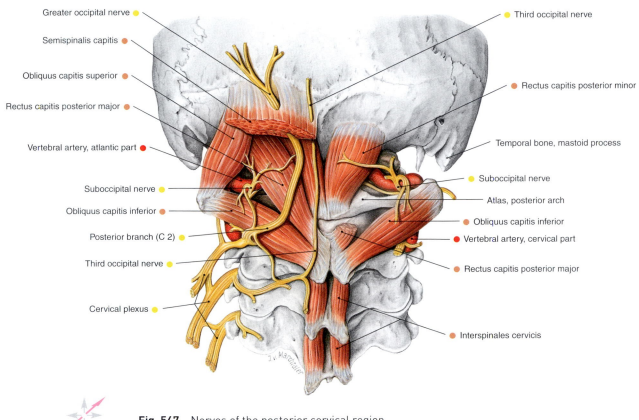

Greater occipital nerve

Semispinalis capitis

Obliquus capitis superior

Rectus capitis posterior major

Vertebral artery, atlantic part

Suboccipital nerve

Obliquus capitis inferior

Posterior branch (C 2)

Third occipital nerve

Cervical plexus

Third occipital nerve

Rectus capitis posterior minor

Temporal bone, mastoid process

Suboccipital nerve

Atlas, posterior arch

Obliquus capitis inferior

Vertebral artery, cervical part

Rectus capitis posterior major

Interspinales cervicis

Fig. 547 Nerves of the posterior cervical region and the vertebral artery.

546

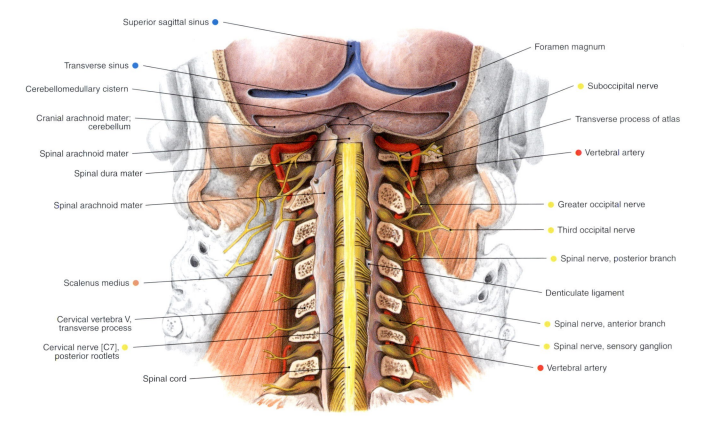

Superior sagittal sinus

Transverse sinus

Cerebellomedullary cistern

Cranial arachnoid mater; cerebellum

Spinal arachnoid mater

Spinal dura mater

Spinal arachnoid mater

Scalenus medius

Cervical vertebra V, transverse process

Cervical nerve [C7], posterior rootlets

Spinal cord

Foramen magnum

Suboccipital nerve

Transverse process of atlas

Vertebral artery

Greater occipital nerve

Third occipital nerve

Spinal nerve, posterior branch

Denticulate ligament

Spinal nerve, anterior branch

Spinal nerve, sensory ganglion

Vertebral artery

Fig. 548 Vessels and nerves of the deep posterior cervical region and the content of the vertebral canal.

Lumbar part of the vertebral canal

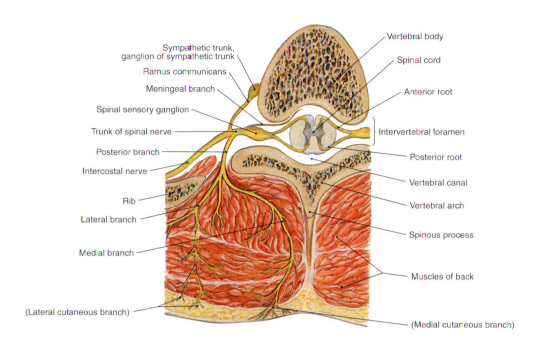

Sympathetic trunk, ganglion of sympathetic trunk
Ramus communicans
Meningeal branch
Spinal sensory ganglion
Trunk of spinal nerve
Posterior branch
Intercostal nerve
Rib
Lateral branch
Medial branch
(Lateral cutaneous branch)

Vertebral body
Spinal cord
Anterior root
Intervertebral foramen
Posterior root
Vertebral canal
Vertebral arch
Spinous process
Muscles of back
(Medial cutaneous branch)

Fig. 549 Spinal nerve; in the thoracic region.

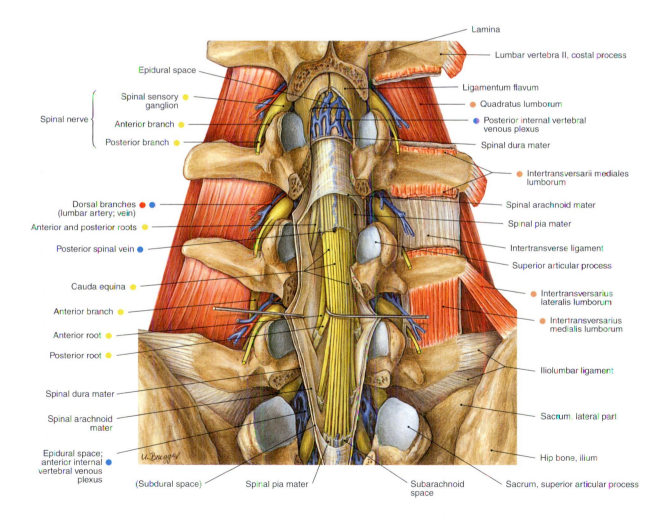

Epidural space
Spinal sensory ganglion
Anterior branch
Posterior branch
Spinal nerve
Dorsal branches (lumbar artery; vein)
Anterior and posterior roots
Posterior spinal vein
Cauda equina
Anterior branch
Anterior root
Posterior root
Spinal dura mater
Spinal arachnoid mater
Epidural space; anterior internal vertebral venous plexus
(Subdural space)
Spinal pia mater

Lamina
Lumbar vertebra II, costal process
Ligamentum flavum
Quadratus lumborum
Posterior internal vertebral venous plexus
Spinal dura mater
Intertransversarii mediales lumborum
Spinal arachnoid mater
Spinal pia mater
Intertransverse ligament
Superior articular process
Intertransversarius lateralis lumborum
Intertransversarius medialis lumborum
Iliolumbar ligament
Sacrum, lateral part
Hip bone, ilium
Subarachnoid space
Sacrum, superior articular process

U. Brügger

Fig. 550 Vessels and nerves of the lumbar part of the vertebral canal.

Veins and nerves of the lumbar part of the vertebral column

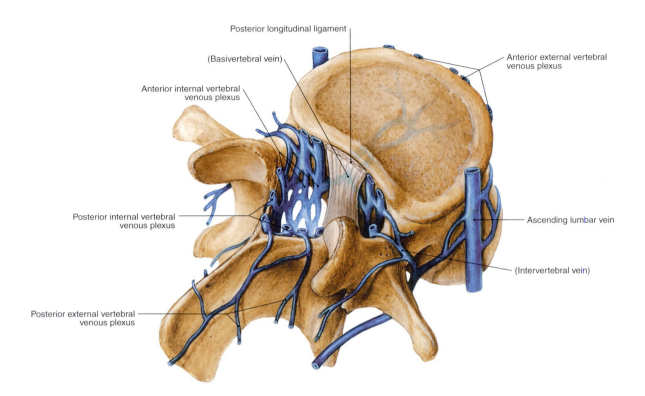

Posterior longitudinal ligament

(Basivertebral vein)

Anterior internal vertebral
venous plexus

Posterior internal vertebral
venous plexus

Posterior external vertebral
venous plexus

Anterior external vertebral
venous plexus

Ascending lumbar vein

(Intervertebral vein)

Fig. 551   Veins of the vertebral canal;
venous plexus.

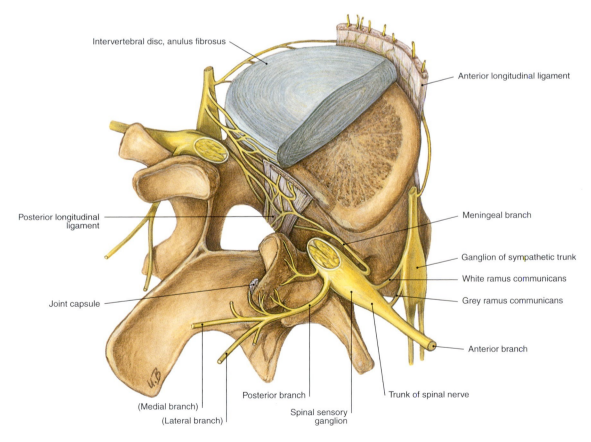

Intervertebral disc, anulus fibrosus

Anterior longitudinal ligament

Posterior longitudinal
ligament

Meningeal branch

Ganglion of sympathetic trunk

White ramus communicans

Grey ramus communicans

Joint capsule

Anterior branch

Trunk of spinal nerve

Posterior branch

(Medial branch)

(Lateral branch)

Spinal sensory
ganglion

Fig. 552   Nerves of the vertebral column;
somatic and autonomous innervation.

Vessels and nerves of the vertebral canal

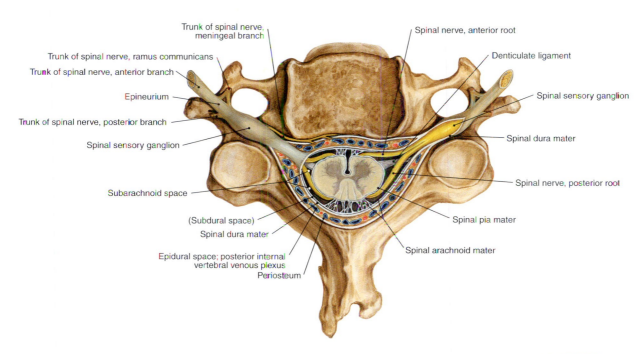

Trunk of spinal nerve, meningeal branch

Trunk of spinal nerve, ramus communicans

Trunk of spinal nerve, anterior branch

Epineurium

Trunk of spinal nerve, posterior branch

Spinal sensory ganglion

Subarachnoid space

(Subdural space)

Spinal dura mater

Epidural space; posterior internal vertebral venous plexus

Periosteum

Spinal nerve, anterior root

Denticulate ligament

Spinal sensory ganglion

Spinal dura mater

Spinal nerve, posterior root

Spinal pia mater

Spinal arachnoid mater

Fig. 553 Content of the vertebral canal; cross-section at the level of the fifth cervical vertebra.

→ 1304 ff

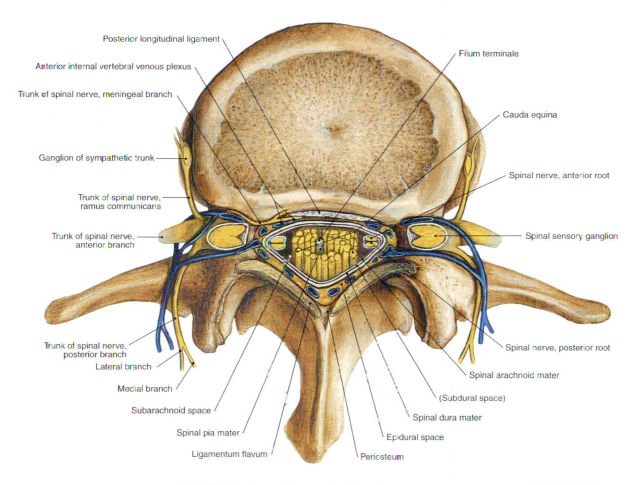

Posterior longitudinal ligament

Anterior internal vertebral venous plexus

Trunk of spinal nerve, meningeal branch

Ganglion of sympathetic trunk

Trunk of spinal nerve, ramus communicans

Trunk of spinal nerve, anterior branch

Trunk of spinal nerve, posterior branch

Lateral branch

Medial branch

Subarachnoid space

Spinal pia mater

Ligamentum flavum

Filum terminale

Cauda equina

Spinal nerve, anterior root

Spinal sensory ganglion

Spinal nerve, posterior root

Spinal arachnoid mater

(Subdural space)

Spinal dura mater

Epidural space

Periosteum

Fig. 554 Content of the vertebral canal; cross-section at the level of the third lumbar vertebra.

→ 1304 ff

Lumbar and sacral puncture

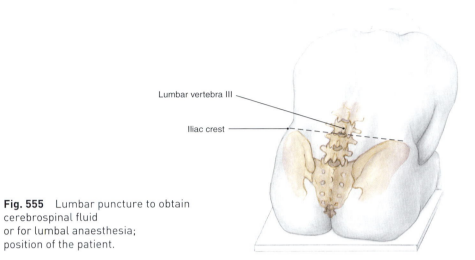

Fig. 555 Lumbar puncture to obtain cerebrospinal fluid or for lumbal anaesthesia; position of the patient.

Lumbar vertebra III

Iliac crest

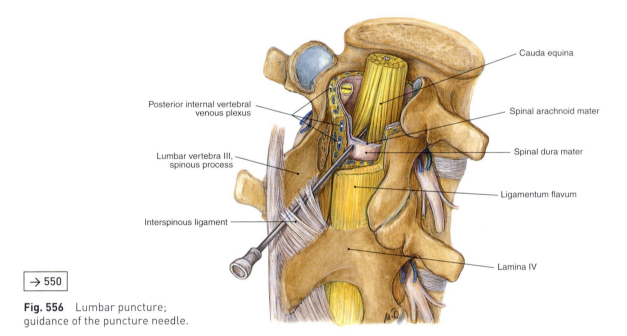

Cauda equina

Posterior internal vertebral venous plexus

Spinal arachnoid mater

Lumbar vertebra III, spinous process

Spinal dura mater

Interspinous ligament

Ligamentum flavum

Lamina IV

→ 550

Fig. 556 Lumbar puncture; guidance of the puncture needle.

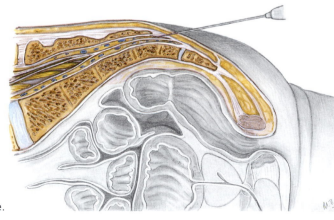

Fig. 557 Sacral puncture; guidance of the puncture needle.

Vessels and nerves of the vertebral canal

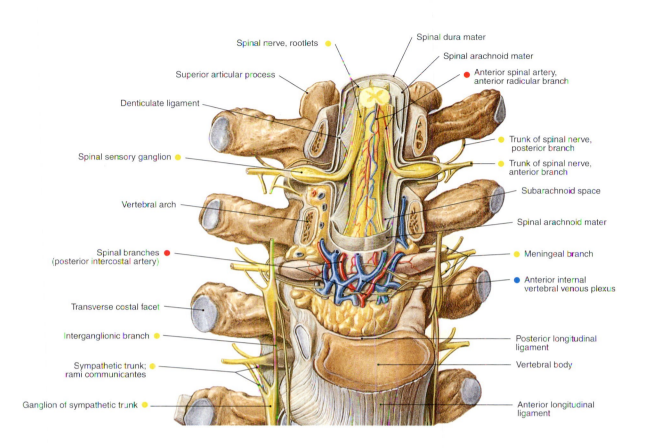

Spinal nerve, rootlets
Spinal dura mater
Superior articular process
Spinal arachnoid mater
Anterior spinal artery, anterior radicular branch
Denticulate ligament
Trunk of spinal nerve, posterior branch
Spinal sensory ganglion
Trunk of spinal nerve, anterior branch
Subarachnoid space
Vertebral arch
Spinal arachnoid mater
Spinal branches (posterior intercostal artery)
Meningeal branch
Anterior internal vertebral venous plexus
Transverse costal facet
Interganglionic branch
Posterior longitudinal ligament
Sympathetic trunk; rami communicantes
Vertebral body
Ganglion of sympathetic trunk
Anterior longitudinal ligament

Fig. 558 Content of the vertebral canal; thoracic portion after stepwise exposure; ventral view.

→ 1304 ff

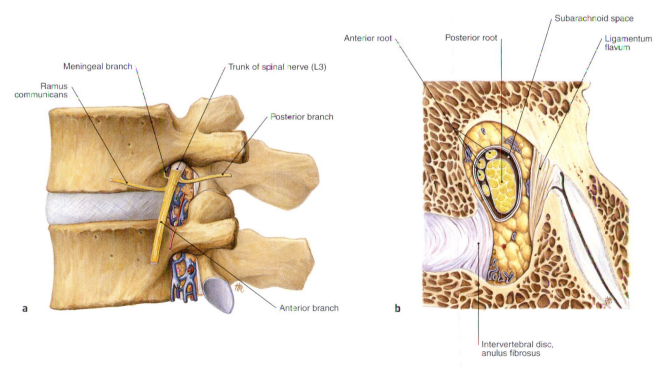

Meningeal branch
Ramus communicans
Trunk of spinal nerve (L3)
Posterior branch
Anterior root
Posterior root
Subarachnoid space
Ligamentum flavum
Anterior branch
Intervertebral disc, anulus fibrosus

a
b

Fig. 559 a, b Intervertebral foramina; lumbar part of the vertebral column.

a Viewed from the left
b Sagittal section

Surface anatomy

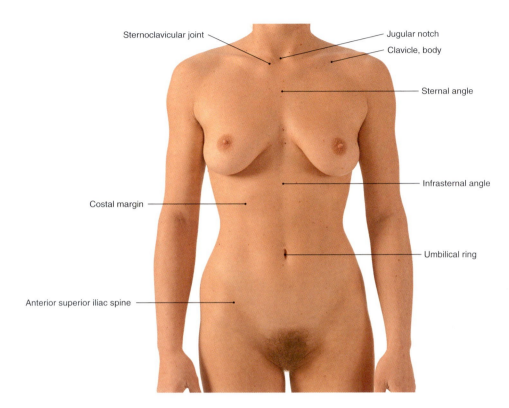

Sternoclavicular joint

Jugular notch

Clavicle, body

Sternal angle

Infrasternal angle

Costal margin

Umbilical ring

Anterior superior iliac spine

Fig. 560 Surface anatomy of the thoracic and abdominal wall of a young woman.

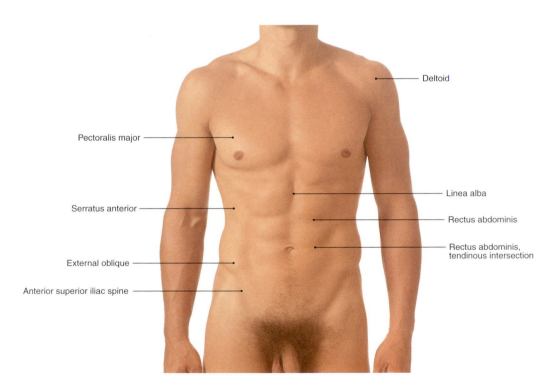

Deltoid

Pectoralis major

Linea alba

Serratus anterior

Rectus abdominis

Rectus abdominis, tendinous intersection

External oblique

Anterior superior iliac spine

Fig. 561 Surface anatomy of the thoracic and abdominal wall of a young man.

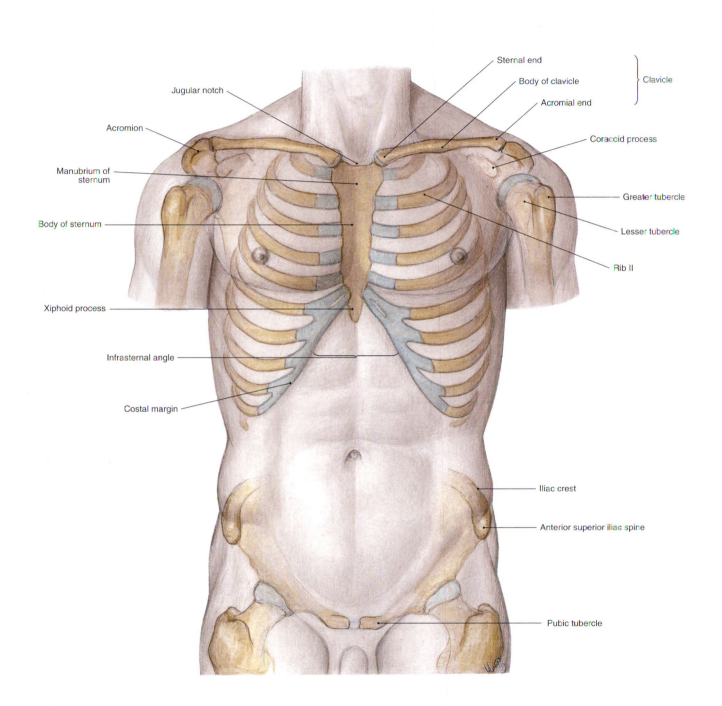

Sternal end

Body of clavicle

Acromial end

Clavicle

Jugular notch

Acromion

Coracoid process

Manubrium of
sternum

Greater tubercle

Body of sternum

Lesser tubercle

Rib II

Xiphoid process

Infrasternal angle

Costal margin

Iliac crest

Anterior superior iliac spine

Pubic tubercle

Fig. 562   Projection of the skeleton
onto the thoracic and abdominal wall.

Skeleton of the trunk

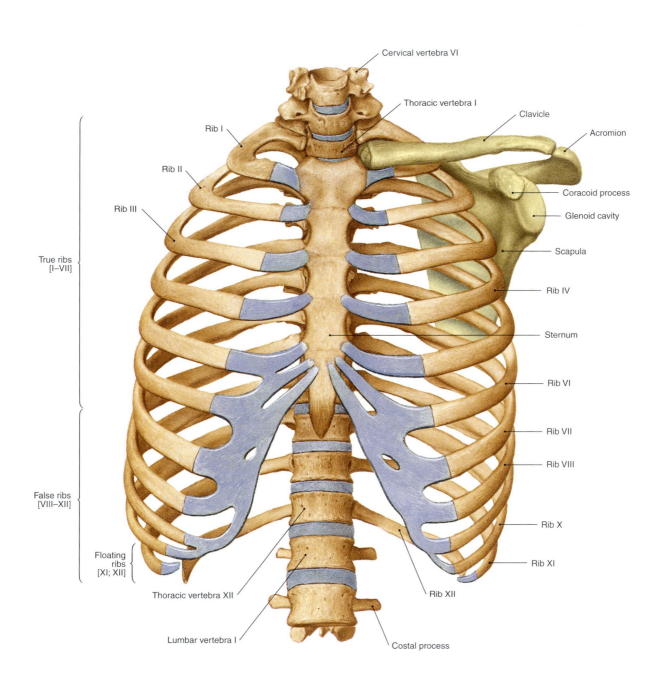

Cervical vertebra VI

Thoracic vertebra I

Clavicle

Acromion

Rib I

Rib II

Coracoid process

Rib III

Glenoid cavity

Scapula

True ribs
[I–VII]

Rib IV

Sternum

Rib VI

Rib VII

Rib VIII

False ribs
[VIII–XII]

Rib X

Floating
ribs
[XI; XII]

Rib XI

Thoracic vertebra XII

Rib XII

Lumbar vertebra I

Costal process

Fig. 563 Thoracic cage and
left shoulder girdle.

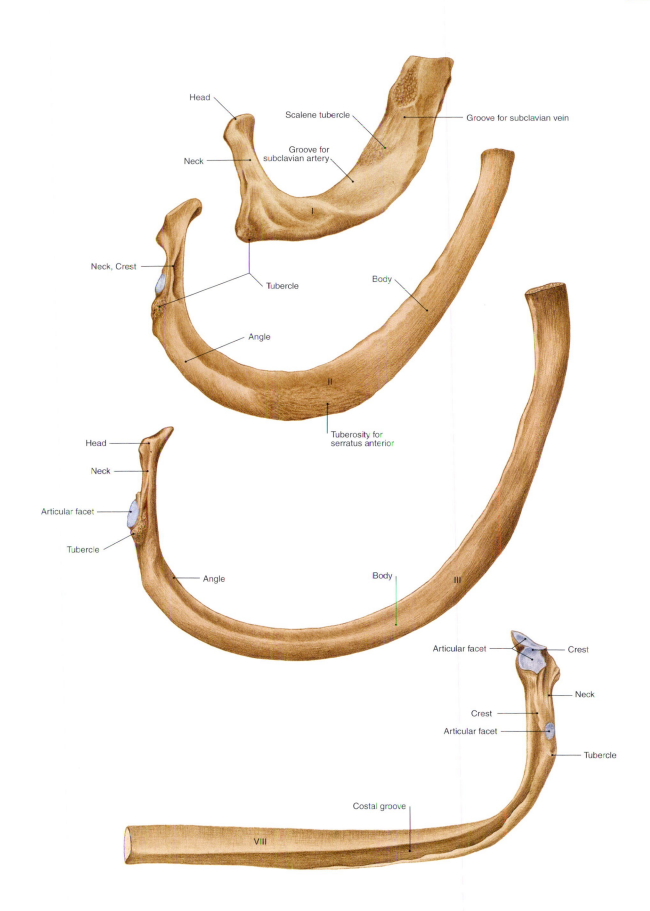

Head

Scalene tubercle

Groove for subclavian vein

Neck

Groove for subclavian artery

I

Neck, Crest

Tubercle

Body

Angle

II

Tuberosity for serratus anterior

Head

Neck

Articular facet

Tubercle

Angle

Body

III

Articular facet

Crest

Neck

Crest

Articular facet

Tubercle

Costal groove

VIII

Fig. 564 Ribs;
I.–III. rib, superior view;
VIII. rib, inferior view.

Sternum

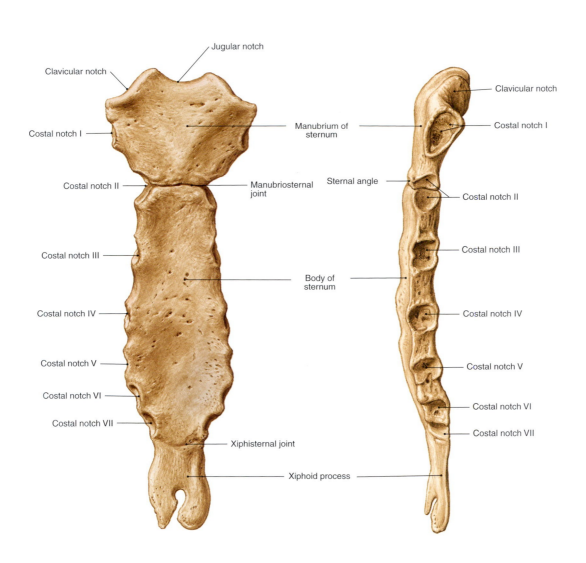

Clavicular notch	Jugular notch
Costal notch I	Manubrium of sternum
Costal notch II	Manubriosternal joint
Costal notch III	Body of sternum
Costal notch IV	
Costal notch V	
Costal notch VI	
Costal notch VII	Xiphisternal joint
	Xiphoid process

Clavicular notch — Costal notch I — Sternal angle — Costal notch II — Costal notch III — Costal notch IV — Costal notch V — Costal notch VI — Costal notch VII

Fig. 565 Sternum.   **Fig. 566** Sternum.

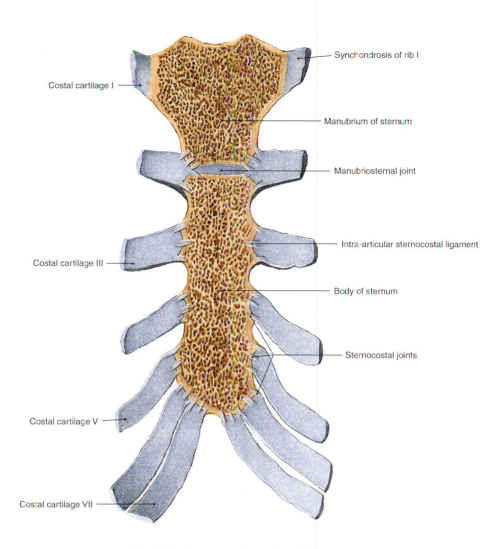

Synchondrosis of rib I

Costal cartilage I

Manubrium of sternum

Manubriosternal joint

Intra-articular sternocostal ligament

Costal cartilage III

Body of sternum

Sternocostal joints

Costal cartilage V

Costal cartilage VII

Fig. 567 Sternum and costal cartilages; section.

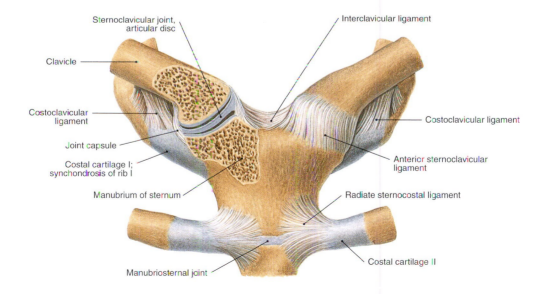

Sternoclavicular joint, articular disc

Interclavicular ligament

Clavicle

Costoclavicular ligament

Joint capsule

Costoclavicular ligament

Costal cartilage I; synchondrosis of rib I

Anterior sternoclavicular ligament

Manubrium of sternum

Radiate sternocostal ligament

Manubriosternal joint

Costal cartilage II

Fig. 568 Sternoclavicular joint.

Muscles of the thoracic and the abdominal wall

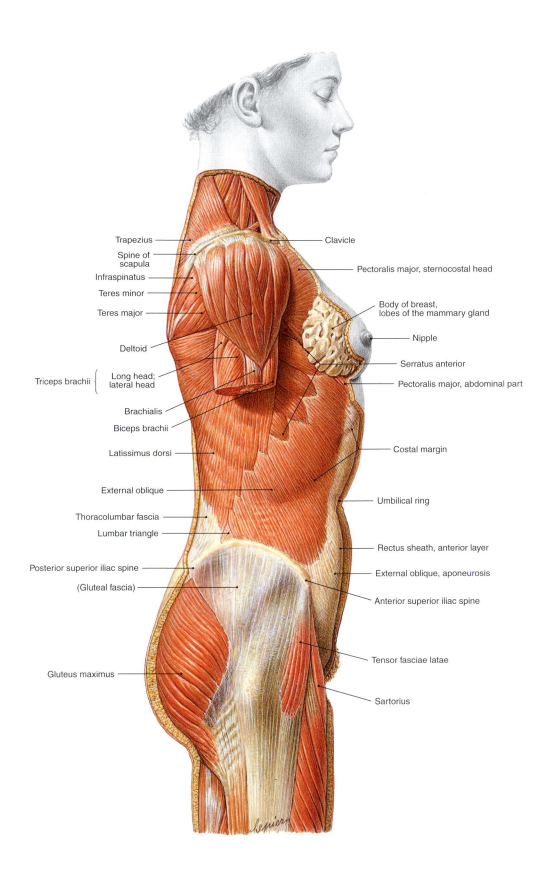

Trapezius

Spine of scapula

Infraspinatus

Teres minor

Teres major

Deltoid

Triceps brachii { Long head; lateral head

Brachialis

Biceps brachii

Latissimus dorsi

External oblique

Thoracolumbar fascia

Lumbar triangle

Posterior superior iliac spine

(Gluteal fascia)

Gluteus maximus

Clavicle

Pectoralis major, sternocostal head

Body of breast, lobes of the mammary gland

Nipple

Serratus anterior

Pectoralis major, abdominal part

Costal margin

Umbilical ring

Rectus sheath, anterior layer

External oblique, aponeurosis

Anterior superior iliac spine

Tensor fasciae latae

Sartorius

→ T 15, T 17, T 18, T 26   **Fig. 569** Muscles of the thoracic and the abdominal wall.

Muscles of the thoracic and the abdominal wall

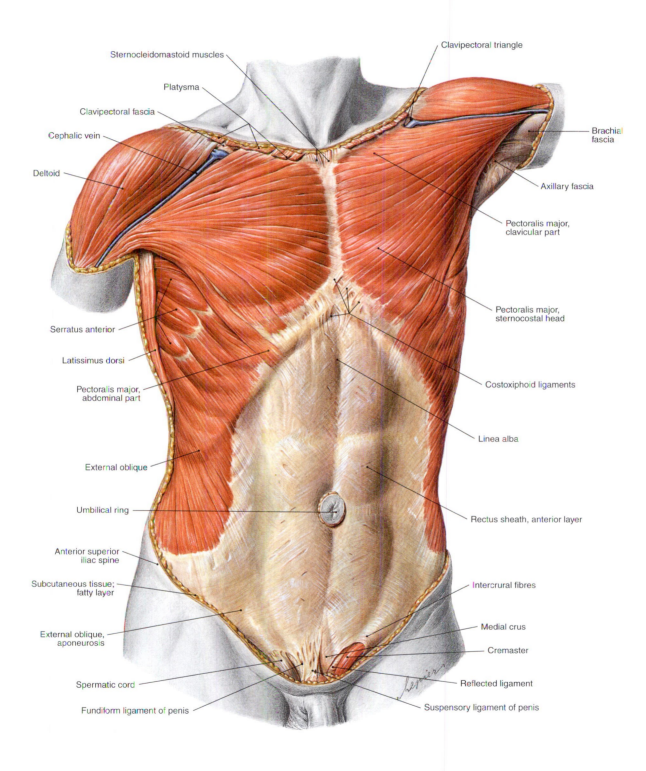

Sternocleidomastoid muscles

Platysma

Clavipectoral fascia

Cephalic vein

Deltoid

Serratus anterior

Latissimus dorsi

Pectoralis major, abdominal part

External oblique

Umbilical ring

Anterior superior iliac spine

Subcutaneous tissue; fatty layer

External oblique, aponeurosis

Spermatic cord

Fundiform ligament of penis

Clavipectoral triangle

Brachial fascia

Axillary fascia

Pectoralis major, clavicular part

Pectoralis major, sternocostal head

Costoxiphoid ligaments

Linea alba

Rectus sheath, anterior layer

Intercrural fibres

Medial crus

Cremaster

Reflected ligament

Suspensory ligament of penis

Fig. 570 Muscles of the thoracic and the abdominal wall; superficial layer.

→ T 15, T 17, T 18, T 26

Muscles of the thoracic and the abdominal wall

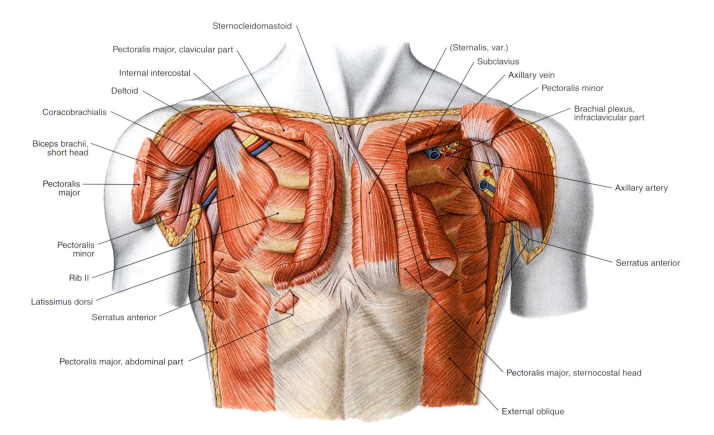

Sternocleidomastoid

Pectoralis major, clavicular part

Internal intercostal

Deltoid

Coracobrachialis

Biceps brachii, short head

Pectoralis major

Pectoralis minor

Rib II

Latissimus dorsi

Serratus anterior

Pectoralis major, abdominal part

(Sternalis, var.)

Subclavius

Axillary vein

Pectoralis minor

Brachial plexus, infraclavicular part

Axillary artery

Serratus anterior

Pectoralis major, sternocostal head

External oblique

→ T 13, T 15, T 26   **Fig. 571**   Muscles of the thoracic wall.

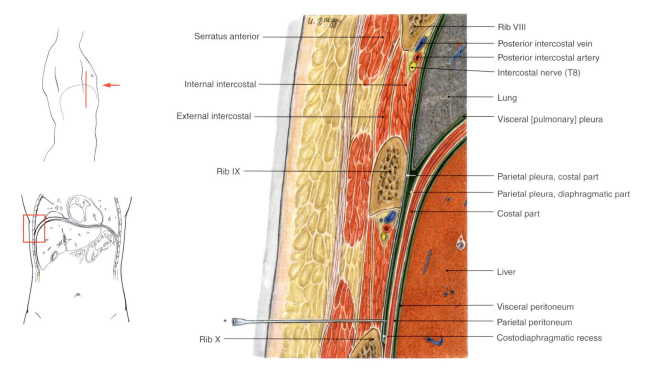

Serratus anterior

Internal intercostal

External intercostal

Rib IX

Rib X

Rib VIII

Posterior intercostal vein

Posterior intercostal artery

Intercostal nerve (T8)

Lung

Visceral [pulmonary] pleura

Parietal pleura, costal part

Parietal pleura, diaphragmatic part

Costal part

Liver

Visceral peritoneum

Parietal peritoneum

Costodiaphragmatic recess

→ T 13   **Fig. 572**   Muscles of the thoracic wall; frontal section.

*   Position of the needle for puncture of the pleural cavity (pleurocentesis)

Muscles of the thoracic wall

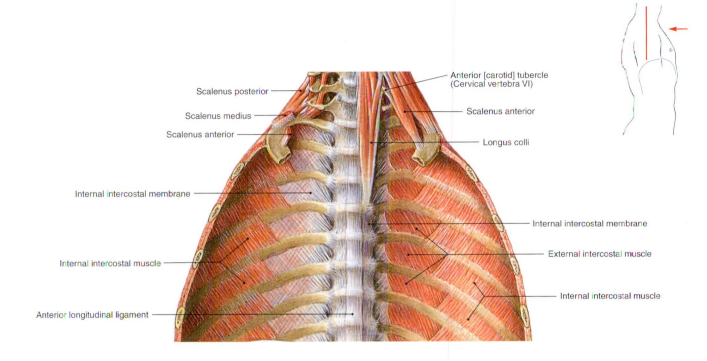

Scalenus posterior

Scalenus medius

Scalenus anterior

Internal intercostal membrane

Internal intercostal muscle

Anterior longitudinal ligament

Anterior [carotid] tubercle
(Cervical vertebra VI)

Scalenus anterior

Longus colli

Internal intercostal membrane

External intercostal muscle

Internal intercostal muscle

Fig. 573 Thoracic cage;
posterior wall.

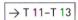 → T 11–T 13

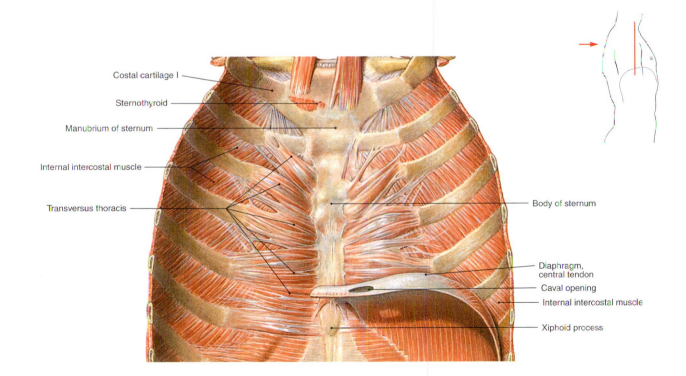

Costal cartilage I

Sternothyroid

Manubrium of sternum

Internal intercostal muscle

Transversus thoracis

Body of sternum

Diaphragm,
central tendon

Caval opening

Internal intercostal muscle

Xiphoid process

Fig. 574 Thoracic cage;
anterior wall.

→ T 13

Abdominal muscles

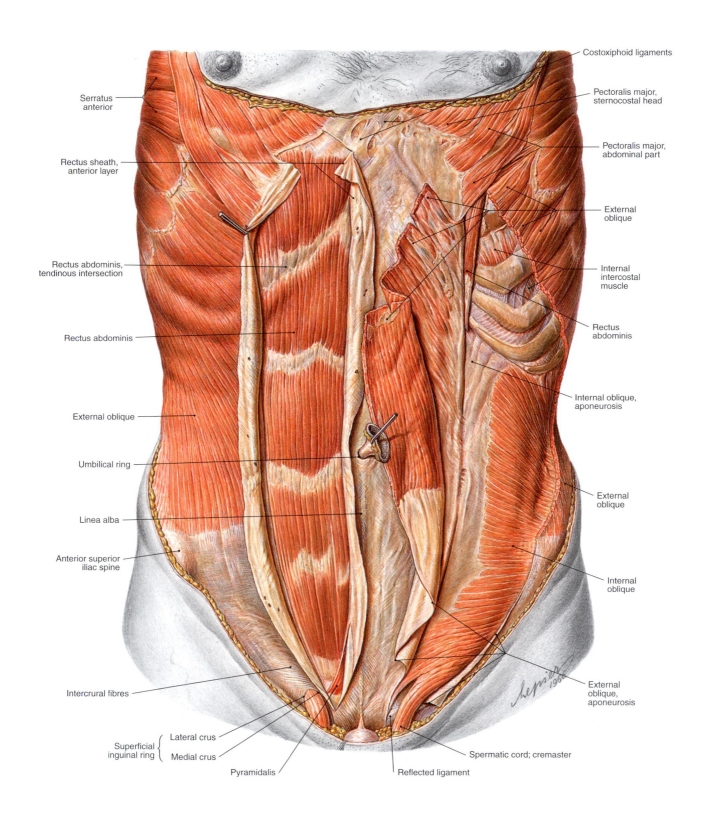

Serratus anterior

Rectus sheath, anterior layer

Rectus abdominis, tendinous intersection

Rectus abdominis

External oblique

Umbilical ring

Linea alba

Anterior superior iliac spine

Intercrural fibres

Superficial inguinal ring { Lateral crus / Medial crus

Pyramidalis

Costoxiphoid ligaments

Pectoralis major, sternocostal head

Pectoralis major, abdominal part

External oblique

Internal intercostal muscle

Rectus abdominis

Internal oblique, aponeurosis

External oblique

Internal oblique

External oblique, aponeurosis

Spermatic cord; cremaster

Reflected ligament

→ T 13–T 15, T 17, T 26

Fig. 575 Muscles of the abdominal wall; superficial and middle layer.

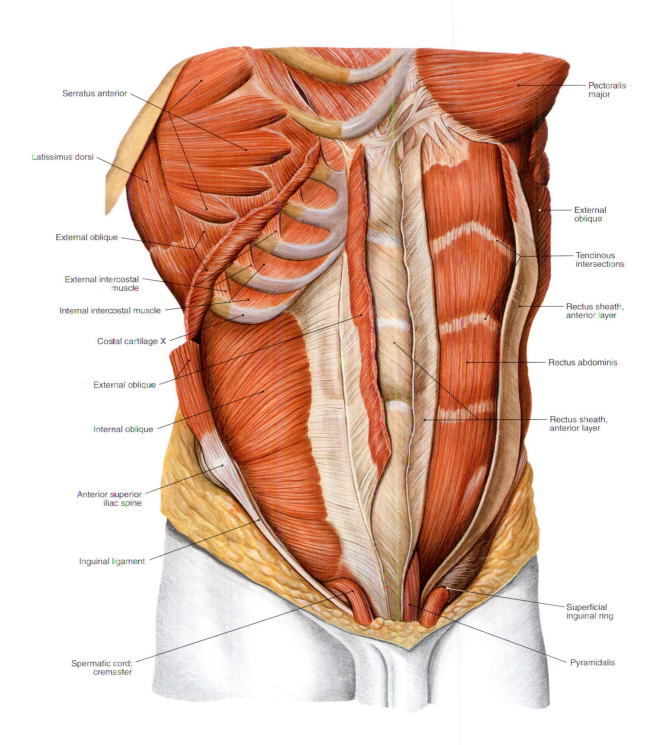

Serratus anterior

Latissimus dorsi

External oblique

External intercostal muscle

Internal intercostal muscle

Costal cartilage X

External oblique

Internal oblique

Anterior superior iliac spine

Inguinal ligament

Spermatic cord; cremaster

Pectoralis major

External oblique

Tendinous intersections

Rectus sheath, anterior layer

Rectus abdominis

Rectus sheath, anterior layer

Superficial inguinal ring

Pyramidalis

Fig. 576 Muscles of the abdominal wall; middle layer.

→ T 13–T 15, T 17

Abdominal muscles

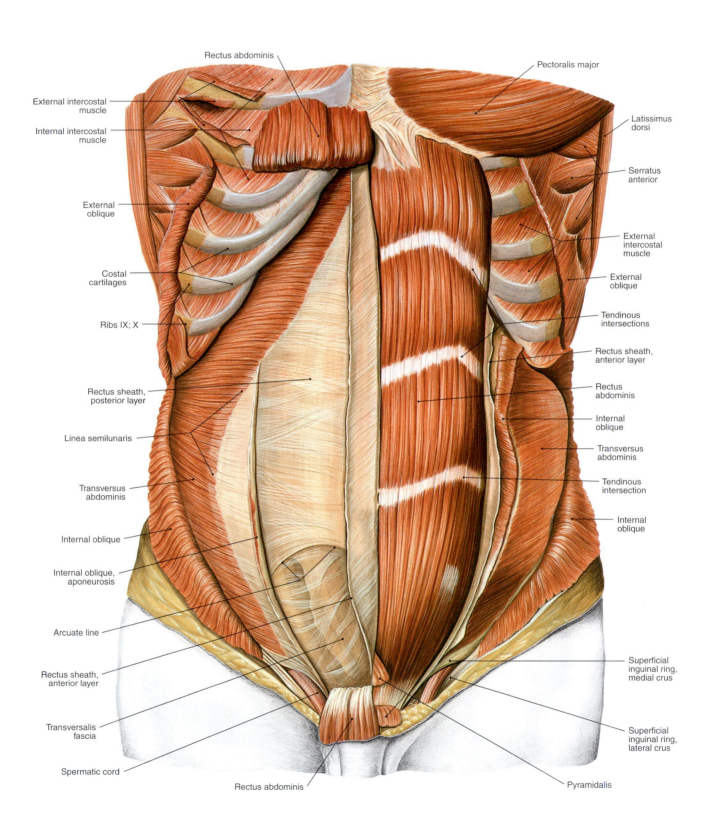

Rectus abdominis

Pectoralis major

External intercostal muscle

Internal intercostal muscle

Latissimus dorsi

Serratus anterior

External oblique

Costal cartilages

External intercostal muscle

Ribs IX; X

External oblique

Tendinous intersections

Rectus sheath, posterior layer

Rectus sheath, anterior layer

Rectus abdominis

Linea semilunaris

Internal oblique

Transversus abdominis

Transversus abdominis

Tendinous intersection

Internal oblique

Internal oblique

Internal oblique, aponeurosis

Arcuate line

Superficial inguinal ring, medial crus

Rectus sheath, anterior layer

Transversalis fascia

Superficial inguinal ring, lateral crus

Spermatic cord

Pyramidalis

Rectus abdominis

→ T 13–T 15

Fig. 577 Muscles of the abdominal wall; deep layer.

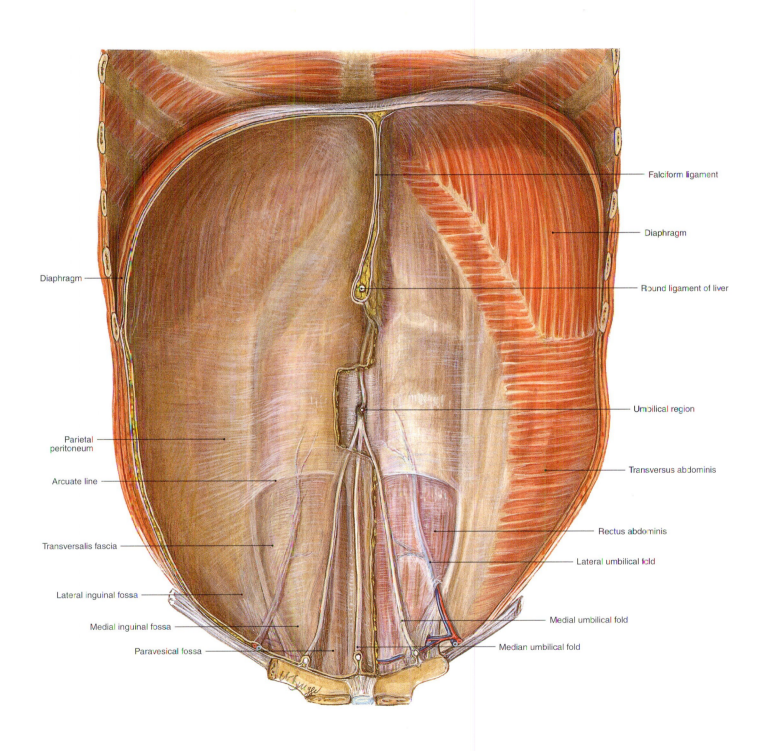

Falciform ligament

Diaphragm

Round ligament of liver

Umbilical region

Transversus abdominis

Rectus abdominis

Lateral umbilical fold

Medial umbilical fold

Median umbilical fold

Diaphragm

Parietal peritoneum

Arcuate line

Transversalis fascia

Lateral inguinal fossa

Medial inguinal fossa

Paravesical fossa

Fig. 578 Internal surface of the anterior abdominal wall.

→ T 14, T 15, T 21

Inguinal canal

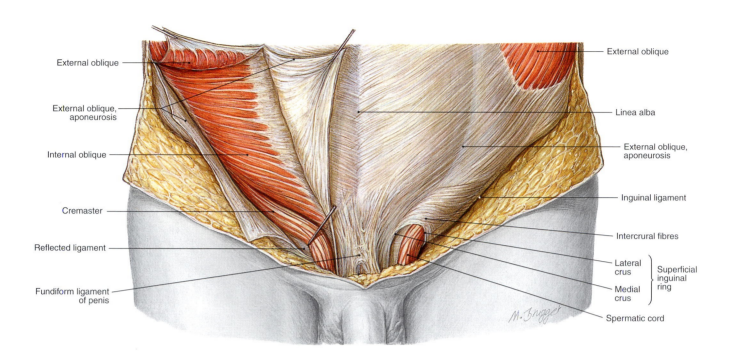

External oblique

External oblique, aponeurosis

Internal oblique

Cremaster

Reflected ligament

Fundiform ligament of penis

External oblique

Linea alba

External oblique, aponeurosis

Inguinal ligament

Intercrural fibres

Lateral crus

Medial crus

Superficial inguinal ring

Spermatic cord

Fig. 579 Superficial inguinal ring.

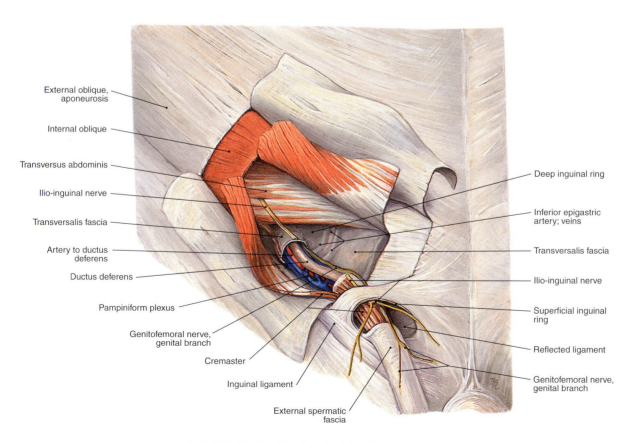

External oblique, aponeurosis

Internal oblique

Transversus abdominis

Ilio-inguinal nerve

Transversalis fascia

Artery to ductus deferens

Ductus deferens

Pampiniform plexus

Genitofemoral nerve, genital branch

Cremaster

Inguinal ligament

External spermatic fascia

Deep inguinal ring

Inferior epigastric artery; veins

Transversalis fascia

Ilio-inguinal nerve

Superficial inguinal ring

Reflected ligament

Genitofemoral nerve, genital branch

Fig. 580 Walls of the inguinal canal.

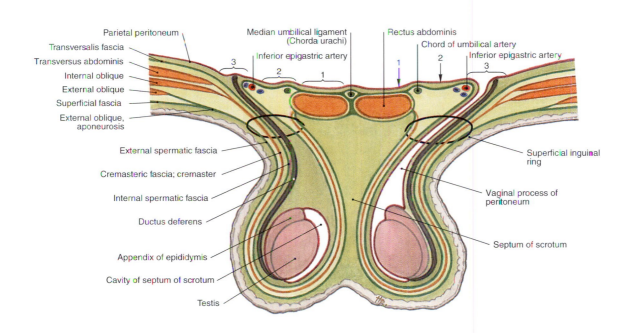

Parietal peritoneum
Transversalis fascia
Transversus abdominis
Internal oblique
External oblique
Superficial fascia
External oblique, aponeurosis

Median umbilical ligament (Chorda urachi)
Inferior epigastric artery

Rectus abdominis
Chord of umbilical artery
Inferior epigastric artery

3
2
1
1
2
3

External spermatic fascia
Cremasteric fascia; cremaster
Internal spermatic fascia
Ductus deferens
Appendix of epididymis
Cavity of septum of scrotum
Testis

Superficial inguinal ring
Vaginal process of peritoneum
Septum of scrotum

Fig. 581   Diagram of the inguinal canal.
The inguinal canal, the spermatic cord and the scrotum are
illustrated in the same plane for didactical reasons.

1 Supravesical fossa
2 Medial inguinal fossa
3 Lateral inguinal fossa

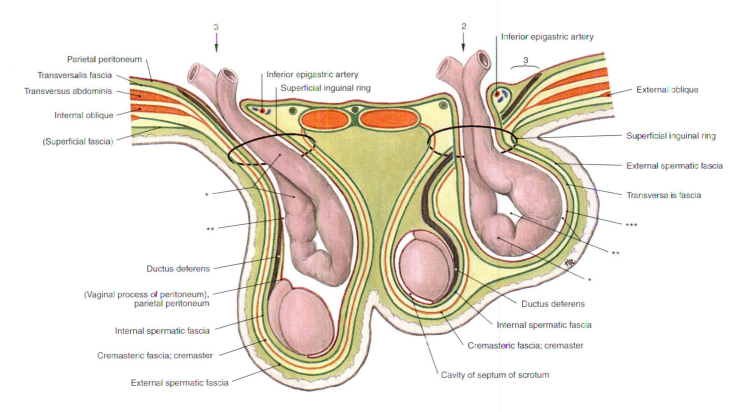

3
2
Inferior epigastric artery
3

Parietal peritoneum
Transversalis fascia
Transversus abdominis
Internal oblique
(Superficial fascia)

Inferior epigastric artery
Superficial inguinal ring

External oblique
Superficial inguinal ring
External spermatic fascia
Transversalis fascia
***
**
*

Ductus deferens
(Vaginal process of peritoneum), parietal peritoneum
Internal spermatic fascia
Cremasteric fascia; cremaster
External spermatic fascia

Ductus deferens
Internal spermatic fascia
Cremasteric fascia; cremaster
Cavity of septum of scrotum

Fig. 582   Diagram of inguinal hernias;
left side: lateral, indirect hernia;
right side: medial, direct hernia.

*   Hernial sac with an intestinal loop
**   Peritoneal space
***   Newly formed peritoneal hernial sac

Diaphragm and posterior abdominal wall

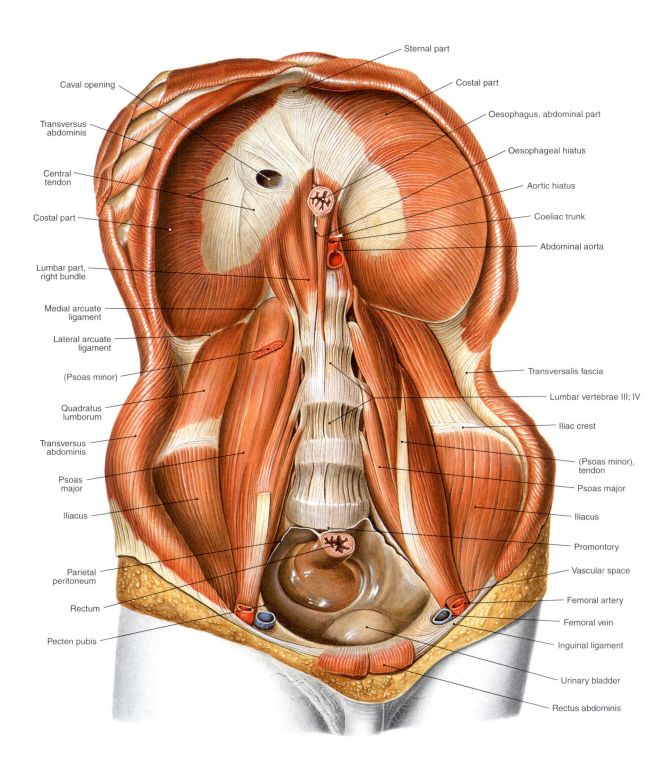

Caval opening

Transversus abdominis

Central tendon

Costal part

Lumbar part, right bundle

Medial arcuate ligament

Lateral arcuate ligament

(Psoas minor)

Quadratus lumborum

Transversus abdominis

Psoas major

Iliacus

Parietal peritoneum

Rectum

Pecten pubis

Sternal part

Costal part

Oesophagus, abdominal part

Oesophageal hiatus

Aortic hiatus

Coeliac trunk

Abdominal aorta

Transversalis fascia

Lumbar vertebrae III; IV

Iliac crest

(Psoas minor), tendon

Psoas major

Iliacus

Promontory

Vascular space

Femoral artery

Femoral vein

Inguinal ligament

Urinary bladder

Rectus abdominis

→ T 15, T 16, T 21, T 42   **Fig. 583** Diaphragm and muscles of the abdominal wall.

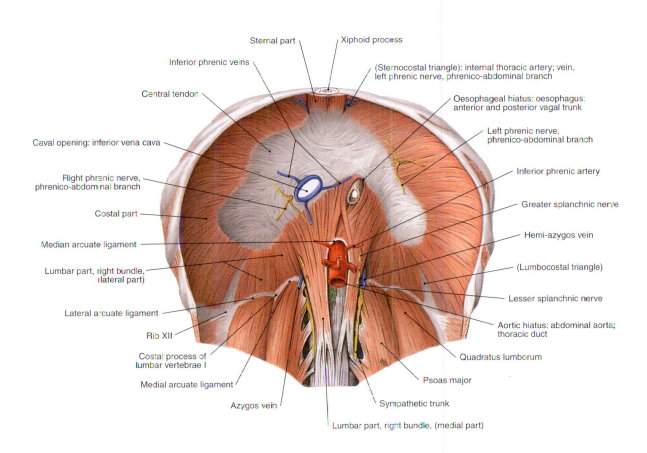

Sternal part
Xiphoid process
Inferior phrenic veins
(Sternocostal triangle): internal thoracic artery; vein, left phrenic nerve, phrenico-abdominal branch
Central tendon
Oesophageal hiatus: oesophagus; anterior and posterior vagal trunk
Left phrenic nerve, phrenico-abdominal branch
Caval opening: inferior vena cava
Inferior phrenic artery
Right phrenic nerve, phrenico-abdominal branch
Greater splanchnic nerve
Costal part
Hemi-azygos vein
Median arcuate ligament
(Lumbocostal triangle)
Lumbar part, right bundle, (lateral part)
Lesser splanchnic nerve
Lateral arcuate ligament
Aortic hiatus: abdominal aorta; thoracic duct
Rib XII
Quadratus lumborum
Costal process of lumbar vertebrae I
Psoas major
Medial arcuate ligament
Azygos vein
Sympathetic trunk
Lumbar part, right bundle, (medial part)

Fig. 584   Diaphragm.

→ T 21

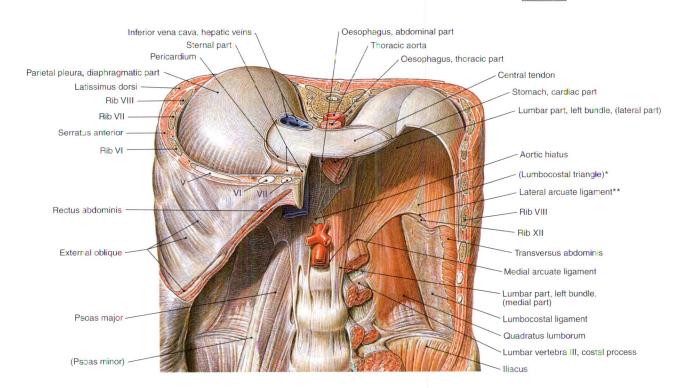

Inferior vena cava, hepatic veins
Oesophagus, abdominal part
Sternal part
Thoracic aorta
Pericardium
Oesophagus, thoracic part
Parietal pleura, diaphragmatic part
Central tendon
Latissimus dorsi
Stomach, cardiac part
Rib VIII
Lumbar part, left bundle, (lateral part)
Rib VII
Serratus anterior
Rib VI
Aortic hiatus
(Lumbocostal triangle)*
Lateral arcuate ligament**
Rib VIII
Rib XII
Rectus abdominis
Transversus abdominis
Medial arcuate ligament
External oblique
Lumbar part, left bundle, (medial part)
Lumbocostal ligament
Psoas major
Quadratus lumborum
Lumbar vertebra III, costal process
(Psoas minor)
Iliacus

Fig. 585   Diaphragm with apertures and muscles of the posterior abdominal wall.

→ T 21

*   Clinical term: BOCHDALEK's triangle
** Psoas arcade

Breast

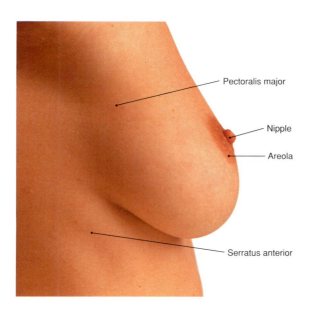

Fig. 586 Breast.

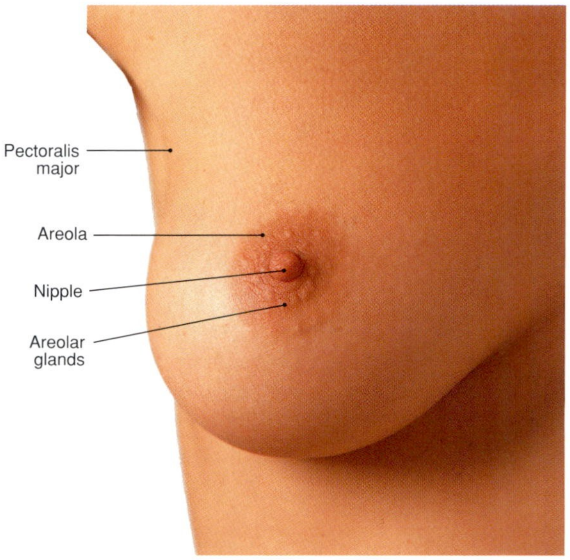

Fig. 587 Breast.

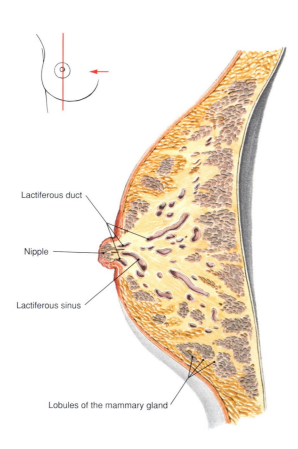

Fig. 588 Breast of a pregnant woman.

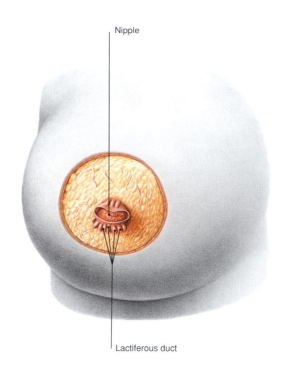

Fig. 589 Breast of a pregnant woman.

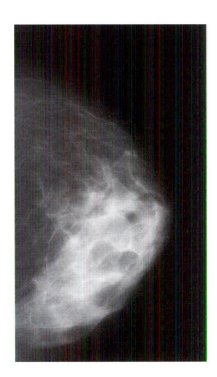

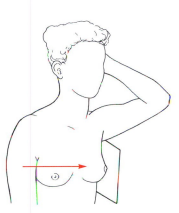

Fig. 590 Radiograph of the breast, mammography, of a 47-year-old woman.

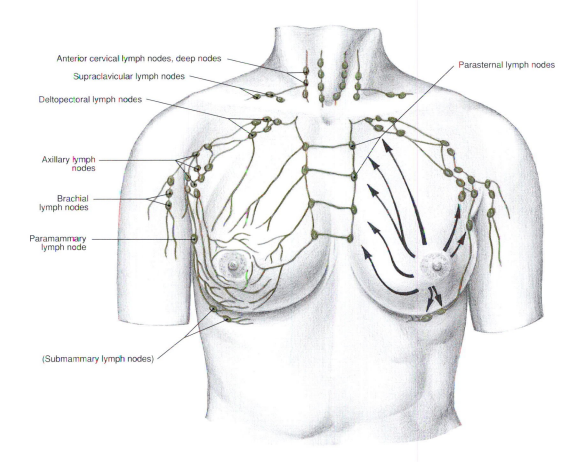

Anterior cervical lymph nodes, deep nodes

Supraclavicular lymph nodes

Deltopectoral lymph nodes

Parasternal lymph nodes

Axillary lymph nodes

Brachial lymph nodes

Paramammary lymph node

(Submammary lymph nodes)

Fig. 591 Lymphatic drainage of the breast and location of the regional lymph nodes.

Vessels and nerves of the wall of the trunk

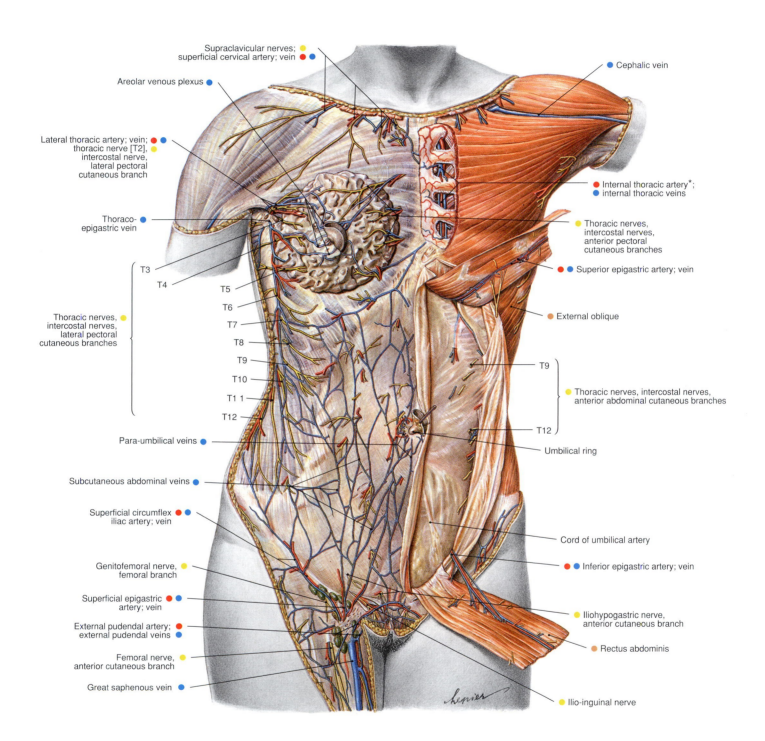

Supraclavicular nerves; ● superficial cervical artery; vein ● ●

● Cephalic vein

Areolar venous plexus ●

Lateral thoracic artery; vein; ● ● thoracic nerve [T2], ● intercostal nerve, lateral pectoral cutaneous branch

● Internal thoracic artery*; ● internal thoracic veins

Thoraco- ● epigastric vein

● Thoracic nerves, intercostal nerves, anterior pectoral cutaneous branches

● ● Superior epigastric artery; vein

T3

T4

T5

T6

● External oblique

T7

T8

Thoracic nerves, ● intercostal nerves, lateral pectoral cutaneous branches

T9

T9

T10

● Thoracic nerves, intercostal nerves, anterior abdominal cutaneous branches

T11

T12

T12

Para-umbilical veins ●

Umbilical ring

Subcutaneous abdominal veins ●

Superficial circumflex ● ● iliac artery; vein

Cord of umbilical artery

● ● Inferior epigastric artery; vein

Genitofemoral nerve, ● femoral branch

Superficial epigastric ● ● artery; vein

● Iliohypogastric nerve, anterior cutaneous branch

External pudendal artery; ● external pudendal veins ●

● Rectus abdominis

Femoral nerve, ● anterior cutaneous branch

Great saphenous vein ●

● Ilio-inguinal nerve

Fig. 592 Vessels and nerves of the thoracic and the abdominal wall.

* Clinical term: internal mammary artery

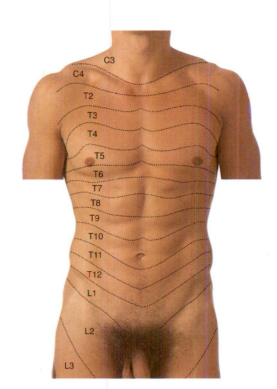

Fig. 593 Segmental sensory innervation of the anterior thoracic and abdominal wall (dermatomes).

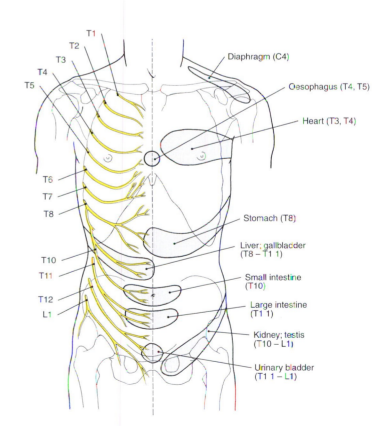

Diaphragm (C4)

Oesophagus (T4, T5)

Heart (T3, T4)

Stomach (T8)

Liver; gallbladder (T8 – T1 1)

Small intestine (T10)

Large intestine (T1 1)

Kidney; testis (T10 – L1)

Urinary bladder (T1 1 – L1)

Fig. 594 Segmental sensory innervation of the anterior thoracic and abdominal wall.
Regions to which pain from diseased viscera (zones of HEAD) is referred to are indicated in grey.

Lumbosacral plexus

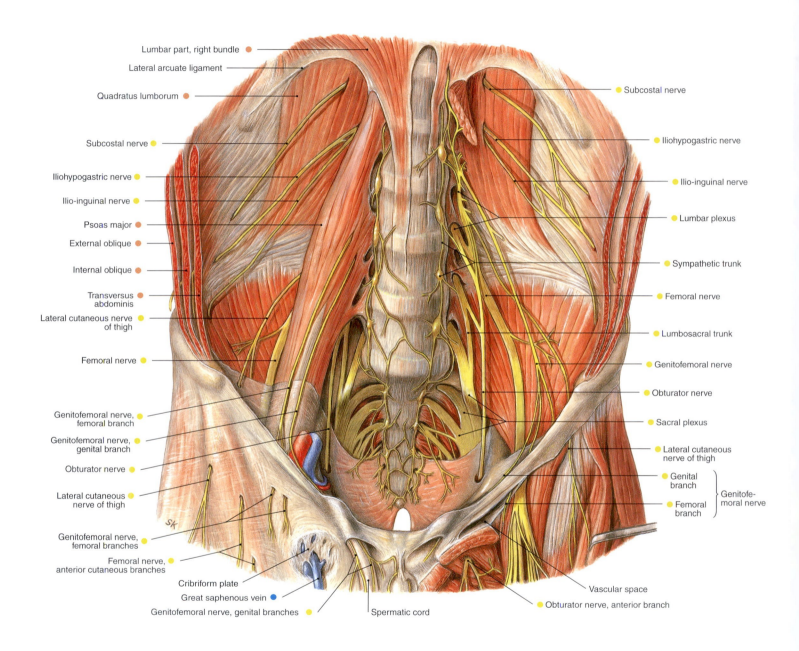

Lumbar part, right bundle

Lateral arcuate ligament

Quadratus lumborum

Subcostal nerve

Iliohypogastric nerve

Ilio-inguinal nerve

Psoas major

External oblique

Internal oblique

Transversus abdominis

Lateral cutaneous nerve of thigh

Femoral nerve

Genitofemoral nerve, femoral branch

Genitofemoral nerve, genital branch

Obturator nerve

Lateral cutaneous nerve of thigh

Genitofemoral nerve, femoral branches

Femoral nerve, anterior cutaneous branches

Cribriform plate

Great saphenous vein

Genitofemoral nerve, genital branches

Subcostal nerve

Iliohypogastric nerve

Ilio-inguinal nerve

Lumbar plexus

Sympathetic trunk

Femoral nerve

Lumbosacral trunk

Genitofemoral nerve

Obturator nerve

Sacral plexus

Lateral cutaneous nerve of thigh

Genital branch

Femoral branch

Genitofemoral nerve

Vascular space

Obturator nerve, anterior branch

Spermatic cord

→ 47, 1102, T 40

Fig. 595 Lumbosacral plexus.

Vessels of the anterior wall of the trunk

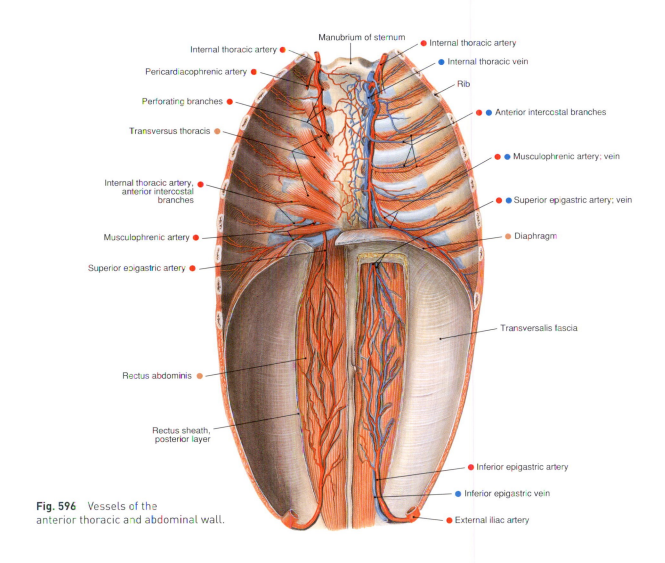

Manubrium of sternum

Internal thoracic artery ●

Pericardiacophrenic artery ●

Perforating branches ●

Transversus thoracis ●

Internal thoracic artery, anterior intercostal branches ●

Musculophrenic artery ●

Superior epigastric artery ●

Rectus abdominis ●

Rectus sheath, posterior layer

● Internal thoracic artery

● Internal thoracic vein

Rib

● ● Anterior intercostal branches

● ● Musculophrenic artery; vein

● ● Superior epigastric artery; vein

● Diaphragm

Transversalis fascia

● Inferior epigastric artery

● Inferior epigastric vein

● External iliac artery

Fig. 596 Vessels of the anterior thoracic and abdominal wall.

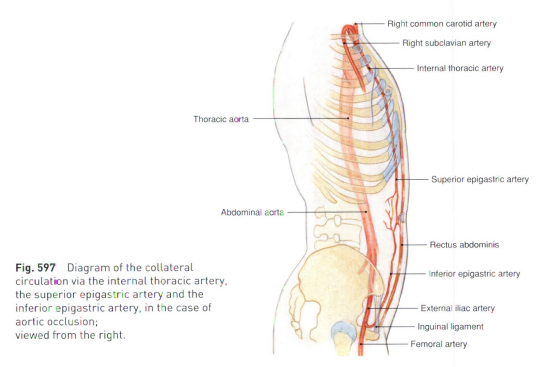

Right common carotid artery

Right subclavian artery

Internal thoracic artery

Thoracic aorta

Superior epigastric artery

Abdominal aorta

Rectus abdominis

Inferior epigastric artery

External iliac artery

Inguinal ligament

Femoral artery

Fig. 597 Diagram of the collateral circulation via the internal thoracic artery, the superior epigastric artery and the inferior epigastric artery, in the case of aortic occlusion; viewed from the right.

Abdominal wall of neonate

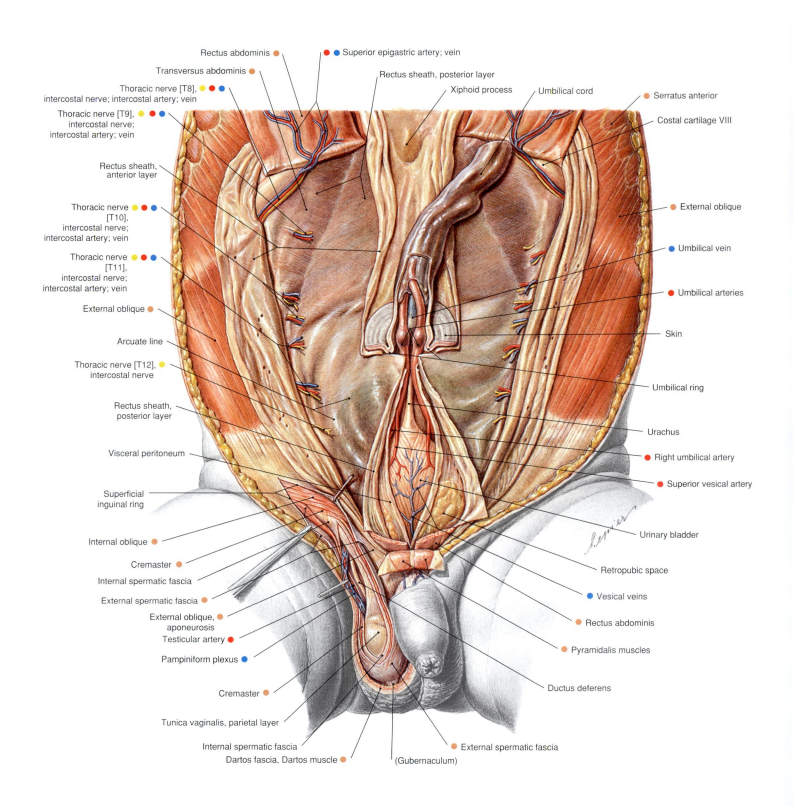

Rectus abdominis

Transversus abdominis

Thoracic nerve [T8], intercostal nerve; intercostal artery; vein

Thoracic nerve [T9], intercostal nerve; intercostal artery; vein

Rectus sheath, anterior layer

Thoracic nerve [T10], intercostal nerve; intercostal artery; vein

Thoracic nerve [T11], intercostal nerve; intercostal artery; vein

External oblique

Arcuate line

Thoracic nerve [T12], intercostal nerve

Rectus sheath, posterior layer

Visceral peritoneum

Superficial inguinal ring

Internal oblique

Cremaster

Internal spermatic fascia

External spermatic fascia

External oblique, aponeurosis

Testicular artery

Pampiniform plexus

Cremaster

Tunica vaginalis, parietal layer

Internal spermatic fascia

Dartos fascia, Dartos muscle

(Gubernaculum)

Superior epigastric artery; vein

Rectus sheath, posterior layer

Xiphoid process

Umbilical cord

Serratus anterior

Costal cartilage VIII

Umbilical vein

Umbilical arteries

Skin

Umbilical ring

Urachus

Right umbilical artery

Superior vesical artery

Urinary bladder

Retropubic space

Vesical veins

Rectus abdominis

Pyramidalis muscles

Ductus deferens

External spermatic fascia

Fig. 598   Anterior abdominal wall of a neonate.

Inner contour of the anterior abdominal wall

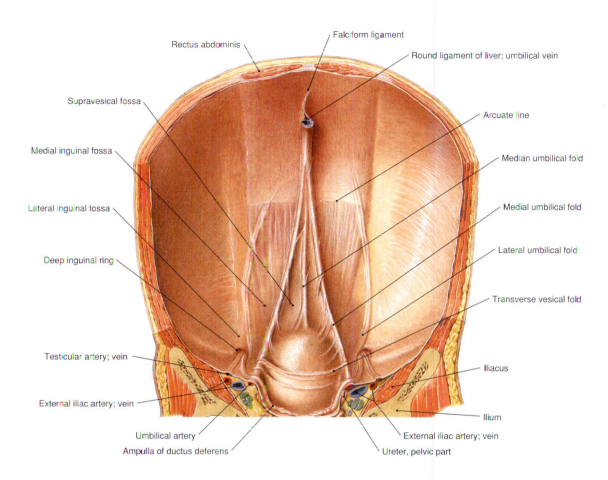

Rectus abdominis

Falciform ligament

Round ligament of liver; umbilical vein

Supravesical fossa

Arcuate line

Medial inguinal fossa

Median umbilical fold

Lateral inguinal fossa

Medial umbilical fold

Deep inguinal ring

Lateral umbilical fold

Transverse vesical fold

Testicular artery; vein

Iliacus

External iliac artery; vein

Ilium

Umbilical artery

External iliac artery; vein

Ampulla of ductus deferens

Ureter, pelvic part

Fig. 599 Anterior abdominal wall of a neonate.

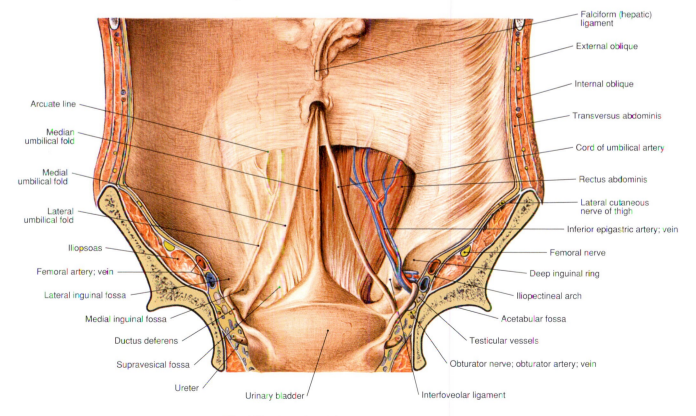

Falciform (hepatic) ligament

External oblique

Arcuate line

Internal oblique

Median umbilical fold

Transversus abdominis

Medial umbilical fold

Cord of umbilical artery

Rectus abdominis

Lateral umbilical fold

Lateral cutaneous nerve of thigh

Iliopsoas

Inferior epigastric artery; vein

Femoral artery; vein

Femoral nerve

Lateral inguinal fossa

Deep inguinal ring

Medial inguinal fossa

Iliopectineal arch

Ductus deferens

Acetabular fossa

Supravesical fossa

Testicular vessels

Ureter

Obturator nerve; obturator artery; vein

Urinary bladder

Interfoveolar ligament

Fig. 600 Anterior abdominal wall, internal aspect.

Abdominal wall, sections

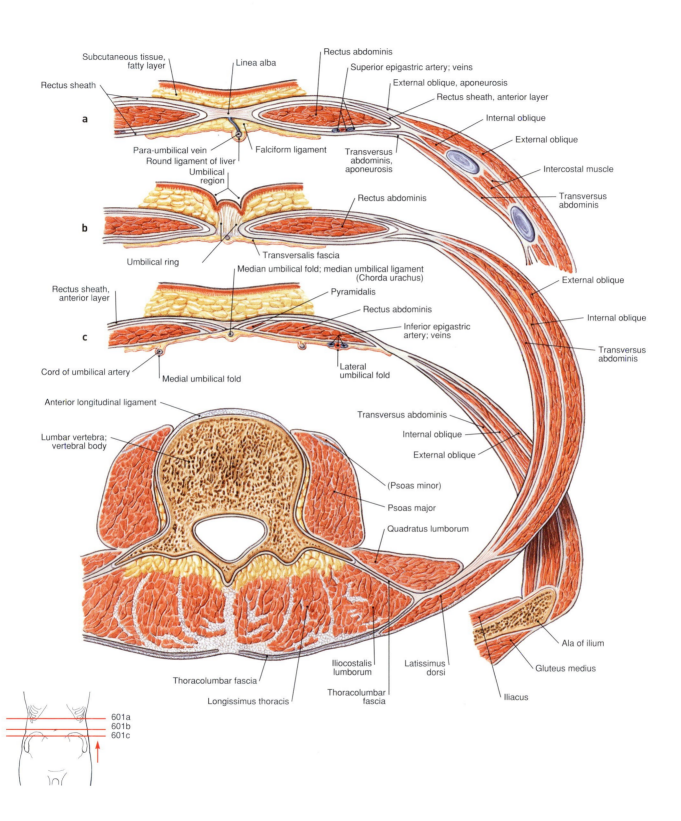

Subcutaneous tissue, fatty layer

Rectus sheath

Linea alba

Rectus abdominis

Superior epigastric artery; veins

External oblique, aponeurosis

Rectus sheath, anterior layer

Internal oblique

External oblique

Intercostal muscle

Transversus abdominis

a

Para-umbilical vein

Round ligament of liver

Falciform ligament

Transversus abdominis, aponeurosis

Umbilical region

Rectus abdominis

b

Umbilical ring

Transversalis fascia

External oblique

Internal oblique

Transversus abdominis

Rectus sheath, anterior layer

Median umbilical fold; median umbilical ligament (Chorda urachus)

Pyramidalis

Rectus abdominis

Inferior epigastric artery; veins

c

Cord of umbilical artery

Medial umbilical fold

Lateral umbilical fold

Anterior longitudinal ligament

Transversus abdominis

Internal oblique

External oblique

Lumbar vertebra; vertebral body

(Psoas minor)

Psoas major

Quadratus lumborum

Ala of ilium

Gluteus medius

Iliacus

Iliocostalis lumborum

Latissimus dorsi

Thoracolumbar fascia

Longissimus thoracis

Thoracolumbar fascia

601a
601b
601c

→ T 14–T 16, T 20a, b, T 42

Fig. 601 a–c Muscles of the abdominal wall; horizontal section.

Abdominal wall, sections

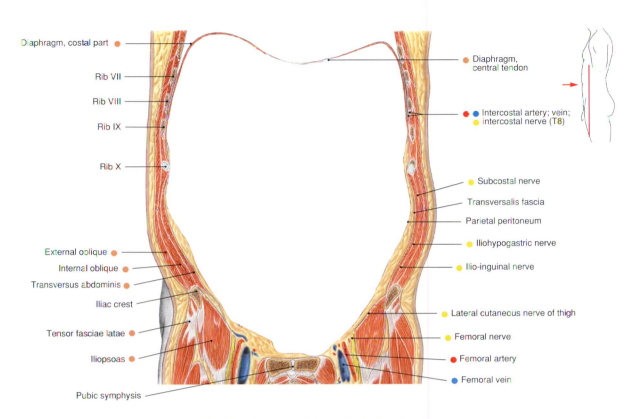

Diaphragm, costal part ●

Rib VII

Rib VIII

Rib IX

Rib X

● Diaphragm, central tendon

● ● Intercostal artery; vein; ● intercostal nerve (T8)

● Subcostal nerve

Transversalis fascia

Parietal peritoneum

● Iliohypogastric nerve

● Ilio-inguinal nerve

External oblique ●

Internal oblique ●

Transversus abdominis ●

Iliac crest

Tensor fasciae latae ●

Iliopsoas ●

Pubic symphysis

● Lateral cutaneous nerve of thigh

● Femoral nerve

● Femoral artery

● Femoral vein

Fig. 602 Muscles of the abdominal wall; frontal section.

603a
603b

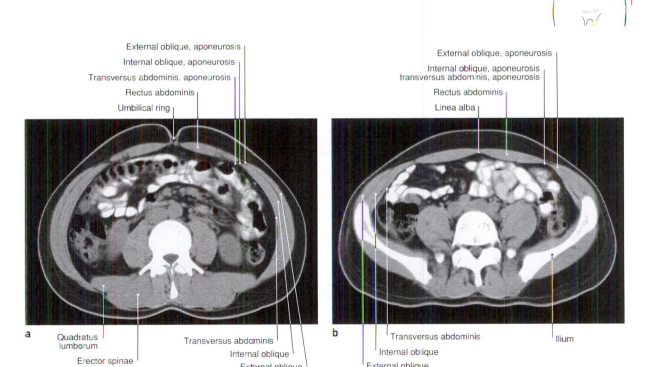

External oblique, aponeurosis

Internal oblique, aponeurosis

Transversus abdominis, aponeurosis

Rectus abdominis

Umbilical ring

External oblique, aponeurosis

Internal oblique, aponeurosis transversus abdominis, aponeurosis

Rectus abdominis

Linea alba

a

Quadratus lumborum

Erector spinae

Transversus abdominis

Internal oblique

External oblique

b

Transversus abdominis

Internal oblique

External oblique

Ilium

Fig. 603 a, b Muscles of the abdominal wall; computed tomographic cross-sections (CT).

Heart

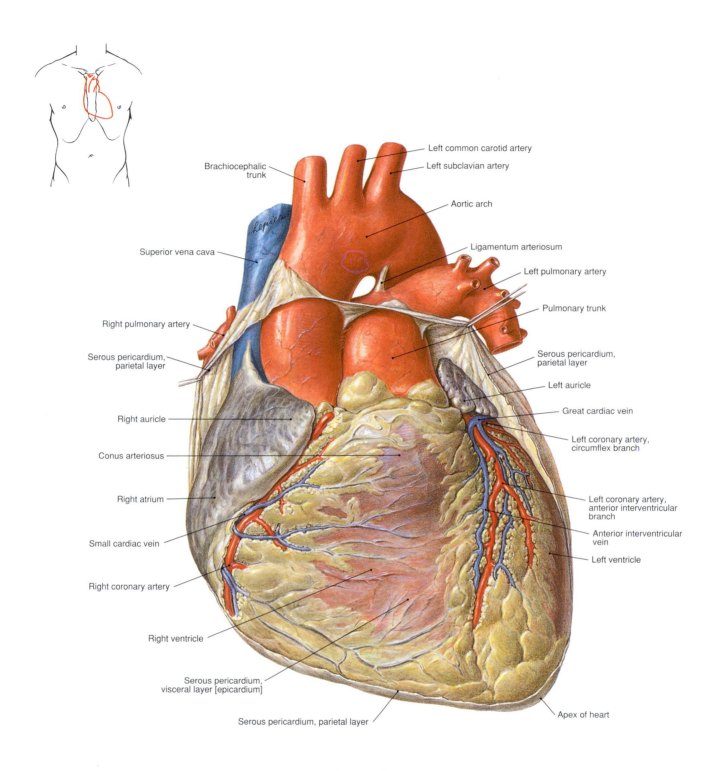

Left common carotid artery

Brachiocephalic trunk

Left subclavian artery

Aortic arch

Superior vena cava

Ligamentum arteriosum

Left pulmonary artery

Right pulmonary artery

Pulmonary trunk

Serous pericardium, parietal layer

Serous pericardium, parietal layer

Left auricle

Right auricle

Great cardiac vein

Left coronary artery, circumflex branch

Conus arteriosus

Right atrium

Left coronary artery, anterior interventricular branch

Anterior interventricular vein

Small cardiac vein

Left ventricle

Right coronary artery

Right ventricle

Serous pericardium, visceral layer [epicardium]

Serous pericardium, parietal layer

Apex of heart

Fig. 604   Heart.

Fibrous pericardium ⎫
Serous pericardium   ⎬ Pericardium
Parietal layer   ⎭

Visceral layer   =   Epicardium

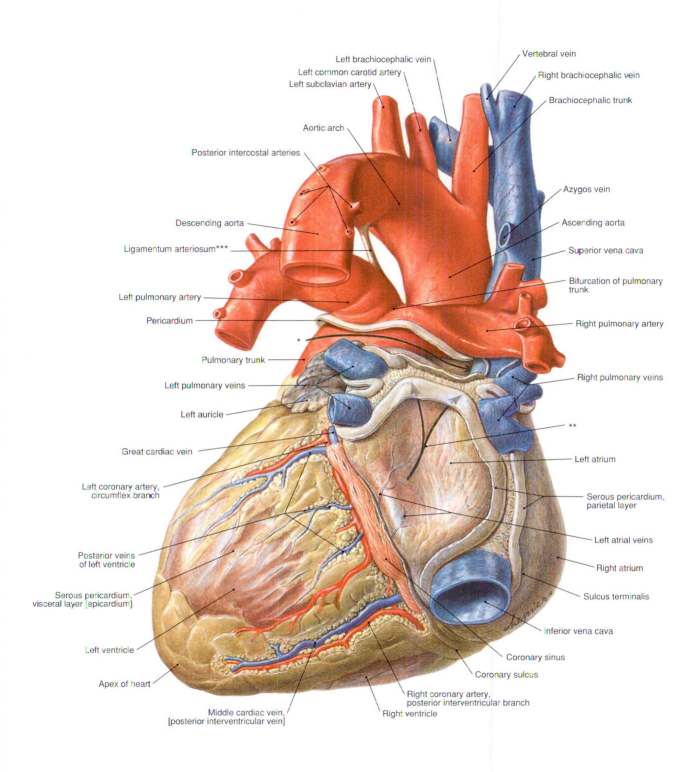

Left brachiocephalic vein
Left common carotid artery
Left subclavian artery

Vertebral vein

Right brachiocephalic vein

Brachiocephalic trunk

Aortic arch

Posterior intercostal arteries

Azygos vein

Descending aorta

Ascending aorta

Ligamentum arteriosum***

Superior vena cava

Left pulmonary artery

Bifurcation of pulmonary trunk

Pericardium

Right pulmonary artery

Pulmonary trunk

Left pulmonary veins

Right pulmonary veins

Left auricle

**

Great cardiac vein

Left atrium

Left coronary artery, circumflex branch

Serous pericardium, parietal layer

Posterior veins of left ventricle

Left atrial veins

Right atrium

Serous pericardium, visceral layer [epicardium]

Sulcus terminalis

Left ventricle

Inferior vena cava

Apex of heart

Coronary sinus

Coronary sulcus

Middle cardiac vein, [posterior interventricular vein]

Right coronary artery, posterior interventricular branch

Right ventricle

Fig. 605 Heart and great vessels; dorsal view.

* Arrow in the transverse pericardial sinus
** Double arrows in the oblique pericardial sinus
*** Remnants of the foetal ductus artericsus (BOTALLO's ligament)

Myocardium

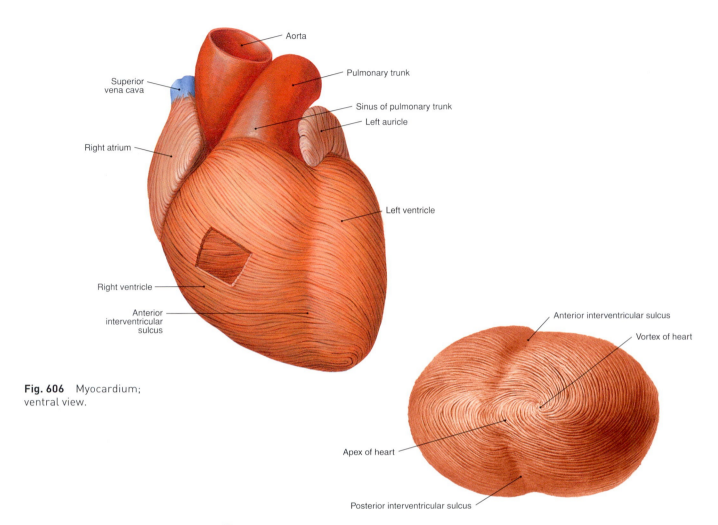

Aorta

Superior
vena cava

Pulmonary trunk

Sinus of pulmonary trunk

Left auricle

Right atrium

Left ventricle

Right ventricle

Anterior
interventricular
sulcus

Fig. 606   Myocardium;
ventral view.

Anterior interventricular sulcus

Vortex of heart

Apex of heart

Posterior interventricular sulcus

Fig. 607   Myocardium;
viewed from the apex of the heart.

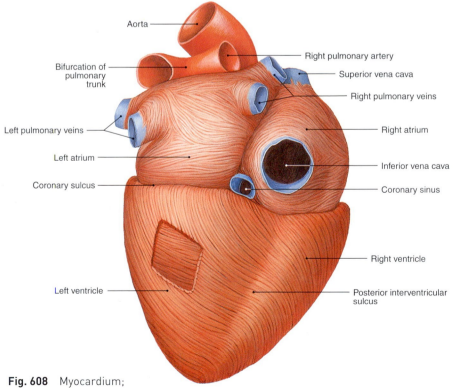

Aorta

Bifurcation of
pulmonary
trunk

Right pulmonary artery

Superior vena cava

Right pulmonary veins

Left pulmonary veins

Right atrium

Left atrium

Inferior vena cava

Coronary sulcus

Coronary sinus

Right ventricle

Left ventricle

Posterior interventricular
sulcus

Fig. 608   Myocardium;
dorsoinferior view.

Valves of the heart

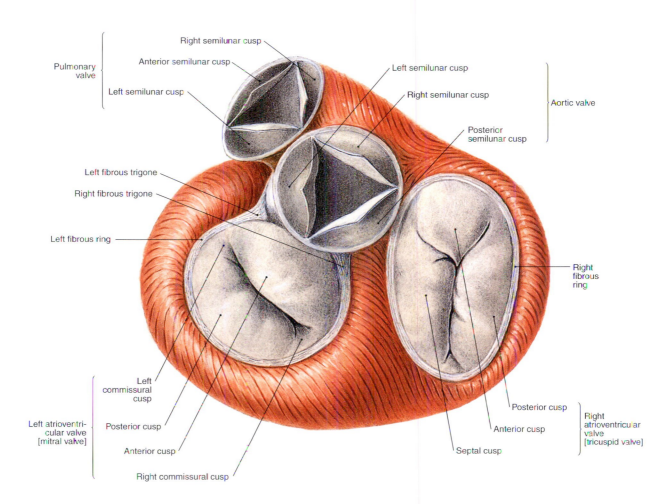

Pulmonary valve
Right semilunar cusp
Anterior semilunar cusp
Left semilunar cusp
Left semilunar cusp
Right semilunar cusp
Aortic valve
Posterior semilunar cusp
Left fibrous trigone
Right fibrous trigone
Left fibrous ring
Right fibrous ring
Left commissural cusp
Posterior cusp
Left atrioventricular valve [mitral valve]
Posterior cusp
Anterior cusp
Septal cusp
Right atrioventricular valve [tricuspid valve]
Anterior cusp
Right commissural cusp

Fig. 609   Valves of the heart; superior view.

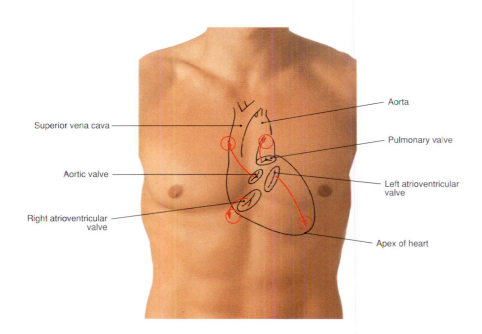

Superior vena cava
Aorta
Pulmonary valve
Aortic valve
Left atrioventricular valve
Right atrioventricular valve
Apex of heart

Fig. 610   Contour of the heart, valves of the heart, and points of auscultation projected onto the anterior thoracic wall (circles).

The heart sounds and (where applicable) the heart murmurs are spreading in the direction of the arrows.

Internal spaces of the heart

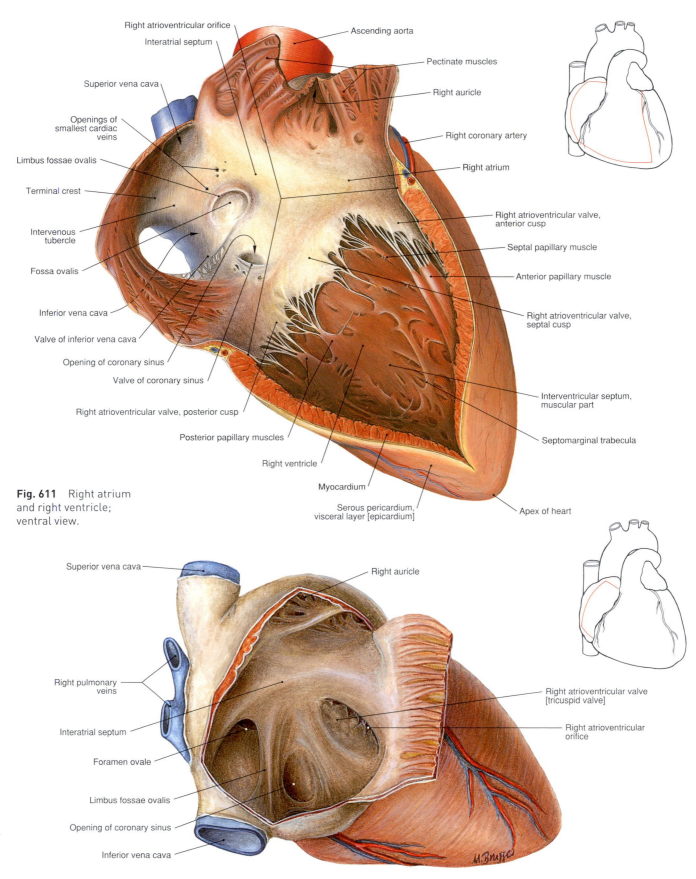

Right atrioventricular orifice
Interatrial septum
Superior vena cava
Openings of smallest cardiac veins
Limbus fossae ovalis
Terminal crest
Intervenous tubercle
Fossa ovalis
Inferior vena cava
Valve of inferior vena cava
Opening of coronary sinus
Valve of coronary sinus
Right atrioventricular valve, posterior cusp
Posterior papillary muscles
Right ventricle
Myocardium
Serous pericardium, visceral layer [epicardium]

Ascending aorta
Pectinate muscles
Right auricle
Right coronary artery
Right atrium
Right atrioventricular valve, anterior cusp
Septal papillary muscle
Anterior papillary muscle
Right atrioventricular valve, septal cusp
Interventricular septum, muscular part
Septomarginal trabecula
Apex of heart

Fig. 611 Right atrium and right ventricle; ventral view.

Superior vena cava
Right auricle
Right pulmonary veins
Interatrial septum
Foramen ovale
Limbus fossae ovalis
Opening of coronary sinus
Inferior vena cava

Right atrioventricular valve [tricuspid valve]
Right atrioventricular orifice

Fig. 612 Right atrium of a neonate; ventral view from the right.

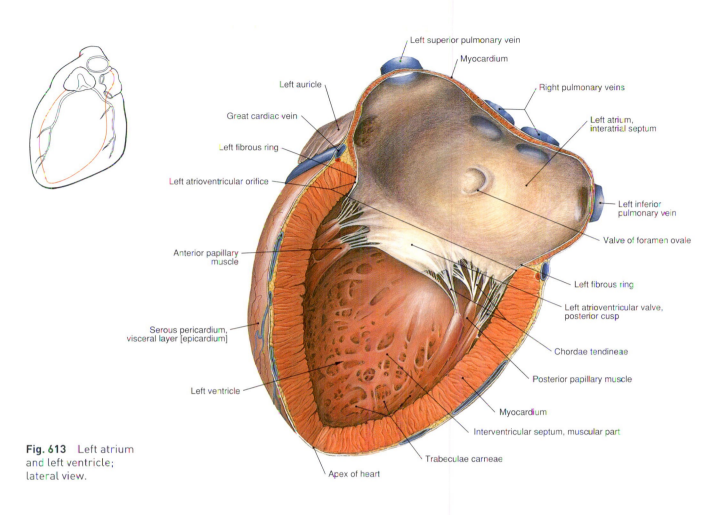

Left superior pulmonary vein
Myocardium
Left auricle
Right pulmonary veins
Great cardiac vein
Left atrium, interatrial septum
Left fibrous ring
Left atrioventricular orifice
Left inferior pulmonary vein
Valve of foramen ovale
Anterior papillary muscle
Left fibrous ring
Left atrioventricular valve, posterior cusp
Serous pericardium, visceral layer [epicardium]
Chordae tendineae
Posterior papillary muscle
Left ventricle
Myocardium
Interventricular septum, muscular part
Trabeculae carneae
Apex of heart

Fig. 613 Left atrium and left ventricle; lateral view.

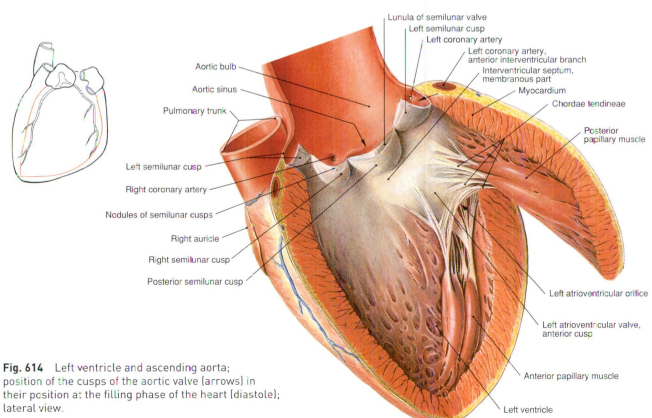

Lunula of semilunar valve
Left semilunar cusp
Left coronary artery
Aortic bulb
Left coronary artery, anterior interventricular branch
Aortic sinus
Interventricular septum, membranous part
Pulmonary trunk
Myocardium
Chordae tendineae
Posterior papillary muscle
Left semilunar cusp
Right coronary artery
Nodules of semilunar cusps
Right auricle
Right semilunar cusp
Posterior semilunar cusp
Left atrioventricular orifice
Left atrioventricular valve, anterior cusp
Anterior papillary muscle
Left ventricle

Fig. 614 Left ventricle and ascending aorta; position of the cusps of the aortic valve (arrows) in their position at the filling phase of the heart (diastole); lateral view.

Internal spaces of the heart

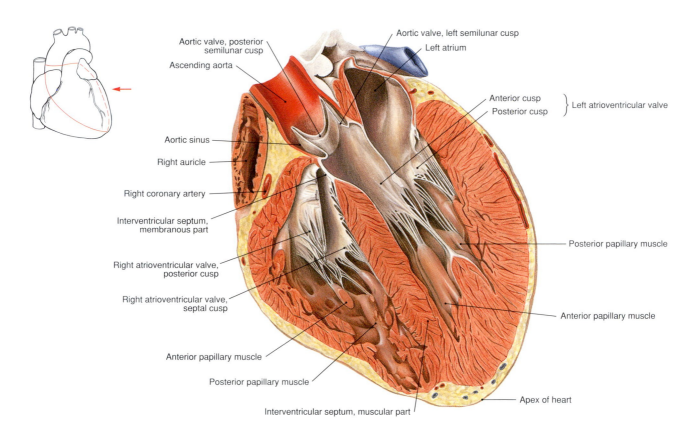

Aortic valve, posterior
semilunar cusp

Aortic valve, left semilunar cusp

Left atrium

Ascending aorta

Anterior cusp
Posterior cusp } Left atrioventricular valve

Aortic sinus

Right auricle

Right coronary artery

Interventricular septum,
membranous part

Posterior papillary muscle

Right atrioventricular valve,
posterior cusp

Right atrioventricular valve,
septal cusp

Anterior papillary muscle

Anterior papillary muscle

Posterior papillary muscle

Apex of heart

Interventricular septum, muscular part

Fig. 615   Left and right ventricle.

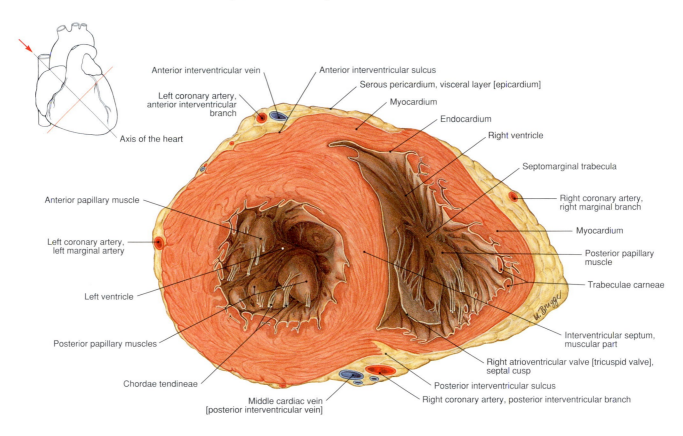

Anterior interventricular vein

Anterior interventricular sulcus

Left coronary artery,
anterior interventricular
branch

Serous pericardium, visceral layer [epicardium]

Myocardium

Endocardium

Right ventricle

Axis of the heart

Septomarginal trabecula

Anterior papillary muscle

Right coronary artery,
right marginal branch

Left coronary artery,
left marginal artery

Myocardium

Posterior papillary
muscle

Left ventricle

Trabeculae carneae

Posterior papillary muscles

Interventricular septum,
muscular part

Chordae tendineae

Right atrioventricular valve [tricuspid valve],
septal cusp

Posterior interventricular sulcus

Middle cardiac vein
[posterior interventricular vein]

Right coronary artery, posterior interventricular branch

Fig. 616   Left and right ventricle;
superior view.

Internal spaces of the heart

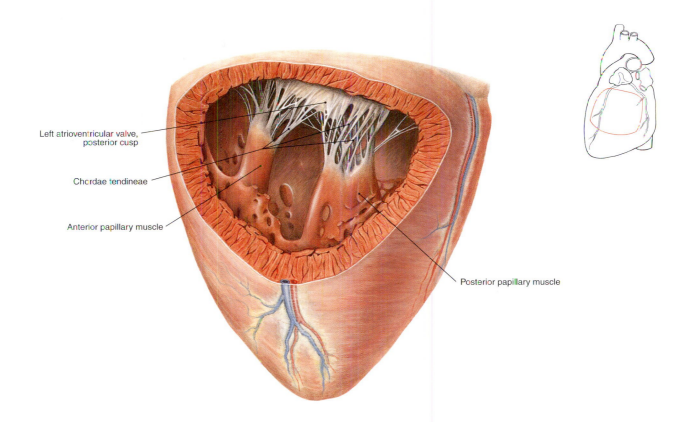

Left atrioventricular valve, posterior cusp

Chordae tendineae

Anterior papillary muscle

Posterior papillary muscle

Fig. 617 Left ventricle; ventrosuperior view from the left.

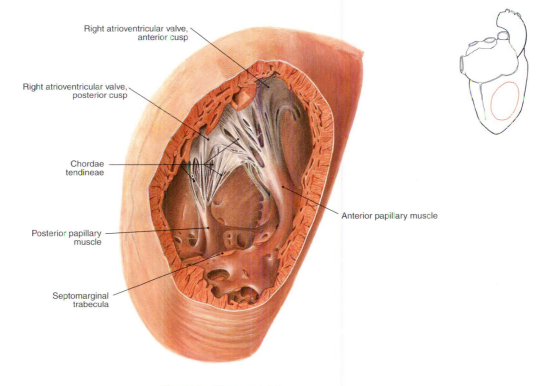

Right atrioventricular valve, anterior cusp

Right atrioventricular valve, posterior cusp

Chordae tendineae

Anterior papillary muscle

Posterior papillary muscle

Septomarginal trabecula

Fig. 618 Right ventricle; dorsal view.

Conducting system

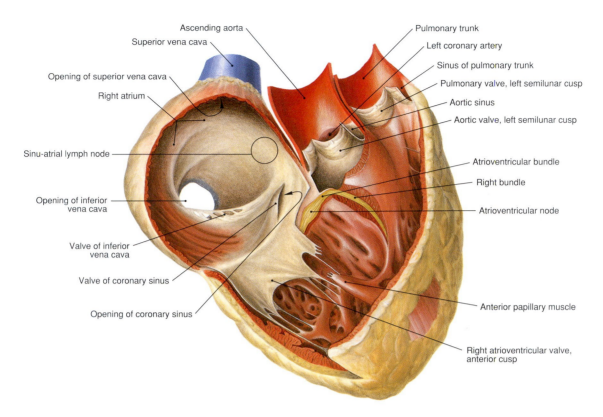

Ascending aorta

Superior vena cava

Opening of superior vena cava

Right atrium

Sinu-atrial lymph node

Opening of inferior vena cava

Valve of inferior vena cava

Valve of coronary sinus

Opening of coronary sinus

Pulmonary trunk

Left coronary artery

Sinus of pulmonary trunk

Pulmonary valve, left semilunar cusp

Aortic sinus

Aortic valve, left semilunar cusp

Atrioventricular bundle

Right bundle

Atrioventricular node

Anterior papillary muscle

Right atrioventricular valve, anterior cusp

Fig. 619   Right atrium
and right ventricle;
conducting system highlighted in yellow;
ventral view.

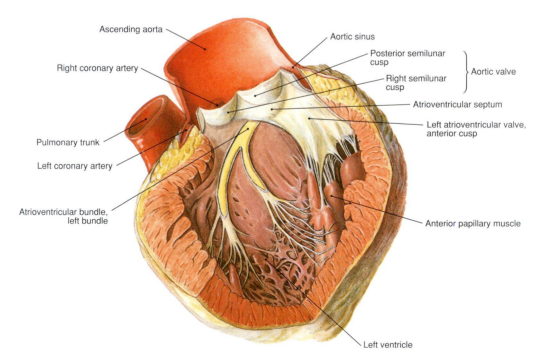

Ascending aorta

Right coronary artery

Pulmonary trunk

Left coronary artery

Atrioventricular bundle, left bundle

Aortic sinus

Posterior semilunar cusp

Right semilunar cusp

} Aortic valve

Atrioventricular septum

Left atrioventricular valve, anterior cusp

Anterior papillary muscle

Left ventricle

Fig. 620   Left ventricle;
conducting system highlighted in yellow;
ventral view from the left.

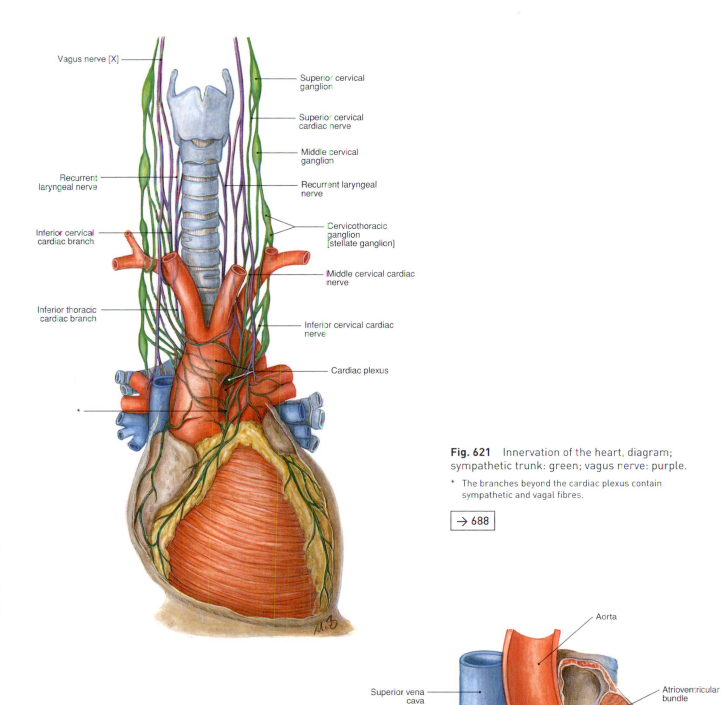

Vagus nerve [X]

Superior cervical
ganglion

Superior cervical
cardiac nerve

Middle cervical
ganglion

Recurrent
laryngeal nerve

Recurrent laryngeal
nerve

Cervicothoracic
ganglion
[stellate ganglion]

Inferior cervical
cardiac branch

Middle cervical cardiac
nerve

Inferior thoracic
cardiac branch

Inferior cervical cardiac
nerve

Cardiac plexus

*

Fig. 621 Innervation of the heart, diagram;
sympathetic trunk: green; vagus nerve: purple.

* The branches beyond the cardiac plexus contain
sympathetic and vagal fibres.

→ 688

Aorta

Superior vena
cava

Atrioventricular
bundle

Sinu-atrial lymph
node

Left
bundle

Atrioventricular
node

Right
bundle

Interventricular
septum

Subendocardial branches

Fig. 622 Conducting system of heart;
section at the plane of the axis of the heart.

Coronary arteries

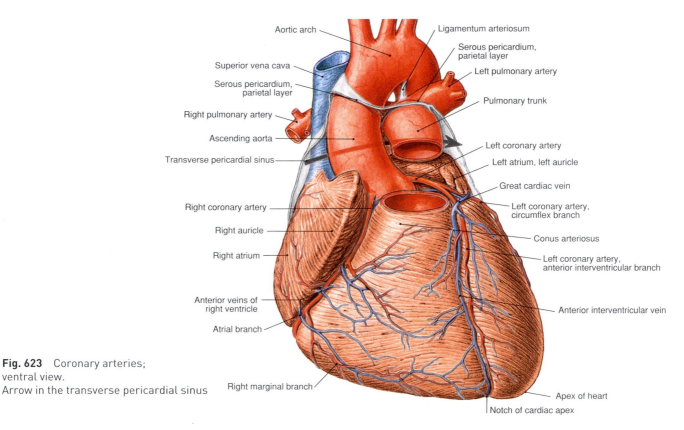

Aortic arch
Ligamentum arteriosum
Serous pericardium, parietal layer
Superior vena cava
Left pulmonary artery
Serous pericardium, parietal layer
Pulmonary trunk
Right pulmonary artery
Ascending aorta
Left coronary artery
Transverse pericardial sinus
Left atrium, left auricle
Great cardiac vein
Right coronary artery
Left coronary artery, circumflex branch
Right auricle
Conus arteriosus
Right atrium
Left coronary artery, anterior interventricular branch
Anterior veins of right ventricle
Anterior interventricular vein
Atrial branch
Right marginal branch
Apex of heart
Notch of cardiac apex

Fig. 623 Coronary arteries; ventral view. Arrow in the transverse pericardial sinus

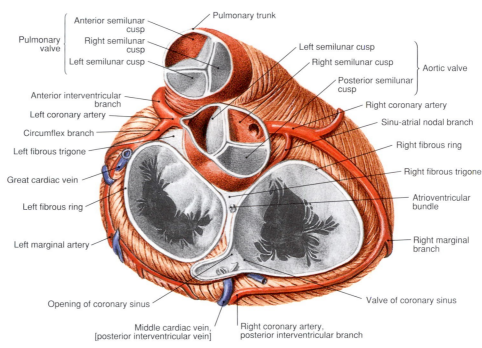

Pulmonary trunk
Anterior semilunar cusp
Pulmonary valve
Right semilunar cusp
Left semilunar cusp
Left semilunar cusp
Right semilunar cusp
Aortic valve
Posterior semilunar cusp
Anterior interventricular branch
Left coronary artery
Right coronary artery
Circumflex branch
Sinu-atrial nodal branch
Left fibrous trigone
Right fibrous ring
Great cardiac vein
Right fibrous trigone
Left fibrous ring
Atrioventricular bundle
Left marginal artery
Right marginal branch
Opening of coronary sinus
Valve of coronary sinus
Middle cardiac vein, [posterior interventricular vein]
Right coronary artery, posterior interventricular branch

Fig. 624 Coronary arteries; superior view.

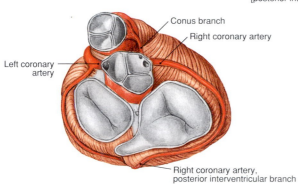

Conus branch
Right coronary artery
Left coronary artery
Right coronary artery, posterior interventricular branch

Fig. 625 Variability of the coronary arteries. The conus arteriosus branch arises from the aorta as an independent artery (~37%).

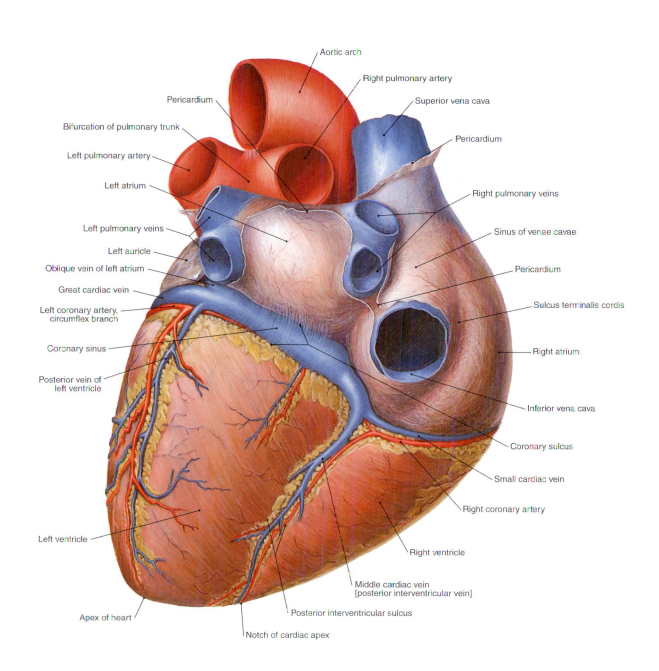

Fig. 626 Veins of the heart.

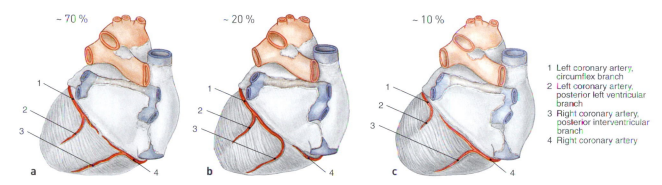

~ 70 %

~ 20 %

~ 10 %

1 Left coronary artery, circumflex branch
2 Left coronary artery, posterior left ventricular branch
3 Right coronary artery, posterior interventricular branch
4 Right coronary artery

Fig. 627 a–c Variations in the arterial supply of the posterior aspect of the heart; dorsal view.

a Balanced coronary artery supply
b Dominant left coronary artery supply
c Dominant right coronary artery supply

Coronary arteries, variability of supply

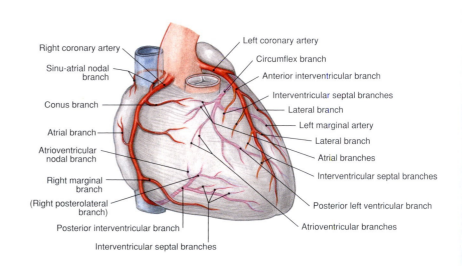

Fig. 628 Coronary arteries;
posterior arterial branches are shown in a
lighter colour;
the posterior interventricular branch arises
from the right coronary artery (balanced coronary
artery supply);
ventral view.

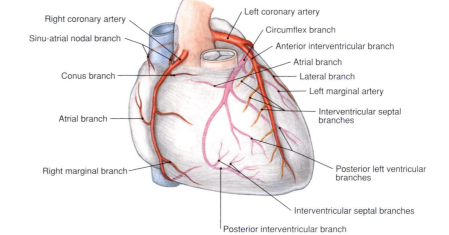

Fig. 629 Coronary arteries;
the posterior interventricular branch arises from
the left coronary artery (dominant left coronary
artery supply);
ventral view.

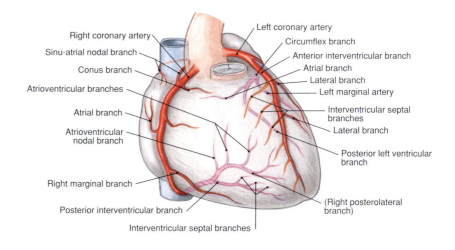

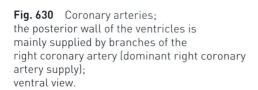

Fig. 630 Coronary arteries;
the posterior wall of the ventricles is
mainly supplied by branches of the
right coronary artery (dominant right coronary
artery supply);
ventral view.

Coronary arteries, radiography

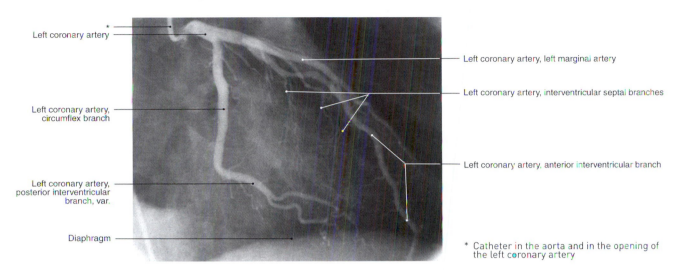

Left coronary artery
*
Left coronary artery, circumflex branch
Left coronary artery, posterior interventricular branch, var.
Diaphragm

Left coronary artery, left marginal artery
Left coronary artery, interventricular septal branches
Left coronary artery, anterior interventricular branch

* Catheter in the aorta and in the opening of the left coronary artery

Fig. 631 Left coronary artery; coronary angiography; the beam is directed obliquely from right anterior to left posterior (RAO).

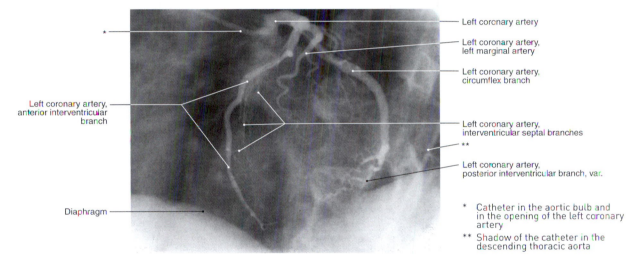

*
Left coronary artery, anterior interventricular branch
Diaphragm

Left coronary artery
Left coronary artery, left marginal artery
Left coronary artery, circumflex branch
Left coronary artery, interventricular septal branches
**
Left coronary artery, posterior interventricular branch, var.

* Catheter in the aortic bulb and in the opening of the left coronary artery
** Shadow of the catheter in the descending thoracic aorta

Fig. 632 Left coronary artery; coronary angiography; the beam is directed obliquely from left anterior to right posterior (LAO).

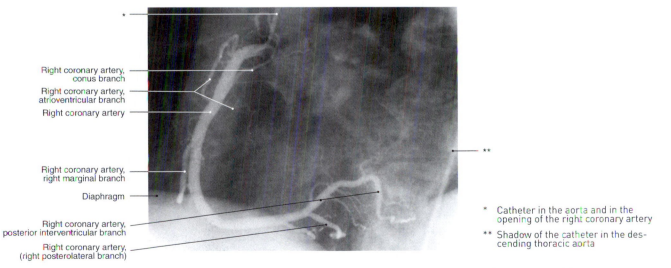

*
Right coronary artery, conus branch
Right coronary artery, atrioventricular branch
Right coronary artery
Right coronary artery, right marginal branch
Diaphragm
Right coronary artery, posterior interventricular branch
Right coronary artery, (right posterolateral branch)

**

* Catheter in the aorta and in the opening of the right coronary artery
** Shadow of the catheter in the descending thoracic aorta

Fig. 633 Right coronary artery; coronary angiography; the beam is directed obliquely from left anterior to right posterior (LAO).

Heart situs

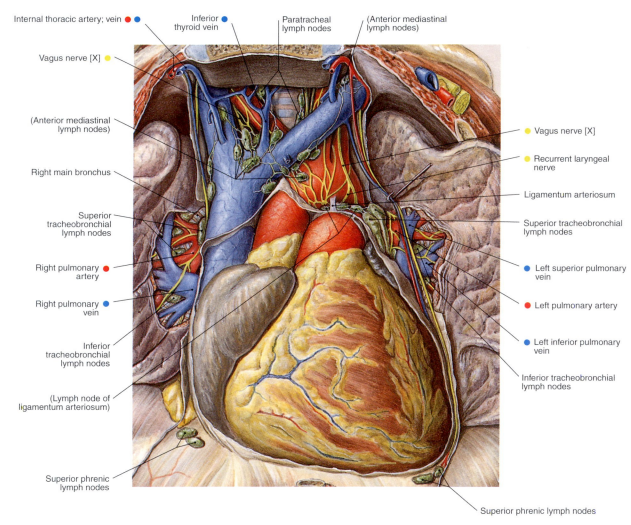

Internal thoracic artery; vein ● ●

Inferior thyroid vein ●

Paratracheal lymph nodes

(Anterior mediastinal lymph nodes)

Vagus nerve [X] ●

(Anterior mediastinal lymph nodes)

Right main bronchus

Superior tracheobronchial lymph nodes

Right pulmonary artery ●

Right pulmonary vein ●

Inferior tracheobronchial lymph nodes

(Lymph node of ligamentum arteriosum)

Superior phrenic lymph nodes

● Vagus nerve [X]

● Recurrent laryngeal nerve

Ligamentum arteriosum

Superior tracheobronchial lymph nodes

● Left superior pulmonary vein

● Left pulmonary artery

● Left inferior pulmonary vein

Inferior tracheobronchial lymph nodes

Superior phrenic lymph nodes

Fig. 634 Position of the heart in the thorax.

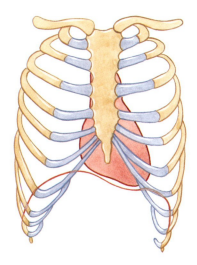

Fig. 635 Position of the heart; inspiration.

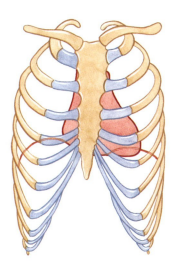

Fig. 636 Position of the heart; expiration.

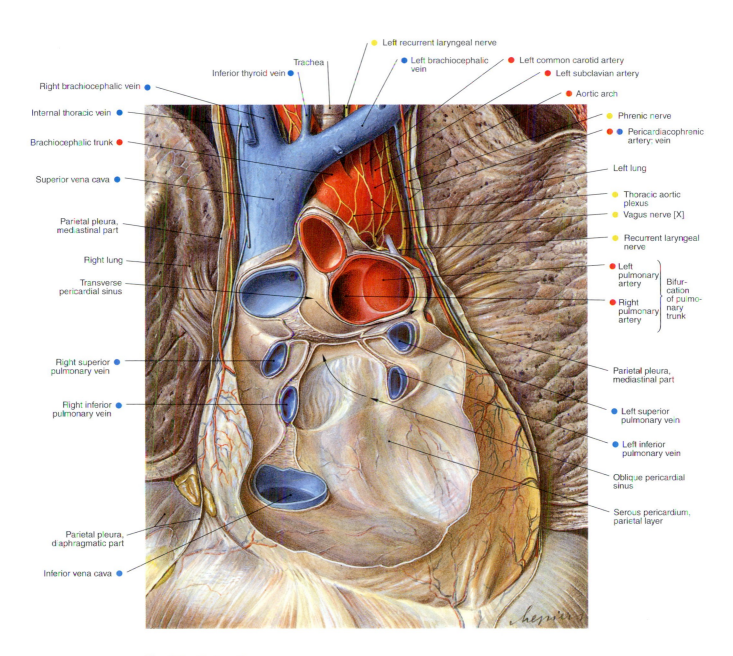

Left recurrent laryngeal nerve

Trachea

Inferior thyroid vein ●

Left brachiocephalic vein ●

Left common carotid artery ●

Left subclavian artery ●

Aortic arch ●

Right brachiocephalic vein ●

Internal thoracic vein ●

Brachiocephalic trunk ●

Superior vena cava ●

Parietal pleura, mediastinal part

Right lung

Transverse pericardial sinus

Right superior pulmonary vein ●

Right inferior pulmonary vein ●

Parietal pleura, diaphragmatic part

Inferior vena cava ●

Phrenic nerve ●

Pericardiacophrenic artery; vein ● ●

Left lung

Thoracic aortic plexus ●

Vagus nerve [X] ●

Recurrent laryngeal nerve ●

Left pulmonary artery ● } Bifurcation of pulmonary trunk

Right pulmonary artery ●

Parietal pleura, mediastinal part

Left superior pulmonary vein ●

Left inferior pulmonary vein ●

Oblique pericardial sinus

Serous pericardium, parietal layer

Fig. 637 Pericardium.

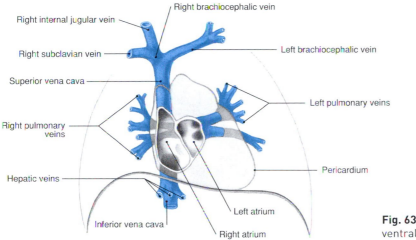

Right internal jugular vein

Right brachiocephalic vein

Right subclavian vein

Left brachiocephalic vein

Superior vena cava

Left pulmonary veins

Right pulmonary veins

Hepatic veins

Pericardium

Left atrium

Inferior vena cava

Right atrium

Fig. 638 Openings of the large veins into the heart; ventral view.

Trachea and bronchi

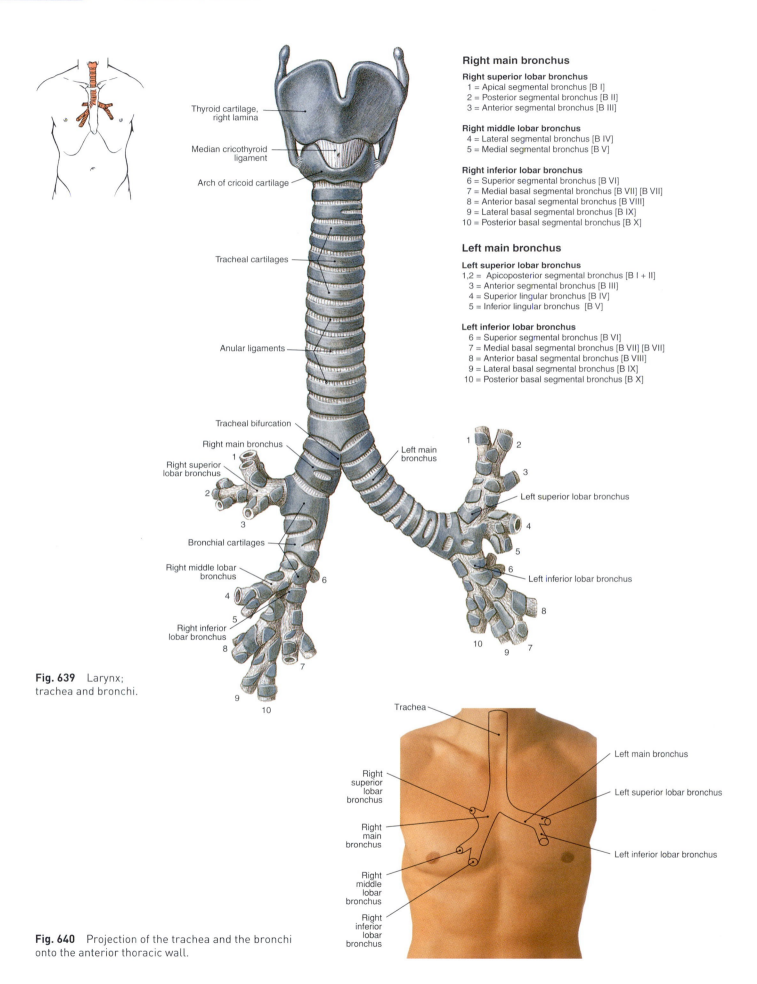

Right main bronchus

Right superior lobar bronchus
1 = Apical segmental bronchus [B I]
2 = Posterior segmental bronchus [B II]
3 = Anterior segmental bronchus [B III]

Right middle lobar bronchus
4 = Lateral segmental bronchus [B IV]
5 = Medial segmental bronchus [B V]

Right inferior lobar bronchus
6 = Superior segmental bronchus [B VI]
7 = Medial basal segmental bronchus [B VII] [B VII]
8 = Anterior basal segmental bronchus [B VIII]
9 = Lateral basal segmental bronchus [B IX]
10 = Posterior basal segmental bronchus [B X]

Left main bronchus

Left superior lobar bronchus
1,2 = Apicoposterior segmental bronchus [B I + II]
3 = Anterior segmental bronchus [B III]
4 = Superior lingular bronchus [B IV]
5 = Inferior lingular bronchus [B V]

Left inferior lobar bronchus
6 = Superior segmental bronchus [B VI]
7 = Medial basal segmental bronchus [B VII] [B VII]
8 = Anterior basal segmental bronchus [B VIII]
9 = Lateral basal segmental bronchus [B IX]
10 = Posterior basal segmental bronchus [B X]

Thyroid cartilage, right lamina
Median cricothyroid ligament
Arch of cricoid cartilage
Tracheal cartilages
Anular ligaments
Tracheal bifurcation
Right main bronchus
Right superior lobar bronchus
Left main bronchus
Left superior lobar bronchus
Left inferior lobar bronchus
Bronchial cartilages
Right middle lobar bronchus
Right inferior lobar bronchus

Fig. 639 Larynx; trachea and bronchi.

Trachea
Right superior lobar bronchus
Right main bronchus
Right middle lobar bronchus
Right inferior lobar bronchus
Left main bronchus
Left superior lobar bronchus
Left inferior lobar bronchus

Fig. 640 Projection of the trachea and the bronchi onto the anterior thoracic wall.

Trachea, structure

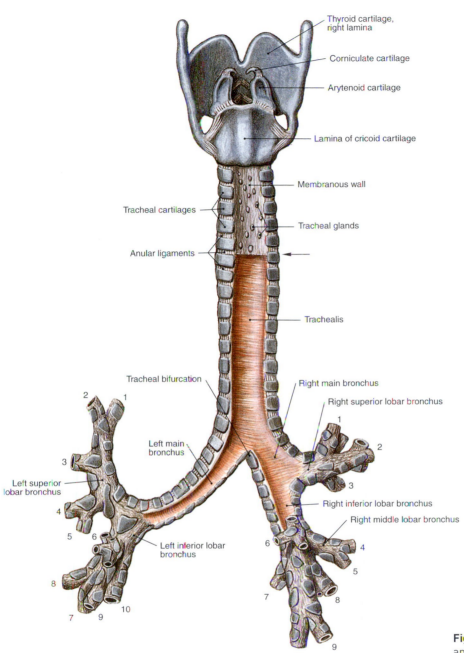

Thyroid cartilage, right lamina

Corniculate cartilage

Arytenoid cartilage

Lamina of cricoid cartilage

Membranous wall

Tracheal cartilages

Tracheal glands

Anular ligaments

Trachealis

Tracheal bifurcation

Right main bronchus

Right superior lobar bronchus

Left main bronchus

Left superior lobar bronchus

Right inferior lobar bronchus

Right middle lobar bronchus

Left inferior lobar bronchus

Fig. 641 Larynx; trachea and bronchi; dorsal view.

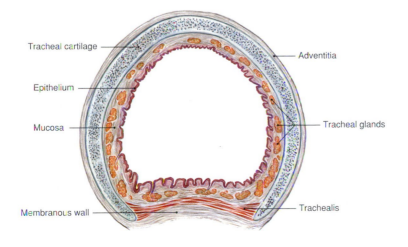

Tracheal cartilage

Adventitia

Epithelium

Mucosa

Tracheal glands

Membranous wall

Trachealis

Fig. 642 Trachea; cross-section; microscopic enlargement at low magnification.

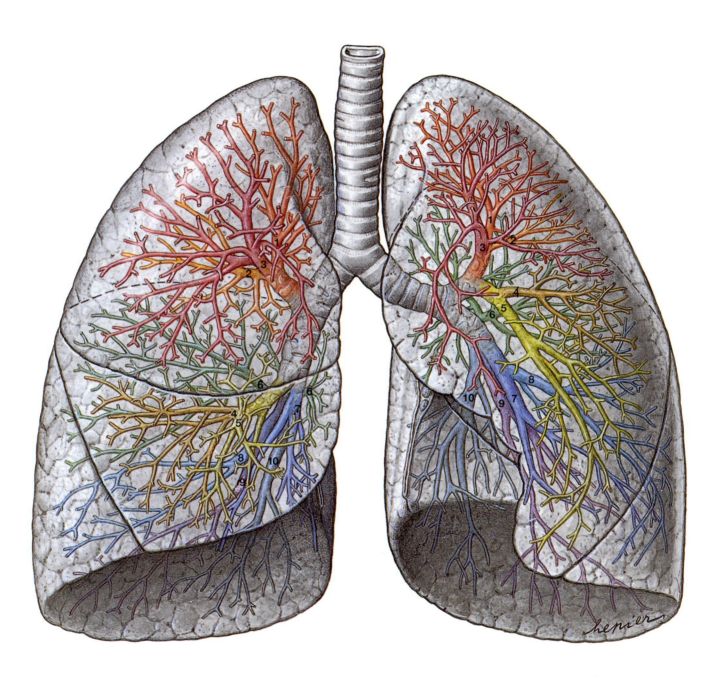

Fig. 643 Bronchi;
the lobar and the segmental bronchi have been projected
onto the lungs and are illustrated with different colours;
ventral view.
Numbers indicate the segmental bronchi (see p. 348).

Bronchial tree, radiography

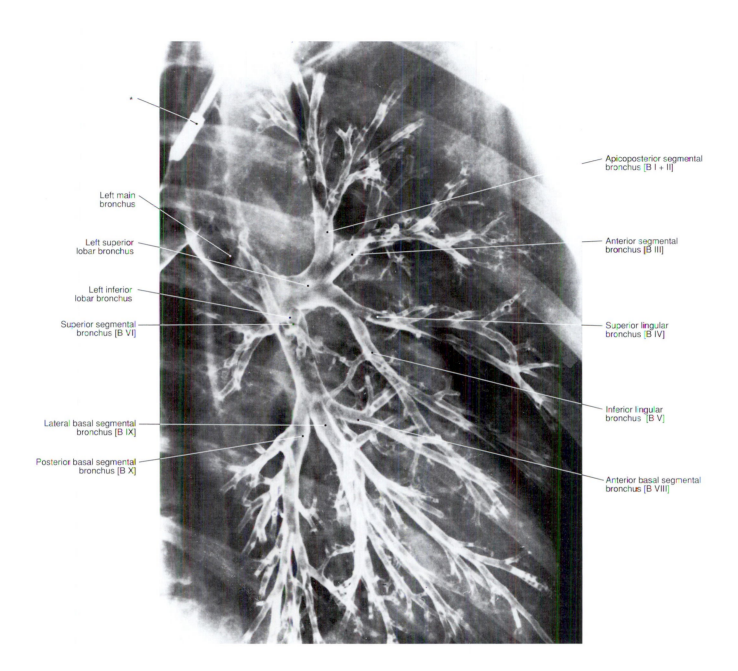

Apicoposterior segmental
bronchus [B I + II]

Left main
bronchus

Left superior
lobar bronchus

Anterior segmental
bronchus [B III]

Left inferior
lobar bronchus

Superior segmental
bronchus [B VI]

Superior lingular
bronchus [B IV]

Inferior lingular
bronchus [B V]

Lateral basal segmental
bronchus [B IX]

Posterior basal segmental
bronchus [B X]

Anterior basal segmental
bronchus [B VIII]

Fig. 644 Bronchi;
AP-radiograph; bronchography of the left lung.

* Bronchography catheter in the trachea

Lungs

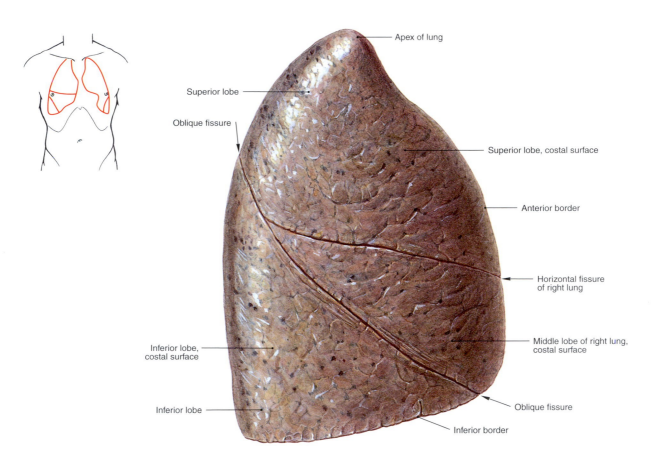

Apex of lung

Superior lobe

Oblique fissure

Superior lobe, costal surface

Anterior border

Horizontal fissure of right lung

Middle lobe of right lung, costal surface

Inferior lobe, costal surface

Oblique fissure

Inferior lobe

Inferior border

Fig. 645   Right lung; lateral view.

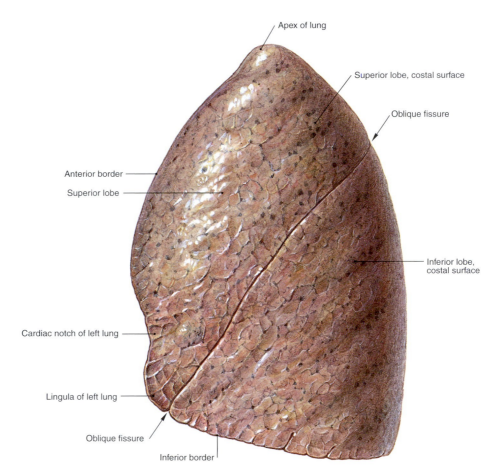

Apex of lung

Superior lobe, costal surface

Oblique fissure

Anterior border

Superior lobe

Inferior lobe, costal surface

Cardiac notch of left lung

Lingula of left lung

Oblique fissure

Inferior border

Fig. 646   Left lung; lateral view.

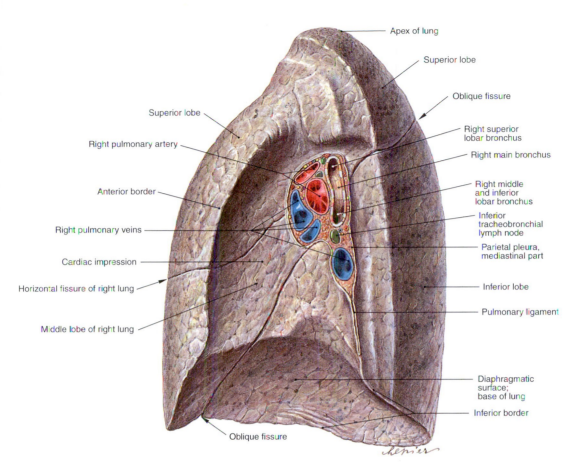

Apex of lung

Superior lobe

Oblique fissure

Superior lobe

Right pulmonary artery

Right superior
lobar bronchus

Right main bronchus

Anterior border

Right middle
and inferior
lobar bronchus

Inferior
tracheobronchial
lymph node

Right pulmonary veins

Parietal pleura,
mediastinal part

Cardiac impression

Horizontal fissure of right lung

Inferior lobe

Middle lobe of right lung

Pulmonary ligament

Diaphragmatic
surface;
base of lung

Inferior border

Oblique fissure

Fig. 647 Right lung;
sagittal section at the plane of the hilum
of the lung;
medial view.

Apex of lung

Oblique fissure

Left pulmonary artery

Left superior
pulmonary vein

Parietal pleura,
mediastinal part

Left main bronchus

Left inferior
pulmonary vein

Anterior border

Costal surface

Pulmonary ligament

Tracheobronchial
lymph nodes

Inferior lobe

Cardiac impression

Cardiac notch of left lung

Inferior border

Lingula of left lung

Diaphragmatic
surface; base of lung

Oblique fissure

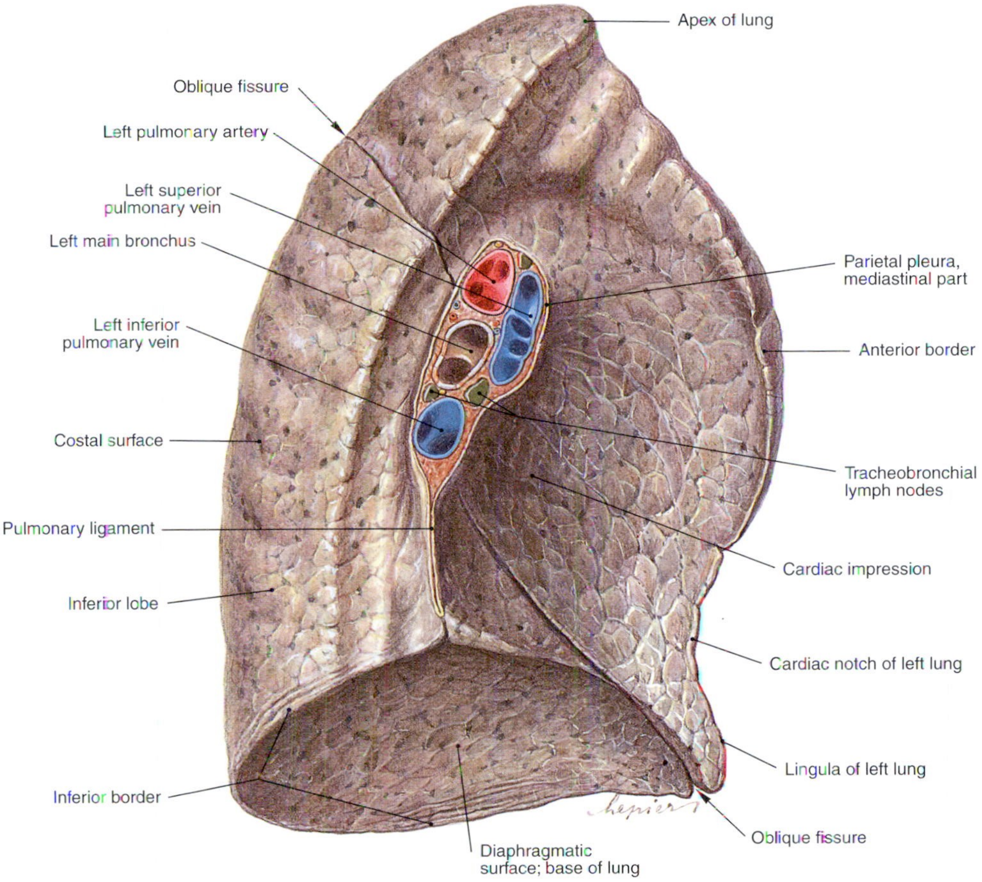

Fig. 648 Left lung;
sagittal section at the plane of the hilum
of the lung;
medial view.

Bronchopulmonary segments

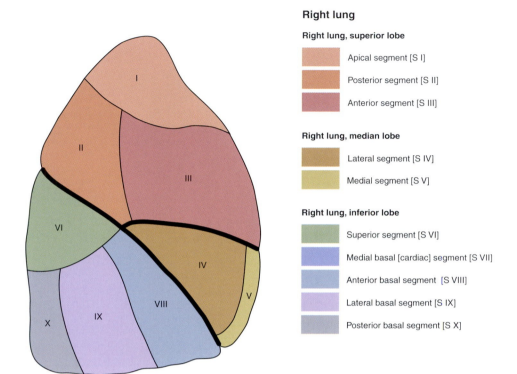

Right lung

Right lung, superior lobe

	Apical segment [S I]
	Posterior segment [S II]
	Anterior segment [S III]

Right lung, median lobe

	Lateral segment [S IV]
	Medial segment [S V]

Right lung, inferior lobe

	Superior segment [S VI]
	Medial basal [cardiac] segment [S VII]
	Anterior basal segment [S VIII]
	Lateral basal segment [S IX]
	Posterior basal segment [S X]

Fig. 649 Right lung; bronchopulmonary segments; lateral view.

Left lung

Left lung, superior lobe

	} Apicoposterior segment [S I + II]
	Anterior segment [S III]
	Superior lingular segment [S IV]
	Inferior lingular segment [S V]

Left lung, inferior lobe

	Superior segment [S VI]
	Medial basal [cardiac] segment [S VII]*
	Anterior basal segment [S VIII]
	Lateral basal segment [S IX]
	Posterior basal segment [S X]

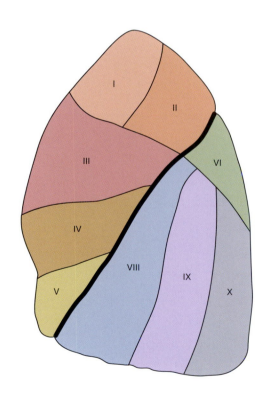

Fig. 650 Left lung; bronchopulmonary segments; lateral view.

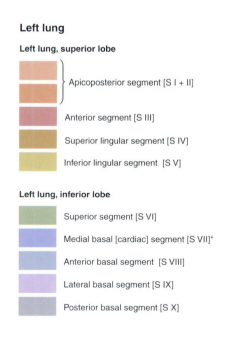

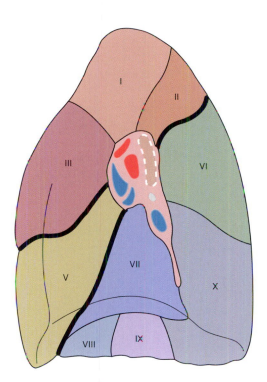

Fig. 651 Right lung;
bronchopulmonary segments;
medial view.

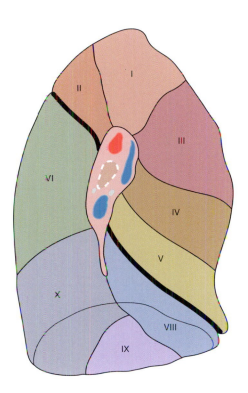

Fig. 652 Left lung;
bronchopulmonary segments;
medial view.

Lungs, structure

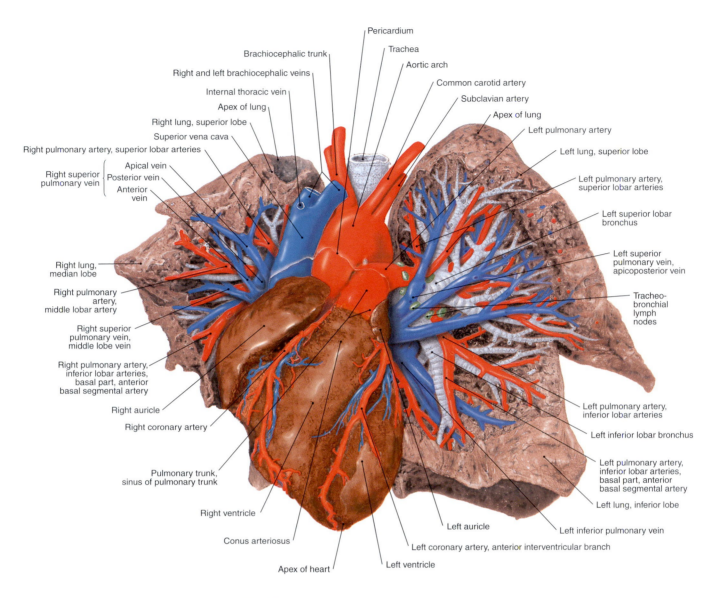

Pericardium
Brachiocephalic trunk
Trachea
Right and left brachiocephalic veins
Aortic arch
Internal thoracic vein
Common carotid artery
Apex of lung
Subclavian artery
Right lung, superior lobe
Apex of lung
Superior vena cava
Left pulmonary artery
Right pulmonary artery, superior lobar arteries
Left lung, superior lobe
Apical vein
Left pulmonary artery, superior lobar arteries
Right superior pulmonary vein
Posterior vein
Anterior vein
Left superior lobar bronchus
Left superior pulmonary vein, apicoposterior vein
Right lung, median lobe
Right pulmonary artery, middle lobar artery
Tracheobronchial lymph nodes
Right superior pulmonary vein, middle lobe vein
Right pulmonary artery, inferior lobar arteries, basal part, anterior basal segmental artery
Left pulmonary artery, inferior lobar arteries
Right auricle
Left inferior lobar bronchus
Right coronary artery
Left pulmonary artery, inferior lobar arteries, basal part, anterior basal segmental artery
Left lung, inferior lobe
Pulmonary trunk, sinus of pulmonary trunk
Left inferior pulmonary vein
Right ventricle
Left auricle
Conus arteriosus
Left coronary artery, anterior interventricular branch
Apex of heart
Left ventricle

Fig. 653 Lungs and heart;
the arteries, the veins and the bronchi have been
dissected up to the external surface of the lungs.

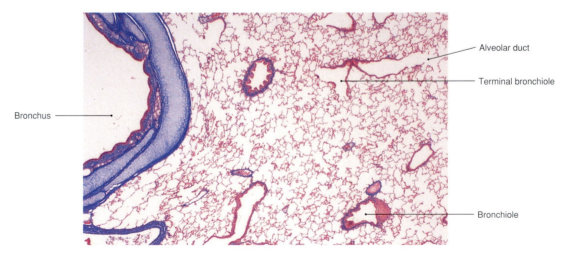

Alveolar duct
Terminal bronchiole
Bronchus
Bronchiole

Fig. 654 Lung;
overview of the lung structure;
microscopic enlargement at low magnification.

Vessels of the lungs and bronchi

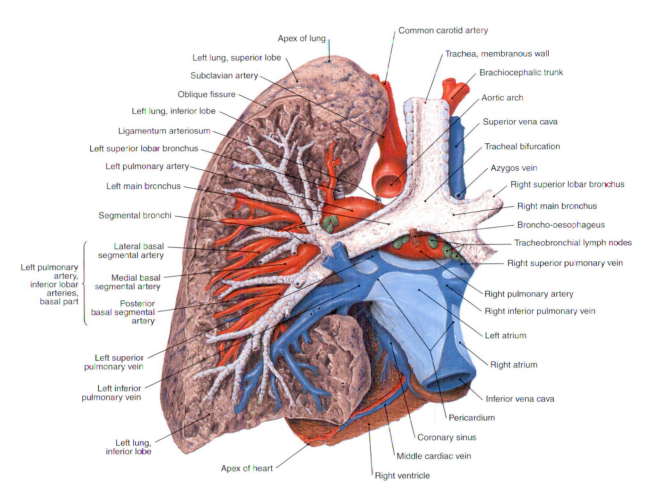

Apex of lung
Common carotid artery
Left lung, superior lobe
Trachea, membranous wall
Subclavian artery
Brachiocephalic trunk
Oblique fissure
Aortic arch
Left lung, inferior lobe
Superior vena cava
Ligamentum arteriosum
Tracheal bifurcation
Left superior lobar bronchus
Azygos vein
Left pulmonary artery
Right superior lobar bronchus
Left main bronchus
Right main bronchus
Segmental bronchi
Broncho-oesophageus
Lateral basal segmental artery
Tracheobronchial lymph nodes
Left pulmonary artery, inferior lobar arteries, basal part
Right superior pulmonary vein
Medial basal segmental artery
Right pulmonary artery
Posterior basal segmental artery
Right inferior pulmonary vein
Left atrium
Left superior pulmonary vein
Right atrium
Left inferior pulmonary vein
Inferior vena cava
Pericardium
Coronary sinus
Left lung, inferior lobe
Middle cardiac vein
Apex of heart
Right ventricle

Fig. 655 Vessels of the left lung; dorsal view.

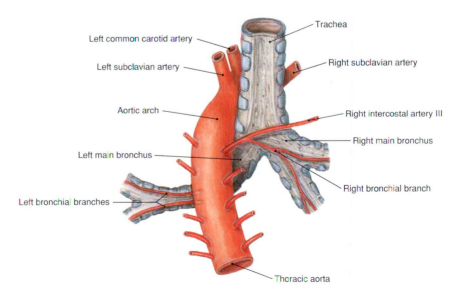

Left common carotid artery
Trachea
Left subclavian artery
Right subclavian artery
Aortic arch
Right intercostal artery III
Right main bronchus
Left main bronchus
Right bronchial branch
Left bronchial branches
Thoracic aorta

Fig. 656 Bronchi; arterial supply.

Vessels of the lung, radiography

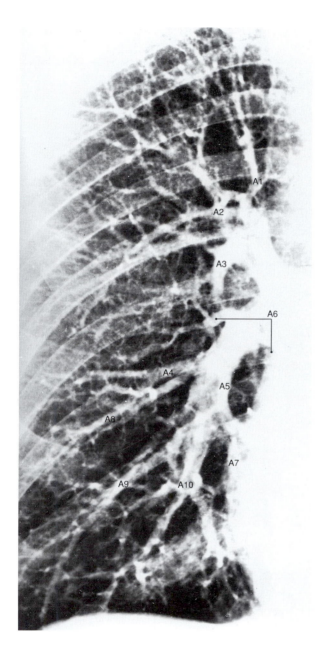

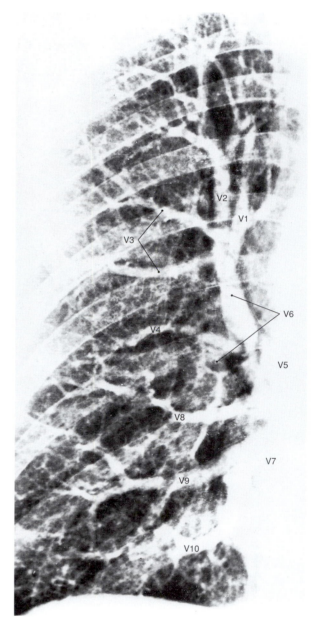

Fig. 657   Arteries of the right lung;
AP-radiograph (pulmonary angiography); after injection
of a contrast medium into the right ventricle;
ventral view.
The numbers designate the segmental arteries
(compare p. 354).

Fig. 658   Veins of the right lung;
AP-radiograph (return via pulmonary veins of the contrast
medium injected into the right ventricle);
ventral view.
Numbers indicate the segmental veins (compare p. 354).

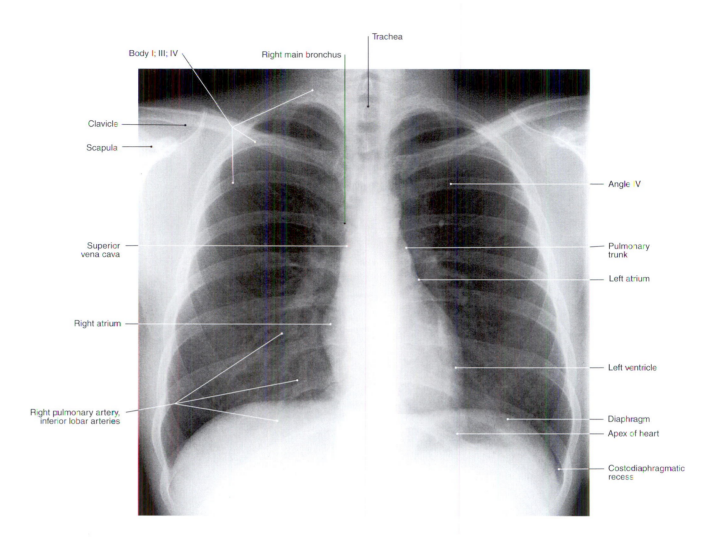

Trachea

Body I; III; IV

Right main bronchus

Clavicle

Scapula

Angle IV

Superior vena cava

Pulmonary trunk

Left atrium

Right atrium

Left ventricle

Right pulmonary artery, inferior lobar arteries

Diaphragm

Apex of heart

Costodiaphragmatic recess

Fig. 659   Thoracic cage and thoracic viscera;
PA-radiograph of a 27-year-old male (thorax radiograph).

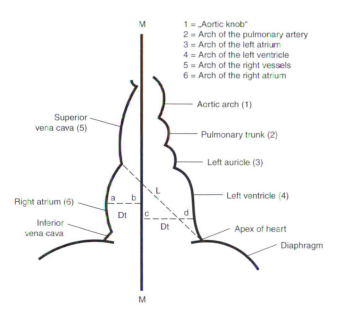

M

1 = „Aortic knob"
2 = Arch of the pulmonary artery
3 = Arch of the left atrium
4 = Arch of the left ventricle
5 = Arch of the right vessels
6 = Arch of the right atrium

Aortic arch (1)

Superior vena cava (5)

Pulmonary trunk (2)

Left auricle (3)

Left ventricle (4)

Right atrium (6)

Inferior vena cava

Apex of heart

Diaphragm

M

Fig. 660   Outline of the heart shadow in the radiograph;
Dt = Transverse diameter,
 ab + cd = 13–14 cm
L = Longitudinal axis of the heart (from the superior border of the right atrial contour to the apex of the heart) = 15–16 cm
M = Median plane of the body

Bronchoscopy

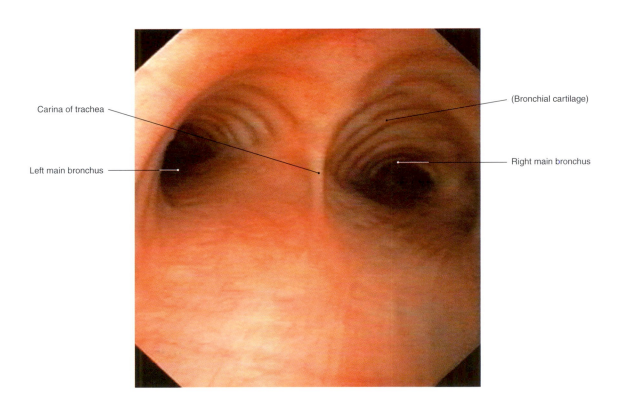

Carina of trachea

Left main bronchus

(Bronchial cartilage)

Right main bronchus

Fig. 661 Bronchi;
bronchoscopy of a healthy individual displaying the tracheal bifurcation and the carina of trachea.

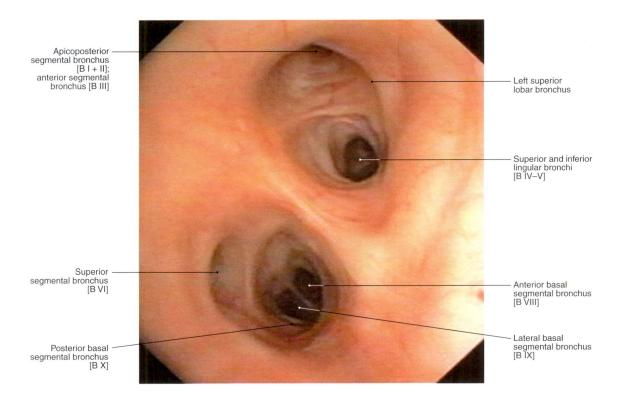

Apicoposterior segmental bronchus [B I + II]; anterior segmental bronchus [B III]

Left superior lobar bronchus

Superior and inferior lingular bronchi [B IV–V]

Superior segmental bronchus [B VI]

Anterior basal segmental bronchus [B VIII]

Posterior basal segmental bronchus [B X]

Lateral basal segmental bronchus [B IX]

Fig. 662 Bronchi;
bronchoscopic view of the left segmental bronchi.

Lungs, surface projections

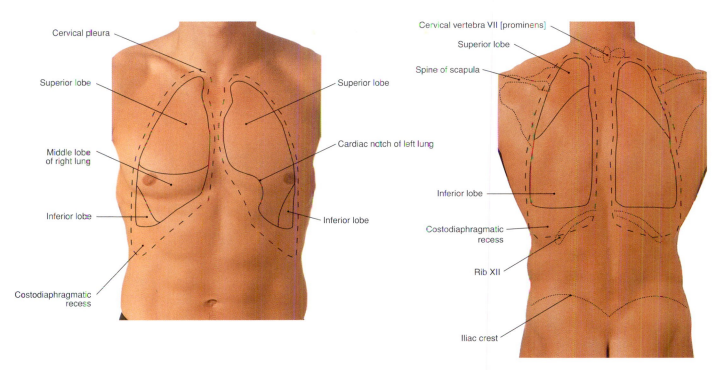

Fig. 663   Projection of the pulmonary and the pleural
borders onto the anterior thoracic wall.

Fig. 664   Projection of the pulmonary and the pleural
borders onto the posterior thoracic wall.

Borders of the lungs – line
Borders of the pleura – dashed line

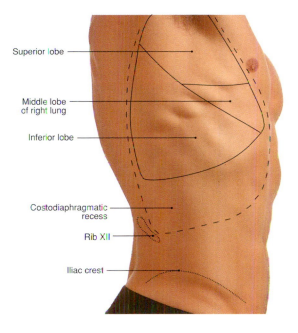

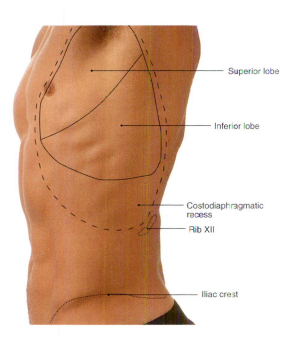

Fig. 665   Projection of the pulmonary and the pleural
borders onto the lateral thoracic wall.

Fig. 666   Projection of the pulmonary and the pleural
borders onto the lateral thoracic wall.

Oesophagus

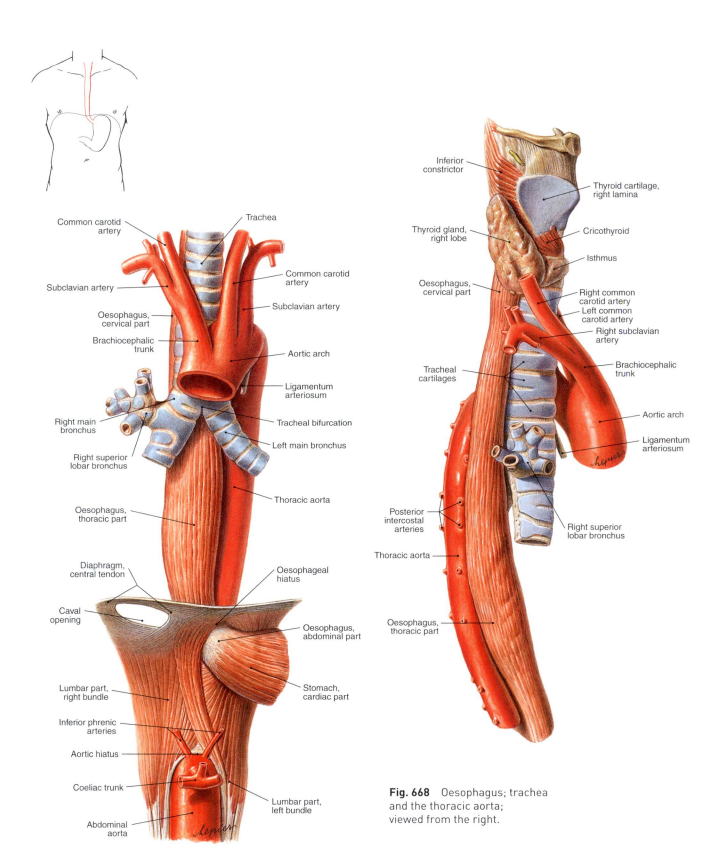

Common carotid artery

Trachea

Subclavian artery

Common carotid artery

Oesophagus, cervical part

Subclavian artery

Brachiocephalic trunk

Aortic arch

Ligamentum arteriosum

Right main bronchus

Tracheal bifurcation

Right superior lobar bronchus

Left main bronchus

Thoracic aorta

Oesophagus, thoracic part

Diaphragm, central tendon

Oesophageal hiatus

Caval opening

Oesophagus, abdominal part

Lumbar part, right bundle

Stomach, cardiac part

Inferior phrenic arteries

Aortic hiatus

Coeliac trunk

Lumbar part, left bundle

Abdominal aorta

Fig. 667 Oesophagus; trachea and the thoracic aorta; ventral view.

Inferior constrictor

Thyroid cartilage, right lamina

Thyroid gland, right lobe

Cricothyroid

Isthmus

Oesophagus, cervical part

Right common carotid artery

Left common carotid artery

Right subclavian artery

Tracheal cartilages

Brachiocephalic trunk

Aortic arch

Ligamentum arteriosum

Posterior intercostal arteries

Right superior lobar bronchus

Thoracic aorta

Oesophagus, thoracic part

Fig. 668 Oesophagus; trachea and the thoracic aorta; viewed from the right.

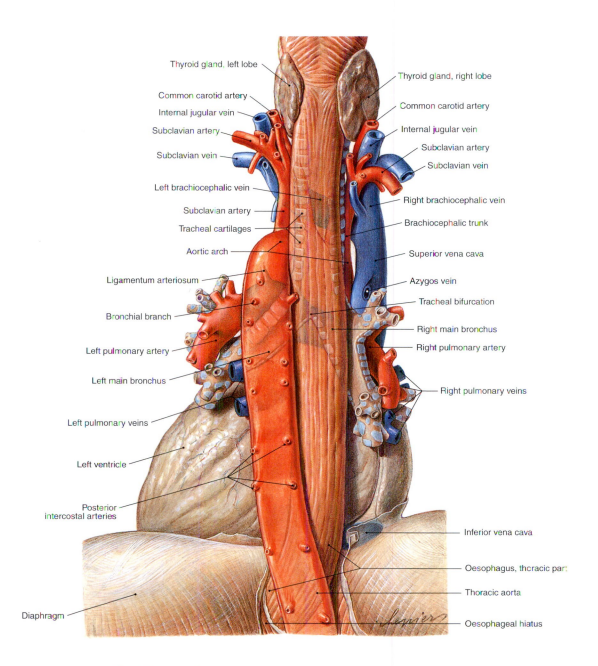

Thyroid gland, left lobe
Common carotid artery
Internal jugular vein
Subclavian artery
Subclavian vein
Left brachiocephalic vein
Subclavian artery
Tracheal cartilages
Aortic arch
Ligamentum arteriosum
Bronchial branch
Left pulmonary artery
Left main bronchus
Left pulmonary veins
Left ventricle
Posterior intercostal arteries
Diaphragm

Thyroid gland, right lobe
Common carotid artery
Internal jugular vein
Subclavian artery
Subclavian vein
Right brachiocephalic vein
Brachiocephalic trunk
Superior vena cava
Azygos vein
Tracheal bifurcation
Right main bronchus
Right pulmonary artery
Right pulmonary veins
Inferior vena cava
Oesophagus, thoracic part
Thoracic aorta
Oesophageal hiatus

Fig. 669 Oesophagus and the thoracic aorta; dorsal view.

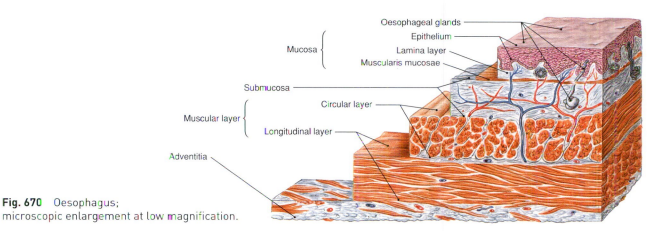

Oesophageal glands
Epithelium
Lamina layer
Muscularis mucosae
Mucosa
Submucosa
Circular layer
Muscular layer
Longitudinal layer
Adventitia

Fig. 670 Oesophagus; microscopic enlargement at low magnification.

Vessels of the oesophagus

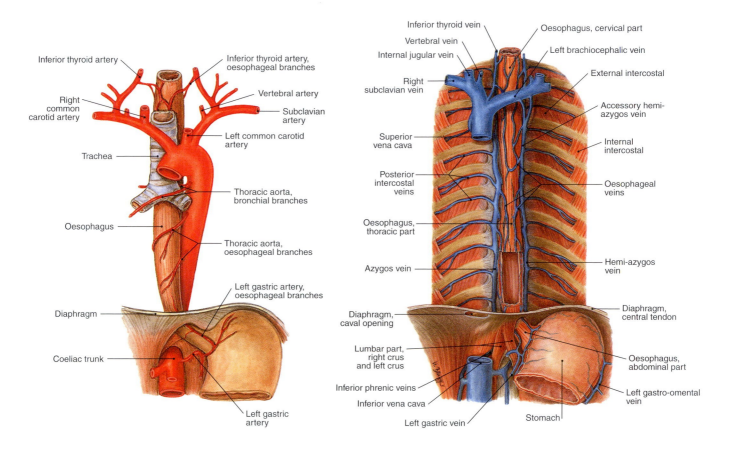

Inferior thyroid artery

Inferior thyroid artery, oesophageal branches

Right common carotid artery

Vertebral artery

Subclavian artery

Left common carotid artery

Trachea

Thoracic aorta, bronchial branches

Oesophagus

Thoracic aorta, oesophageal branches

Left gastric artery, oesophageal branches

Diaphragm

Coeliac trunk

Left gastric artery

Inferior thyroid vein

Oesophagus, cervical part

Vertebral vein

Left brachiocephalic vein

Internal jugular vein

Right subclavian vein

External intercostal

Accessory hemi-azygos vein

Superior vena cava

Internal intercostal

Posterior intercostal veins

Oesophageal veins

Oesophagus, thoracic part

Azygos vein

Hemi-azygos vein

Diaphragm, caval opening

Diaphragm, central tendon

Lumbar part, right crus and left crus

Oesophagus, abdominal part

Inferior phrenic veins

Inferior vena cava

Left gastro-omental vein

Left gastric vein

Stomach

Fig. 671   Oesophagus; supplying arteries; ventral view.

Fig. 672   Veins of the oesophagus.

→ 809, 810

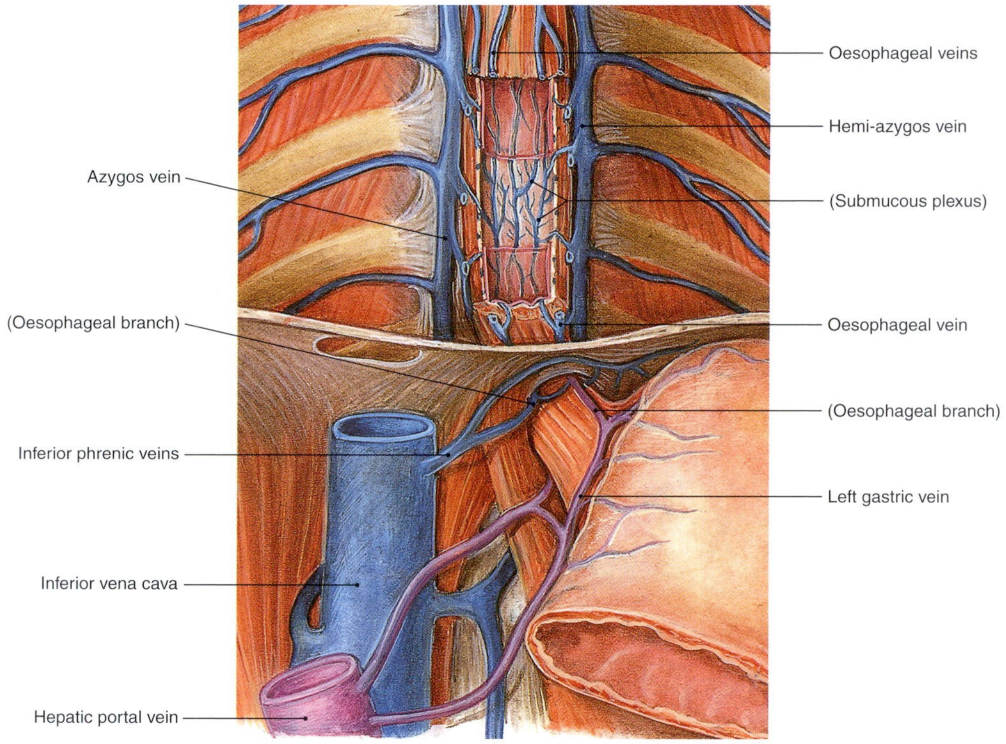

Azygos vein

Oesophageal veins

Hemi-azygos vein

(Submucous plexus)

(Oesophageal branch)

Oesophageal vein

Inferior phrenic veins

(Oesophageal branch)

Inferior vena cava

Left gastric vein

Hepatic portal vein

→ 810

Fig. 673   Veins of the oesophagus; magnification of Fig. 672; demonstration of anastomoses between branches of the hepatic portal vein and the superior vena cava.

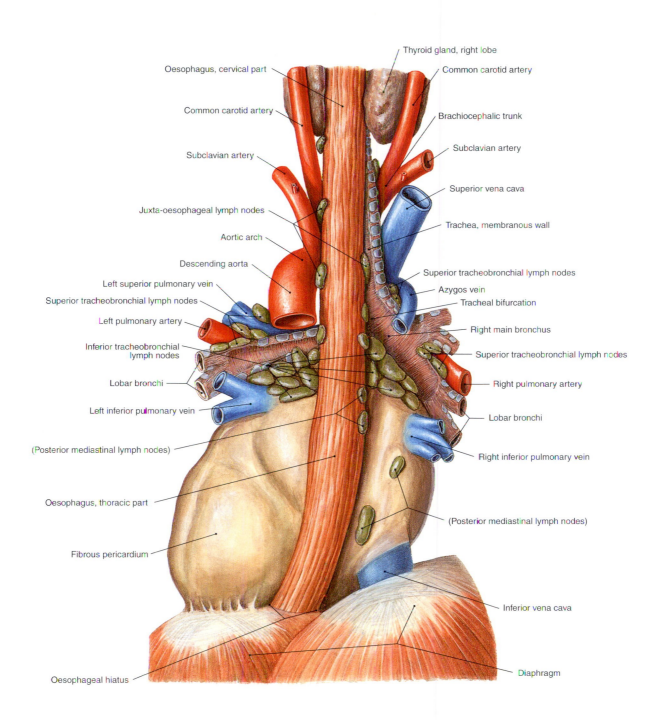

Thyroid gland, right lobe
Oesophagus, cervical part
Common carotid artery
Common carotid artery
Brachiocephalic trunk
Subclavian artery
Subclavian artery
Superior vena cava
Juxta-oesophageal lymph nodes
Trachea, membranous wall
Aortic arch
Descending aorta
Superior tracheobronchial lymph nodes
Left superior pulmonary vein
Azygos vein
Superior tracheobronchial lymph nodes
Tracheal bifurcation
Left pulmonary artery
Right main bronchus
Inferior tracheobronchial lymph nodes
Superior tracheobronchial lymph nodes
Lobar bronchi
Right pulmonary artery
Left inferior pulmonary vein
Lobar bronchi
(Posterior mediastinal lymph nodes)
Right inferior pulmonary vein
Oesophagus, thoracic part
(Posterior mediastinal lymph nodes)
Fibrous pericardium
Inferior vena cava
Oesophageal hiatus
Diaphragm

Fig. 674 Thoracic lymph nodes; dorsal view.

Oesophagus, radiography and oesophagoscopy

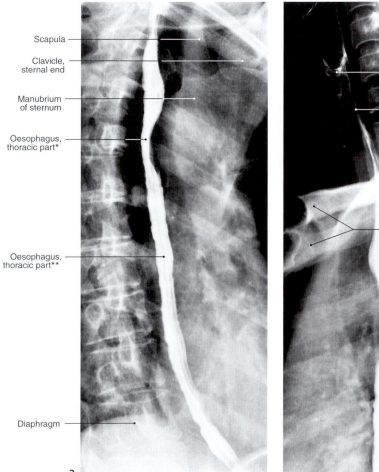

Scapula

Clavicle, sternal end

Manubrium of sternum

Oesophagus, thoracic part*

Oesophagus, thoracic part**

Diaphragm

a

Piriform fossa

Oesophagus, cervical part***

Clavicles

Aortic arch

Oesophagus, thoracic part

b

Fig. 675 a, b   Oesophagus;
radiograph after swallowing of a contrast medium.
a   Right anterior oblique position, oblique diameter I (beam directed from left anterior to right posterior)
b   Left anterior oblique position, oblique diameter II (beam directed from right anterior to left posterior)

*   Oesophageal constriction caused by the aortic arch
**   Retrocardial portion of the oesophagus
*** Oesophageal constriction at the junction of the pharynx with the oesophagus

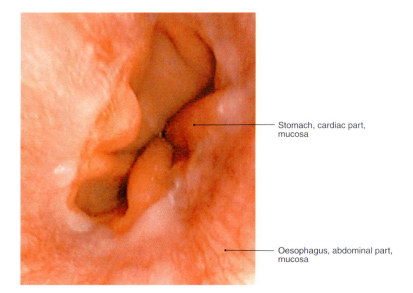

Stomach, cardiac part, mucosa

Oesophagus, abdominal part, mucosa

Fig. 676   Oesophagus;
oesophagoscopy (technical details see Fig. 718);
superior view.

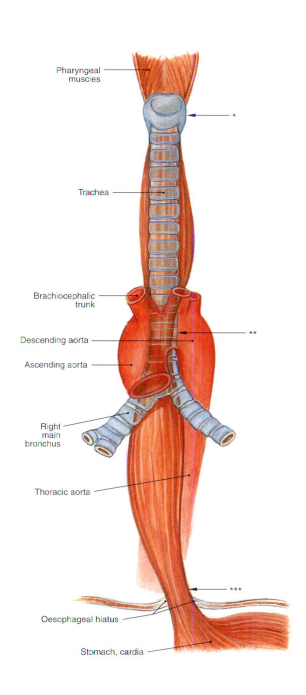

Fig. 677 Oesophagus;
constrictions.

* Upper cesophageal sphincter
** Narrowing caused by the aortic arch
*** Diaphragmatic constriction

Pharyngeal muscles

Trachea

Brachiocephalic trunk

Descending aorta

Ascending aorta

Right main bronchus

Thoracic aorta

Oesophageal hiatus

Stomach, cardia

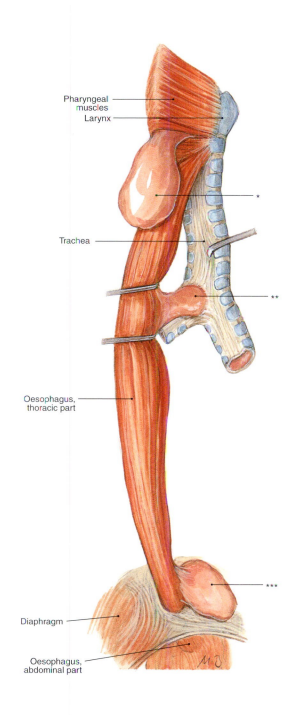

Fig. 678 Oesophagus;
typical location and frequency of diverticula.

* Cervical diverticulum
(ZENKER's diverticulum), (~70%)
** Mid-oesophageal diverticulum (~22%)
*** Epiphrenic diverticulum (~8%)

Pharyngeal muscles
Larynx

Trachea

Oesophagus, thoracic part

Diaphragm

Oesophagus, abdominal part

Thymus

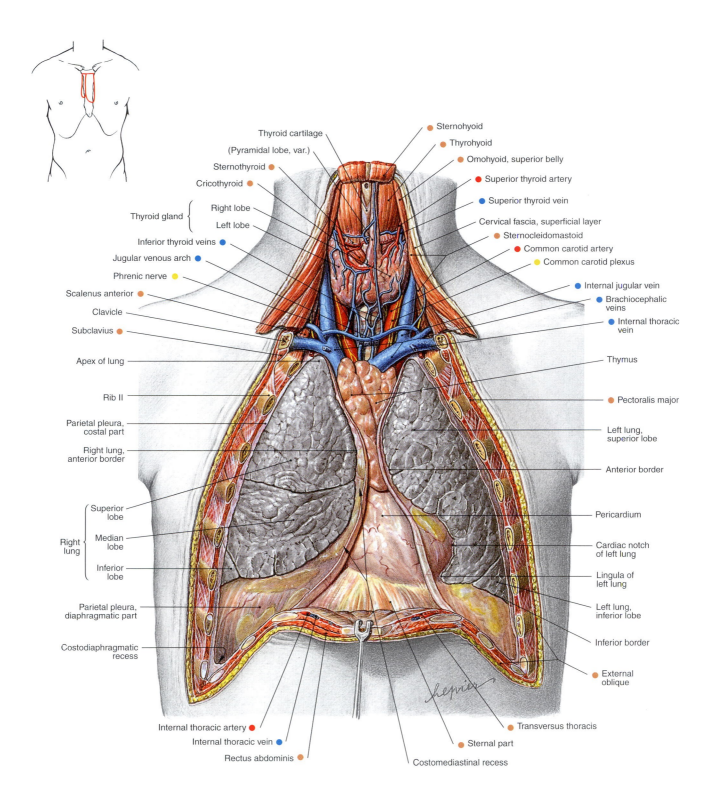

Thyroid cartilage

(Pyramidal lobe, var.)

Sternothyroid ●

Cricothyroid ●

Thyroid gland { Right lobe
Left lobe

Inferior thyroid veins ●

Jugular venous arch ●

Phrenic nerve ●

Scalenus anterior ●

Clavicle

Subclavius ●

Apex of lung

Rib II

Parietal pleura, costal part

Right lung, anterior border

Right lung { Superior lobe
Median lobe
Inferior lobe

Parietal pleura, diaphragmatic part

Costodiaphragmatic recess

● Sternohyoid

● Thyrohyoid

● Omohyoid, superior belly

● Superior thyroid artery

● Superior thyroid vein

Cervical fascia, superficial layer

● Sternocleidomastoid

● Common carotid artery

● Common carotid plexus

● Internal jugular vein

● Brachiocephalic veins

● Internal thoracic vein

Thymus

● Pectoralis major

Left lung, superior lobe

Anterior border

Pericardium

Cardiac notch of left lung

Lingula of left lung

Left lung, inferior lobe

Inferior border

● External oblique

Internal thoracic artery ●

Internal thoracic vein ●

Rectus abdominis ●

Costomediastinal recess

● Transversus thoracis

● Sternal part

→ 781

Fig. 679 Thymus; pericardium and lungs of an adolescent.
Note the size of the adolescent thymus. In older individuals,
the thymic tissue is almost entirely replaced by adipose tissue

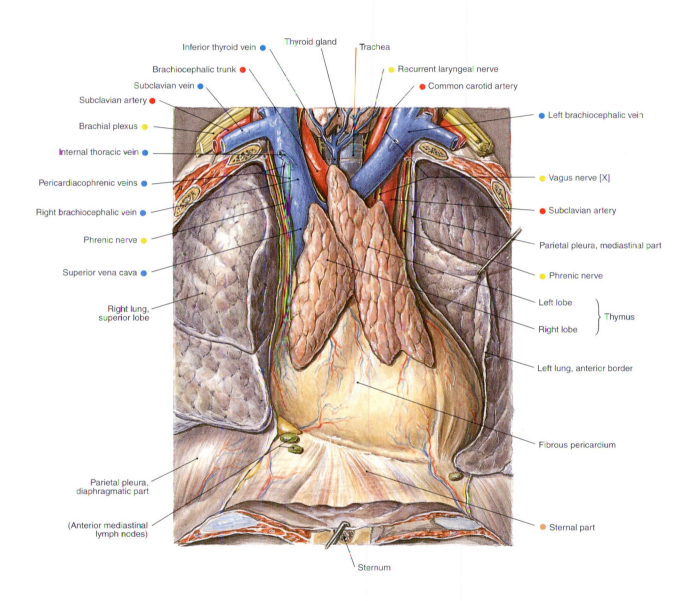

Inferior thyroid vein ●
Thyroid gland
Trachea
Brachiocephalic trunk ●
Subclavian vein ●
Recurrent laryngeal nerve ●
Subclavian artery ●
Common carotid artery ●
Brachial plexus ●
Left brachiocephalic vein ●
Internal thoracic vein ●
Pericardiacophrenic veins ●
Vagus nerve [X] ●
Right brachiocephalic vein ●
Subclavian artery ●
Phrenic nerve ●
Parietal pleura, mediastinal part
Superior vena cava ●
Phrenic nerve ●
Right lung, superior lobe
Left lobe
Right lobe
Thymus
Left lung, anterior border
Fibrous pericardium
Parietal pleura, diaphragmatic part
(Anterior mediastinal lymph nodes)
Sternal part ●
Sternum

Fig. 680 Thymus of an adolescent.

→ 781

Pleural cavity

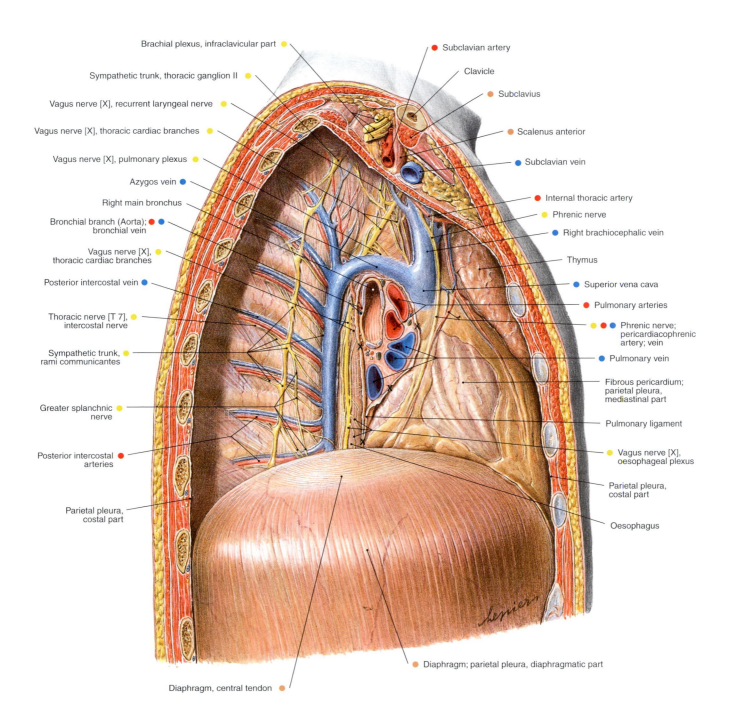

Brachial plexus, infraclavicular part

Sympathetic trunk, thoracic ganglion II

Vagus nerve [X], recurrent laryngeal nerve

Vagus nerve [X], thoracic cardiac branches

Vagus nerve [X], pulmonary plexus

Azygos vein

Right main bronchus

Bronchial branch (Aorta); bronchial vein

Vagus nerve [X], thoracic cardiac branches

Posterior intercostal vein

Thoracic nerve [T 7], intercostal nerve

Sympathetic trunk, rami communicantes

Greater splanchnic nerve

Posterior intercostal arteries

Parietal pleura, costal part

Diaphragm, central tendon

Subclavian artery

Clavicle

Subclavius

Scalenus anterior

Subclavian vein

Internal thoracic artery

Phrenic nerve

Right brachiocephalic vein

Thymus

Superior vena cava

Pulmonary arteries

Phrenic nerve; pericardiacophrenic artery; vein

Pulmonary vein

Fibrous pericardium; parietal pleura, mediastinal part

Pulmonary ligament

Vagus nerve [X], oesophageal plexus

Parietal pleura, costal part

Oesophagus

Diaphragm; parietal pleura, diaphragmatic part

Fig. 681   Pleural cavity and mediastinum of an adolescent; lateral thoracic wall and right lung have been removed; viewed from the right.
The x indicate the areas at the root of the lung and the pulmonary ligament, respectively, where the visceral pleura folds back into the parietal pleura.

Pleural cavity

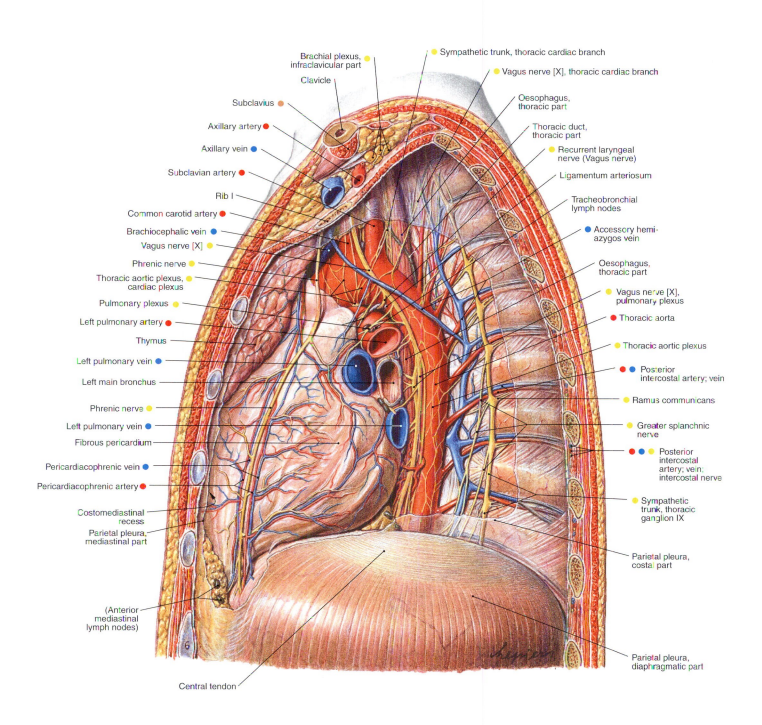

Brachial plexus, infraclavicular part
Clavicle
Subclavius
Axillary artery
Axillary vein
Subclavian artery
Rib I
Common carotid artery
Brachiocephalic vein
Vagus nerve [X]
Phrenic nerve
Thoracic aortic plexus, cardiac plexus
Pulmonary plexus
Left pulmonary artery
Thymus
Left pulmonary vein
Left main bronchus
Phrenic nerve
Left pulmonary vein
Fibrous pericardium
Pericardiacophrenic vein
Pericardiacophrenic artery
Costomediastinal recess
Parietal pleura, mediastinal part
(Anterior mediastinal lymph nodes)
Central tendon

Sympathetic trunk, thoracic cardiac branch
Vagus nerve [X], thoracic cardiac branch
Oesophagus, thoracic part
Thoracic duct, thoracic part
Recurrent laryngeal nerve (Vagus nerve)
Ligamentum arteriosum
Tracheobronchial lymph nodes
Accessory hemi-azygos vein
Oesophagus, thoracic part
Vagus nerve [X], pulmonary plexus
Thoracic aorta
Thoracic aortic plexus
Posterior intercostal artery; vein
Ramus communicans
Greater splanchnic nerve
Posterior intercostal artery; vein; intercostal nerve
Sympathetic trunk, thoracic ganglion IX
Parietal pleura, costal part
Parietal pleura, diaphragmatic part

Fig. 682 Pleural cavity and mediastinum of an adolescent; viewed from the left.
In older individuals, the thymic tissue is almost entirely replaced by adipose tissue.

Aortic arch

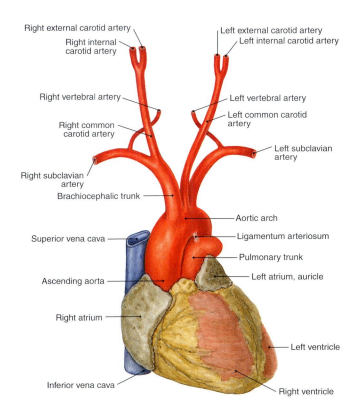

Fig. 683   Heart and aortic arch
with the origins of the major arteries;
ventral view.

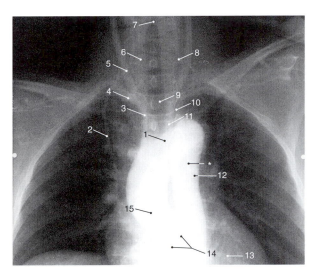

Fig. 684   Aortic arch and branches;
AP-radiograph after injection of a contrast medium
into the aortic bulb;
ventral view.

* Catheter

1	Aortic arch	9	Trachea
2	Internal thoracic artery	10	Left subclavian artery
3	Brachiocephalic trunk	11	Left common carotid artery
4	Right subclavian artery	12	Descending aorta
5	Right common carotid artery	13	Heart
6	Right vertebral artery	14	Aortic valve
7	Rima glottidis	15	Ascending aorta
8	Left vertebral artery		

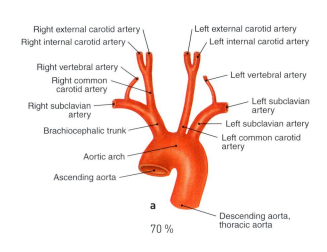

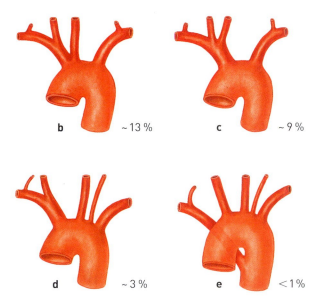

Fig. 685 a–e   Variability of the origin of the major arteries
from the aortic arch.
a   "Textbook case"
b   Common origin of the brachiocephalic trunk and the left
   common carotid artery
c   Common trunk for the brachiocephalic trunk and the left
   common carotid artery

d   Left vertebral artery branching off the aortic arch
   independently
e   Right subclavian artery as the ultimate branch of the
   aortic arch
   This abnormal artery frequently passes behind the
   oesophagus to the right, which can result in swallowing
   difficulties (Dysphagia lusoria).

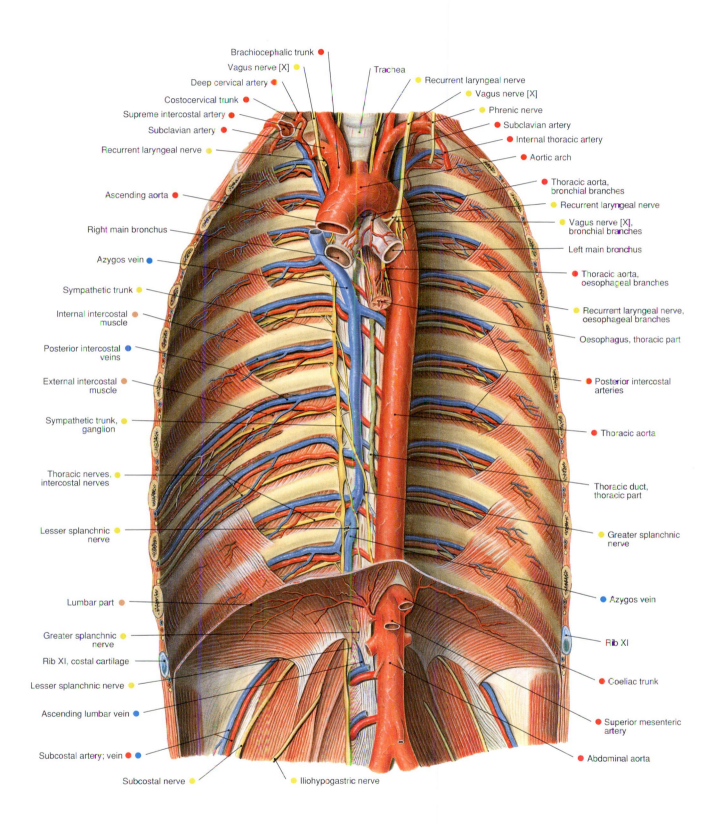

Brachiocephalic trunk ●
Vagus nerve [X] ●
Deep cervical artery ●
Costocervical trunk ●
Supreme intercostal artery ●
Subclavian artery ●
Recurrent laryngeal nerve ●
Trachea
Recurrent laryngeal nerve ●
Vagus nerve [X] ●
Phrenic nerve ●
Subclavian artery ●
Internal thoracic artery ●
Aortic arch ●
Thoracic aorta, bronchial branches ●
Recurrent laryngeal nerve ●
Vagus nerve [X], bronchial branches ●
Left main bronchus

Ascending aorta ●
Right main bronchus
Azygos vein ●
Sympathetic trunk ●
Internal intercostal muscle ●
Posterior intercostal veins ●
External intercostal muscle ●
Sympathetic trunk, ganglion ●
Thoracic nerves, intercostal nerves ●
Lesser splanchnic nerve ●

Thoracic aorta, oesophageal branches ●
Recurrent laryngeal nerve, oesophageal branches ●
Oesophagus, thoracic part
Posterior intercostal arteries ●
Thoracic aorta ●
Thoracic duct, thoracic part
Greater splanchnic nerve ●

Lumbar part ●
Greater splanchnic nerve ●
Rib XI, costal cartilage ●
Lesser splanchnic nerve ●
Ascending lumbar vein ●
Subcostal artery; vein ● ●
Subcostal nerve ●
Iliohypogastric nerve ●

Azygos vein ●
Rib XI
Coeliac trunk ●
Superior mesenteric artery ●
Abdominal aorta ●

Fig. 686 Thoracic and abdominal aorta.

Posterior mediastinum

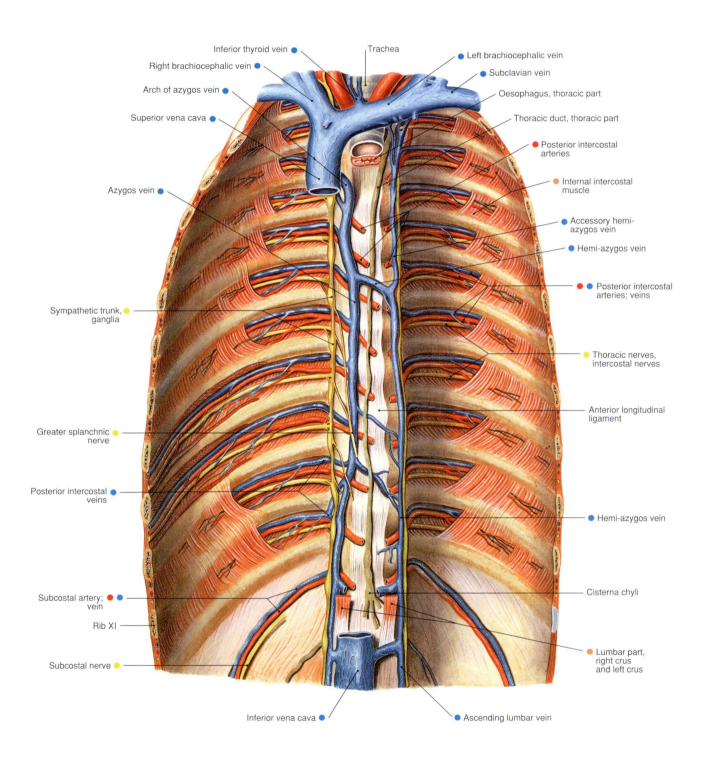

Inferior thyroid vein ●

Trachea

● Left brachiocephalic vein

Right brachiocephalic vein ●

● Subclavian vein

Arch of azygos vein ●

Oesophagus, thoracic part

Superior vena cava ●

Thoracic duct, thoracic part

● Posterior intercostal arteries

● Internal intercostal muscle

Azygos vein ●

● Accessory hemi-azygos vein

● Hemi-azygos vein

● ● Posterior intercostal arteries; veins

Sympathetic trunk, ganglia ●

● Thoracic nerves, intercostal nerves

Anterior longitudinal ligament

Greater splanchnic nerve ●

Posterior intercostal veins ●

● Hemi-azygos vein

Subcostal artery; ● ● vein

Cisterna chyli

Rib XI

● Lumbar part, right crus and left crus

Subcostal nerve ●

Inferior vena cava ●

● Ascending lumbar vein

Fig. 687 Vessels and nerves of the posterior mediastinum.

Posterior mediastinum

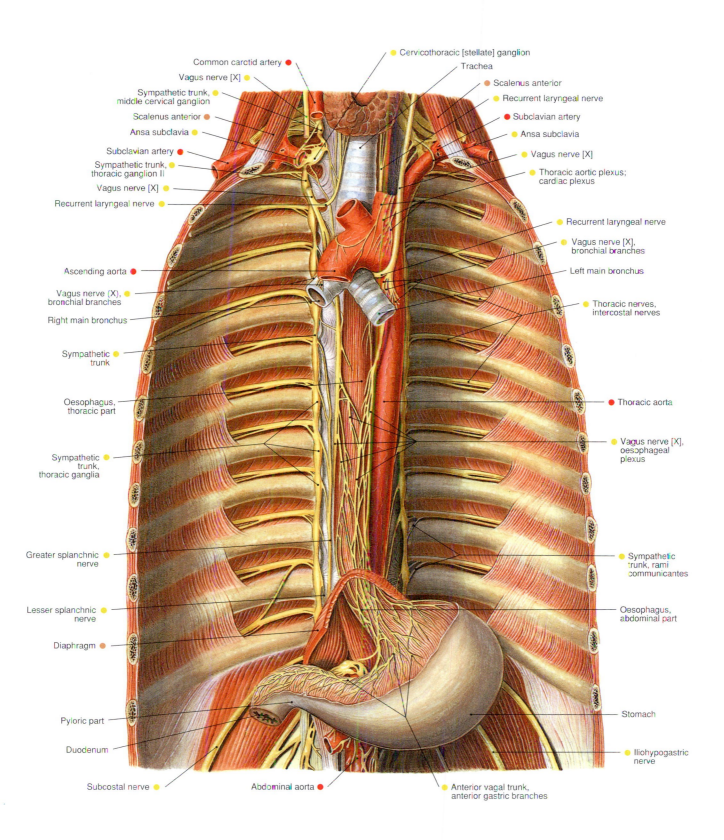

Common carotid artery ●
Vagus nerve [X] ●
Sympathetic trunk, middle cervical ganglion ●
Scalenus anterior ●
Ansa subclavia ●
Subclavian artery ●
Sympathetic trunk, thoracic ganglion II ●
Vagus nerve [X] ●
Recurrent laryngeal nerve ●

Cervicothoracic [stellate] ganglion ●
Trachea
Scalenus anterior ●
Recurrent laryngeal nerve ●
Subclavian artery ●
Ansa subclavia ●
Vagus nerve [X] ●
Thoracic aortic plexus; cardiac plexus ●

Ascending aorta ●
Vagus nerve (X), bronchial branches ●
Right main bronchus
Sympathetic trunk ●
Oesophagus, thoracic part
Sympathetic trunk, thoracic ganglia ●
Greater splanchnic nerve ●
Lesser splanchnic nerve ●
Diaphragm ●
Pyloric part
Duodenum
Subcostal nerve ●

Recurrent laryngeal nerve ●
Vagus nerve [X], bronchial branches ●
Left main bronchus
Thoracic nerves, intercostal nerves ●
Thoracic aorta ●
Vagus nerve [X], oesophageal plexus ●
Sympathetic trunk, rami communicantes ●
Oesophagus, abdominal part
Stomach
Iliohypogastric nerve ●
Anterior vagal trunk, anterior gastric branches
Abdominal aorta ●

Fig. 688 Autonomous nervous system of the thoracic cavity.

→ 49, 50

Phrenic nerve

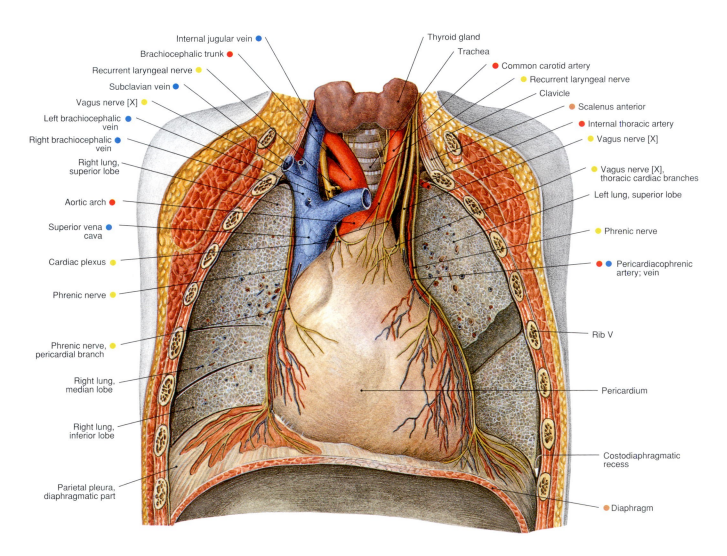

Internal jugular vein ●
Brachiocephalic trunk ●
Recurrent laryngeal nerve ●
Subclavian vein ●
Vagus nerve [X] ●
Left brachiocephalic vein ●
Right brachiocephalic vein ●
Right lung, superior lobe
Aortic arch ●
Superior vena cava ●
Cardiac plexus ●
Phrenic nerve ●
Phrenic nerve, pericardial branch ●
Right lung, median lobe
Right lung, inferior lobe
Parietal pleura, diaphragmatic part

Thyroid gland
Trachea
● Common carotid artery
● Recurrent laryngeal nerve
Clavicle
● Scalenus anterior
● Internal thoracic artery
● Vagus nerve [X]
● Vagus nerve [X], thoracic cardiac branches
Left lung, superior lobe
● Phrenic nerve
● ● Pericardiacophrenic artery; vein
Rib V
Pericardium
Costodiaphragmatic recess
● Diaphragm

Fig. 689   Thoracic viscera of an adult; the anterior thoracic wall has been removed, and the right and the left lung have been sectioned in the frontal plane; ventral view.

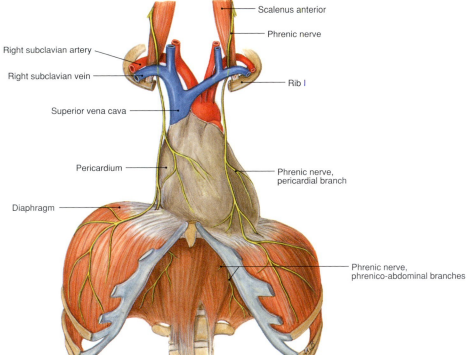

Scalenus anterior
Phrenic nerve
Right subclavian artery
Right subclavian vein
Rib I
Superior vena cava
Pericardium
Phrenic nerve, pericardial branch
Diaphragm
Phrenic nerve, phrenico-abdominal branches

Fig. 690   Course of the phrenic nerve.

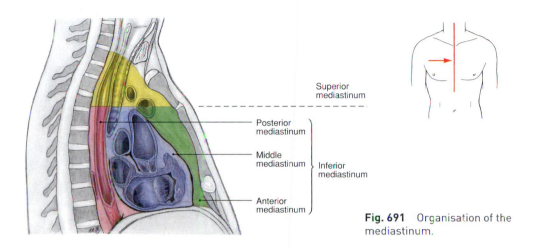

Fig. 691 Organisation of the mediastinum.

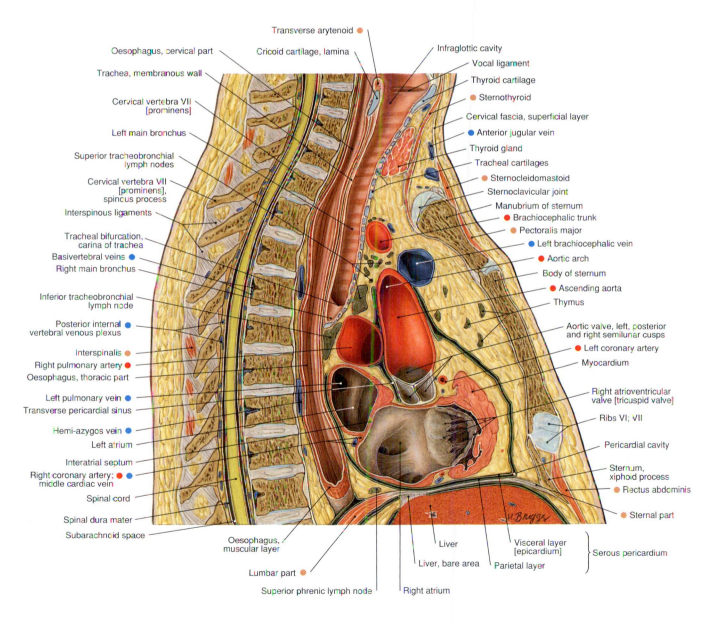

Fig. 692 Thoracic cavity and mediastinum; median sagittal section through the neck and the thorax; lateral view from the right.

Thorax, frontal sections

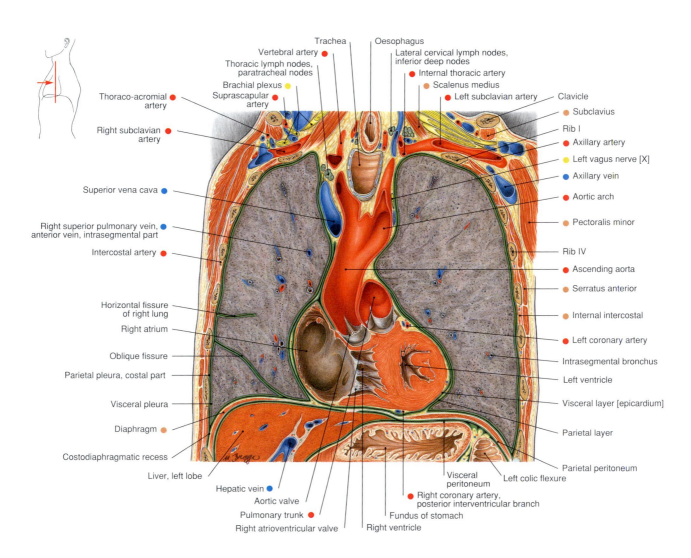

Trachea
Vertebral artery ●
Thoracic lymph nodes, paratracheal nodes
Brachial plexus ●
Suprascapular artery ●
Thoraco-acromial artery ●
Right subclavian artery ●

Oesophagus
Lateral cervical lymph nodes, inferior deep nodes
Internal thoracic artery ●
Scalenus medius ●
Left subclavian artery ●
Clavicle
Subclavius ●
Rib I
Axillary artery ●
Left vagus nerve [X] ●
Axillary vein ●
Aortic arch ●
Pectoralis minor ●
Rib IV
Ascending aorta ●
Serratus anterior ●
Internal intercostal ●
Left coronary artery ●
Intrasegmental bronchus
Left ventricle
Visceral layer [epicardium]
Parietal layer
Parietal peritoneum
Left colic flexure

Superior vena cava ●
Right superior pulmonary vein, anterior vein, intrasegmental part ●
Intercostal artery ●
Horizontal fissure of right lung
Right atrium
Oblique fissure
Parietal pleura, costal part
Visceral pleura
Diaphragm ●
Costodiaphragmatic recess
Liver, left lobe
Hepatic vein ●
Aortic valve
Pulmonary trunk ●
Right atrioventricular valve

Visceral peritoneum
Right coronary artery, posterior interventricular branch ●
Fundus of stomach
Right ventricle

Fig. 693 Thoracic cavity.

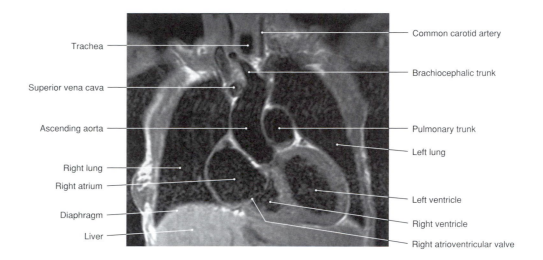

Trachea
Superior vena cava
Ascending aorta
Right lung
Right atrium
Diaphragm
Liver

Common carotid artery
Brachiocephalic trunk
Pulmonary trunk
Left lung
Left ventricle
Right ventricle
Right atrioventricular valve

Fig. 694 Thoracic cavity;
magnetic resonance tomographic image (MRI);
frontal section at the level of the superior vena cava;
ventral view.

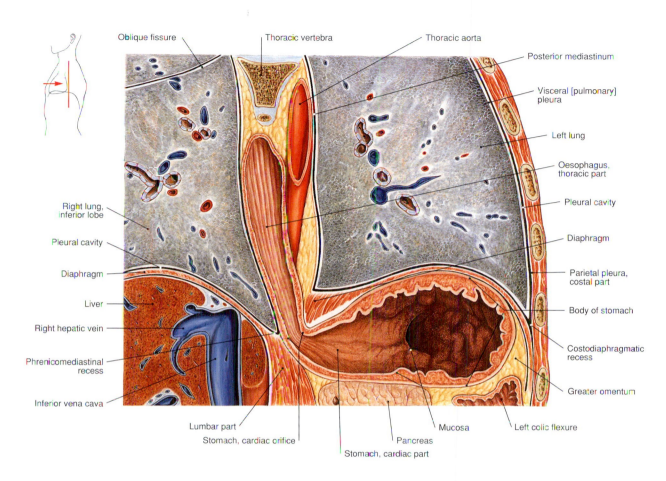

Oblique fissure

Thoracic vertebra

Thoracic aorta

Posterior mediastinum

Visceral [pulmonary] pleura

Left lung

Oesophagus, thoracic part

Pleural cavity

Diaphragm

Parietal pleura, costal part

Body of stomach

Costodiaphragmatic recess

Greater omentum

Left colic flexure

Right lung, inferior lobe

Pleural cavity

Diaphragm

Liver

Right hepatic vein

Phrenicomediastinal recess

Inferior vena cava

Lumbar part

Stomach, cardiac orifice

Stomach, cardiac part

Pancreas

Mucosa

Fig. 695 Diaphragm and oesophagus with its transition into the stomach;
frontal section through the lower part of the thoracic cavity and the upper part of the abdominal cavity.

→ 919

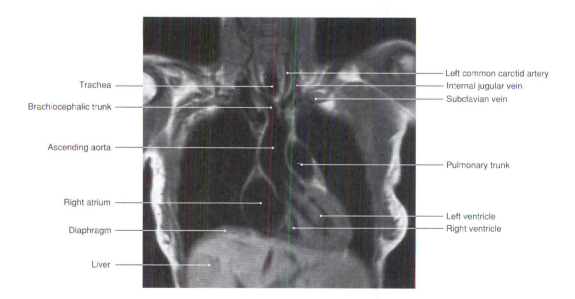

Trachea

Brachiocephalic trunk

Ascending aorta

Right atrium

Diaphragm

Liver

Left common carotid artery

Internal jugular vein

Subclavian vein

Pulmonary trunk

Left ventricle

Right ventricle

Fig. 696 Thoracic cavity;
magnetic resonance tomographic image (MRI);
frontal section at the level of the aortic valve;
ventral view.

Thorax, frontal sections

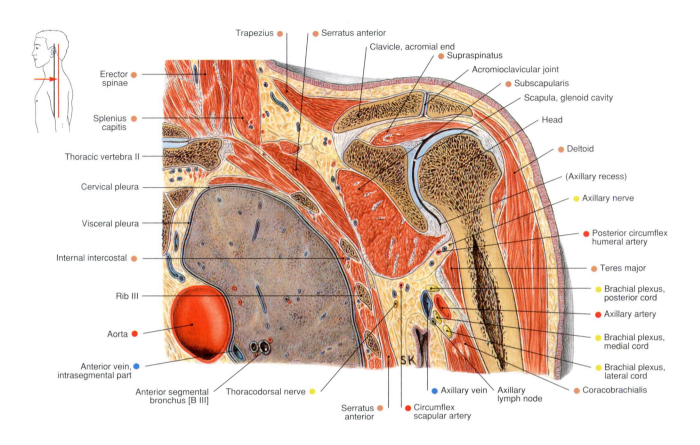

Trapezius — Serratus anterior — Clavicle, acromial end — Supraspinatus — Acromioclavicular joint — Subscapularis — Scapula, glenoid cavity — Head

Erector spinae — Splenius capitis — Thoracic vertebra II — Cervical pleura — Visceral pleura — Internal intercostal — Rib III — Aorta — Anterior vein, intrasegmental part

Deltoid — (Axillary recess) — Axillary nerve — Posterior circumflex humeral artery — Teres major — Brachial plexus, posterior cord — Axillary artery — Brachial plexus, medial cord — Brachial plexus, lateral cord — Coracobrachialis

Anterior segmental bronchus [B III] — Thoracodorsal nerve — Serratus anterior — Circumflex scapular artery — Axillary vein — Axillary lymph node

SK

Fig. 697 Thoracic cavity; axilla and shoulder joint.

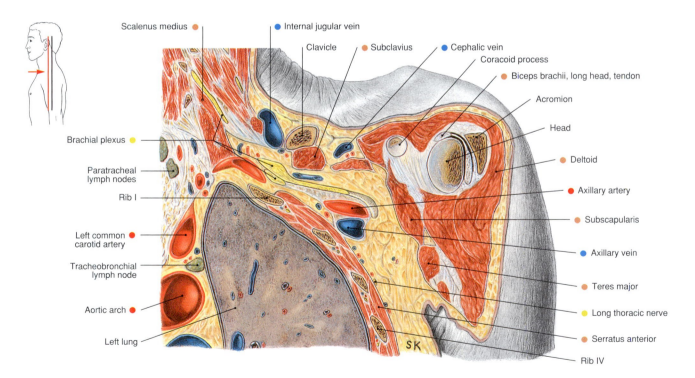

Scalenus medius — Internal jugular vein — Clavicle — Subclavius — Cephalic vein — Coracoid process — Biceps brachii, long head, tendon — Acromion — Head — Deltoid — Axillary artery — Subscapularis — Axillary vein — Teres major — Long thoracic nerve — Serratus anterior — Rib IV

Brachial plexus — Paratracheal lymph nodes — Rib I — Left common carotid artery — Tracheobronchial lymph node — Aortic arch — Left lung

SK

Fig. 698 Thoracic cavity; axilla and shoulder joint.

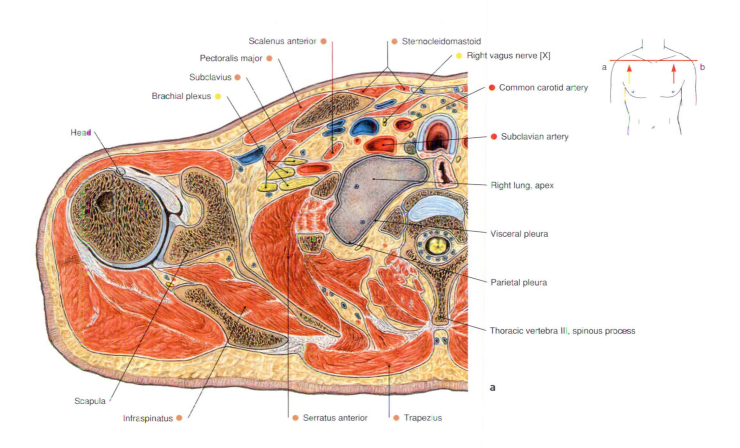

Scalenus anterior ●
Pectoralis major ●
Subclavius ●
Brachial plexus ●
Head
Scalenus anterior ●
Sternocleidomastoid ●
Right vagus nerve [X] ●
● Common carotid artery
● Subclavian artery
Right lung, apex
Visceral pleura
Parietal pleura
Thoracic vertebra III, spinous process
Scapula
Infraspinatus ●
Serratus anterior ●
Trapezius ●

a

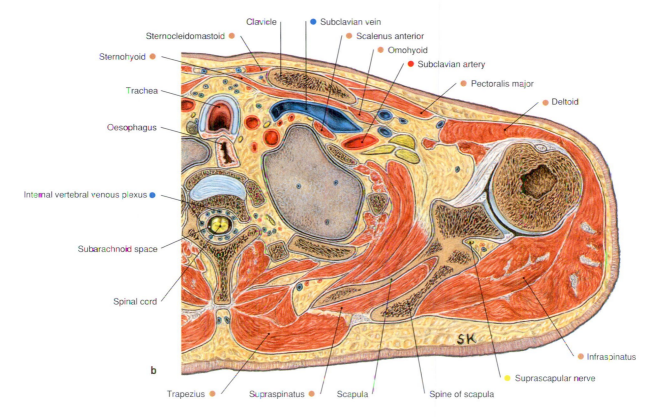

Sternohyoid ●
Sternocleidomastoid ●
Trachea
Oesophagus
Internal vertebral venous plexus ●
Subarachnoid space
Spinal cord
Clavicle
● Subclavian vein
Scalenus anterior ●
Omohyoid ●
● Subclavian artery
Pectoralis major ●
Deltoid ●
Infraspinatus ●
Suprascapular nerve ●
Spine of scapula
Scapula
Supraspinatus ●
Trapezius ●

b

Fig. 699 a, b Thoracic cavity; axilla and shoulder joint.

a Right part of the body
b Left part of the body

→ 294

Thorax, transverse sections

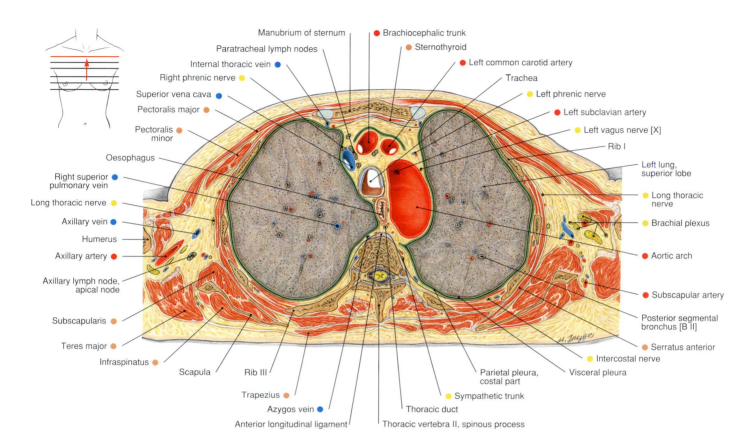

Manubrium of sternum
Paratracheal lymph nodes
Internal thoracic vein ●
Right phrenic nerve ●
Superior vena cava ●
Pectoralis major ●
Pectoralis minor ●
Oesophagus
Right superior pulmonary vein ●
Long thoracic nerve ●
Axillary vein ●
Humerus
Axillary artery ●
Axillary lymph node, apical node
Subscapularis ●
Teres major ●
Infraspinatus ●
Scapula
Rib III
Trapezius ●
Azygos vein ●
Anterior longitudinal ligament

Brachiocephalic trunk ●
Sternothyroid ●
Left common carotid artery ●
Trachea
Left phrenic nerve ●
Left subclavian artery ●
Left vagus nerve [X] ●
Rib I
Left lung, superior lobe
Long thoracic nerve ●
Brachial plexus ●
Aortic arch ●
Subscapular artery ●
Posterior segmental bronchus [B II]
Serratus anterior ●
Intercostal nerve ●
Visceral pleura
Parietal pleura, costal part
Sympathetic trunk ●
Thoracic duct
Thoracic vertebra II, spinous process

Fig. 700 Thoracic cavity.

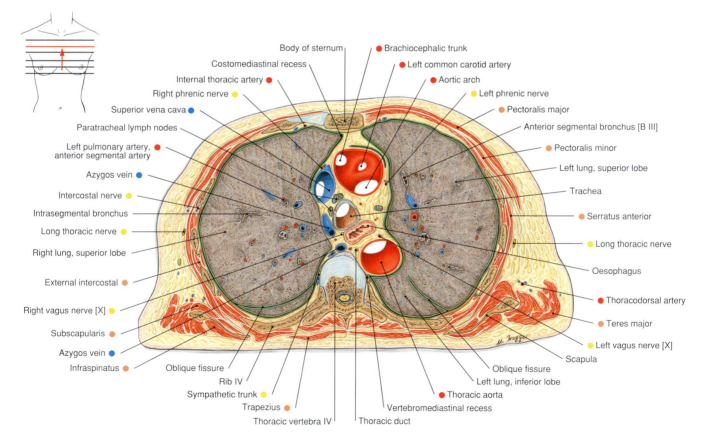

Body of sternum
Costomediastinal recess
Internal thoracic artery ●
Right phrenic nerve ●
Superior vena cava ●
Paratracheal lymph nodes
Left pulmonary artery, anterior segmental artery ●
Azygos vein ●
Intercostal nerve ●
Intrasegmental bronchus
Long thoracic nerve ●
Right lung, superior lobe
External intercostal
Right vagus nerve [X] ●
Subscapularis ●
Azygos vein ●
Infraspinatus ●
Oblique fissure
Rib IV
Sympathetic trunk ●
Trapezius ●
Thoracic vertebra IV

Brachiocephalic trunk ●
Left common carotid artery ●
Aortic arch ●
Left phrenic nerve ●
Pectoralis major ●
Anterior segmental bronchus [B III]
Pectoralis minor ●
Left lung, superior lobe
Trachea
Serratus anterior ●
Long thoracic nerve ●
Oesophagus
Thoracodorsal artery ●
Teres major ●
Left vagus nerve [X] ●
Scapula
Oblique fissure
Left lung, inferior lobe
Thoracic aorta ●
Vertebromediastinal recess
Thoracic duct

Fig. 701 Thoracic cavity.

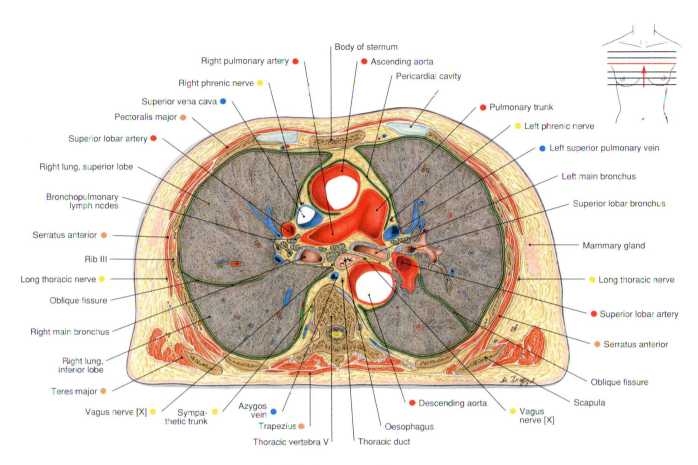

Right pulmonary artery ●
Right phrenic nerve ●
Superior vena cava ●
Pectoralis major ●
Superior lobar artery ●
Right lung, superior lobe
Bronchopulmonary lymph nodes
Serratus anterior ●
Rib III
Long thoracic nerve ●
Oblique fissure
Right main bronchus
Right lung, inferior lobe
Teres major ●
Vagus nerve [X] ●
Sympa-thetic trunk ●
Azygos vein ●
Trapezius ●
Thoracic vertebra V
Thoracic duct

Body of sternum
● Ascending aorta
Pericardial cavity
● Pulmonary trunk
● Left phrenic nerve
● Left superior pulmonary vein
Left main bronchus
Superior lobar bronchus
Mammary gland
● Long thoracic nerve
● Superior lobar artery
● Serratus anterior
Oblique fissure
Scapula
● Descending aorta
● Vagus nerve [X]
Oesophagus

Fig. 702 Thoracic cavity.

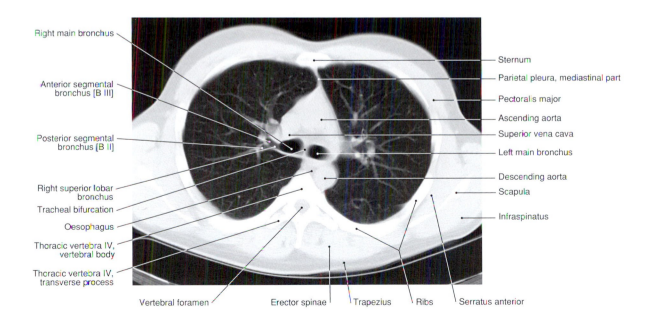

Right main bronchus
Anterior segmental bronchus [B III]
Posterior segmental bronchus [B II]
Right superior lobar bronchus
Tracheal bifurcation
Oesophagus
Thoracic vertebra IV, vertebral body
Thoracic vertebra IV, transverse process

Sternum
Parietal pleura, mediastinal part
Pectoralis major
Ascending aorta
Superior vena cava
Left main bronchus
Descending aorta
Scapula
Infraspinatus

Vertebral foramen
Erector spinae
Trapezius
Ribs
Serratus anterior

Fig. 703 Thoracic cavity; computed tomographic cross-section (CT).

Thorax, transverse sections

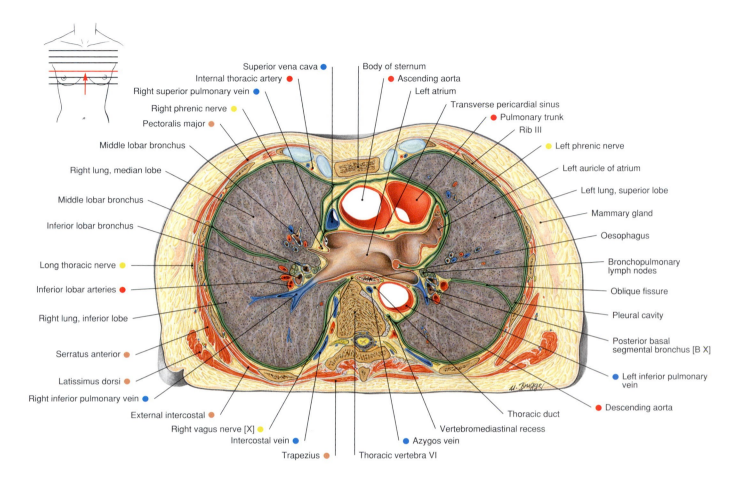

Superior vena cava ●
Internal thoracic artery ●
Right superior pulmonary vein ●
Right phrenic nerve ●
Pectoralis major ●
Middle lobar bronchus
Right lung, median lobe
Middle lobar bronchus
Inferior lobar bronchus
Long thoracic nerve ●
Inferior lobar arteries ●
Right lung, inferior lobe
Serratus anterior ●
Latissimus dorsi ●
Right inferior pulmonary vein ●
External intercostal ●
Right vagus nerve [X] ●
Intercostal vein ●
Trapezius ●

Body of sternum
Ascending aorta ●
Left atrium
Transverse pericardial sinus
Pulmonary trunk ●
Rib III
● Left phrenic nerve
Left auricle of atrium
Left lung, superior lobe
Mammary gland
Oesophagus
Bronchopulmonary lymph nodes
Oblique fissure
Pleural cavity
Posterior basal segmental bronchus [B X]
● Left inferior pulmonary vein
● Descending aorta
Thoracic duct
Vertebromediastinal recess
● Azygos vein
Thoracic vertebra VI

Fig. 704 Thoracic cavity.

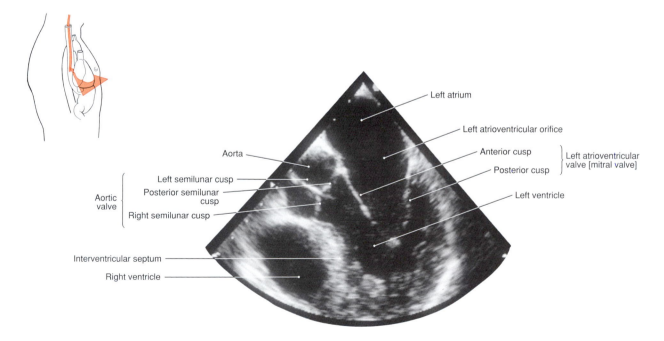

Aorta
Left semilunar cusp
Posterior semilunar cusp
Right semilunar cusp
Aortic valve
Interventricular septum
Right ventricle

Left atrium
Left atrioventricular orifice
Anterior cusp
Posterior cusp
Left atrioventricular valve [mitral valve]
Left ventricle

Fig. 705 Heart;
ultrasound image viewed from the oesophagus (transoesophageal echocardiography).

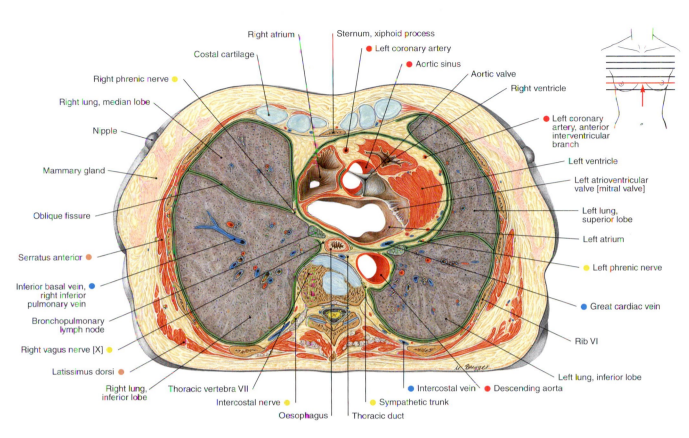

Right atrium
Costal cartilage
Right phrenic nerve
Right lung, median lobe
Nipple
Mammary gland
Oblique fissure
Serratus anterior
Inferior basal vein, right inferior pulmonary vein
Bronchopulmonary lymph node
Right vagus nerve [X]
Latissimus dorsi
Right lung, inferior lobe
Thoracic vertebra VII
Intercostal nerve
Oesophagus
Thoracic duct
Sympathetic trunk
Intercostal vein
Descending aorta
Left lung, inferior lobe
Rib VI
Great cardiac vein
Left phrenic nerve
Left atrium
Left lung, superior lobe
Left atrioventricular valve [mitral valve]
Left ventricle
Left coronary artery, anterior interventricular branch
Right ventricle
Aortic valve
Aortic sinus
Left coronary artery
Sternum, xiphoid process

Fig. 706 Thoracic cavity.

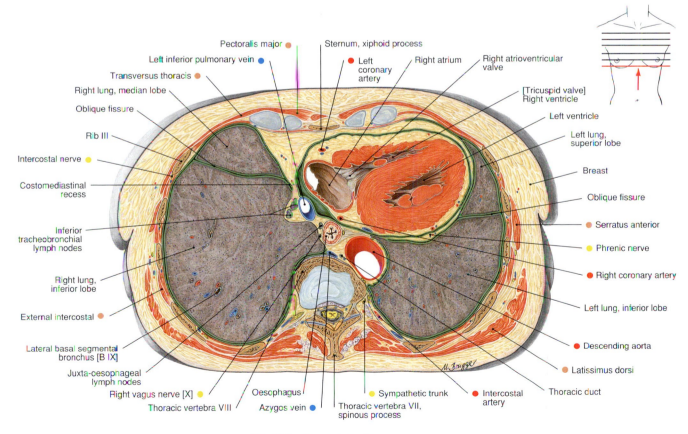

Pectoralis major
Left inferior pulmonary vein
Transversus thoracis
Right lung, median lobe
Oblique fissure
Rib III
Intercostal nerve
Costomediastinal recess
Inferior tracheobronchial lymph nodes
Right lung, inferior lobe
External intercostal
Lateral basal segmental bronchus [B IX]
Juxta-oesopnageal lymph nodes
Right vagus nerve [X]
Thoracic vertebra VIII
Oesophagus
Azygos vein
Thoracic vertebra VII, spinous process
Sympathetic trunk
Intercostal artery
Thoracic duct
Latissimus dorsi
Descending aorta
Left lung, inferior lobe
Right coronary artery
Phrenic nerve
Serratus anterior
Oblique fissure
Breast
Left lung, superior lobe
Left ventricle
[Tricuspid valve] Right ventricle
Right atrioventricular valve
Right atrium
Left coronary artery
Sternum, xiphoid process

Fig. 707 Thoracic cavity.

Stomach

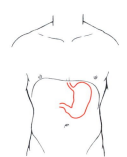

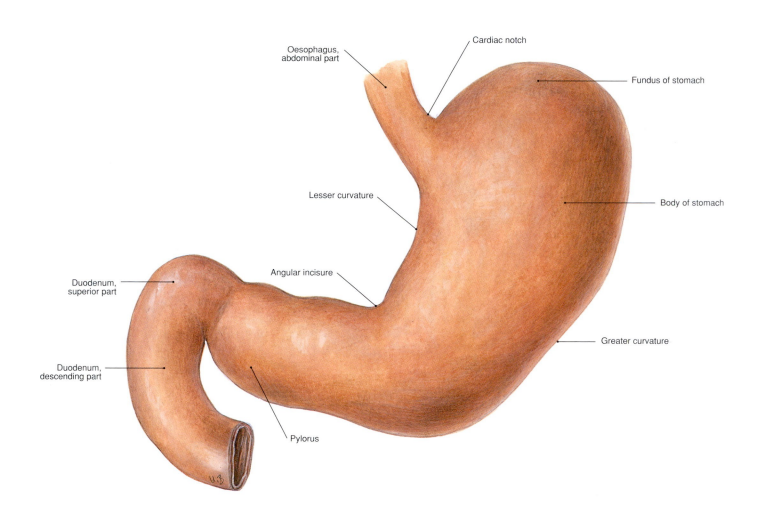

Oesophagus, abdominal part

Cardiac notch

Fundus of stomach

Lesser curvature

Body of stomach

Duodenum, superior part

Angular incisure

Duodenum, descending part

Greater curvature

Pylorus

Fig. 708 Stomach; ventral view.

Muscles of the stomach

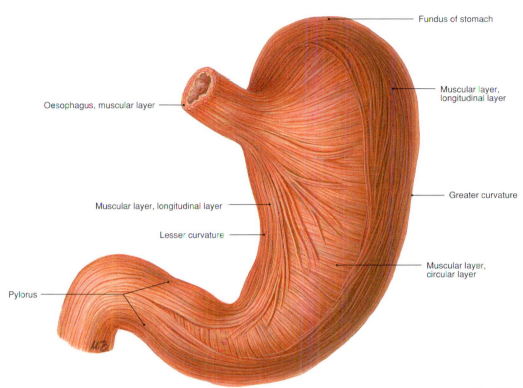

Fundus of stomach

Muscular layer,
longitudinal layer

Oesophagus, muscular layer

Muscular layer, longitudinal layer

Lesser curvature

Greater curvature

Muscular layer,
circular layer

Pylorus

Fig. 709 Stomach;
external muscle layers;
ventral view.

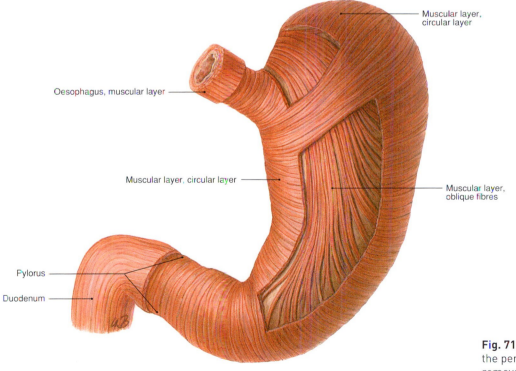

Muscular layer,
circular layer

Oesophagus, muscular layer

Muscular layer, circular layer

Muscular layer,
oblique fibres

Pylorus

Duodenum

Fig. 710 Stomach;
the peritoneum has been
removed to demonstrate the
internal muscle layers;
ventral view.

Stomach, structure

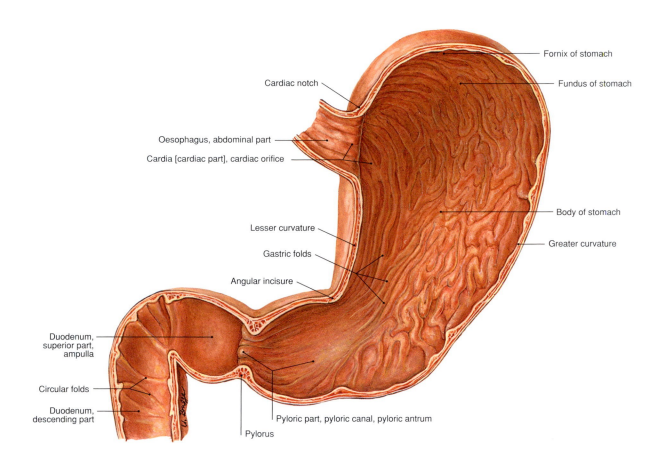

Cardiac notch

Oesophagus, abdominal part

Cardia [cardiac part], cardiac orifice

Lesser curvature

Gastric folds

Angular incisure

Duodenum, superior part, ampulla

Circular folds

Duodenum, descending part

Pylorus

Pyloric part, pyloric canal, pyloric antrum

Fornix of stomach

Fundus of stomach

Body of stomach

Greater curvature

Fig. 711   Stomach and duodenum; ventral view.

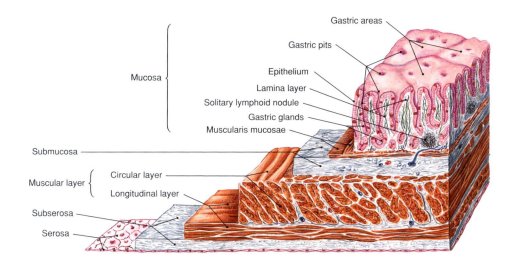

Gastric areas

Gastric pits

Epithelium

Lamina layer

Solitary lymphoid nodule

Gastric glands

Muscularis mucosae

Mucosa

Submucosa

Muscular layer
— Circular layer
— Longitudinal layer

Subserosa

Serosa

Fig. 712   Diagram of the stomach wall; the layers of the wall have been removed stepwise; microscopic enlargement at low magnification.

Vessels of the stomach

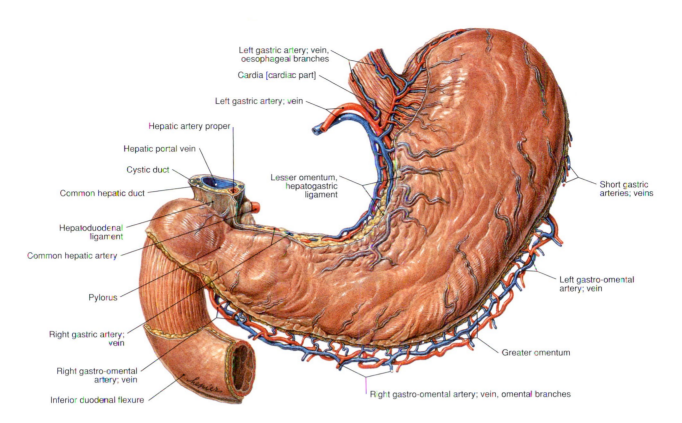

Left gastric artery; vein, oesophageal branches

Cardia [cardiac part]

Left gastric artery; vein

Hepatic artery proper

Hepatic portal vein

Cystic duct

Common hepatic duct

Hepatoduodenal ligament

Common hepatic artery

Pylorus

Right gastric artery; vein

Right gastro-omental artery; vein

Inferior duodenal flexure

Lesser omentum, hepatogastric ligament

Short gastric arteries; veins

Left gastro-omental artery; vein

Greater omentum

Right gastro-omental artery; vein, omental branches

Fig. 713 Blood vessels of the stomach; ventral view.

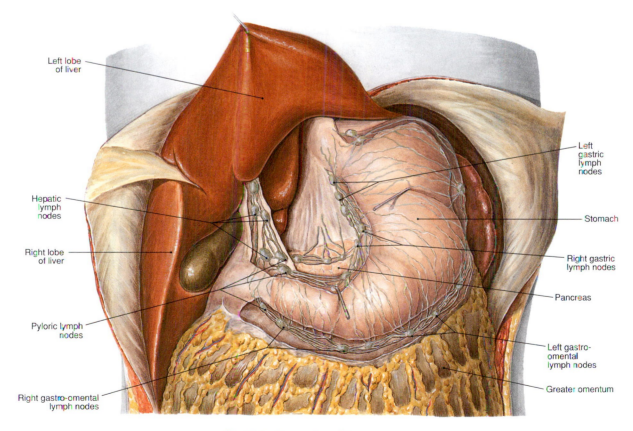

Left lobe of liver

Hepatic lymph nodes

Right lobe of liver

Pyloric lymph nodes

Right gastro-omental lymph nodes

Left gastric lymph nodes

Stomach

Right gastric lymph nodes

Pancreas

Left gastro-omental lymph nodes

Greater omentum

Fig. 714 Stomach and liver with lymph nodes; ventral view.

Stomach, radiography

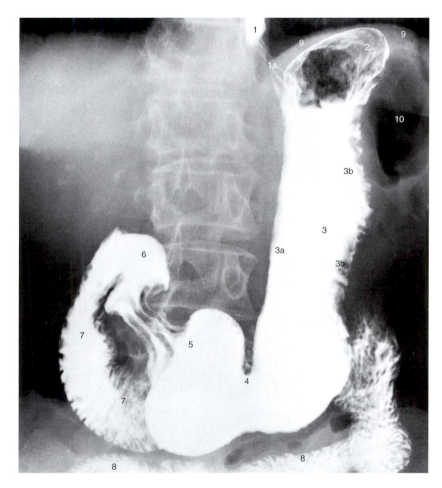

1 = Oesophagus with contrast medium.
At the transition (1a) into the fundus
of stomach, the grooves between
the folds appear as dark striations.
2 = Fundus of stomach with air bubble
3 = Body of stomach
3a = Lesser curvature
3b = Greater curvature.
In the linings of the latter, notches
corresponding to the contour
of the mucous are visible.
4 = Peristaltic constriction at
the angular notch
5 = Pyloric part prior to the progression of
a portion of the stomach's content
6 = Ampulla of duodenum
7 = Descending part of the duodenum
with circular folds
8 = Jejunum
9 = Left „dome" of diaphragm
10 = Left colic flexure (filled with air)

Fig. 715 Stomach and
duodenum;
AP-radiograph after oral
administration of a contrast medium;
upright position;
ventral view.

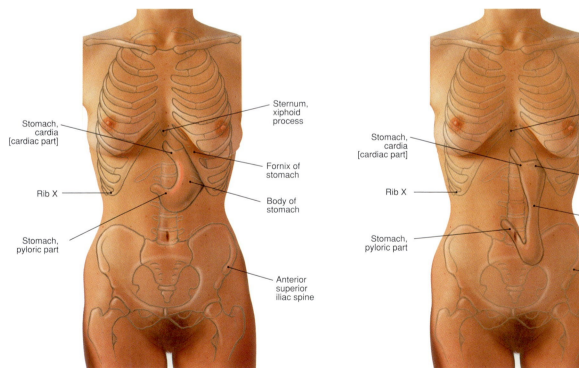

Stomach,
cardia
[cardiac part]

Rib X

Stomach,
pyloric part

Sternum,
xiphoid
process

Fornix of
stomach

Body of
stomach

Anterior
superior
iliac spine

Fig. 716 Stomach;
projection of a „normal" stomach onto the anterior abdominal
wall;
upright position.

Stomach,
cardia
[cardiac part]

Rib X

Stomach,
pyloric part

Sternum,
xiphoid
process

Fornix of
stomach

Body of
stomach

Anterior
superior
iliac spine

Fig. 717 Stomach;
projection of a „long" stomach onto the anterior abdominal
wall;
upright position.

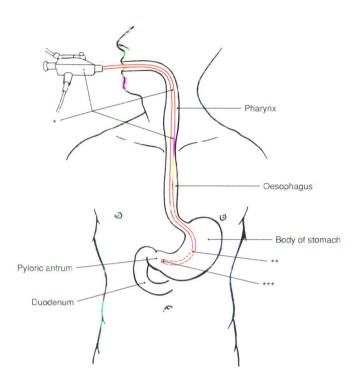

Fig. 718 Technical procedure of oesophagoscopy and gastroscopy.

* Gastroscope
** The gastroscope's tip located in the body of stomach (compare Fig. 719 a)
*** The gastroscope's tip located in the pyloric antrum (compare Fig. 719 b)

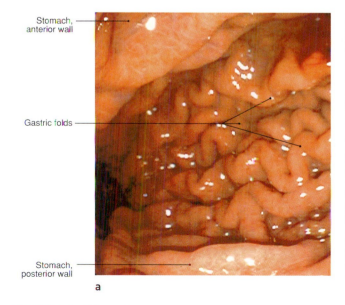

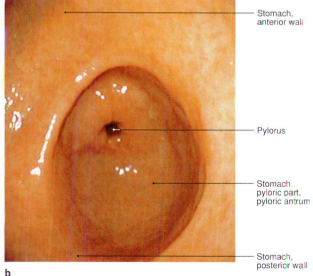

Fig. 719 a, b Stomach; endoscopic image of the stomach (gastroscopy); superior view.

a View of the body of stomach with distinct longitudinal folds of the mucosa (Plica gastricae)
b View of the pyloric antrum predominantly covered with smooth mucosa

Duodenum

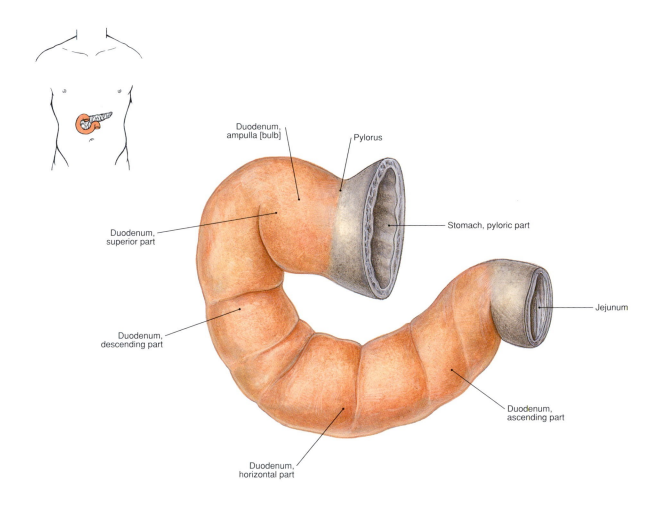

Duodenum, ampulla [bulb]

Pylorus

Duodenum, superior part

Stomach, pyloric part

Duodenum, descending part

Jejunum

Duodenum, ascending part

Duodenum, horizontal part

Fig. 720 Duodenum.

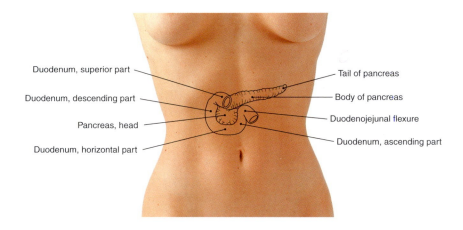

Duodenum, superior part

Tail of pancreas

Duodenum, descending part

Body of pancreas

Pancreas, head

Duodenojejunal flexure

Duodenum, ascending part

Duodenum, horizontal part

Fig. 721 Duodenum and pancreas;
projected onto the anterior abdominal wall.

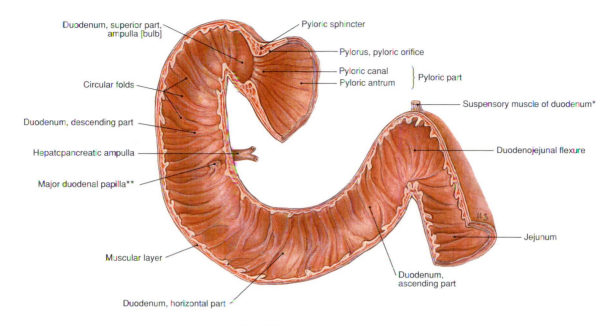

Duodenum, superior part, ampulla [bulb]
Pyloric sphincter
Pylorus, pyloric orifice
Pyloric canal
Pyloric antrum
Pyloric part
Circular folds
Suspensory muscle of duodenum*
Duodenum, descending part
Duodenojejunal flexure
Hepatopancreatic ampulla
Major duodenal papilla**
Jejunum
Muscular layer
Duodenum, ascending part
Duodenum, horizontal part

Fig. 722 Duodenum; ventral view.

* Clinical term: muscle of TREITZ
** Clinical term: papilla of VATER

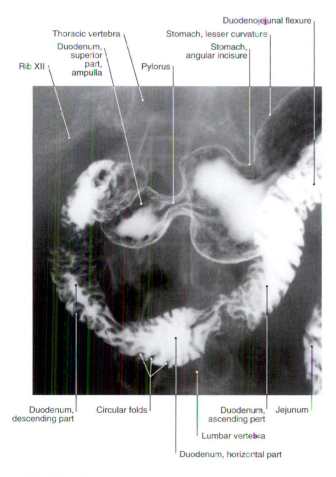

Rib XII
Thoracic vertebra
Duodenum, superior part, ampulla
Pylorus
Duodenojejunal flexure
Stomach, lesser curvature
Stomach, angular incisure

Duodenum, descending part
Circular folds
Duodenum, ascending part
Jejunum
Lumbar vertebra
Duodenum, horizontal part

Fig. 723 Duodenum;
AP-radiograph after oral administration of a contrast medium;
upright position;
ventral view.

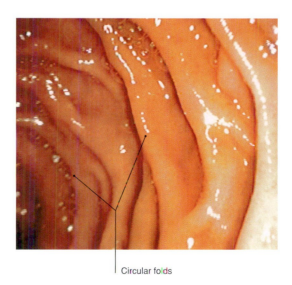

Circular folds

Fig. 724 Duodenum;
endoscopic image.

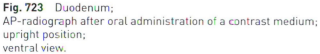

Small intestine, structure

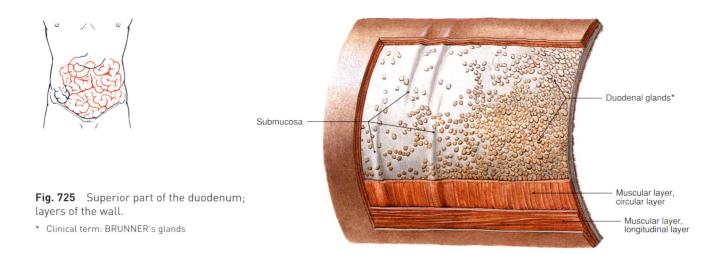

Fig. 725 Superior part of the duodenum; layers of the wall.

* Clinical term: BRUNNER's glands

Submucosa

Duodenal glands*

Muscular layer, circular layer

Muscular layer, longitudinal layer

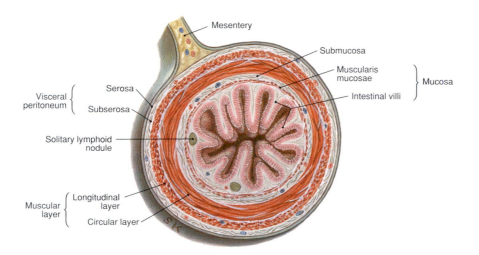

Mesentery

Submucosa

Muscularis mucosae

Mucosa

Intestinal villi

Serosa

Visceral peritoneum

Subserosa

Solitary lymphoid nodule

Longitudinal layer

Muscular layer

Circular layer

Fig. 726 Small intestine; cross-section through the upper small intestine.

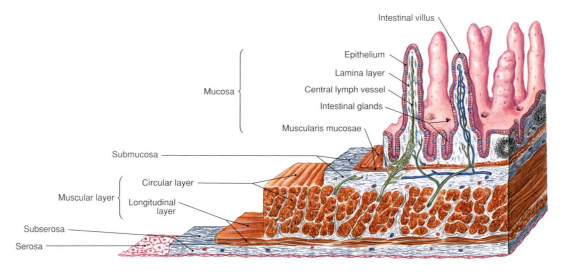

Intestinal villus

Epithelium

Lamina layer

Central lymph vessel

Intestinal glands

Muscularis mucosae

Mucosa

Submucosa

Circular layer

Muscular layer

Longitudinal layer

Subserosa

Serosa

Fig. 727 Small intestine; layers of the wall; microscopic enlargement at low magnification.

Mucosa of the small intestine

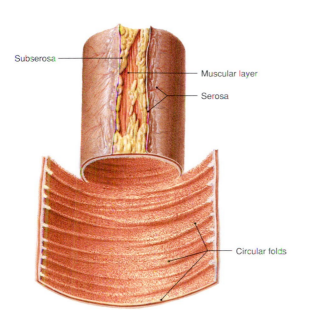

Fig. 728   Jejunum.

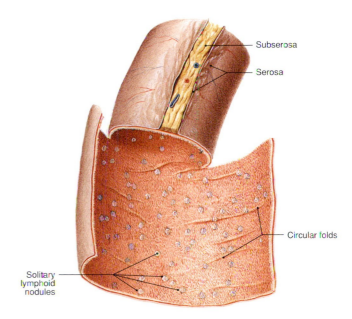

Fig. 729   Ileum.

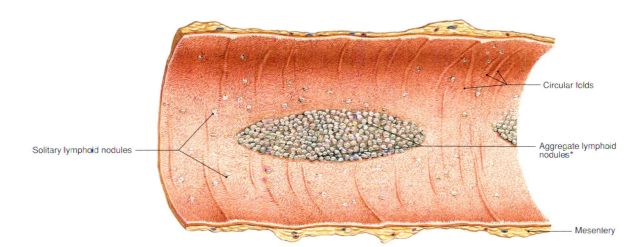

Fig. 730   Terminal ileum.

* Clinical term: PEYER's patches

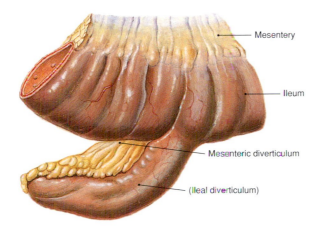

Fig. 731   MECKEL's diverticulum (ileal diverticulum). This vestige of the yolk stalk (omphalomesenteric duct) occurs in 1–3% of cases. It is located 30–70 cm oral to the ileocaecal junction opposite to the attachment of the mesentery.

Large intestine

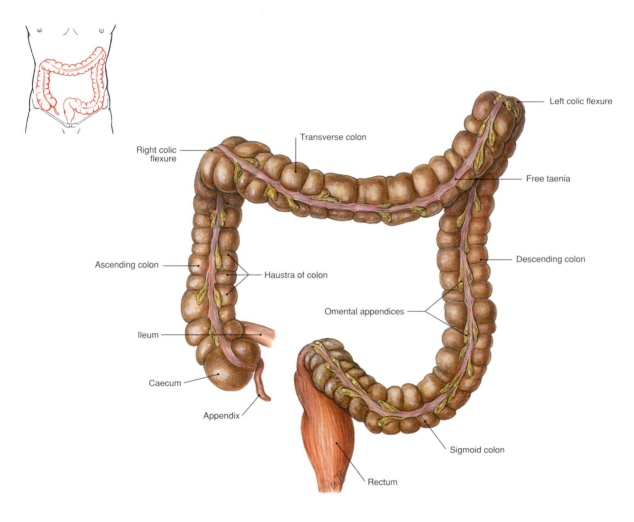

Left colic flexure

Transverse colon

Right colic flexure

Free taenia

Ascending colon

Haustra of colon

Descending colon

Omental appendices

Ileum

Caecum

Appendix

Sigmoid colon

Rectum

Fig. 732 Large intestine;
ventral view.

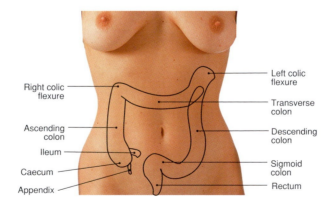

Right colic flexure

Left colic flexure

Transverse colon

Ascending colon

Descending colon

Ileum

Caecum

Sigmoid colon

Appendix

Rectum

Fig. 733 Large intestine;
projected onto the anterior abdominal wall.
The positions of the transverse colon and of the sigmoid
colon are highly variable (compare Fig. 742).

Large intestine, structure

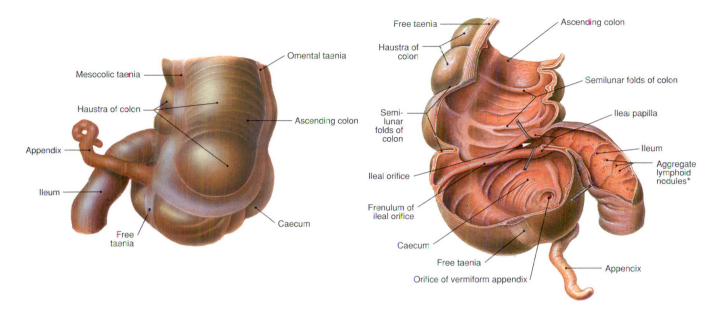

Fig. 734   Caecum; vermiform appendix and terminal ileum; dorsal view.

Fig. 735   Ascending colon; caecum, and vermiform appendix; ventral view.

* Clinical term: PEYER's patches

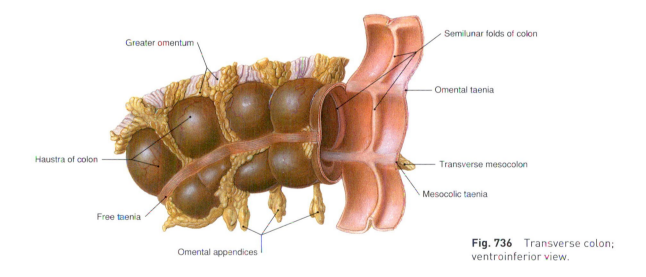

Fig. 736   Transverse colon; ventroinferior view.

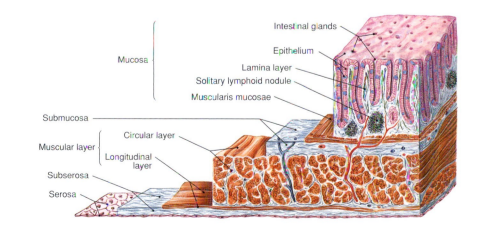

Fig. 737   Colon; layers of the wall; microscopic enlargement at low magnification.

Vermiform appendix

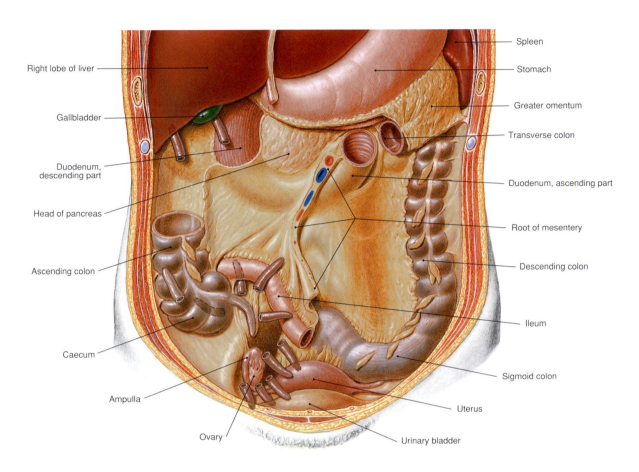

Fig. 738 Vermiform appendix; variations in its position; ventral view.

Right lobe of liver

Gallbladder

Duodenum, descending part

Head of pancreas

Ascending colon

Caecum

Ampulla

Ovary

Spleen

Stomach

Greater omentum

Transverse colon

Duodenum, ascending part

Root of mesentery

Descending colon

Ileum

Sigmoid colon

Uterus

Urinary bladder

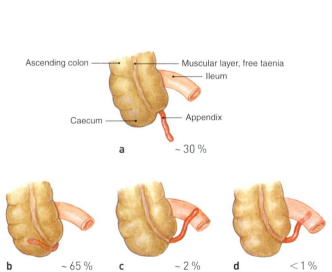

Ascending colon

Muscular layer, free taenia

Ileum

Caecum

Appendix

a ~ 30 %

b ~ 65 %   **c** ~ 2 %   **d** < 1 %

Fig. 739 Vermiform appendix; variations in its position.
a Descending into the lesser pelvis
b Behind the caecum
c In front of the ileum
d Behind the ileum

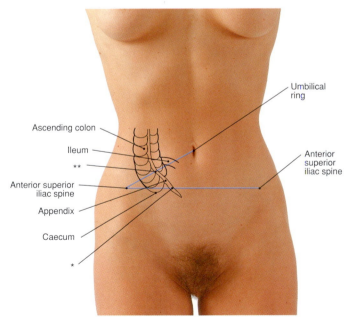

Umbilical ring

Ascending colon

Ileum

**

Anterior superior iliac spine

Anterior superior iliac spine

Appendix

Caecum

*

Fig. 740 Caecum and vermiform appendix; projection onto the anterior abdominal wall.

* Clinical term: v. LANZ's point, at the right third of a line connecting the anterior superior iliac spines, locates the tip of the vermiform appendix

** Clinical term: McBURNEY's point, at the outer third of a line connecting the right anterior superior iliac spine and the umbilicus, locates the base of the vermiform appendix

Large intestine, imaging

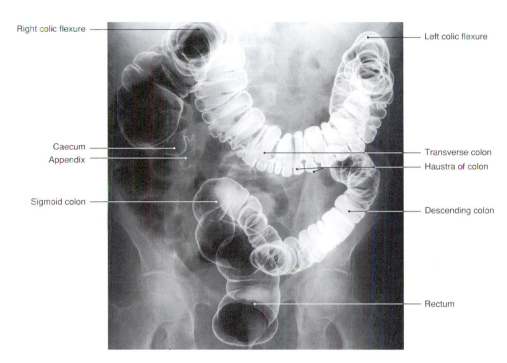

Right colic flexure
Left colic flexure
Caecum
Appendix
Transverse colon
Haustra of colon
Sigmoid colon
Descending colon
Rectum

Fig. 741 Colon and rectum;
AP-radiograph after filling with a contrast medium
and air (double contrast method).

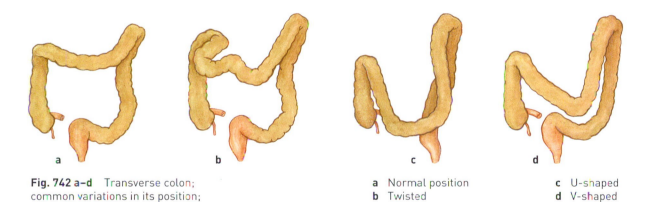

a
b
c
d

Fig. 742 a–d Transverse colon;
common variations in its position;
ventral view.

a Normal position	**c** U-shaped
b Twisted	**d** V-shaped

Haustra of colon
Semilunar folds of colon

Fig. 743 Ascending colon;
endoscopic image after passage of the rectum,
the sigmoid colon, the descending colon
and the transverse colon (colonoscopy).

Liver

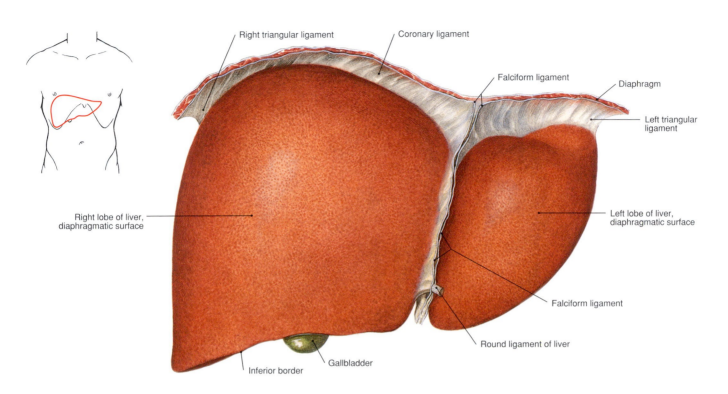

Right triangular ligament

Coronary ligament

Falciform ligament

Diaphragm

Left triangular ligament

Right lobe of liver, diaphragmatic surface

Left lobe of liver, diaphragmatic surface

Falciform ligament

Round ligament of liver

Inferior border

Gallbladder

Fig. 744   Liver; ventral view.

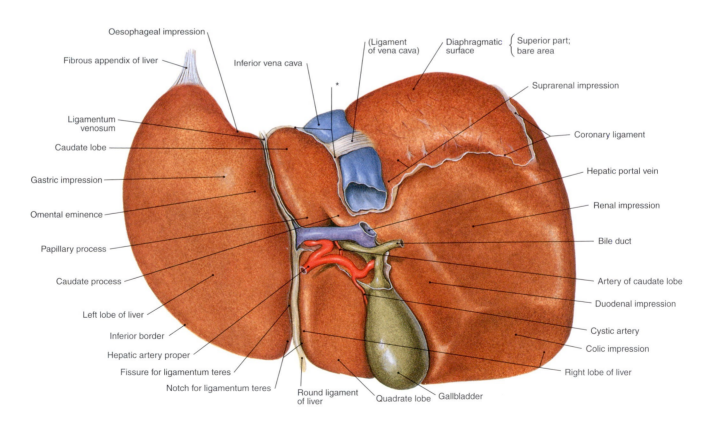

Oesophageal impression

Fibrous appendix of liver

Inferior vena cava

(Ligament of vena cava)

Diaphragmatic surface

Superior part; bare area

Ligamentum venosum

Caudate lobe

Suprarenal impression

Coronary ligament

Gastric impression

Hepatic portal vein

Omental eminence

Renal impression

Papillary process

Bile duct

Caudate process

Artery of caudate lobe

Left lobe of liver

Duodenal impression

Inferior border

Cystic artery

Hepatic artery proper

Colic impression

Fissure for ligamentum teres

Right lobe of liver

Notch for ligamentum teres

Round ligament of liver

Quadrate lobe

Gallbladder

Fig. 745   Liver and porta hepatis; dorsal view.

* Borders of the superior recess of the omental bursa

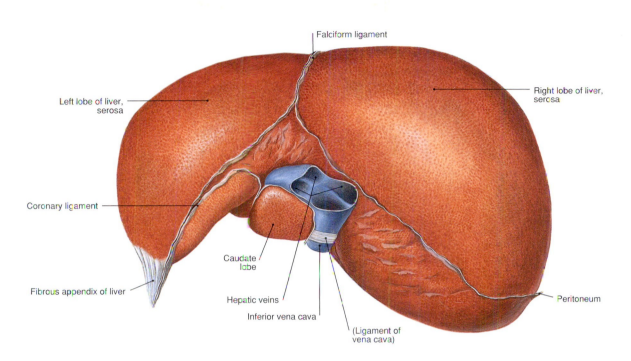

Falciform ligament

Left lobe of liver, serosa

Right lobe of liver, serosa

Coronary ligament

Caudate lobe

Fibrous appendix of liver

Hepatic veins

Inferior vena cava

(Ligament of vena cava)

Peritoneum

Fig. 746 Liver; superior view.

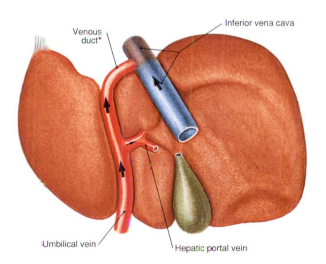

Venous duct*

Inferior vena cava

Umbilical vein

Hepatic portal vein

Fig. 747 Liver of a foetus; oxygen content of the blood is shown by different colours and the direction of flow by arrows; dorsal view.

* Also: Ductus ARANTII

Liver puncture

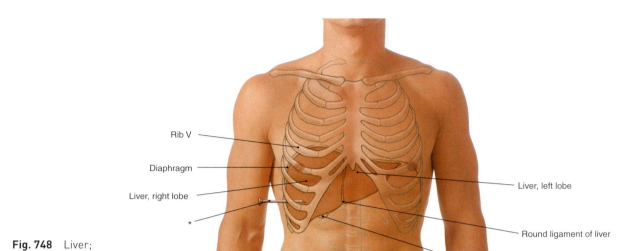

Rib V

Diaphragm

Liver, right lobe

*

Liver, left lobe

Round ligament of liver

Gallbladder

Fig. 748 Liver;
projection onto the anterior
abdominal wall;
intermediate position between
inspiration and expiration.

* Position of the needle for liver puncture

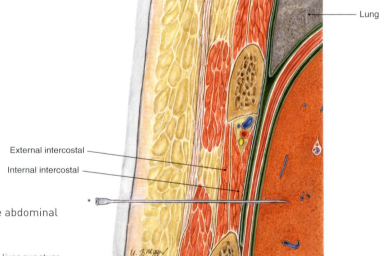

Lung

External intercostal

Internal intercostal

*

Fig. 749 Layers of the abdominal
wall and the liver;
frontal section.

* Position of the needle for liver puncture

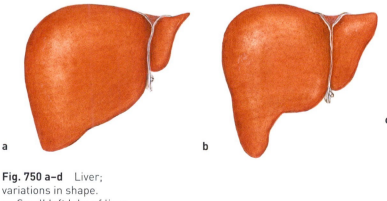

a

b

c

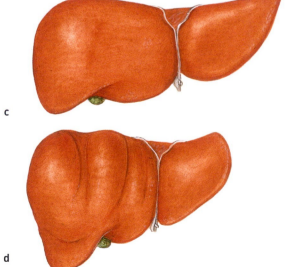

d

Fig. 750 a–d Liver;
variations in shape.
a Small left lobe of liver
b Tongue-shaped process of the right lobe of liver
c Bridged flat shape
d Diaphragmatic furrows

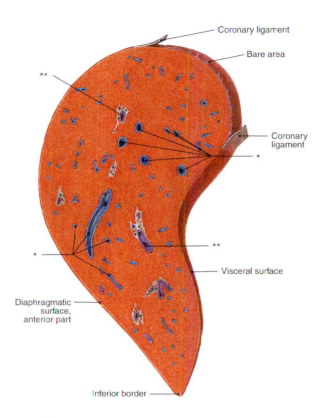

Coronary ligament

Bare area

Coronary ligament

**

*

Visceral surface

Diaphragmatic surface, anterior part

**

Inferior border

Fig. 751   Liver;
sagittal section through the right lobe of liver to demonstrate
the branches of the hepatic veins and the hepatic portal vein.

*   Intrahepatic branches of the hepatic veins
** Intrahepatic branches of the hepatic portal vein and the hepatic artery

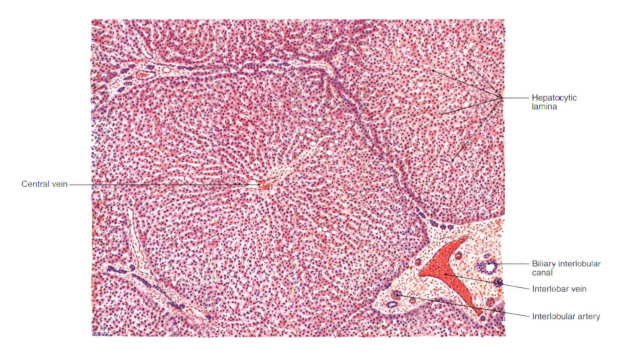

Hepatocytic lamina

Central vein

Biliary interlobular canal

Interlobar vein

Interlobular artery

Fig. 752   Liver;
microscopic structure (microscopic enlargement at low
magnification);

trias of GLISSON (consists of a branch of the hepatic portal
vein, a branch of the hepatic artery proper and a small bile duct),
and a small liver lobule surrounding a central vein.

Liver puncture

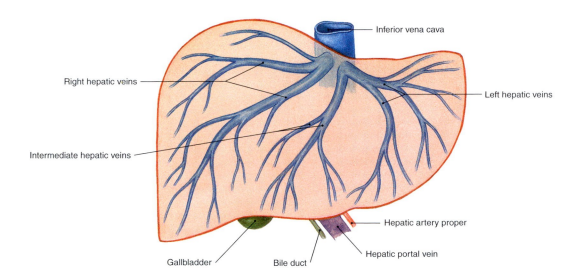

Fig. 753   Liver and hepatic veins;
ventral view.

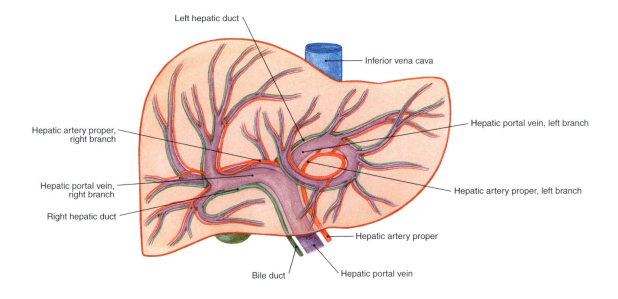

Fig. 754   Liver and the hepatic portal vein;
ventral view.

Segments of the liver

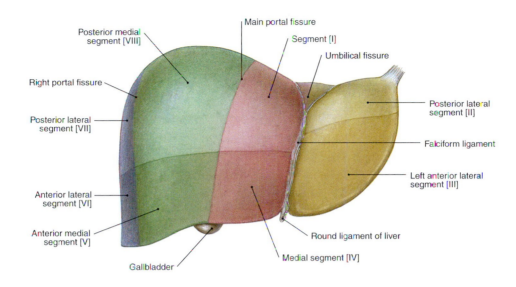

Main portal fissure
Posterior medial segment [VIII]
Segment [I]
Umbilical fissure
Right portal fissure
Posterior lateral segment [II]
Posterior lateral segment [VII]
Falciform ligament
Left anterior lateral segment [III]
Anterior lateral segment [VI]
Anterior medial segment [V]
Round ligament of liver
Medial segment [IV]
Gallbladder

Fig. 755 Liver;
the segments of the lobes are shown in different colours;
ventral view.

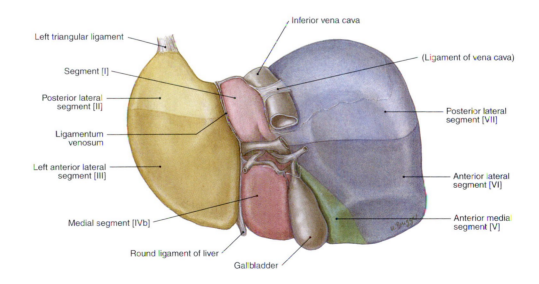

Inferior vena cava
Left triangular ligament
(Ligament of vena cava)
Segment [I]
Posterior lateral segment [II]
Posterior lateral segment [VII]
Ligamentum venosum
Left anterior lateral segment [III]
Anterior lateral segment [VI]
Medial segment [IVb]
Anterior medial segment [V]
Round ligament of liver
Gallbladder

Fig. 756 Liver;
the segments of the lobes are shown in different colours;
dorsal view.

Liver, ultrasound

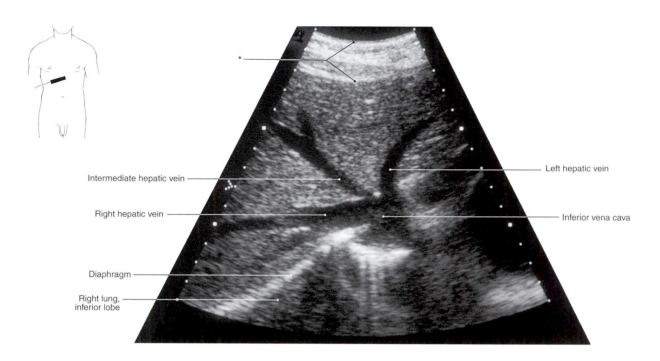

Intermediate hepatic vein

Right hepatic vein

Diaphragm

Right lung,
inferior lobe

Left hepatic vein

Inferior vena cava

→ 753

Fig. 757 Hepatic veins;
ultrasound image showing the opening of the hepatic veins
into the inferior vena cava;
inferior view.

* Abdominal wall

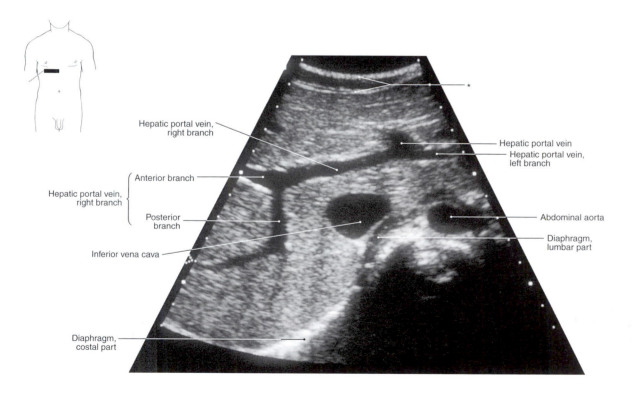

Hepatic portal vein,
right branch

Anterior branch

Hepatic portal vein,
right branch

Posterior
branch

Inferior vena cava

Diaphragm,
costal part

Hepatic portal vein

Hepatic portal vein,
left branch

Abdominal aorta

Diaphragm,
lumbar part

→ 754

Fig. 758 Hepatic portal vein;
ultrasound image showing the division of the hepatic portal vein
into the main branches;
inferior view.

* Abdominal wall

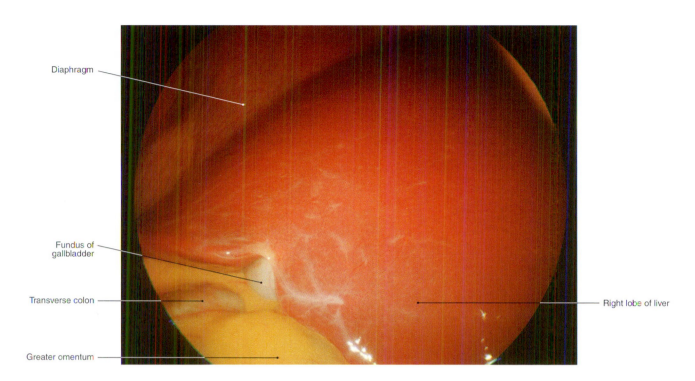

Diaphragm

Fundus of gallbladder

Transverse colon

Greater omentum

Right lobe of liver

Fig. 759 Liver and gallbladder;
laparoscopy;
oblique inferior view from the left.

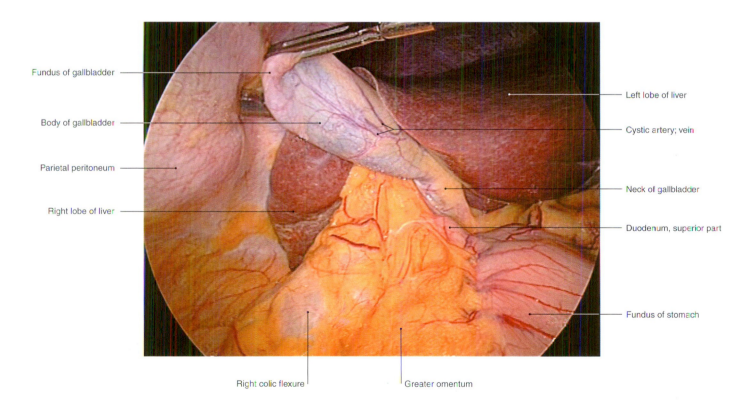

Fundus of gallbladder

Body of gallbladder

Parietal peritoneum

Right lobe of liver

Left lobe of liver

Cystic artery; vein

Neck of gallbladder

Duodenum, superior part

Fundus of stomach

Right colic flexure

Greater omentum

Fig. 760 Gallbladder and liver;
laparoscopy;
ventral view.

Gallbladder and bile duct system

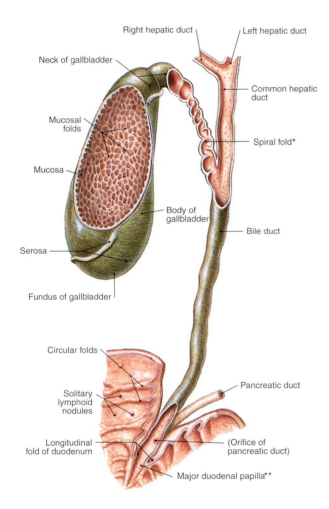

Fig. 761 Gallbladder
and bile duct system;
ventral view.

* Clinical term: HEISTER's valve
** Clinical term: tubercle of VATER

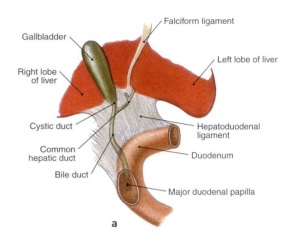

a

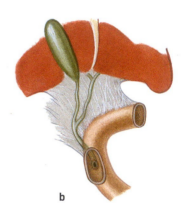

b

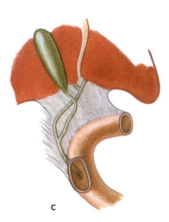

c

Fig. 762 a–c Variations in the bile duct system:
common hepatic duct and bile duct.
a High union of the common hepatic duct and the cystic duct
b Low union of the common hepatic duct and the cystic duct
c Low union after the cystic duct crosses
over the common hepatic duct

Bile duct system, radiography

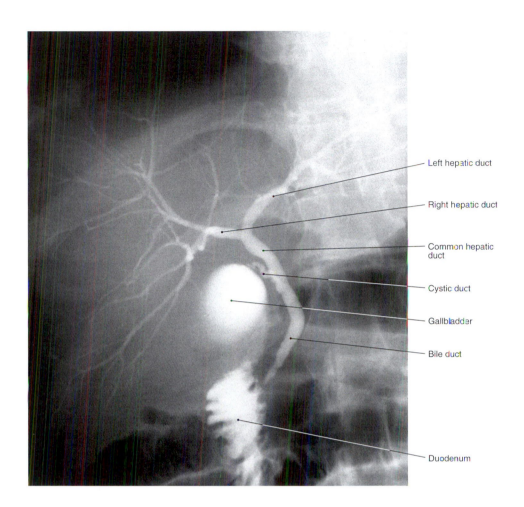

- Left hepatic duct
- Right hepatic duct
- Common hepatic duct
- Cystic duct
- Gallbladder
- Bile duct
- Duodenum

Fig. 763 Bile duct system;
AP-radiograph after administration of a contrast medium;
upright position;
ventral view.

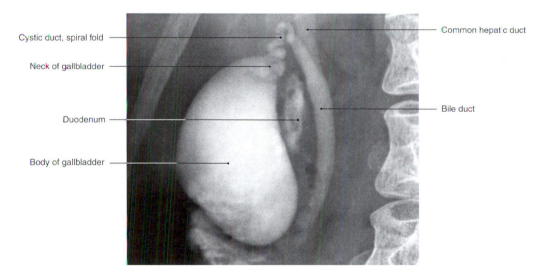

- Cystic duct, spiral fold
- Neck of gallbladder
- Duodenum
- Body of gallbladder
- Common hepatic duct
- Bile duct

Fig. 764 Gallbladder and bile duct system;
AP-radiograph after administration of a contrast medium;
upright position;
ventral view.

Pancreas

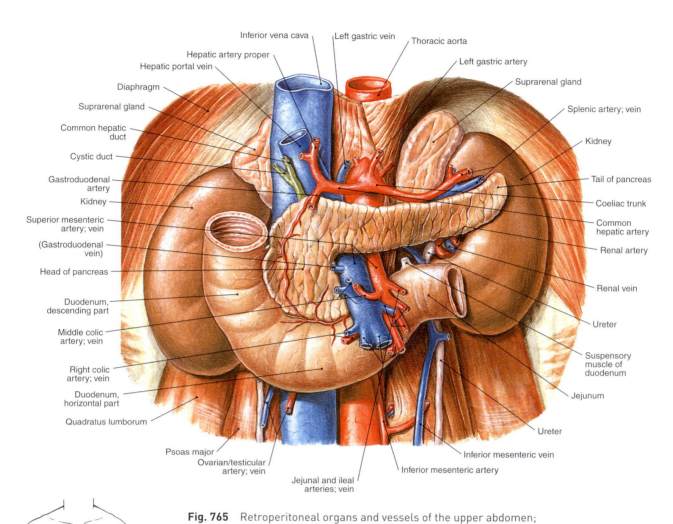

Inferior vena cava
Left gastric vein
Thoracic aorta
Hepatic artery proper
Left gastric artery
Hepatic portal vein
Suprarenal gland
Diaphragm
Suprarenal gland
Splenic artery; vein
Common hepatic duct
Kidney
Cystic duct
Tail of pancreas
Gastroduodenal artery
Coeliac trunk
Kidney
Common hepatic artery
Superior mesenteric artery; vein
Renal artery
(Gastroduodenal vein)
Renal vein
Head of pancreas
Duodenum, descending part
Ureter
Middle colic artery; vein
Suspensory muscle of duodenum
Right colic artery; vein
Jejunum
Duodenum, horizontal part
Quadratus lumborum
Ureter
Psoas major
Inferior mesenteric vein
Ovarian/testicular artery; vein
Inferior mesenteric artery
Jejunal and ileal arteries; vein

Fig. 765 Retroperitoneal organs and vessels of the upper abdomen; ventral view.

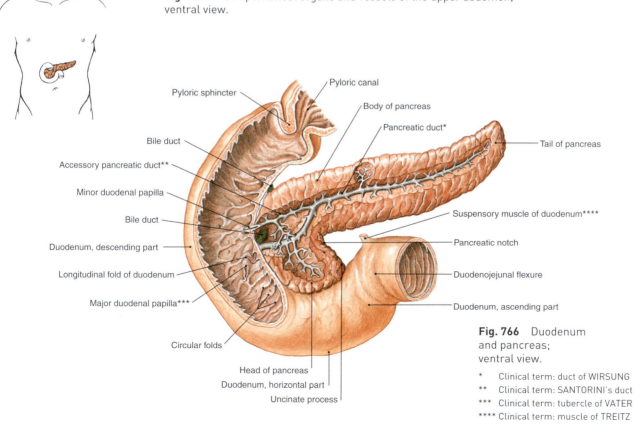

Pyloric sphincter
Pyloric canal
Body of pancreas
Pancreatic duct*
Bile duct
Tail of pancreas
Accessory pancreatic duct**
Minor duodenal papilla
Bile duct
Suspensory muscle of duodenum****
Duodenum, descending part
Pancreatic notch
Longitudinal fold of duodenum
Duodenojejunal flexure
Major duodenal papilla***
Duodenum, ascending part
Circular folds

Fig. 766 Duodenum and pancreas; ventral view.

Head of pancreas
Duodenum, horizontal part
Uncinate process

*   Clinical term: duct of WIRSUNG
**   Clinical term: SANTORINI's duct
***   Clinical term: tubercle of VATER
**** Clinical term: muscle of TREITZ

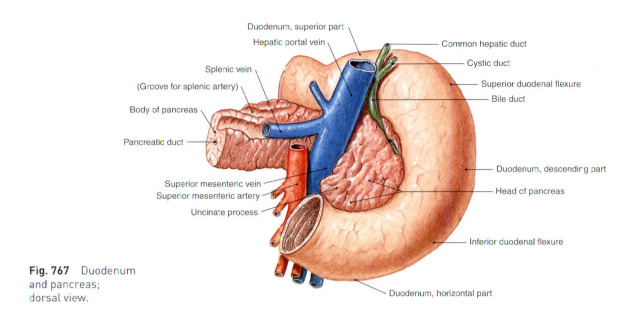

Duodenum, superior part
Hepatic portal vein
Common hepatic duct
Cystic duct
Splenic vein
Superior duodenal flexure
(Groove for splenic artery)
Bile duct
Body of pancreas
Pancreatic duct
Duodenum, descending part
Superior mesenteric vein
Head of pancreas
Superior mesenteric artery
Uncinate process
Inferior duodenal flexure

Fig. 767 Duodenum and pancreas; dorsal view.

Duodenum, horizontal part

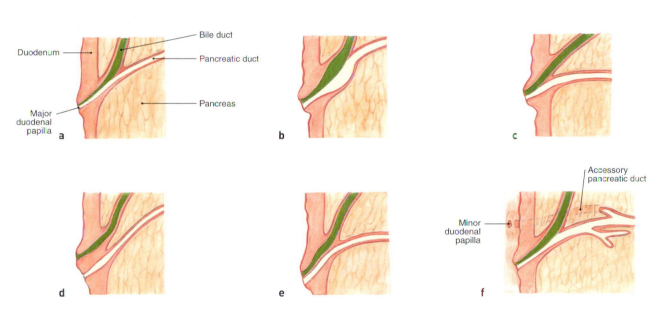

Bile duct
Duodenum
Pancreatic duct
Pancreas
Major duodenal papilla **a**

b

c

d

e

Accessory pancreatic duct
Minor duodenal papilla
f

Fig. 768 a–f Variations in the opening of the bile duct and the pancreatic duct.
a Long common part
b Ampullary enlargement at the terminal part
c Short common part
d Separate opening
e Single opening with a septum dividing the common duct
f Accessory pancreatic duct

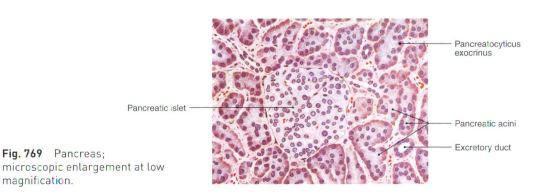

Pancreatocyticus exocrinus
Pancreatic islet
Pancreatic acini
Excretory duct

Fig. 769 Pancreas; microscopic enlargement at low magnification.

Pancreas, imaging

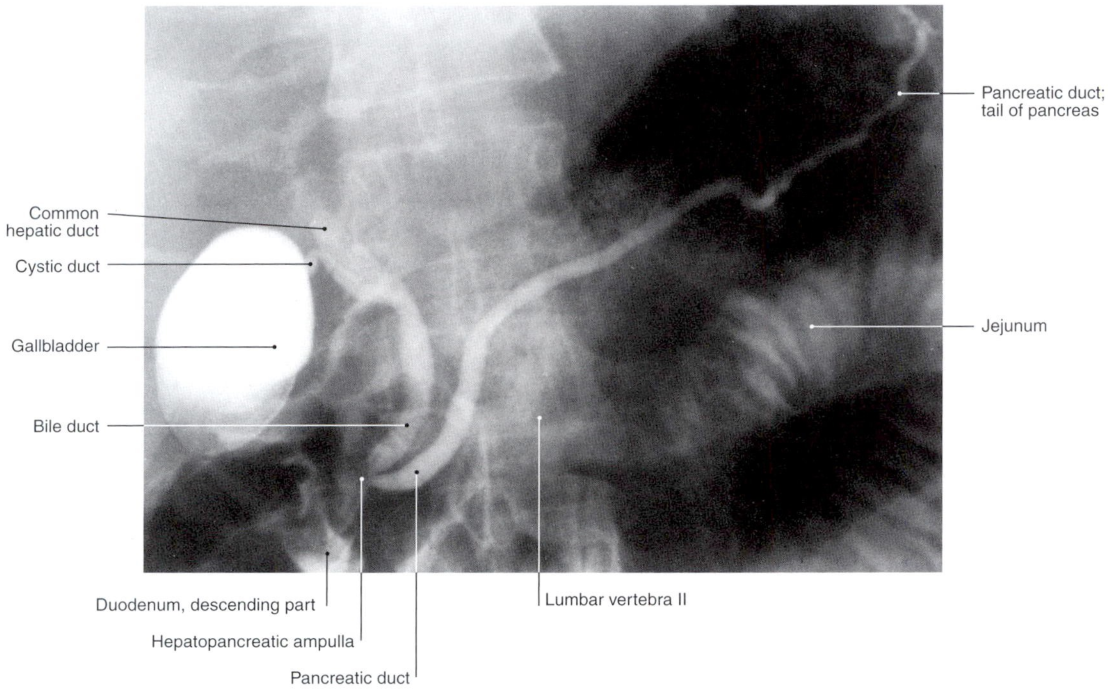

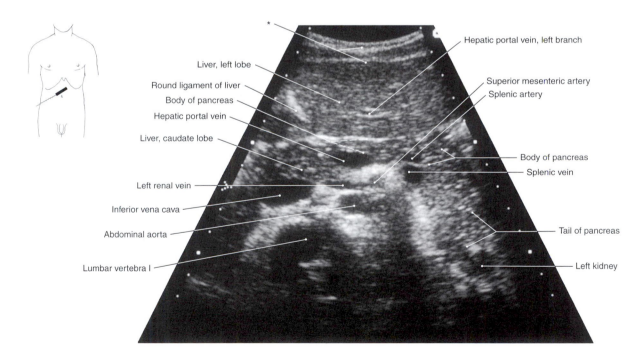

Common hepatic duct

Cystic duct

Gallbladder

Bile duct

Pancreatic duct;
tail of pancreas

Jejunum

Duodenum, descending part

Hepatopancreatic ampulla

Pancreatic duct

Lumbar vertebra II

Fig. 770 Pancreatic duct;
bile duct and gallbladder;
AP-radiograph; supine position; after endoscopic
intubation of the common excretory duct of the liver
and the pancreas, as well as injection of a contrast medium;
ventral view.
Clinical term: ERCP (endoscopic retrograde cholangio-
pancreaticography).

Liver, left lobe

Round ligament of liver

Body of pancreas

Hepatic portal vein

Liver, caudate lobe

Left renal vein

Inferior vena cava

Abdominal aorta

Lumbar vertebra I

Hepatic portal vein, left branch

Superior mesenteric artery

Splenic artery

Body of pancreas

Splenic vein

Tail of pancreas

Left kidney

Fig. 771 Pancreas;
ultrasound image showing the pancreas and adjacent
large vessels in deep inspiration;

oblique inferior view.

* Abdominal wall

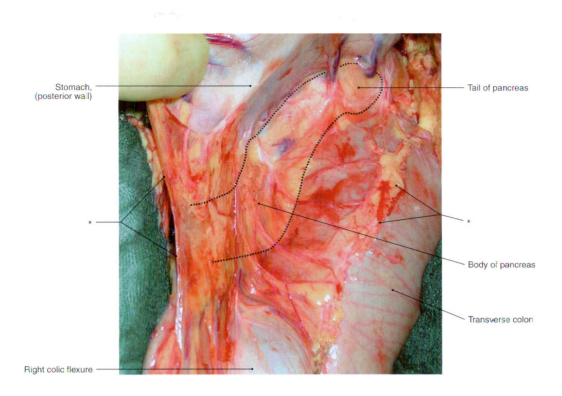

Stomach, (posterior wall)

Tail of pancreas

*

*

Body of pancreas

Transverse colon

Right colic flexure

Fig. 772 Pancreas;
the gastrocolic ligament of the greater omentum has been
dissected to expose the omental bursa;
photograph taken during surgery.

* Dissection line at the greater omentum

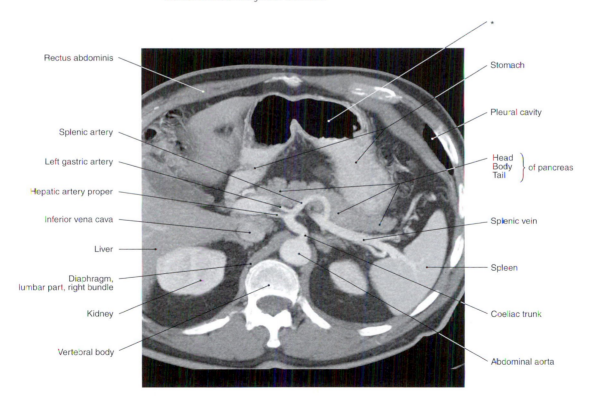

*

Rectus abdominis

Stomach

Pleural cavity

Splenic artery

Left gastric artery

Head
Body } of pancreas
Tail

Hepatic artery proper

Inferior vena cava

Splenic vein

Liver

Spleen

Diaphragm,
lumbar part, right bundle

Kidney

Coeliac trunk

Vertebral body

Abdominal aorta

Fig. 773 Pancreas;
computed tomographic horizontal section (CT);

inferior view.
In this subject, the coeliac trunk is located remarkably low.

* Air bubble in the stomach

Spleen

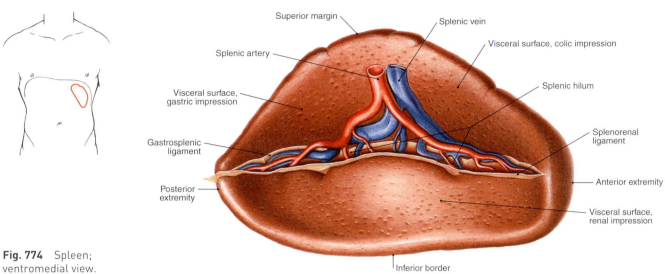

Fig. 774   Spleen;
ventromedial view.

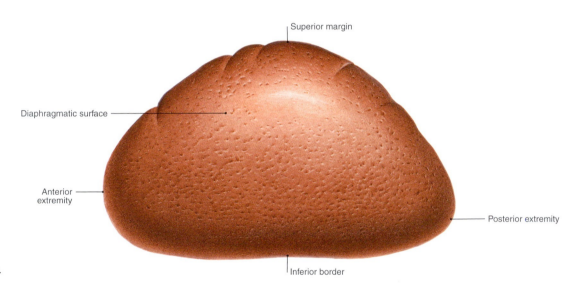

Fig. 775   Spleen;
superolateral view.

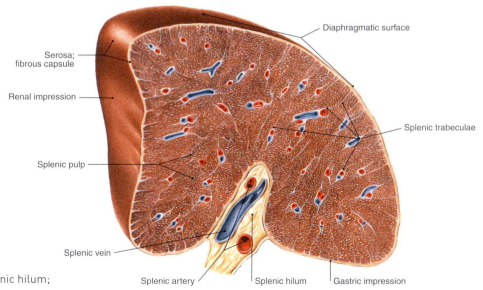

Fig. 776   Spleen;
cross-section through the splenic hilum;
superomedial view.

Development of the intestines

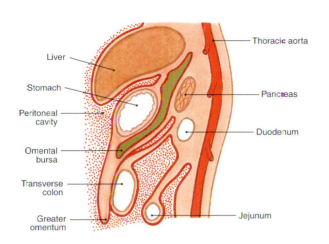

Fig. 777 Development of the peritoneal cavity
and the visceral relationships;
schematic median section;
lateral view.

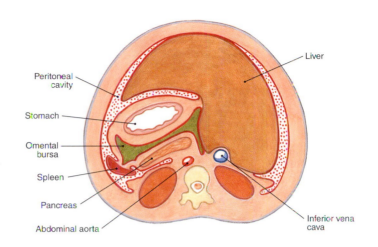

Fig. 778 Development of the peritoneal cavity;
schematic horizontal section;
superior view.

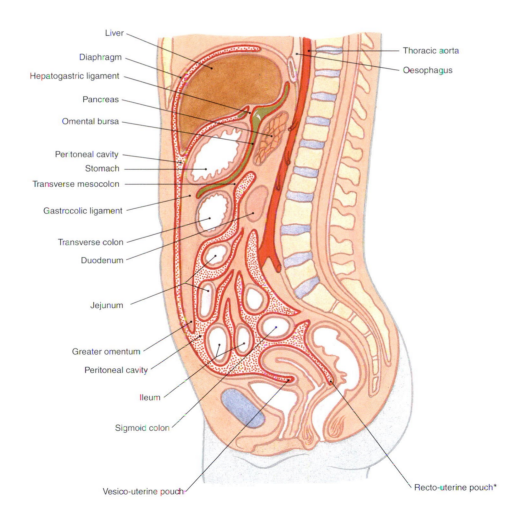

Fig. 779 Development of the peritoneal cavity and the
visceral relationships of the female;
final state of the peritoneal cavity with adhesion of the
greater omentum to the transverse colon;

schematic median section;
lateral view.
The omental bursa corresponds with the peritoneal cavity via
the omental foramen.

* Clinical term: pouch of DOUGLAS

Greater omentum

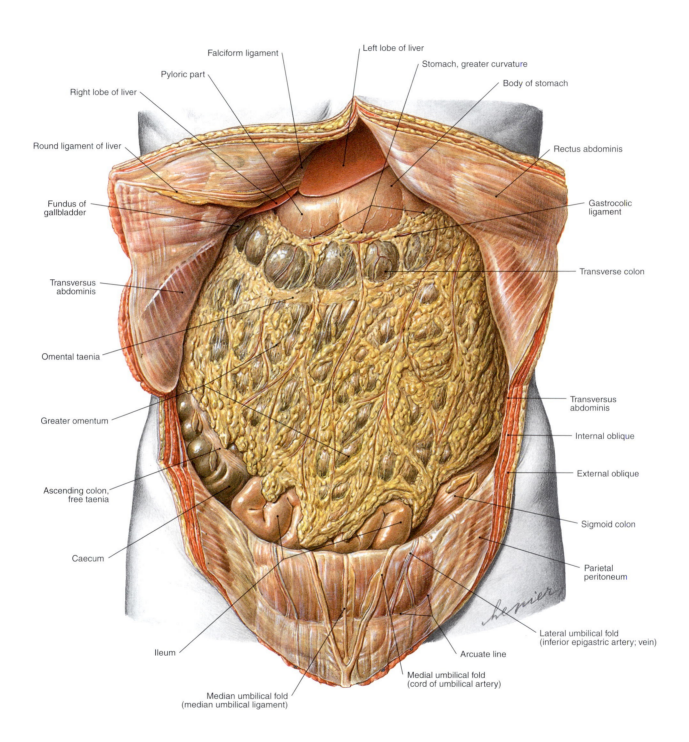

Falciform ligament

Left lobe of liver

Pyloric part

Stomach, greater curvature

Right lobe of liver

Body of stomach

Round ligament of liver

Rectus abdominis

Fundus of gallbladder

Gastrocolic ligament

Transversus abdominis

Transverse colon

Omental taenia

Greater omentum

Transversus abdominis

Internal oblique

Ascending colon, free taenia

External oblique

Caecum

Sigmoid colon

Parietal peritoneum

Ileum

Lateral umbilical fold (inferior epigastric artery; vein)

Arcuate line

Medial umbilical fold (cord of umbilical artery)

Median umbilical fold (median umbilical ligament)

→ 578

Fig. 780 Position of the abdominal viscera and greater omentum.

Abdominal viscera of the neonate

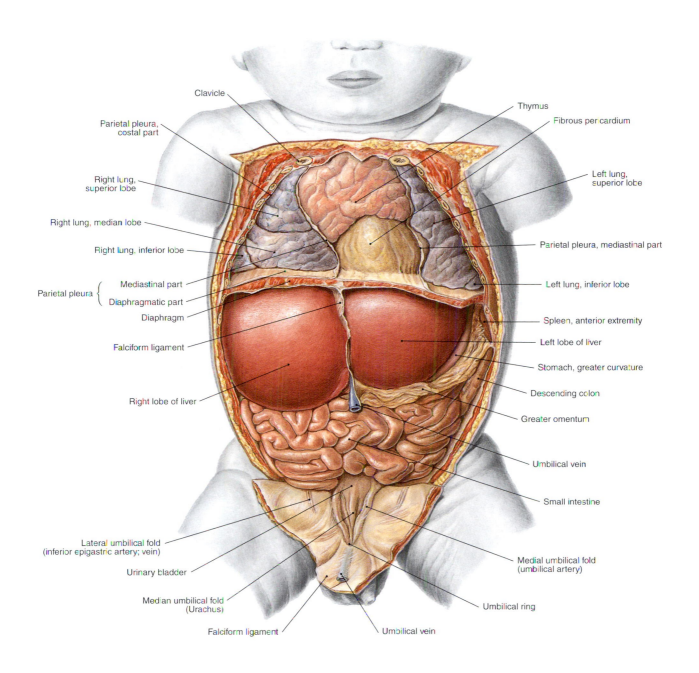

Clavicle

Parietal pleura,
costal part

Right lung,
superior lobe

Right lung, median lobe

Right lung, inferior lobe

Parietal pleura {
Mediastinal part

Diaphragmatic part

Diaphragm

Falciform ligament

Right lobe of liver

Lateral umbilical fold
(inferior epigastric artery; vein)

Urinary bladder

Median umbilical fold
(Urachus)

Falciform ligament

Thymus

Fibrous pericardium

Left lung,
superior lobe

Parietal pleura, mediastinal part

Left lung, inferior lobe

Spleen, anterior extremity

Left lobe of liver

Stomach, greater curvature

Descending colon

Greater omentum

Umbilical vein

Small intestine

Medial umbilical fold
(umbilical artery)

Umbilical ring

Umbilical vein

Fig. 781   Position of the abdominal viscera of the neonate

Abdominal viscera in the upper abdomen

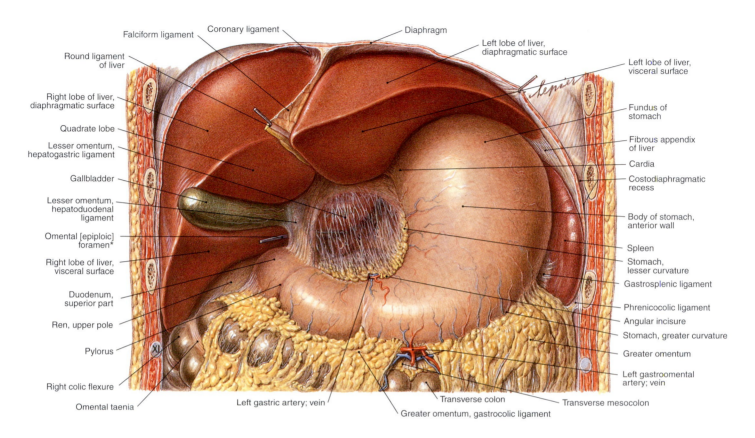

Falciform ligament
Coronary ligament
Diaphragm
Left lobe of liver, diaphragmatic surface
Round ligament of liver
Left lobe of liver, visceral surface
Right lobe of liver, diaphragmatic surface
Fundus of stomach
Quadrate lobe
Fibrous appendix of liver
Lesser omentum, hepatogastric ligament
Cardia
Gallbladder
Costodiaphragmatic recess
Lesser omentum, hepatoduodenal ligament
Body of stomach, anterior wall
Omental [epiploic] foramen*
Spleen
Right lobe of liver, visceral surface
Stomach, lesser curvature
Duodenum, superior part
Gastrosplenic ligament
Ren, upper pole
Phrenicocolic ligament
Angular incisure
Pylorus
Stomach, greater curvature
Greater omentum
Right colic flexure
Left gastroomental artery; vein
Omental taenia
Left gastric artery; vein
Transverse colon
Transverse mesocolon
Greater omentum, gastrocolic ligament

Fig. 782 Position of the abdominal viscera in the upper abdomen; ventral view.

* Also: foramen of WINSLOW

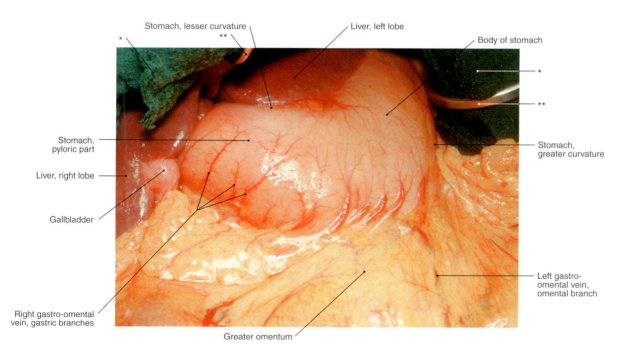

Stomach, lesser curvature
Liver, left lobe
Body of stomach
*
**
*
Stomach, pyloric part
**
Liver, right lobe
Stomach, greater curvature
Gallbladder
Left gastro-omental vein, omental branch
Right gastro-omental vein, gastric branches
Greater omentum

Fig. 783 Stomach and greater omentum; photograph taken during surgery; ventral view.

* Surgical drape
** Surgical retractor

Abdominal viscera in the upper abdomen

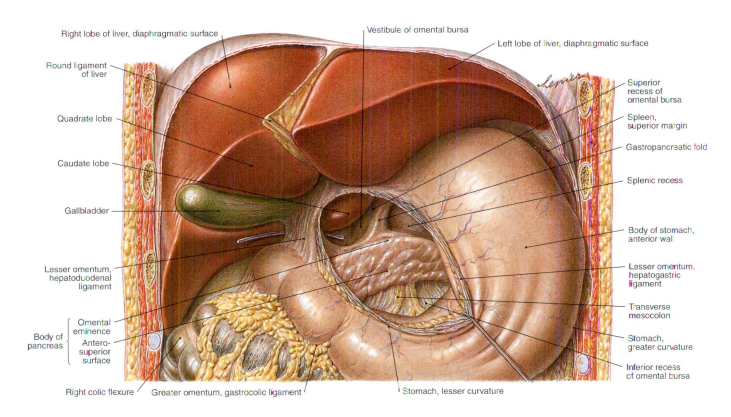

Right lobe of liver, diaphragmatic surface

Vestibule of omental bursa

Left lobe of liver, diaphragmatic surface

Round ligament of liver

Superior recess of omental bursa

Quadrate lobe

Spleen, superior margin

Caudate lobe

Gastropancreatic fold

Gallbladder

Splenic recess

Body of stomach, anterior wall

Lesser omentum, hepatoduodenal ligament

Lesser omentum, hepatogastric ligament

Omental eminence

Body of pancreas

Antero-superior surface

Transverse mesocolon

Stomach, greater curvature

Inferior recess of omental bursa

Right colic flexure

Greater omentum, gastrocolic ligament

Stomach, lesser curvature

Fig. 784 Abdominal viscera in the upper abdomen;
parts of the lesser omentum have been removed to expose
the omental bursa and the pancreas;
oblique view from superior.

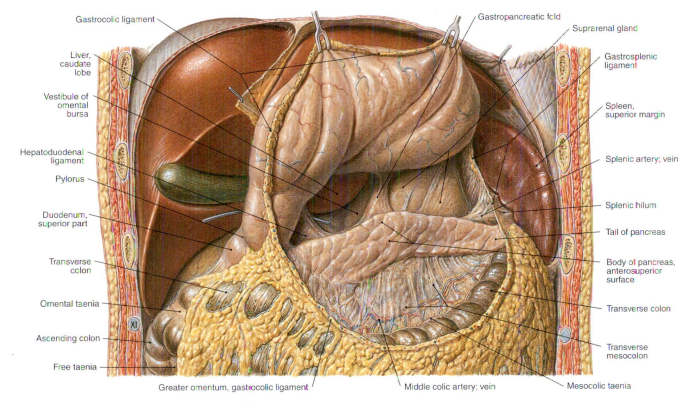

Gastrocolic ligament

Gastropancreatic fold

Suprarenal gland

Liver, caudate lobe

Gastrosplenic ligament

Vestibule of omental bursa

Spleen, superior margin

Hepatoduodenal ligament

Splenic artery; vein

Pylorus

Splenic hilum

Duodenum, superior part

Tail of pancreas

Transverse colon

Body of pancreas, anterosuperior surface

Omental taenia

Transverse colon

Ascending colon

Transverse mesocolon

Free taenia

Greater omentum, gastrocolic ligament

Middle colic artery; vein

Mesocolic taenia

Fig. 785 Omental bursa;
after dissection of the gastrocolic ligament;
oblique view from inferior.

Abdominal viscera in the lower abdomen

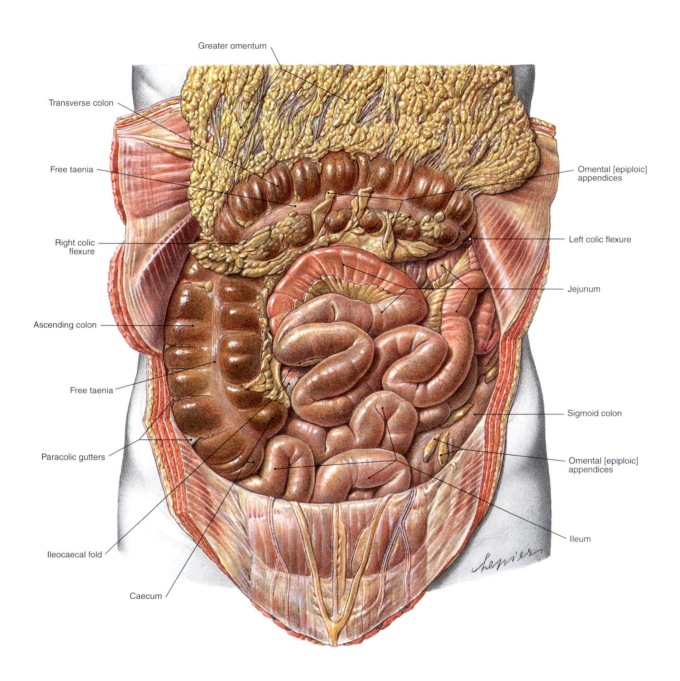

Greater omentum

Transverse colon

Free taenia

Omental [epiploic] appendices

Right colic flexure

Left colic flexure

Jejunum

Ascending colon

Free taenia

Sigmoid colon

Paracolic gutters

Omental [epiploic] appendices

Ileocaecal fold

Ileum

Caecum

Fig. 786　Position of the abdominal viscera.

Abdominal viscera in the lower abdomen

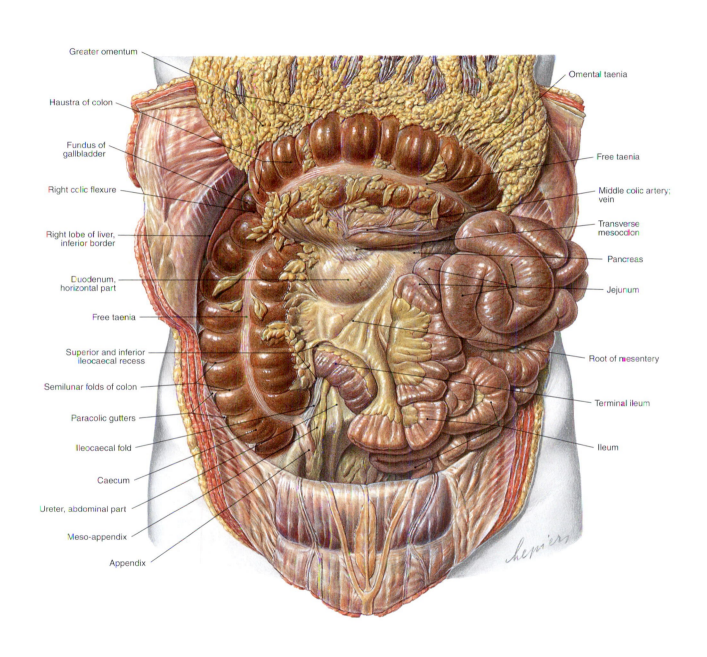

Greater omentum
Haustra of colon
Fundus of gallbladder
Right colic flexure
Right lobe of liver, inferior border
Duodenum, horizontal part
Free taenia
Superior and inferior ileocaecal recess
Semilunar folds of colon
Paracolic gutters
Ileocaecal fold
Caecum
Ureter, abdominal part
Meso-appendix
Appendix

Omental taenia
Free taenia
Middle colic artery; vein
Transverse mesocolon
Pancreas
Jejunum
Root of mesentery
Terminal ileum
Ileum

Fig. 787   Small intestine and large intestine.

Abdominal viscera in the lower abdomen

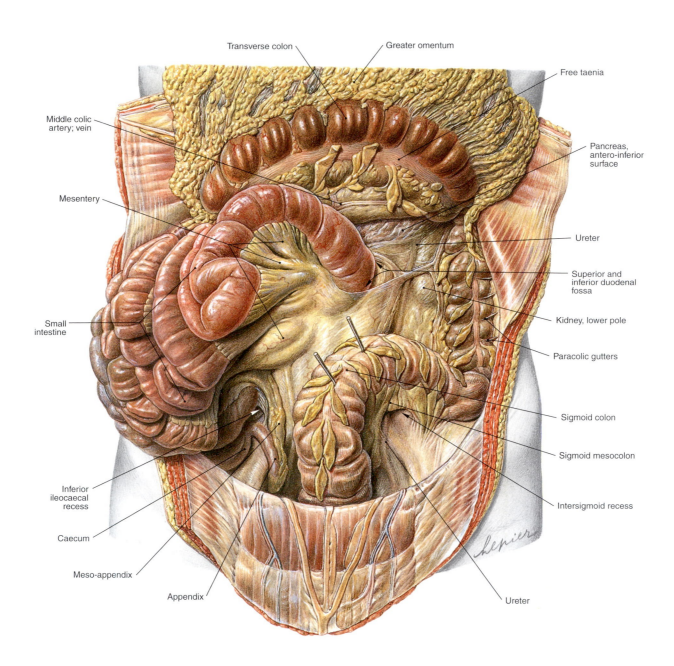

Transverse colon

Greater omentum

Free taenia

Middle colic
artery; vein

Pancreas,
antero-inferior
surface

Mesentery

Ureter

Superior and
inferior duodenal
fossa

Kidney, lower pole

Paracolic gutters

Small
intestine

Sigmoid colon

Sigmoid mesocolon

Intersigmoid recess

Inferior
ileocaecal
recess

Caecum

Ureter

Meso-appendix

Appendix

Fig. 788   Small intestine
and large intestine.

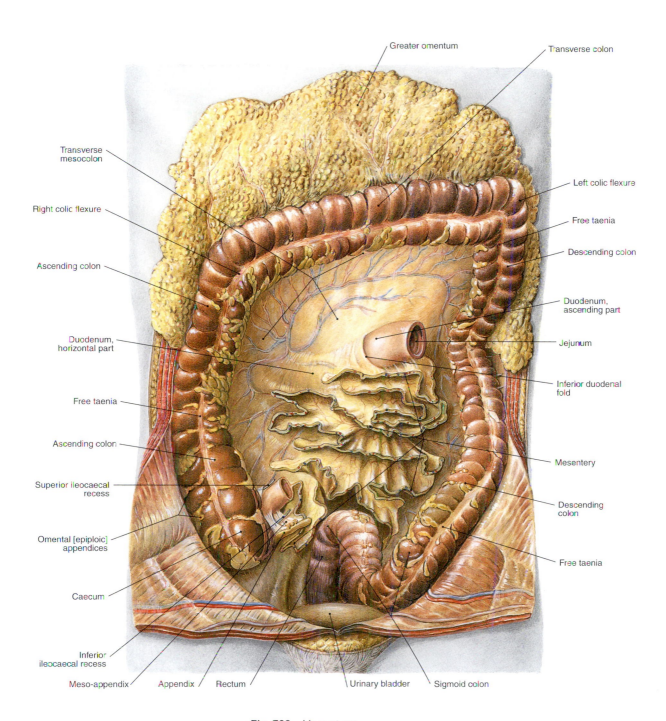

Greater omentum

Transverse colon

Transverse mesocolon

Left colic flexure

Right colic flexure

Free taenia

Descending colon

Ascending colon

Duodenum, ascending part

Duodenum, horizontal part

Jejunum

Free taenia

Inferior duodenal fold

Ascending colon

Mesentery

Superior ileocaecal recess

Descending colon

Omental [epiploic] appendices

Free taenia

Caecum

Inferior ileocaecal recess

Meso-appendix | Appendix | Rectum | Urinary bladder | Sigmoid colon

Fig. 789 Mesentery and large intestine.

Mesenteric root and retroperitoneal space

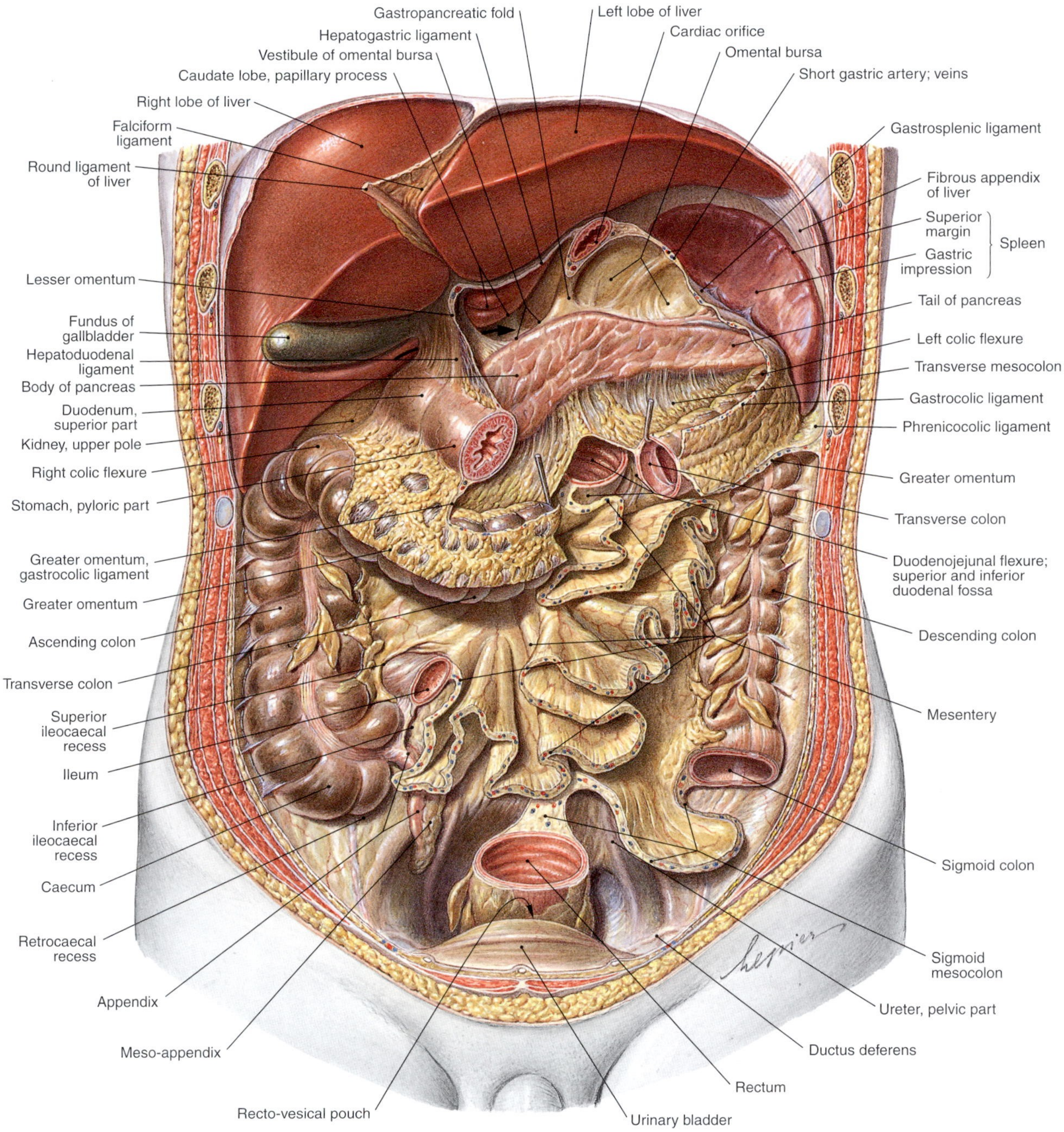

Gastropancreatic fold
Hepatogastric ligament
Vestibule of omental bursa
Caudate lobe, papillary process
Right lobe of liver
Falciform ligament
Round ligament of liver
Lesser omentum
Fundus of gallbladder
Hepatoduodenal ligament
Body of pancreas
Duodenum, superior part
Kidney, upper pole
Right colic flexure
Stomach, pyloric part
Greater omentum, gastrocolic ligament
Greater omentum
Ascending colon
Transverse colon
Superior ileocaecal recess
Ileum
Inferior ileocaecal recess
Caecum
Retrocaecal recess
Appendix
Meso-appendix
Recto-vesical pouch

Left lobe of liver
Cardiac orifice
Omental bursa
Short gastric artery; veins
Gastrosplenic ligament
Fibrous appendix of liver
Superior margin
Gastric impression
Spleen
Tail of pancreas
Left colic flexure
Transverse mesocolon
Gastrocolic ligament
Phrenicocolic ligament
Greater omentum
Transverse colon
Duodenojejunal flexure; superior and inferior duodenal fossa
Descending colon
Mesentery
Sigmoid colon
Sigmoid mesocolon
Ureter, pelvic part
Ductus deferens
Rectum
Urinary bladder

Fig. 790 Position of the abdominal viscera and the omental bursa.
An arrow indicates the omental [epiploic] foramen.

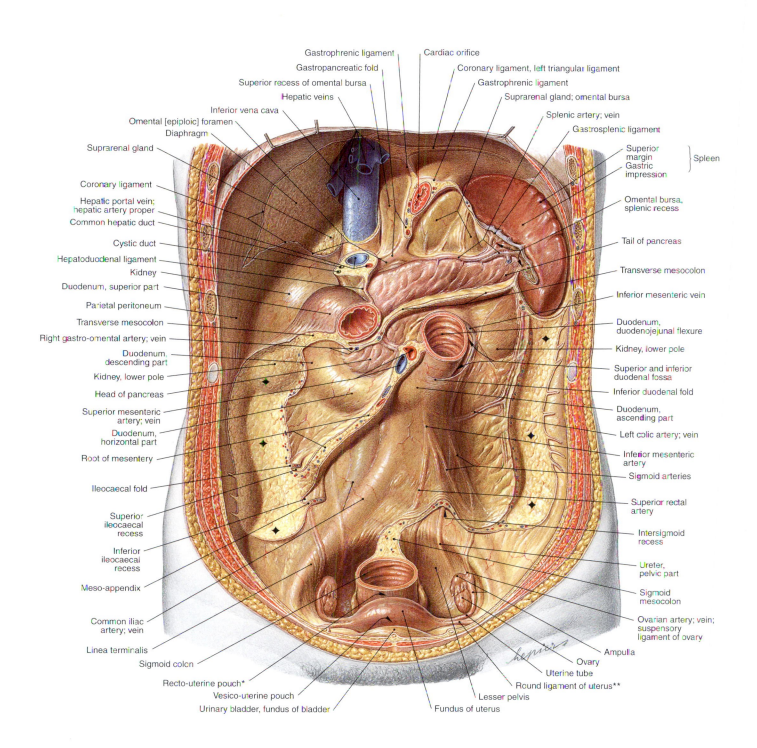

Gastrophrenic ligament
Gastropancreatic fold
Superior recess of omental bursa
Hepatic veins
Inferior vena cava
Omental [epiploic] foramen
Diaphragm
Suprarenal gland
Coronary ligament
Hepatic portal vein; hepatic artery proper
Common hepatic duct
Cystic duct
Hepatoduodenal ligament
Kidney
Duodenum, superior part
Parietal peritoneum
Transverse mesocolon
Right gastro-omental artery; vein
Duodenum, descending part
Kidney, lower pole
Head of pancreas
Superior mesenteric artery; vein
Duodenum, horizontal part
Root of mesentery
Ileocaecal fold
Superior ileocaecal recess
Inferior ileocaecal recess
Meso-appendix
Common iliac artery; vein
Linea terminalis
Sigmoid colon
Recto-uterine pouch*
Vesico-uterine pouch
Urinary bladder, fundus of bladder

Cardiac orifice
Coronary ligament, left triangular ligament
Gastrophrenic ligament
Suprarenal gland; omental bursa
Splenic artery; vein
Gastrosplenic ligament
Superior margin
Gastric impression
} Spleen
Omental bursa, splenic recess
Tail of pancreas
Transverse mesocolon
Inferior mesenteric vein
Duodenum, duodenojejunal flexure
Kidney, lower pole
Superior and inferior duodenal fossa
Inferior duodenal fold
Duodenum, ascending part
Left colic artery; vein
Inferior mesenteric artery
Sigmoid arteries
Superior rectal artery
Intersigmoid recess
Ureter, pelvic part
Sigmoid mesocolon
Ovarian artery; vein; suspensory ligament of ovary
Ampulla
Ovary
Uterine tube
Round ligament of uterus**
Lesser pelvis
Fundus of uterus

Fig. 791 Posterior wall of the peritoneal cavity and spleen of the female.
Sites of attachment of the ascending and descending colon are indicated (◆).

*   Clinical term: pouch of DOUGLAS
** Clinical term: round ligament

Abdominal arteries, overview

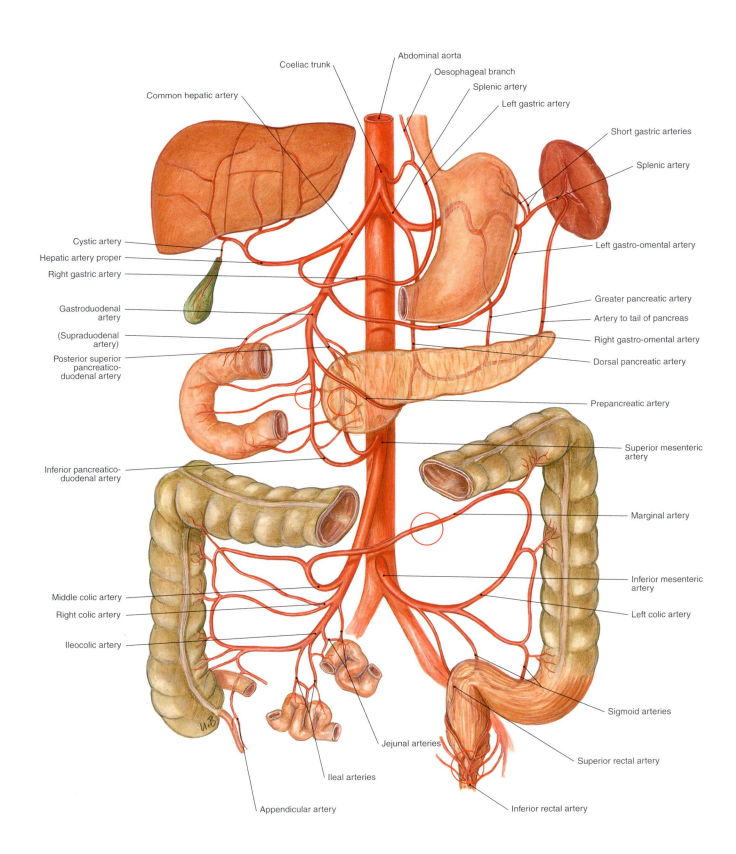

Abdominal aorta
Coeliac trunk
Oesophageal branch
Splenic artery
Left gastric artery
Common hepatic artery
Short gastric arteries
Splenic artery
Cystic artery
Hepatic artery proper
Right gastric artery
Left gastro-omental artery
Gastroduodenal artery
Greater pancreatic artery
Artery to tail of pancreas
(Supraduodenal artery)
Right gastro-omental artery
Posterior superior pancreatico-duodenal artery
Dorsal pancreatic artery
Prepancreatic artery
Inferior pancreatico-duodenal artery
Superior mesenteric artery
Marginal artery
Middle colic artery
Inferior mesenteric artery
Right colic artery
Left colic artery
Ileocolic artery
Sigmoid arteries
Jejunal arteries
Superior rectal artery
Ileal arteries
Appendicular artery
Inferior rectal artery

Fig. 792 Arteries of the abdominal viscera; semi-schematic; possible anastomoses are indicated (O).

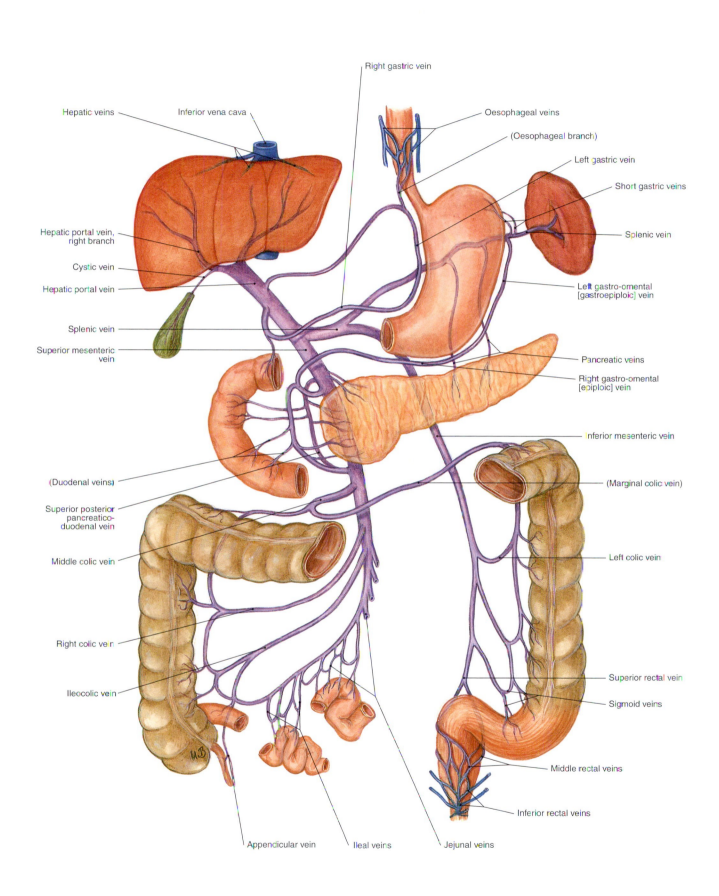

Right gastric vein

Hepatic veins

Inferior vena cava

Oesophageal veins

(Oesophageal branch)

Left gastric vein

Short gastric veins

Hepatic portal vein, right branch

Cystic vein

Hepatic portal vein

Splenic vein

Superior mesenteric vein

Splenic vein

Left gastro-omental [gastroepiploic] vein

Pancreatic veins

Right gastro-omental [epiploic] vein

Inferior mesenteric vein

(Duodenal veins)

(Marginal colic vein)

Superior posterior pancreatico-duodenal vein

Middle colic vein

Left colic vein

Right colic vein

Ileocolic vein

Superior rectal vein

Sigmoid veins

Middle rectal veins

Inferior rectal veins

Appendicular vein

Ileal veins

Jejunal veins

Fig. 793 Hepatic portal vein with tributaries; semi-schematic.

Coeliac trunk

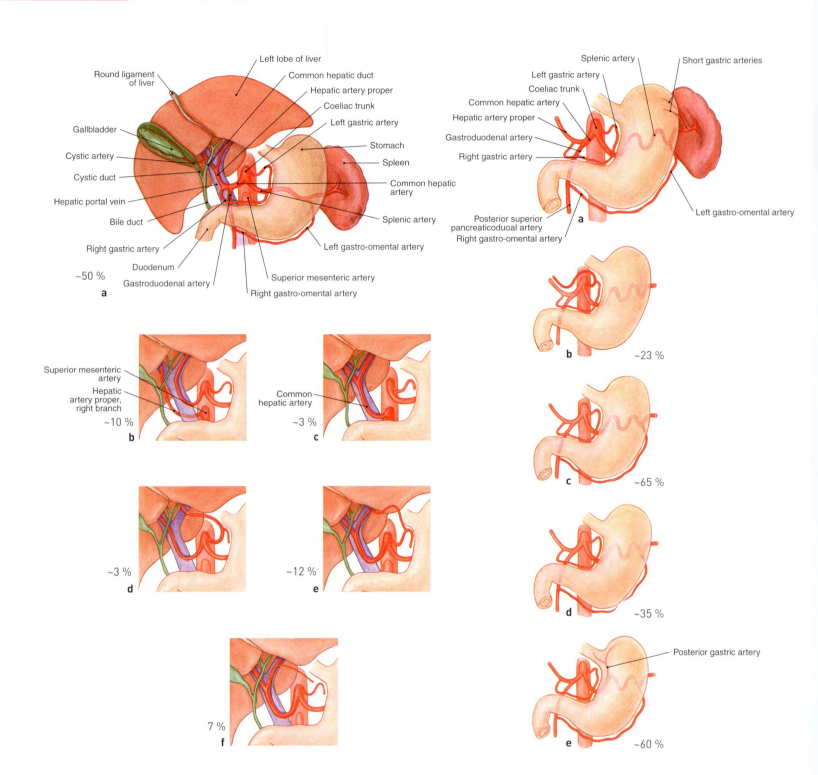

Fig. 794 a–f   Variability of the arterial blood supply of the liver.
a   "Textbook case"
b   The superior mesenteric artery participates in the supply of the right lobe of the liver.
c   The common hepatic artery arises from the superior mesenteric artery.
d   The left lobe of the liver is supplied by the left gastric artery.
e   A branch of the left gastric artery supplies the left lobe of the liver along with the left branch of the hepatic artery proper.
f   An accessory branch of the hepatic artery proper supplies the lesser curvature of the stomach.

Fig. 795 a–e   Variability of the arterial blood supply of the stomach.
a   "Textbook case", closed arterial arcade supplying both the lesser and the greater curvature
b   The left gastric artery participates in the supply of the left lobe of the liver.
c   Anastomosis between the right and left gastro-omental arteries at the greater curvature
d   Absence of an anastomosis between the right and left gastro-omental arteries at the greater curvature
e   An accessory posterior gastric artery arising from the splenic artery supplies the posterior wall of the stomach.

Arteries of the upper abdomen, radiography

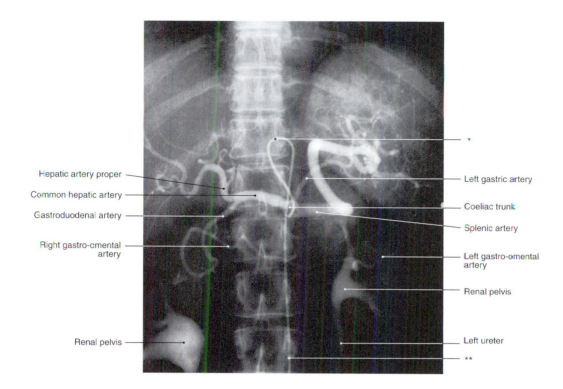

Hepatic artery proper

Common hepatic artery

Gastroduodenal artery

Right gastro-omental artery

Renal pelvis

*

Left gastric artery

Coeliac trunk

Splenic artery

Left gastro-omental artery

Renal pelvis

Left ureter

**

Fig. 796 Arteries of the stomach; the spleen and the liver; AP-radiograph after selective injection of a contrast medium into the coeliac trunk (coeliacography) with concomitant visualization of the renal pelvis due to the renal excretion of the medium; ventral view.

* Catheter loop in the aorta
** Catheter in the aorta

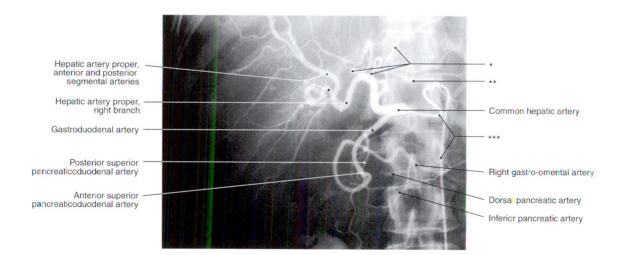

Hepatic artery proper, anterior and posterior segmental arteries

Hepatic artery proper, right branch

Gastroduodenal artery

Posterior superior pancreaticoduodenal artery

Anterior superior pancreaticoduodenal artery

*

**

Common hepatic artery

***

Right gastro-omental artery

Dorsal pancreatic artery

Inferior pancreatic artery

Fig. 797 Common hepatic artery; AP-radiograph after selective injection of a contrast medium into the common hepatic artery; ventral view.

* Branches to the left lobe of the liver replacing a single left branch of the hepatic artery proper
** An accessory branch of the hepatic artery to the lesser curvature of the stomach
*** Catheter in the aorta

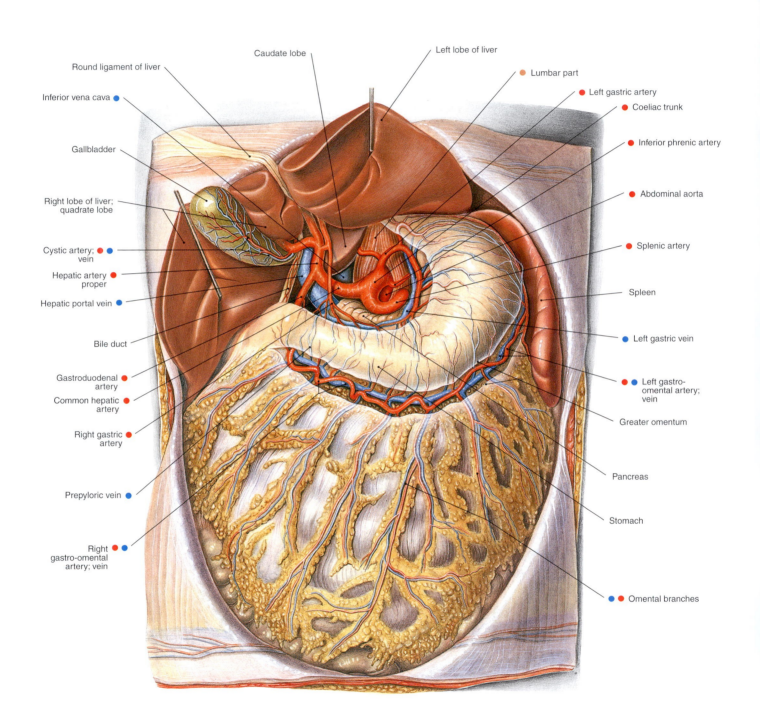

Round ligament of liver

Caudate lobe

Left lobe of liver

● Lumbar part

Inferior vena cava ●

● Left gastric artery

● Coeliac trunk

Gallbladder

● Inferior phrenic artery

Right lobe of liver; quadrate lobe

● Abdominal aorta

Cystic artery; ● ● vein

● Splenic artery

Hepatic artery ● proper

Spleen

Hepatic portal vein ●

Bile duct

● Left gastric vein

Gastroduodenal ● artery

● ● Left gastro-omental artery; vein

Common hepatic ● artery

Greater omentum

Right gastric ● artery

Pancreas

Prepyloric vein ●

Stomach

Right ● ● gastro-omental artery; vein

● ● Omental branches

Fig. 798   Vessels of the upper abdomen.

Vessels of the upper abdomen

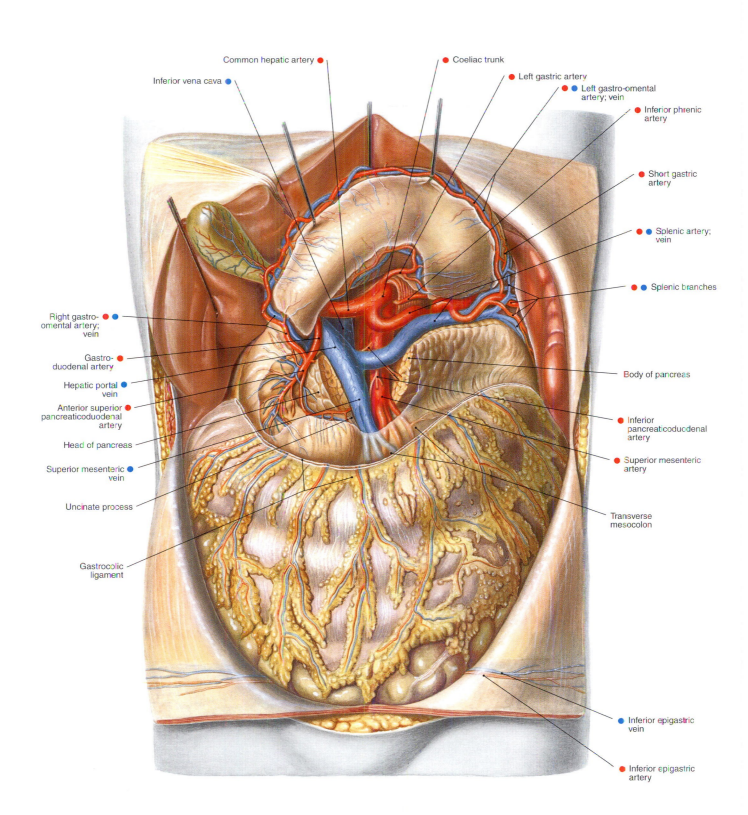

Common hepatic artery ●   ● Coeliac trunk

Inferior vena cava ●

● Left gastric artery

● ● Left gastro-omental artery; vein

● Inferior phrenic artery

● Short gastric artery

● ● Splenic artery; vein

● ● Splenic branches

Right gastro- ● ●
omental artery;
vein

Gastro- ●
duodenal artery

Hepatic portal ●
vein

Anterior superior ●
pancreaticoduodenal
artery

Head of pancreas

Superior mesenteric ●
vein

Uncinate process

Gastrocolic
ligament

Body of pancreas

● Inferior pancreaticoduodenal artery

● Superior mesenteric artery

Transverse mesocolon

● Inferior epigastric vein

● Inferior epigastric artery

Fig. 799 Vessels of the upper abdomen.

Superior mesenteric artery

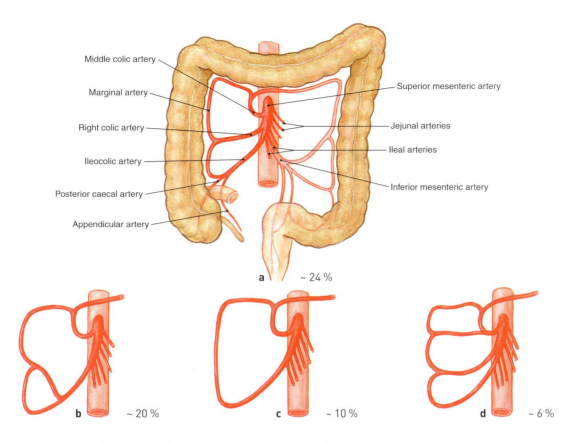

Fig. 800 a–d Variability of the branches of the superior mesenteric artery supplying the large intestine.
a „Textbook case", the ascending and the transverse colon are supplied by three branches.

b The ileocolic artery and the right colic artery form a common trunk.
c Only two branches arise from the mesenteric artery while the right colic artery is absent.
d Duplication of the right colic artery.

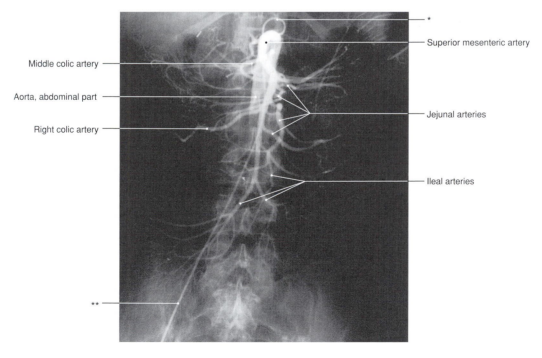

Fig. 801 Superior mesenteric artery;
AP-radiograph after injection of a contrast medium into the origin of the superior mesenteric artery;
ventral view.

* Catheter in the aorta
** Catheter in the common iliac artery

Vessels of the lower abdomen

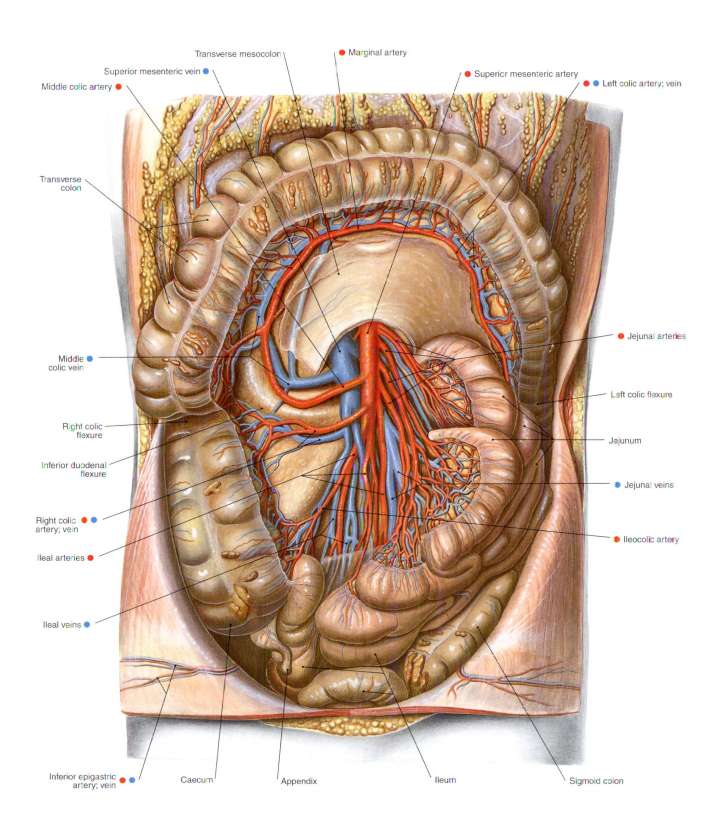

Transverse mesocolon

Superior mesenteric vein ●

Middle colic artery ●

● Marginal artery

● Superior mesenteric artery

● ● Left colic artery; vein

Transverse colon

● Jejunal arteries

Middle colic vein ●

Left colic flexure

Right colic flexure

Jejunum

Inferior duodenal flexure

● Jejunal veins

Right colic artery; vein ● ●

Ileal arteries ●

● Ileocolic artery

Ileal veins ●

Inferior epigastric artery; vein ● ●

Caecum

Appendix

Ileum

Sigmoid colon

Fig. 802 Superior mesenteric artery and vein.
The arteries supplying the small intestine form a series of arcades.

Inferior mesenteric artery

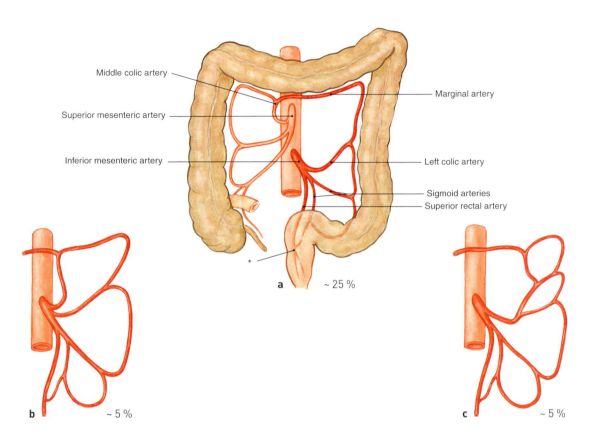

Middle colic artery

Superior mesenteric artery

Inferior mesenteric artery

Marginal artery

Left colic artery

Sigmoid arteries

Superior rectal artery

*

a ~ 25 %

b ~ 5 %

c ~ 5 %

Fig. 803 a–c Variations in the branches of the inferior mesenteric artery.
a The inferior mesenteric artery divides into three parts supplying the descending and sigmoid colon, as well as the rectum.

b An accessory middle colic artery arises from the inferior mesenteric artery.
c An accessory middle colic artery arises from the left colic artery.

* Clinical term: SUDECK's point

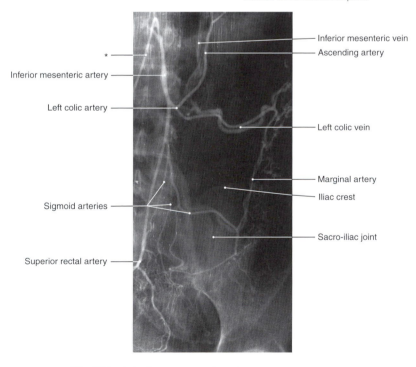

*

Inferior mesenteric artery

Left colic artery

Sigmoid arteries

Superior rectal artery

Inferior mesenteric vein

Ascending artery

Left colic vein

Marginal artery

Iliac crest

Sacro-iliac joint

Fig. 804 Inferior mesenteric artery;
AP-radiograph after selective injection of a contrast medium into the origin of the inferior mesenteric artery;
ventral view.

* Catheter in the aorta

Vessels of the lower abdomen

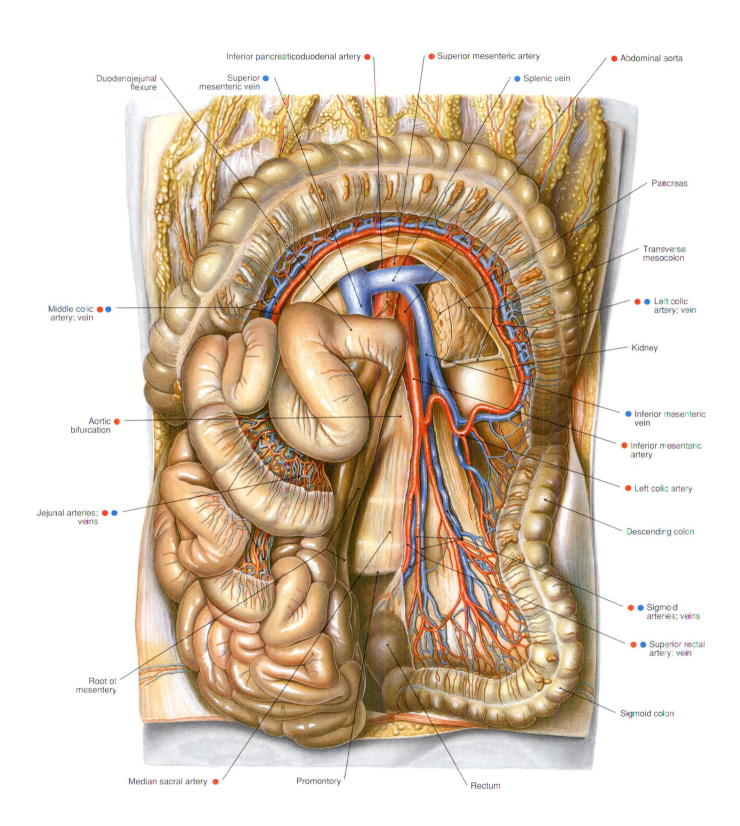

Inferior pancreaticoduodenal artery ●

Superior mesenteric artery ●

Abdominal aorta ●

Duodenojejunal flexure

Superior ● mesenteric vein

Splenic vein ●

Pancreas

Transverse mesocolon

Middle colic ● ● artery; vein

● ● Left colic artery; vein

Kidney

Aortic ● bifurcation

● Inferior mesenteric vein

● Inferior mesenteric artery

Jejunal arteries; ● ● veins

● Left colic artery

Descending colon

Root of mesentery

● ● Sigmoid arteries; veins

● ● Superior rectal artery; vein

Sigmoid colon

Median sacral artery ●

Promontory

Rectum

Fig. 805   Inferior mesenteric artery and vein.

Coeliac trunk

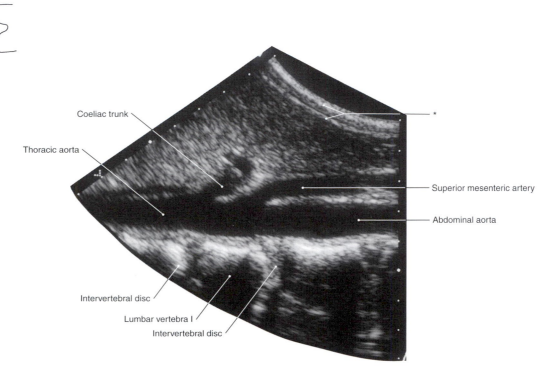

Fig. 806   Abdominal aorta with the coeliac trunk
and the superior mesenteric artery;
ultrasound image; almost in the sagittal plane.

* Abdominal wall

Coeliac trunk

Thoracic aorta

*

Superior mesenteric artery

Abdominal aorta

Intervertebral disc

Lumbar vertebra I

Intervertebral disc

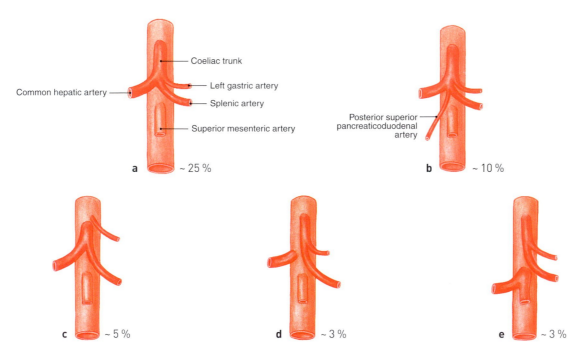

Coeliac trunk

Common hepatic artery

Left gastric artery

Splenic artery

Superior mesenteric artery

a   ~ 25 %

Posterior superior
pancreaticoduodenal
artery

b   ~ 10 %

c   ~ 5 %

d   ~ 3 %

e   ~ 3 %

Fig. 807 a–e   Variability of the coeliac trunk.
a   „Textbook case", division of the trunk into three branches
b   Division of the trunk into four branches
c   Development of a hepatosplenic trunk
d   Development of a gastrosplenic trunk
e   Development of a gastrosplenic trunk
    and a hepatomesenteric trunk

Vessels of the retroperitoneal space

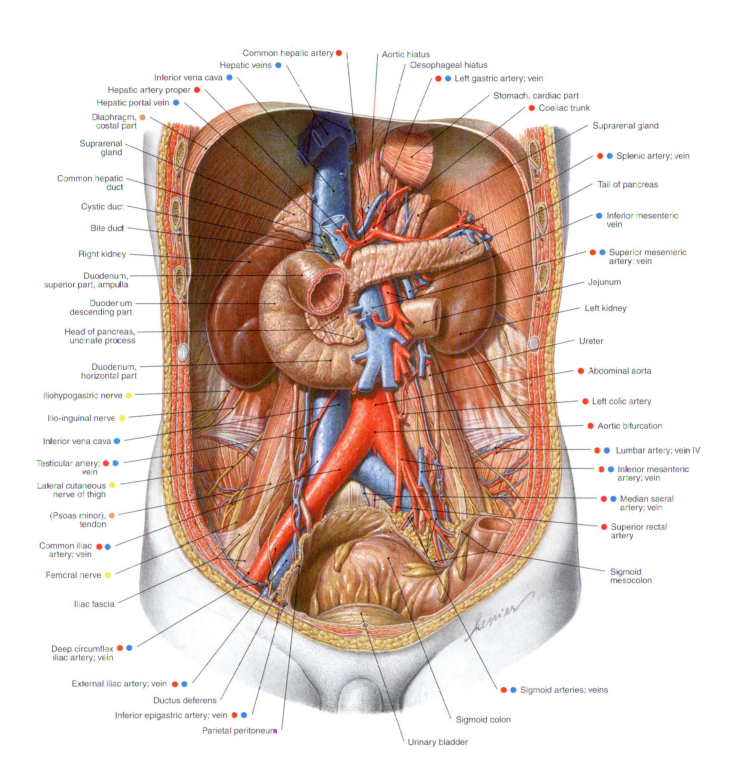

Fig. 808 Vessels of the retroperitoneal space of the male.

Hepatic portal vein, overview

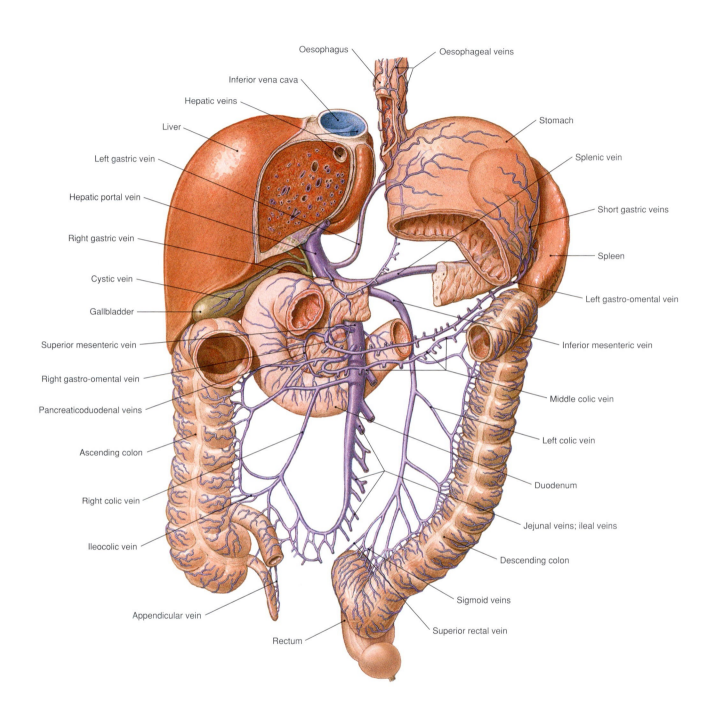

Oesophagus

Oesophageal veins

Inferior vena cava

Hepatic veins

Liver

Stomach

Left gastric vein

Splenic vein

Hepatic portal vein

Right gastric vein

Short gastric veins

Cystic vein

Spleen

Gallbladder

Left gastro-omental vein

Superior mesenteric vein

Inferior mesenteric vein

Right gastro-omental vein

Middle colic vein

Pancreaticoduodenal veins

Left colic vein

Ascending colon

Duodenum

Right colic vein

Jejunal veins; ileal veins

Ileocolic vein

Descending colon

Appendicular vein

Sigmoid veins

Rectum

Superior rectal vein

Fig. 809   Hepatic portal vein;
ventral view.

Portocaval anastomoses

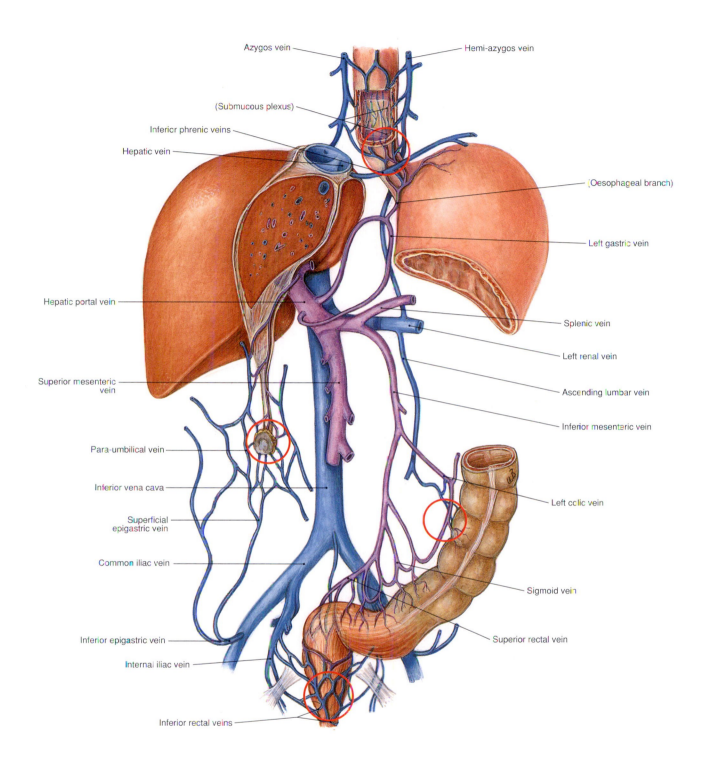

Azygos vein

Hemi-azygos vein

(Submucous plexus)

Inferior phrenic veins

Hepatic vein

(Oesophageal branch)

Left gastric vein

Hepatic portal vein

Splenic vein

Left renal vein

Superior mesenteric vein

Ascending lumbar vein

Inferior mesenteric vein

Para-umbilical vein

Left colic vein

Inferior vena cava

Superficial epigastric vein

Common iliac vein

Sigmoid vein

Inferior epigastric vein

Superior rectal vein

Internal iliac vein

Inferior rectal veins

Fig. 810 Hepatic portal vein and inferior vena cava;
semi-schematic;
tributaries of the inferior vena cava in blue;
tributaries of the hepatic portal vein in purple;
potential portocaval anastomoses are indicated
by circles.

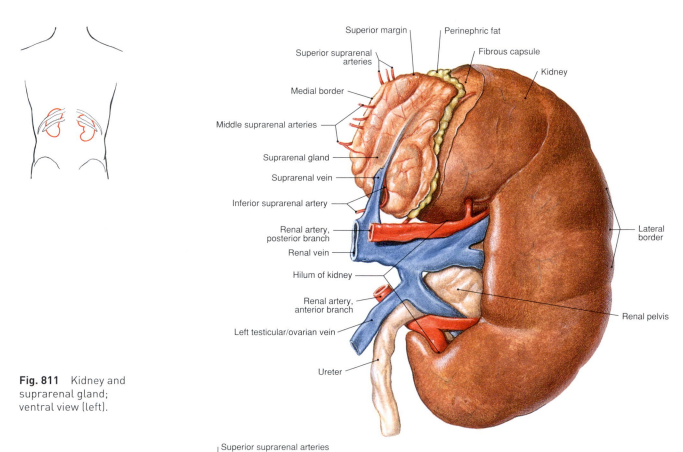

Fig. 811 Kidney and suprarenal gland; ventral view (left).

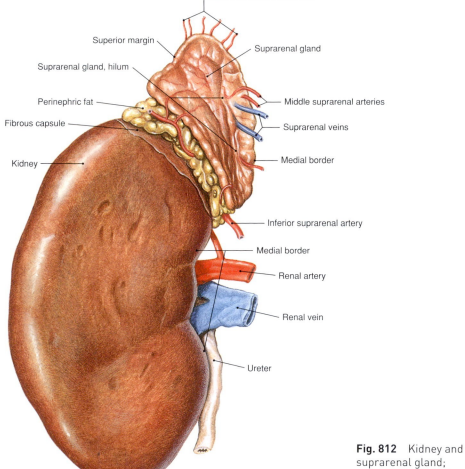

Fig. 812 Kidney and suprarenal gland; ventral view (right).

Kidney

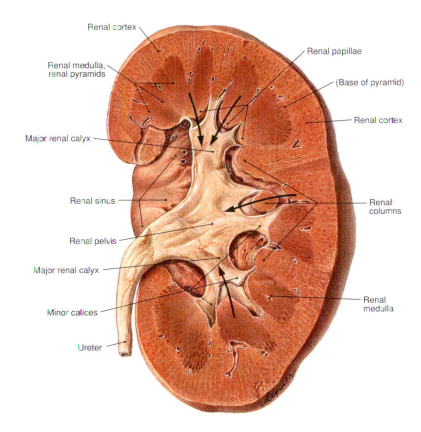

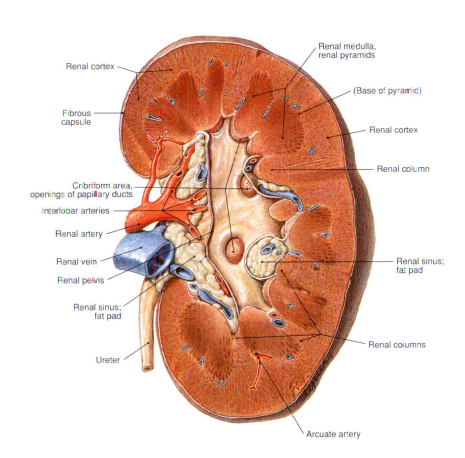

Fig. 813 Kidney;
oblique and vertical hemisection
displaying the renal cortex, the medulla
and the pelvis;
ventral view (left).
Arrows point from the pyramids to the
calyces.

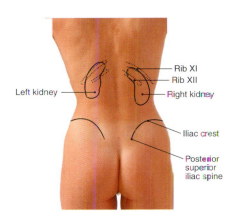

Fig. 814 Projection of the kidneys
onto the back.

Fig. 815 Kidney;
oblique and vertical hemisection;
ventral view (left).

Kidney, structure

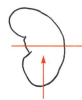

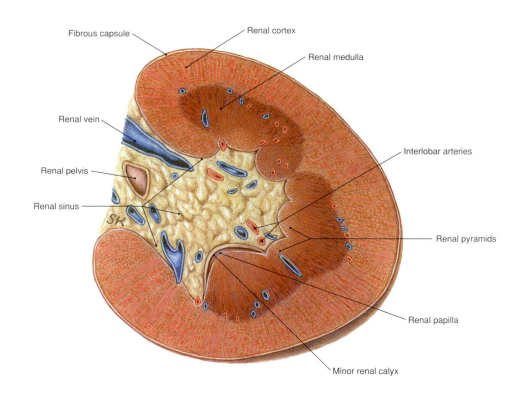

Fibrous capsule

Renal cortex

Renal medulla

Renal vein

Renal pelvis

Renal sinus

Interlobar arteries

Renal pyramids

Renal papilla

Minor renal calyx

Fig. 816   Kidney;
transverse section through the renal sinus;
inferior view (left).

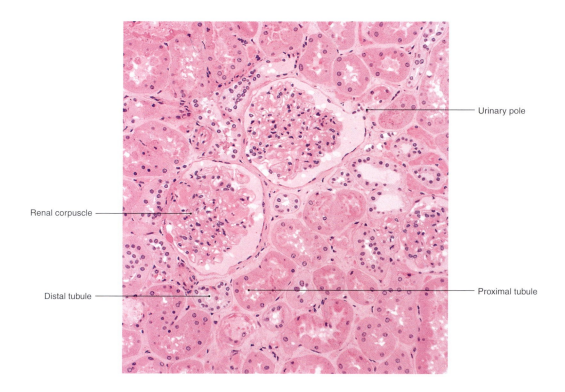

Urinary pole

Renal corpuscle

Distal tubule

Proximal tubule

Fig. 817   Kidney;
microscopic section of the cortex (100 x).

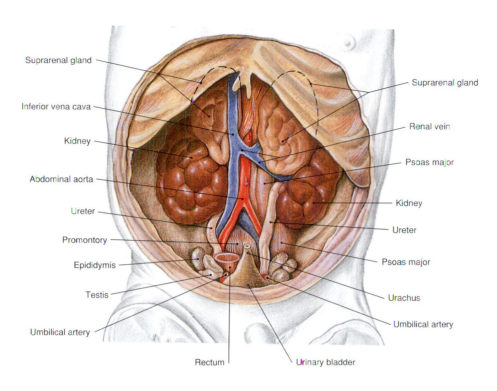

Suprarenal gland

Inferior vena cava

Kidney

Abdominal aorta

Ureter

Promontory

Epididymis

Testis

Umbilical artery

Suprarenal gland

Renal vein

Psoas major

Kidney

Ureter

Psoas major

Urachus

Umbilical artery

Rectum

Urinary bladder

Fig. 818 Kidney and the suprarenal gland
of a ~ 5-month-old foetus.

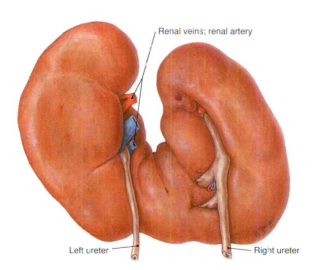

Renal veins; renal artery

Left ureter

Right ureter

Fig. 819 Kidney;
dorsal view.
The lower poles of both kidneys are fused
(= horseshoe kidney).

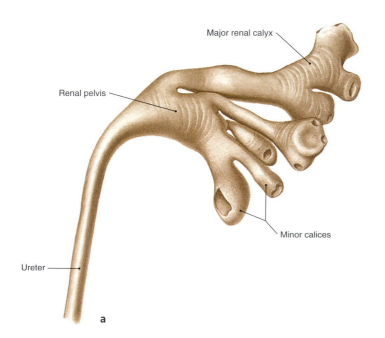

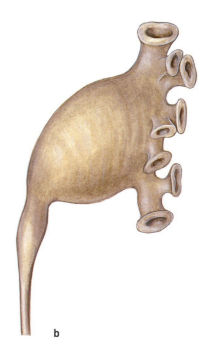

Major renal calyx

Renal pelvis

Minor calices

Ureter

a

b

Fig. 820 a, b Renal pelvis;
corrosion casts;
ventral view (left).
a Dendritic type
b Ampullar type

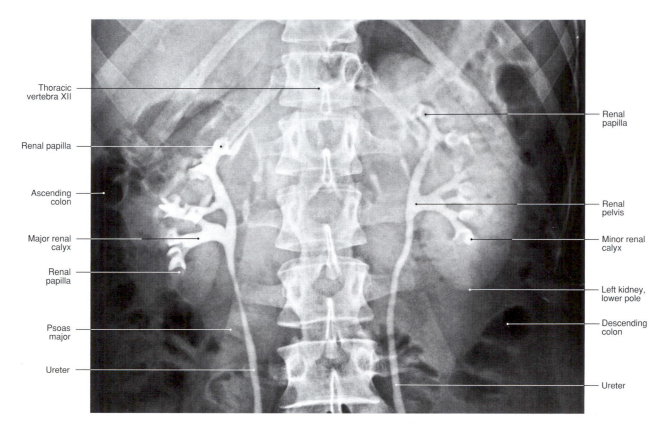

Thoracic
vertebra XII

Renal papilla

Ascending
colon

Major renal
calyx

Renal
papilla

Psoas
major

Ureter

Renal
papilla

Renal
pelvis

Minor renal
calyx

Left kidney,
lower pole

Descending
colon

Ureter

Fig. 821 Kidney;
renal pelvis and ureter;
AP-radiograph after retrograde injection of a
contrast medium via both ureters.

Areas of contact and renal segments

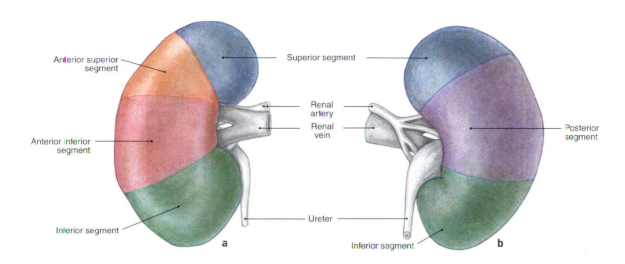

Fig. 822 a, b Renal segments.

a Ventral view (right)
b Dorsal view (right)

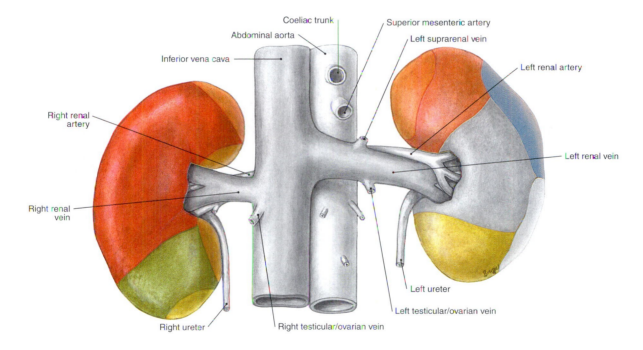

Fig. 823 Kidney;
areas of contact with adjacent organs;
ventral view.

Areas of contact of the Kidneys

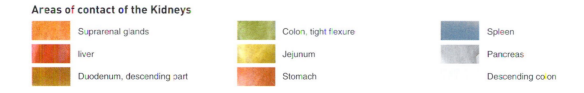

Suprarenal glands

liver

Duodenum, descending part

Colon, tight flexure

Jejunum

Stomach

Spleen

Pancreas

Descending colon

Kidney, imaging

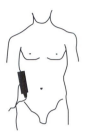

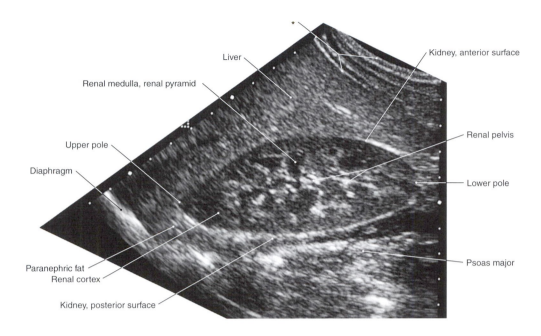

Fig. 824 Kidney;
ultrasound image;
the transducer is directed from ventroinferior to dorsosuperior;
lateral view (right).

* Abdominal wall

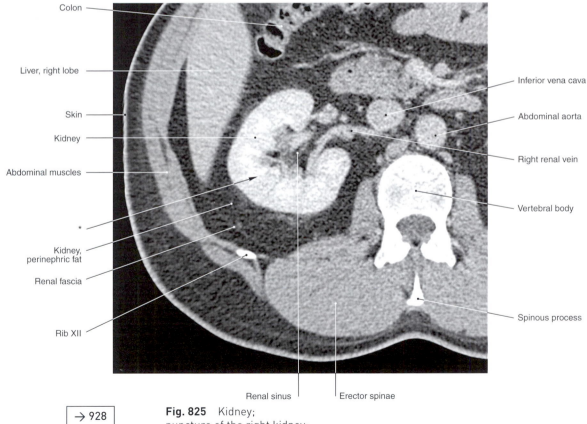

→ 928

Fig. 825 Kidney;
puncture of the right kidney;
computed tomographic cross-section (CT);
inferior view.

* Guidance of a needle for kidney biopsy

Suprarenal gland

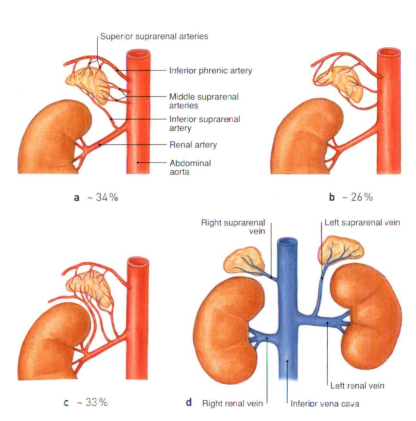

Fig. 827 a–d Variability of the suprarenal arteries and course of the suprarenal veins.
a Arterial supply by three arteries („textbook case")
b Arterial supply without a branch from the renal artery
c Arterial supply without a direct branch from the aorta
d Course of the suprarenal veins

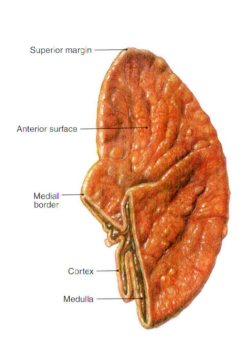

Fig. 826 Suprarenal gland; ventral view (right).

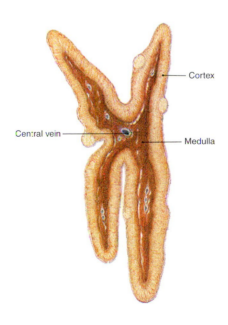

Fig. 828 Suprarenal gland; sagittal section; lateral view (right).

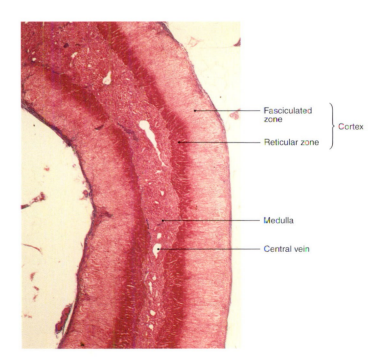

Fig. 829 Suprarenal gland; microscopic enlargement at low magnification.

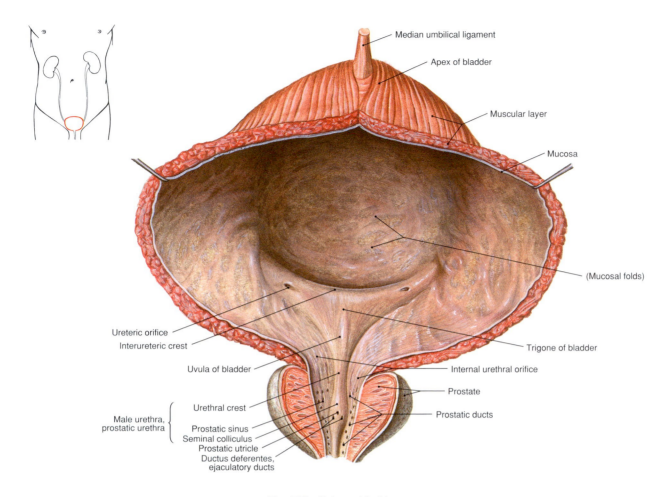

Median umbilical ligament

Apex of bladder

Muscular layer

Mucosa

(Mucosal folds)

Ureteric orifice

Interureteric crest

Uvula of bladder

Trigone of bladder

Internal urethral orifice

Prostate

Prostatic ducts

Male urethra,
prostatic urethra

Urethral crest

Prostatic sinus

Seminal colliculus

Prostatic utricle

Ductus deferentes,
ejaculatory ducts

Fig. 830   Urinary bladder;
prostate and urethra;
ventral view.

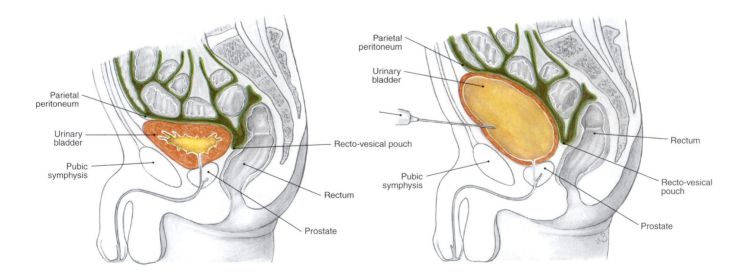

Parietal
peritoneum

Urinary
bladder

Pubic
symphysis

Recto-vesical pouch

Rectum

Prostate

Parietal
peritoneum

Urinary
bladder

Pubic
symphysis

Rectum

Recto-vesical
pouch

Prostate

Fig. 831   Urinary bladder almost
completely voided.

Fig. 832   Urinary bladder filled.
In this situation, the bladder can be punctured from just above
the pubic bone without passing through the peritoneal cavity.

*   Puncture needle

Urinary bladder, ductus deferens and seminal vesicle

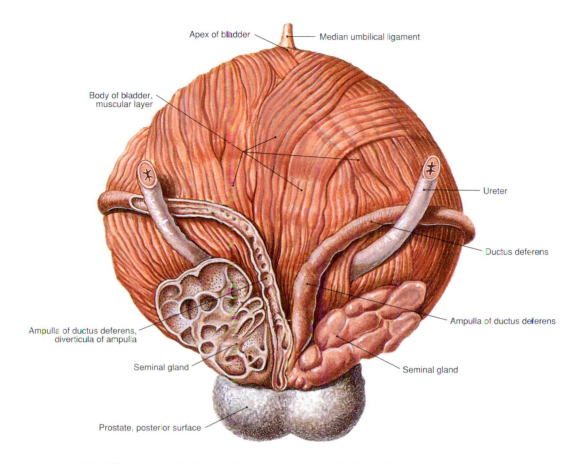

Apex of bladder — Median umbilical ligament

Body of bladder, muscular layer

Ureter

Ductus deferens

Ampulla of ductus deferens

Ampulla of ductus deferens, diverticula of ampulla

Seminal gland

Seminal gland

Prostate, posterior surface

Fig. 833 Urinary bladder, ductus deferentes, seminal vesicles and prostate; dorsal view.

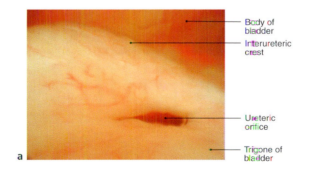

a

Body of bladder

Interureteric crest

Ureteric orifice

Trigone of bladder

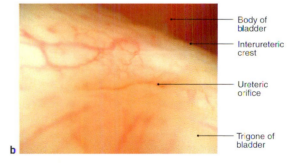

b

Body of bladder

Interureteric crest

Ureteric orifice

Trigone of bladder

Fig. 834 a, b Urinary bladder; endoscopic view of the opening of the ureter (cystoscopy).
a Open ostium of the ureter with a peristaltic wave transporting urine into the bladder
b Closed ostium of the ureter

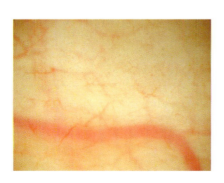

Fig. 835 Urinary bladder; endoscopic view of the mucosa in the body of the bladder (cystoscopy); inferior view.

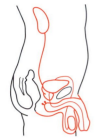

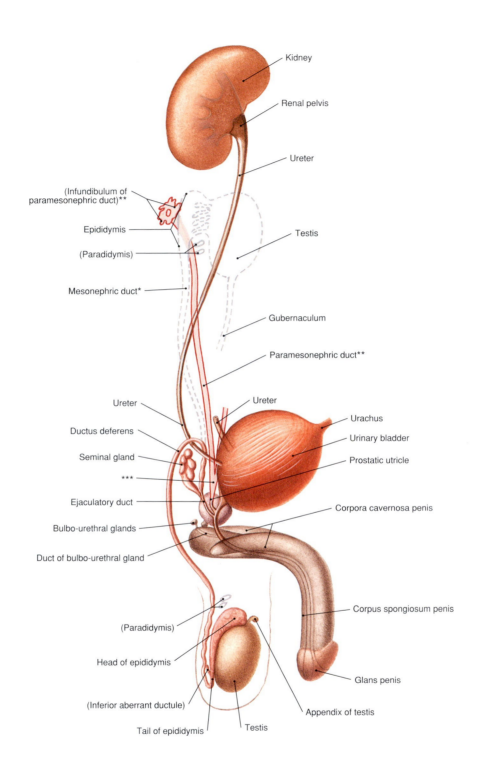

Kidney

Renal pelvis

Ureter

(Infundibulum of paramesonephric duct)**

Epididymis

(Paradidymis)

Testis

Mesonephric duct*

Gubernaculum

Paramesonephric duct**

Ureter

Ureter

Urachus

Ductus deferens

Urinary bladder

Seminal gland

Prostatic utricle

***

Ejaculatory duct

Corpora cavernosa penis

Bulbo-urethral glands

Duct of bulbo-urethral gland

(Paradidymis)

Corpus spongiosum penis

Head of epididymis

(Inferior aberrant ductule)

Glans penis

Appendix of testis

Tail of epididymis

Testis

→ 851

Fig. 836 Male urinary and genital organs; diagram of the development: the parts that degenerate are displayed in pale pink, and the position of the testis prior to its descent is indicated by the dashed line; viewed from the right.

Epididymis = genital part of the mesonephros;
Paradidymis = remnants of tubules of the mesonephros

*   WOLFFian duct
** MÜLLERian duct
*** Junction of the MÜLLERian ducts, paramesonephric duct

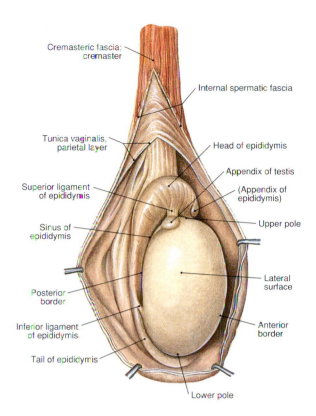

Cremasteric fascia; cremaster
Internal spermatic fascia
Tunica vaginalis, parietal layer
Head of epididymis
Appendix of testis
Superior ligament of epididymis
(Appendix of epididymis)
Sinus of epididymis
Upper pole
Posterior border
Lateral surface
Inferior ligament of epididymis
Anterior border
Tail of epididymis
Lower pole

Fig. 837 Testis and epididymis; viewed from the right.

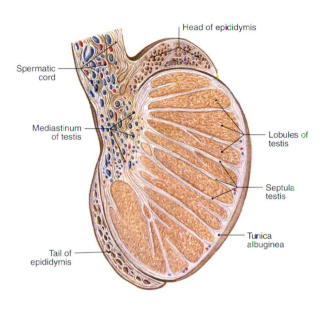

Head of epididymis
Spermatic cord
Mediastinum of testis
Lobules of testis
Septula testis
Tail of epididymis
Tunica albuginea

Fig. 838 Testis and epididymis; viewed from the right.

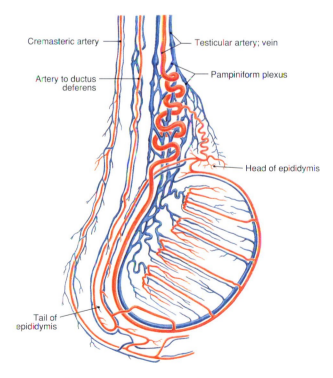

Cremasteric artery
Testicular artery; vein
Artery to ductus deferens
Pampiniform plexus
Head of epididymis
Tail of epididymis

Fig. 839 Blood vessels of the testis, the epididymis and the spermatic cord; viewed from the right.

452

► **Pelvic viscera
and retroperitoneal space**

Testis and epididymis

►► | Kidney | Suprarenal gland | Urinary bladde

►►► **Male genital**

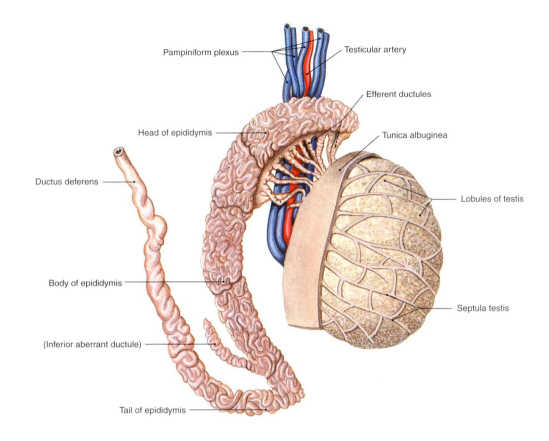

Pampiniform plexus

Testicular artery

Efferent ductules

Head of epididymis

Tunica albuginea

Ductus deferens

Lobules of testis

Body of epididymis

Septula testis

(Inferior aberrant ductule)

Tail of epididymis

Fig. 840 Testis; epididymis
and ductus deferens (vas deferens);
lateral view.

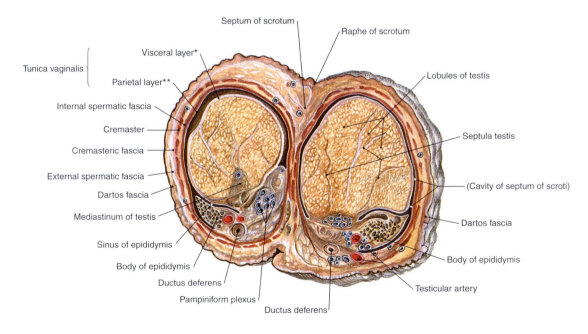

Septum of scrotum

Raphe of scrotum

Visceral layer*

Tunica vaginalis

Parietal layer**

Lobules of testis

Internal spermatic fascia

Cremaster

Cremasteric fascia

Septula testis

External spermatic fascia

Dartos fascia

(Cavity of septum of scroti)

Mediastinum of testis

Sinus of epididymis

Dartos fascia

Body of epididymis

Body of epididymis

Ductus deferens

Pampiniform plexus

Testicular artery

Ductus deferens

Fig. 841 Testis; epididymis and scrotum;
superior view.

* Also: Epiorchium
** Also: Periorchium

Ductus deferens and seminal vesicle

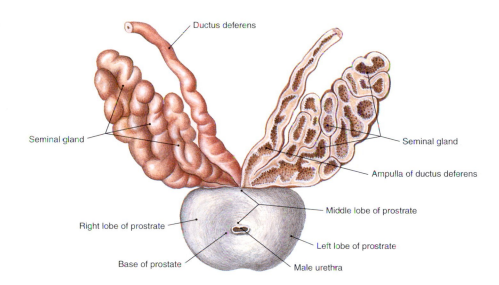

Fig. 842 Ductus deferentes, seminal vesicles and prostate;
superior view.

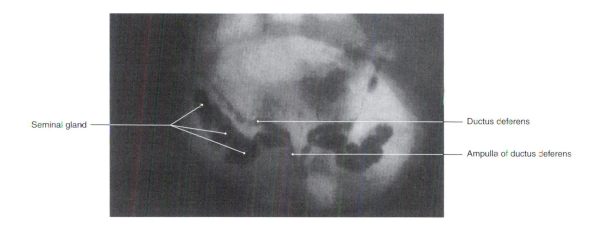

Fig. 843 Ductus deferentes and seminal vesicles;
AP-radiograph after injection of a contrast medium via
the ejaculatory ducts;
ventral view.

Though this technique demonstrates size and position
of the seminal vesicles, it is no more applied under clinical
circumstances.

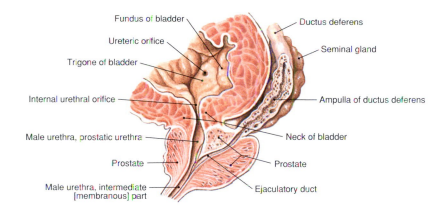

Fig. 844 Urinary bladder; prostate;
ductus deferens (vas deferens) and seminal vesicle;
viewed from the right.

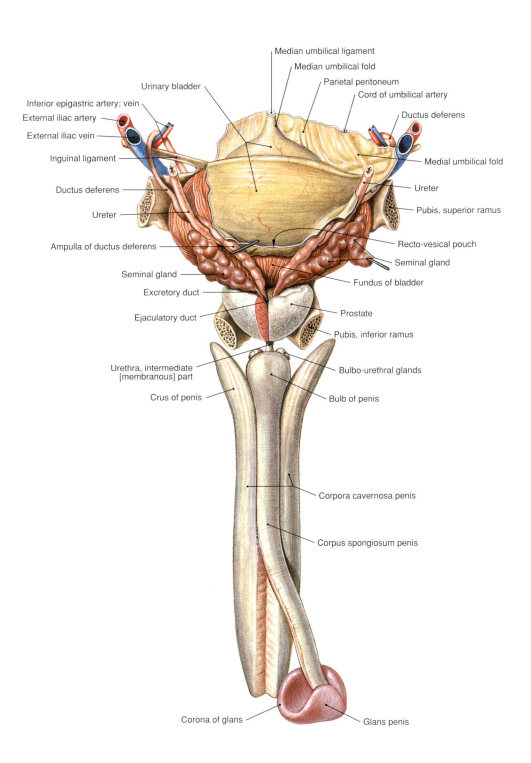

Median umbilical ligament

Median umbilical fold

Urinary bladder

Parietal peritoneum

Cord of umbilical artery

Inferior epigastric artery; vein

Ductus deferens

External iliac artery

External iliac vein

Medial umbilical fold

Inguinal ligament

Ureter

Ductus deferens

Pubis, superior ramus

Ureter

Recto-vesical pouch

Ampulla of ductus deferens

Seminal gland

Seminal gland

Fundus of bladder

Excretory duct

Ejaculatory duct

Prostate

Pubis, inferior ramus

Urethra, intermediate [membranous] part

Bulbo-urethral glands

Crus of penis

Bulb of penis

Corpora cavernosa penis

Corpus spongiosum penis

Corona of glans

Glans penis

Fig. 845 Urinary bladder; ductus deferentes; seminal vesicles; prostate and male urethra; dorsal view.

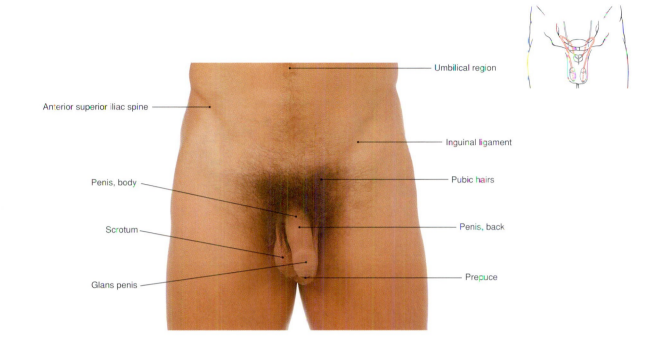

Umbilical region

Anterior superior iliac spine

Inguinal ligament

Penis, body

Pubic hairs

Scrotum

Penis, back

Glans penis

Prepuce

Fig. 846 Male external genitalia.

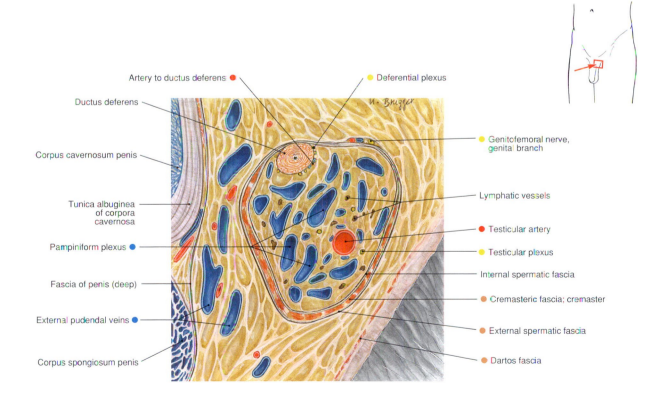

Artery to ductus deferens

Deferential plexus

Ductus deferens

Genitofemoral nerve, genital branch

Corpus cavernosum penis

Tunica albuginea of corpora cavernosa

Lymphatic vessels

Pampiniform plexus

Testicular artery

Testicular plexus

Fascia of penis (deep)

Internal spermatic fascia

Cremasteric fascia; cremaster

External pudendal veins

External spermatic fascia

Corpus spongiosum penis

Dartos fascia

Fig. 847 Spermatic cord;
frontal section;
ventral view (left, 250%).

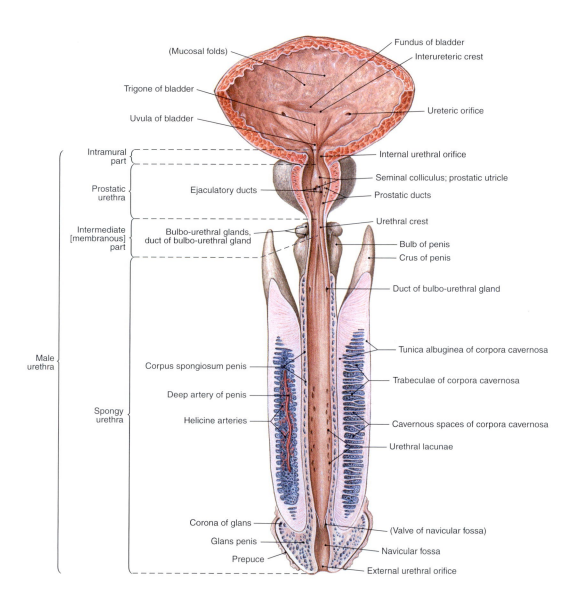

(Mucosal folds)

Fundus of bladder

Interureteric crest

Trigone of bladder

Uvula of bladder

Ureteric orifice

Intramural part

Prostatic urethra

Intermediate [membranous] part

Male urethra

Spongy urethra

Internal urethral orifice

Seminal colliculus; prostatic utricle

Ejaculatory ducts

Prostatic ducts

Urethral crest

Bulbo-urethral glands, duct of bulbo-urethral gland

Bulb of penis

Crus of penis

Duct of bulbo-urethral gland

Corpus spongiosum penis

Deep artery of penis

Helicine arteries

Tunica albuginea of corpora cavernosa

Trabeculae of corpora cavernosa

Cavernous spaces of corpora cavernosa

Urethral lacunae

Corona of glans

Glans penis

Prepuce

(Valve of navicular fossa)

Navicular fossa

External urethral orifice

→ 931

Fig. 848 Urinary bladder; prostate and male urethra; ventral view.

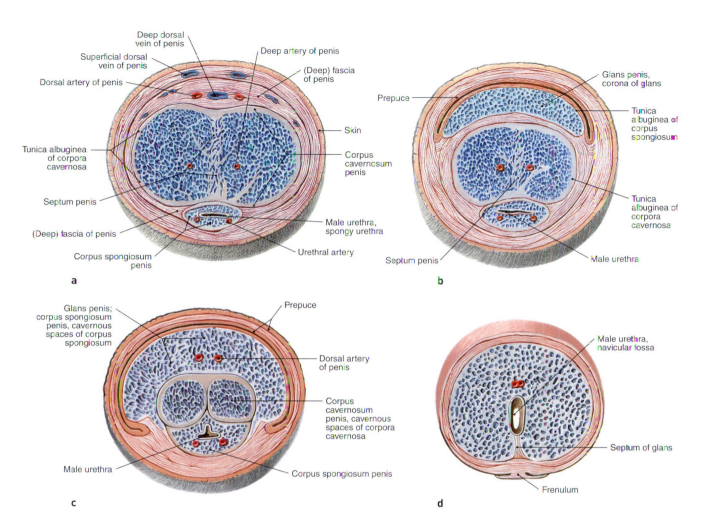

Fig. 849 a–d Penis;
cross-sections; planes indicated in Fig. 850;
ventral view.

a Cross-section through the middle of the shaft
b Cross-section at the level of the proximal part of the glans penis
c Cross-section through the middle of the glans penis
d Cross-section at the level of the distal part of the glans penis

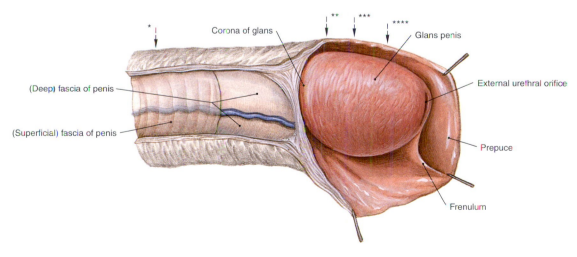

Fig. 850 Penis with glans penis
and prepuce.

*   Level of section of Fig. 849 a
**   Level of section of Fig. 849 b
***   Level of section of Fig. 849 c
**** Level of section of Fig. 849 d

458

► **Pelvic viscera
and retroperitoneal space**

Female urinary and genital organs, overview

►► Kidney | Suprarenal gland | Urinary bladd

►►► Male genita

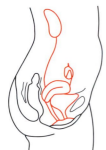

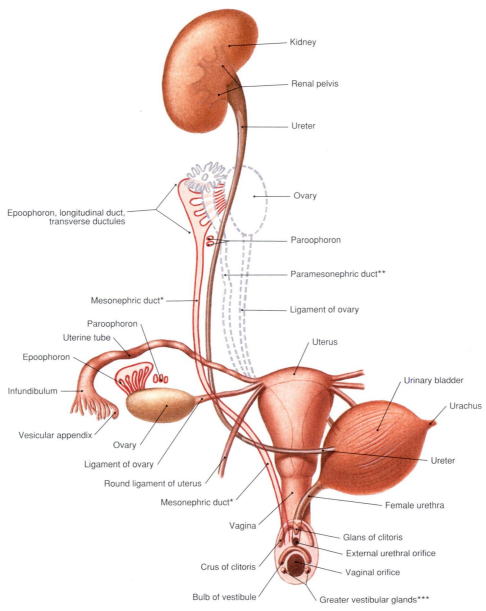

Kidney

Renal pelvis

Ureter

Ovary

Epoophoron, longitudinal duct,
transverse ductules

Paroophoron

Paramesonephric duct**

Mesonephric duct*

Ligament of ovary

Paroophoron

Uterine tube

Uterus

Epoophoron

Urinary bladder

Infundibulum

Urachus

Ureter

Vesicular appendix

Ovary

Female urethra

Ligament of ovary

Round ligament of uterus

Mesonephric duct*

Glans of clitoris

Vagina

External urethral orifice

Crus of clitoris

Vaginal orifice

Bulb of vestibule

Greater vestibular glands***

→ 836

Fig. 851 Female urinary and genital organs;
diagram of the development: the parts that degenerate are
displayed in pale pink, and the retro position of the ovary prior to its
descent is indicated by the dashed line;
ventral view.

Epoophoron = genital part of the mesonephros;
Paroophoron = remnants of the tubules of the mesonephros

*   WOLFFian duct
**   MÜLLERian duct
*** BARTHOLIN's glands

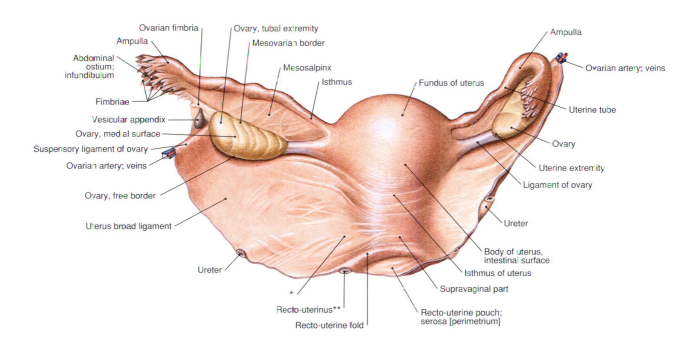

Ovarian fimbria
Ampulla
Abdominal ostium; infundibulum
Fimbriae
Vesicular appendix
Ovary, medial surface
Suspensory ligament of ovary
Ovarian artery; veins
Ovary, free border
Uterus broad ligament
Ureter

Ovary, tubal extremity
Mesovarian border
Mesosalpinx
Isthmus
Fundus of uterus

Ampulla
Ovarian artery; veins
Uterine tube
Ovary
Uterine extremity
Ligament of ovary
Ureter
Body of uterus, intestinal surface
Isthmus of uterus
Supravaginal part
Recto-uterine pouch; serosa [perimetrium]

*
Recto-uterinus**
Recto-uterine fold

Fig. 852 Uterus; ovary and uterine tube; dorsal view.

* Clinical term: cardinal ligament
** Clinical term: sacrouterine ligament

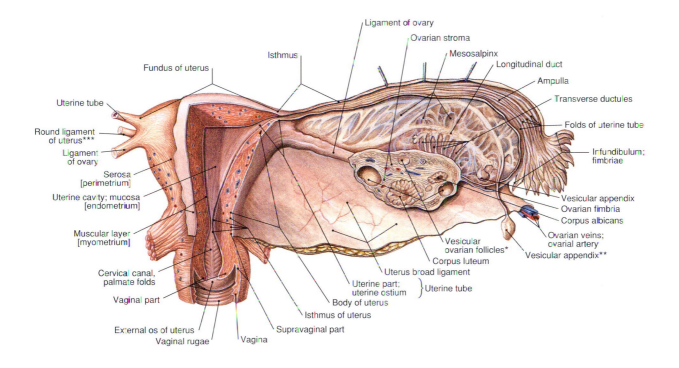

Ligament of ovary
Ovarian stroma
Mesosalpinx
Longitudinal duct
Ampulla
Transverse ductules

Isthmus
Fundus of uterus
Uterine tube
Round ligament of uterus***
Ligament of ovary
Serosa [perimetrium]
Uterine cavity; mucosa [endometrium]
Muscular layer [myometrium]

Folds of uterine tube
Infundibulum; fimbriae
Vesicular appendix
Ovarian fimbria
Corpus albicans
Ovarian veins; ovarial artery
Vesicular appendix**

Cervical canal, palmate folds
Vaginal part
External os of uterus
Vaginal rugae
Vagina

Vesicular ovarian follicles*
Corpus luteum
Uterus broad ligament
Uterine part; uterine ostium } Uterine tube
Body of uterus
Isthmus of uterus
Supravaginal part

Fig. 853 Uterus; ovary and uterine tube; dorsal view.

* Clinical term: GRAAFian follicle
** Stalked hydatid
*** Clinical term: round ligament

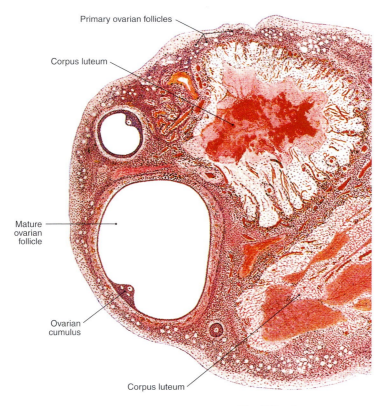
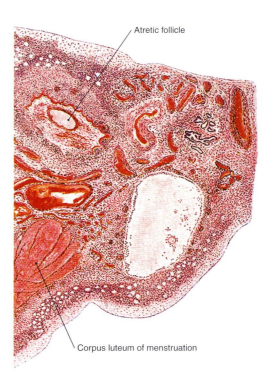

Fig. 854 Ovary;
microscopic enlargement at low magnification.

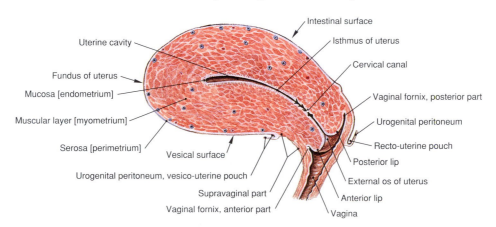

Fig. 855 Uterus and vagina;
viewed from the right.

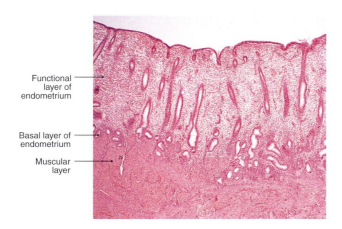

Fig. 856 Mucosa of the uterus;
early phase of proliferation.

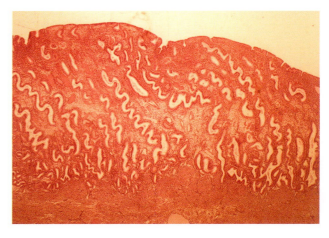

Fig. 857 Mucosa of the uterus;
late phase of proliferation with excretory glands.

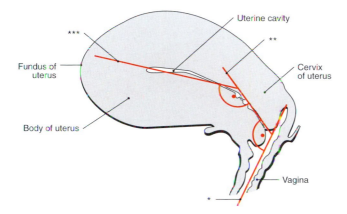

Fig. 858 Uterus and vagina;
normal angles between the vagina, the cervix, and the
body of uterus;
viewed from the right.

*   Longitudinal axis of the vagina
**   Longitudinal axis of the cervix of uterus
*** Longitudinal axis of the body of uterus

Angle between vagina and cervix of uterus = version
Angle between cervix and body of uterus = flexion
Normal topographical situation of the uterus:
anteversion, anteflexion
Relation to the median plane = position

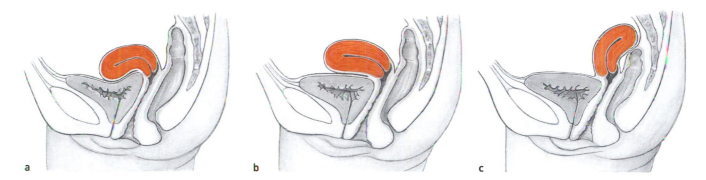

a   b   c

Fig. 859 a–c Uterus and vagina.
a Anteversion, anteflexion = normal position
b Anteversion, but no anteflexion
c Retroversion, retroflexion

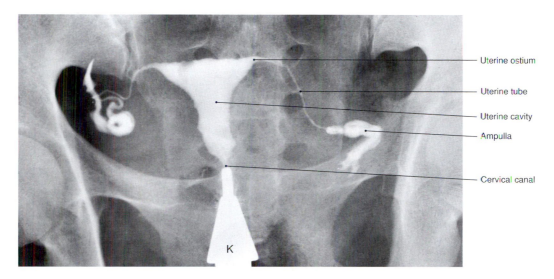

Uterine ostium

Uterine tube

Uterine cavity

Ampulla

Cervical canal

K

Fig. 860 Uterus and uterine tube;
AP-radiograph after injection of to contrast medium into the
cervix of uterus (hysterosalpingography);
uterus in dextroposition;
ventral view.

This formerly clinically applied technique allows to determine
the position of the organs and the patency of the tubes.
K = tube adaptor for injection of the contrast medium

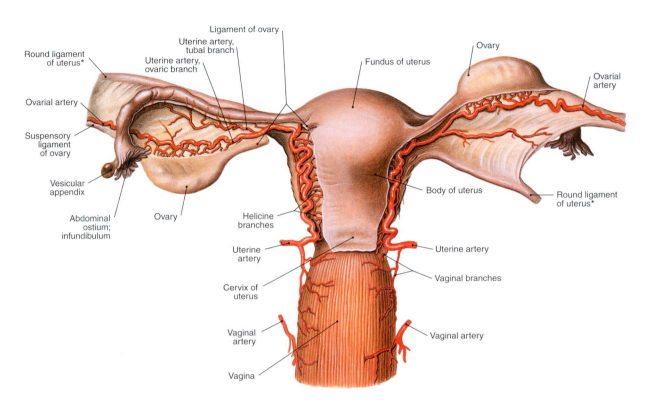

Fig. 861 Arteries of the female internal genitalia; dorsal view.

* Clinical term: round ligament

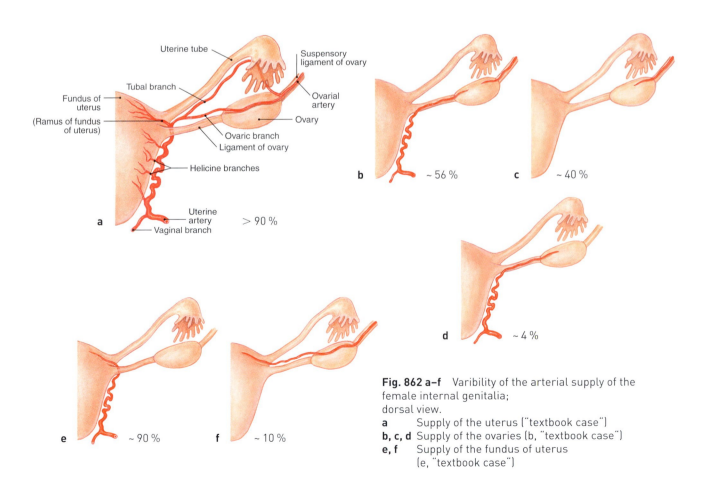

Fig. 862 a–f Varibility of the arterial supply of the female internal genitalia; dorsal view.

a Supply of the uterus ("textbook case")

b, c, d Supply of the ovaries (b, "textbook case")

e, f Supply of the fundus of uterus (e, "textbook case")

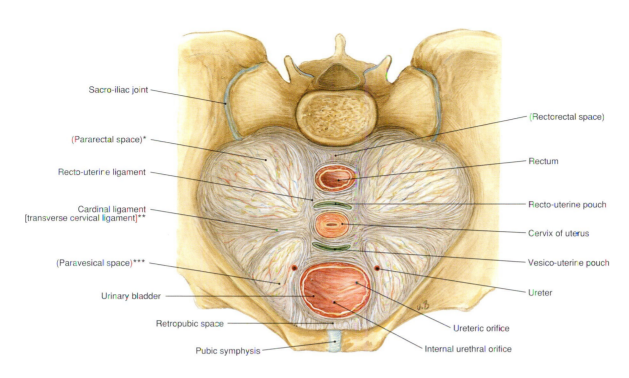

Fig. 863 Uterus;
uterine ligaments and connective tissue spaces;
semi-schematic transverse section at the
level of the cervix of uterus;
superior view.

* Clinical term: Paraproctium
** Clinical term: Parametrium
(existence of this structure is controversial)
*** Clinical term: Paracystium

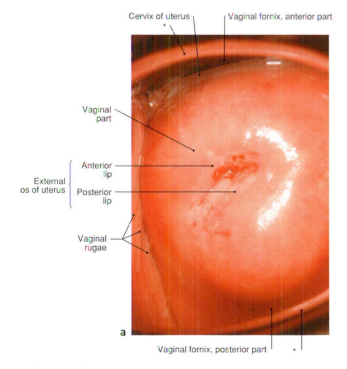

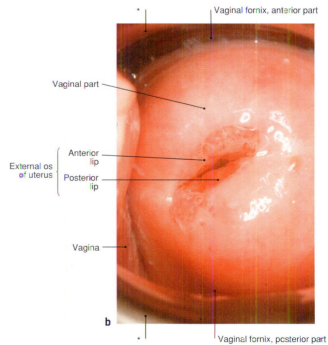

Fig. 864 Vaginal portion of the cervix of uterus.
a Photograph of the cervix of a young nulliparous woman
b Photograph of the cervix of a young woman who has given
birth to two children

For the inspection of the vaginal portion of the cervix the
normally slit-like vagina is spreaded by means of a bivalve
speculum (*);
inferior view.

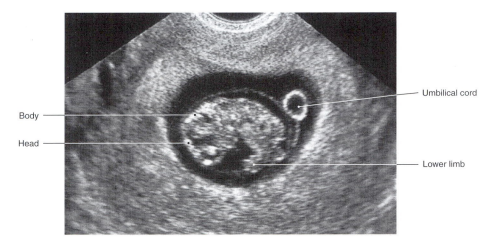

Fig. 865 Uterus with an embryo;
ultrasound image taken in the eighth week of pregnancy;
lateral view (right).

The embryo is immersed in the amniotic fluid of
the chorionic cavity.

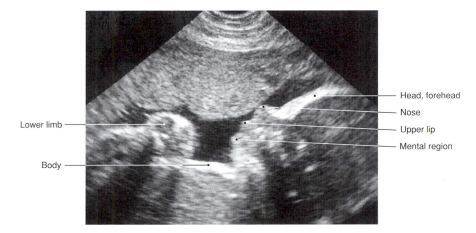

Fig. 866 Uterus with a foetus;
ultrasound image taken in the 28th week of pregnancy;
lateral view (left).

Ultrasound examination allows the visualization of movements
of the extremities and the opening of the mouth.

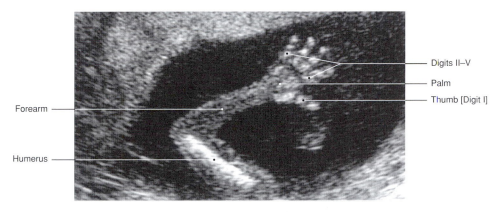

Fig. 867 Hand of a foetus;
ultrasound image taken in the 18th week of pregnancy;
lateral view.

Details such as fingers can be observed.

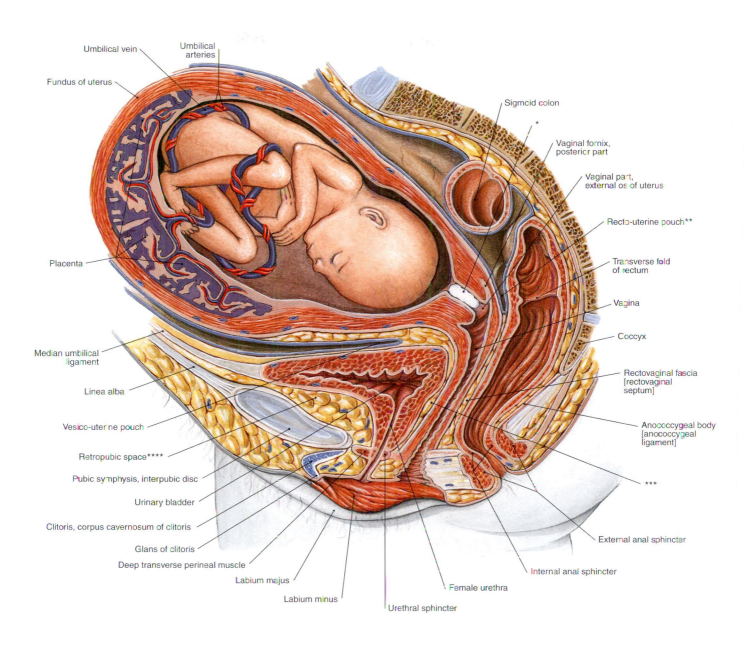

Umbilical vein
Umbilical arteries
Fundus of uterus
Placenta
Median umbilical ligament
Linea alba
Vesico-uterine pouch
Retropubic space****
Pubic symphysis, interpubic disc
Urinary bladder
Clitoris, corpus cavernosum of clitoris
Glans of clitoris
Deep transverse perineal muscle
Labium majus
Labium minus
Urethral sphincter
Female urethra
Internal anal sphincter
External anal sphincter
***
Anococcygeal body [anococcygeal ligament]
Rectovaginal fascia [rectovaginal septum]
Coccyx
Vagina
Transverse fold of rectum
Recto-uterine pouch**
Vaginal part, external os of uterus
Vaginal fornix, posterior part
*
Sigmoid colon

Fig. 868 Uterus with a foetus;
the pelvis has been sectioned in the median plane.

*   Mucous plug (of KRISTELLER) in the cervical canal of the uterus
**   Clinical term: pouch of DOUGLAS
***   Clinical term: vesicovaginal septum
**** Clinical term: cave of RETZIUS

Sternum, xiphoid process
Costal margin
Anterior superior iliac spine

9
8
10
7
10
6
5
4
3

Fig. 869 Uterus;
position of the fundus of uterus during pregnancy.
Numbers refer to the end of the respective
month of pregnancy (= 28 days).

466

► **Pelvic viscera
and retroperitoneal space**

►► Kidney | Suprarenal gland | Urinary bladder

►►► Male genital

Placenta

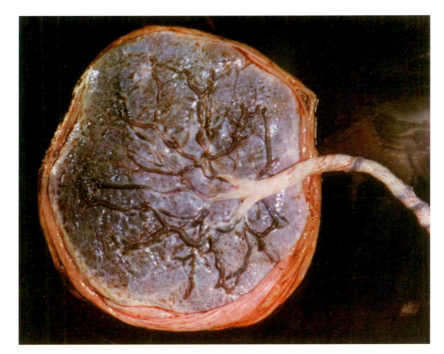

a

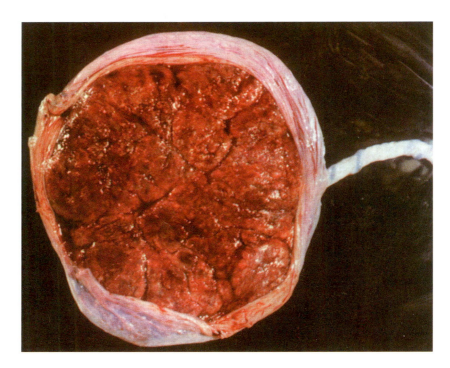

b

Fig. 870 a, b Placenta and umbilical cord.
a View of the foetal surface
b View of the maternal surface of a
parturient placenta

Ovaries and uterine tubes

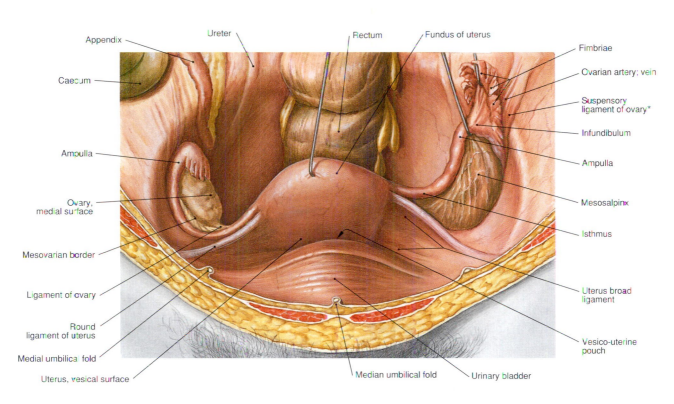

Fig. 871   Female internal genitalia;
ventral view.

*   Clinical term: infundibulopelvic ligament

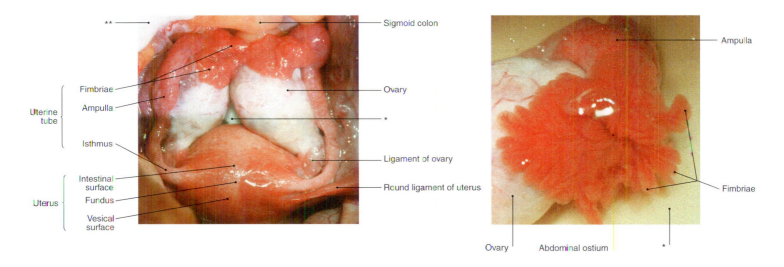

Fig. 872   Female internal genitalia;
surgical exposure in a young woman;
ovaries displaced both medially and superiorly by
compresses (*) in the pouch of DOUGLAS;
ventrosuperior view.

** Swab

Fig. 873   Abdominal ostium of the uterine tube;
surgical exposure in a young woman;
the pelvic cavity is filled with saline to demonstrate
the fimbria;
dorsosuperior view.

*   Plastic tray to support the uterine tube

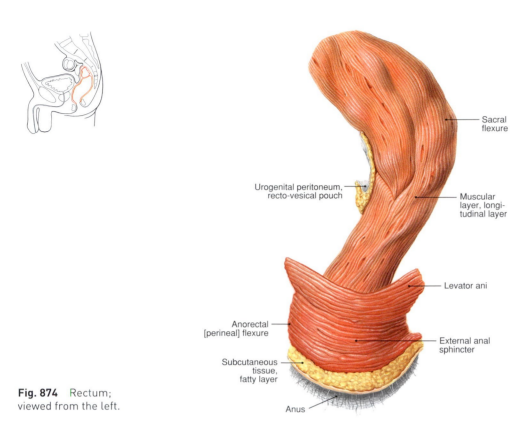

Sacral flexure

Urogenital peritoneum, recto-vesical pouch

Muscular layer, longi-tudinal layer

Levator ani

Anorectal [perineal] flexure

External anal sphincter

Subcutaneous tissue, fatty layer

Anus

Fig. 874 Rectum; viewed from the left.

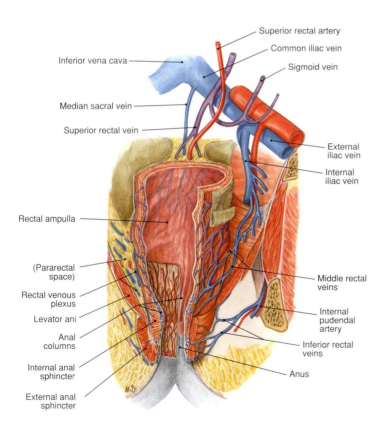

Superior rectal artery

Common iliac vein

Inferior vena cava

Sigmoid vein

Median sacral vein

Superior rectal vein

External iliac vein

Internal iliac vein

Rectal ampulla

(Pararectal space)

Rectal venous plexus

Levator ani

Anal columns

Middle rectal veins

Internal pudendal artery

Inferior rectal veins

Internal anal sphincter

External anal sphincter

Anus

Fig. 875 Rectum; blood supply; the mucosa and the pararectal adipose tissues have been partly removed; openings into the hepatic portal vein in purple.

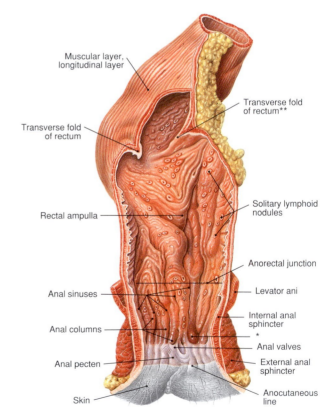

Muscular layer, longitudinal layer

Transverse fold of rectum

Transverse fold of rectum**

Rectal ampulla

Solitary lymphoid nodules

Anorectal junction

Anal sinuses

Levator ani

Anal columns

Internal anal sphincter

*

Anal valves

Anal pecten

External anal sphincter

Skin

Anocutaneous line

Fig. 876 Rectum and anus; ventral view.

* Haemorrhoidal node
** KOHLRAUSCH's fold

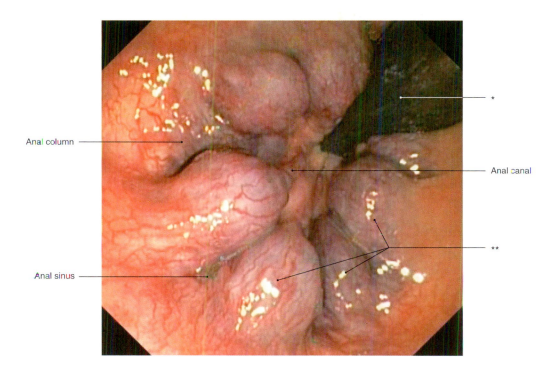

Anal column

Anal canal

Anal sinus

*

**

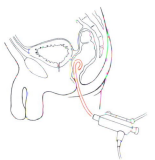

Fig. 877 Rectum;
endoscopic image of the anal canal with six enlarged
nodes of the cavernous rectal body, haemorrhoids;
superior view.

* Colonoscope
** Three haemorrhoidal nodes

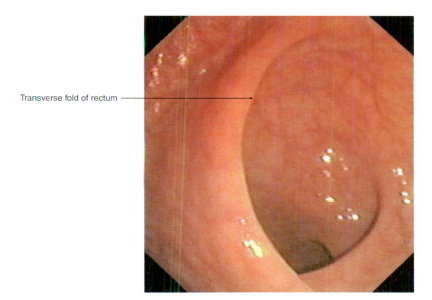

Transverse fold of rectum

Fig. 878 Rectum;
endoscopic image of the rectal ampulla (rectoscopy);
inferior view.

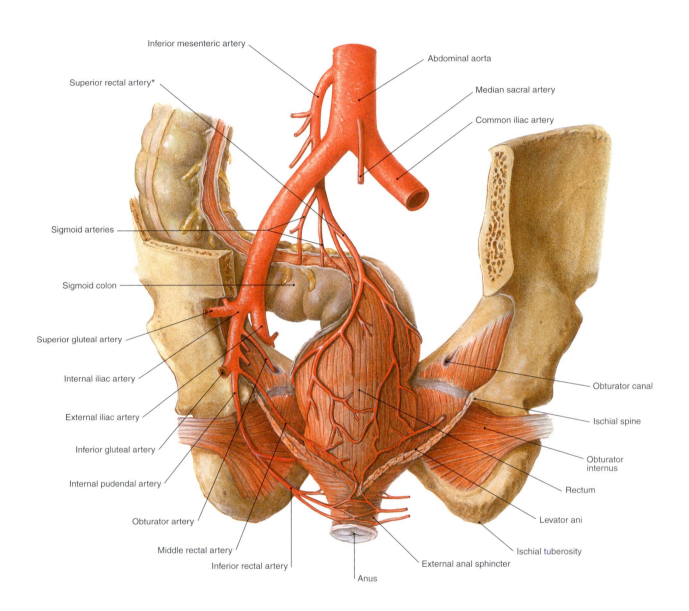

Inferior mesenteric artery

Superior rectal artery*

Sigmoid arteries

Sigmoid colon

Superior gluteal artery

Internal iliac artery

External iliac artery

Inferior gluteal artery

Internal pudendal artery

Obturator artery

Middle rectal artery

Inferior rectal artery

Anus

Abdominal aorta

Median sacral artery

Common iliac artery

Obturator canal

Ischial spine

Obturator internus

Rectum

Levator ani

Ischial tuberosity

External anal sphincter

Fig. 879   Rectal arteries; dorsal view.

*   Clinical term: SUDECK's point (from this point on there are no further anastomoses with the sigmoid arteries)

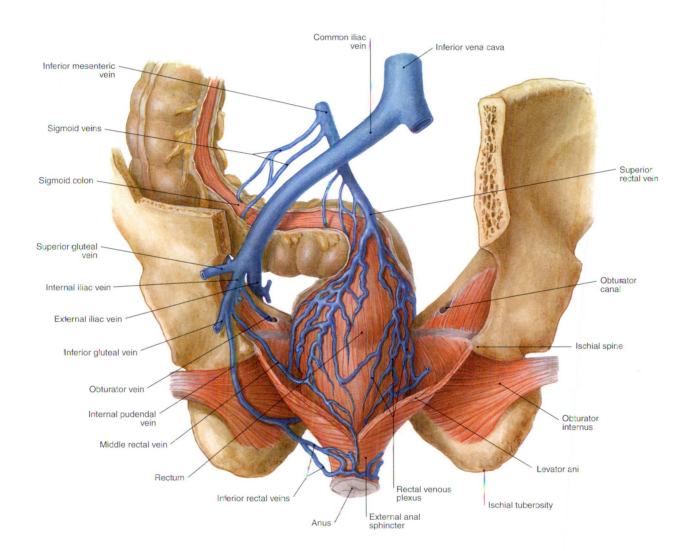

Fig. 880   Rectal veins;
diagram with parts of the pelvis and the pelvic diaphragm;
dorsal view.
There are numerous connections between the veins
draining into the hepatic portal vein (superior
rectal vein) and those draining into the inferior vena
cava (middle and inferior rectal veins). They form
the portocaval anastomoses, which are of particular
clinical importance.

→ 809, 810

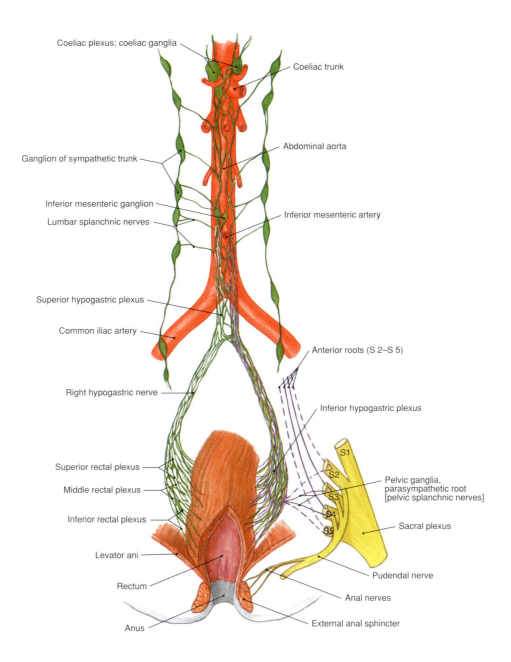

Coeliac plexus; coeliac ganglia

Coeliac trunk

Ganglion of sympathetic trunk

Abdominal aorta

Inferior mesenteric ganglion

Lumbar splanchnic nerves

Inferior mesenteric artery

Superior hypogastric plexus

Common iliac artery

Anterior roots (S 2–S 5)

Right hypogastric nerve

Inferior hypogastric plexus

S1
S2
S3
S4
S5

Superior rectal plexus

Pelvic ganglia, parasympathetic root [pelvic splanchnic nerves]

Middle rectal plexus

Inferior rectal plexus

Sacral plexus

Levator ani

Rectum

Pudendal nerve

Anal nerves

Anus

External anal sphincter

Fig. 881 Rectum;
schematic overview of the innervation;
ventral view.
Green = sympathetic nervous system
Purple = parasympathetic nervous system

Rectum, radiography

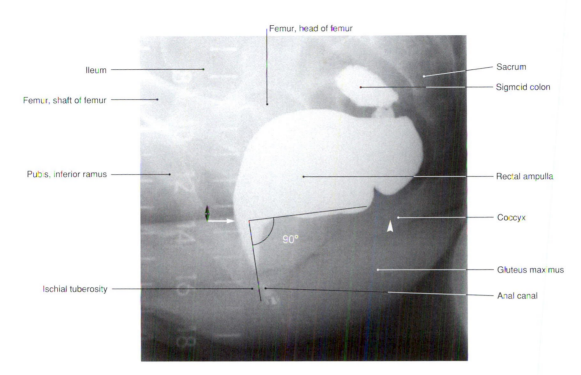

Fig. 882   Rectum;
lateral radiograph in voluntary closure of the anus after filling with a contrast medium (defaecography).

The transitional zone between the anus and the rectum (arrow) is located at the level of the tip of the coccyx (triangle). The angle between the axes of the anus and the rectum (∡) is approximately 90° and depends upon the curvature of the levator ani muscle (puborectal muscle). Scale in cm.

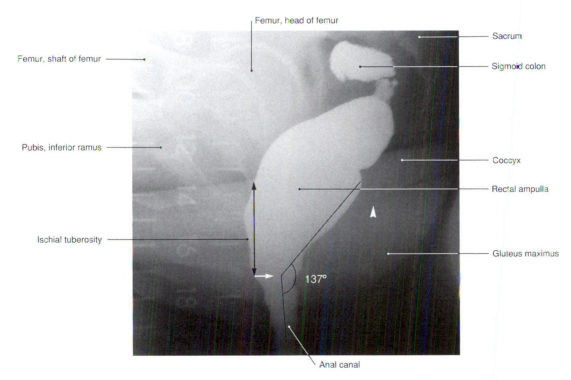

Fig. 883   Rectum;
lateral radiograph of the defaecation after filling with a contrast medium (defaecography).

In comparison to Fig. 882, the anorectal transitional zone has descended and the angle (∡) increased to 137° due to the relaxation of the curvature of the levator ani muscle. As the bending acts like a valve, the elongation results in an unimpeded pressure of the faeces on the anal canal leading to defaecation.

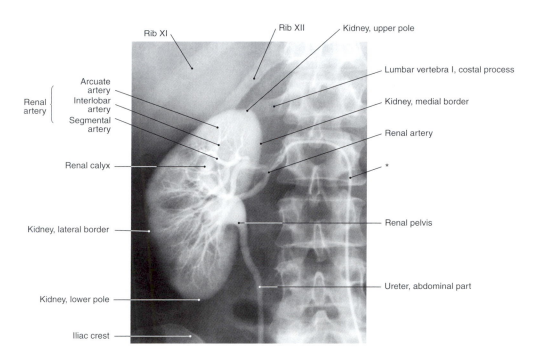

Rib XI · Rib XII · Kidney, upper pole

Arcuate artery
Renal artery {
Interlobar artery
Segmental artery

Lumbar vertebra I, costal process

Kidney, medial border

Renal artery

Renal calyx

*

Kidney, lateral border

Renal pelvis

Kidney, lower pole

Ureter, abdominal part

Iliac crest

Fig. 884 Kidney;
AP-radiograph after intravenous injection of a contrast medium which is excreted via the kidneys to demonstrate the renal pelvis and the ureters (intravenous pyelography); concomitant visualization of the arteries by injection of a contrast medium into the renal artery through a catheter* introduced into the aorta (arteriography).

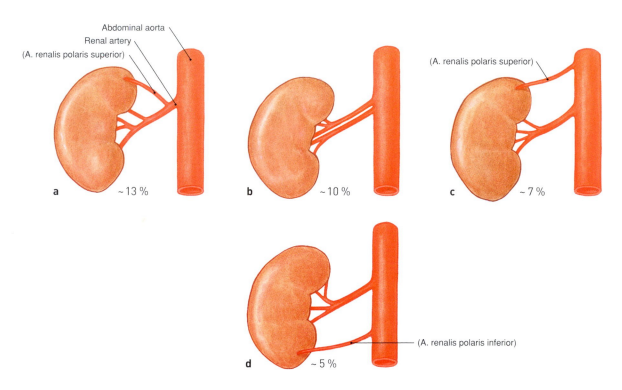

Abdominal aorta
Renal artery
(A. renalis polaris superior)

(A. renalis polaris superior)

a ~ 13 %   **b** ~ 10 %   **c** ~ 7 %

d ~ 5 %   (A. renalis polaris inferior)

Fig. 885 a–d Variations in the arterial supply of the kidney.
a One renal artery with a branch to the superior pole
b Two renal arteries to the renal hilum
c Two renal arteries, one of which supplies the superior pole
d Two renal arteries, one of which supplies the inferior pole

Retroperitoneal space, overview

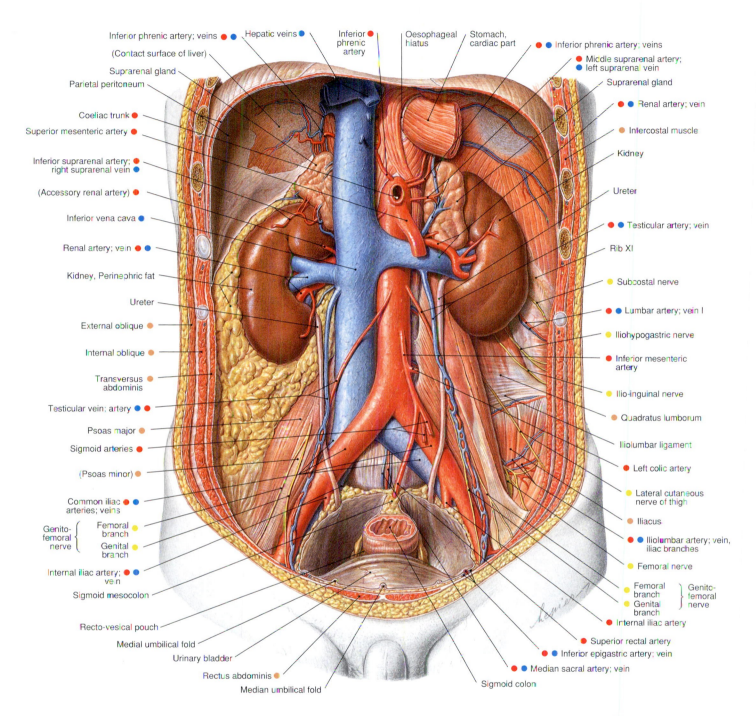

Inferior phrenic artery; veins ● ●
Hepatic veins ●
Inferior phrenic artery ●
Oesophageal hiatus
Stomach, cardiac part
● ● Inferior phrenic artery; veins

(Contact surface of liver)
● Middle suprarenal artery;
● left suprarenal vein

Suprarenal gland
Parietal peritoneum
Suprarenal gland

Coeliac trunk ●
● ● Renal artery; vein

Superior mesenteric artery ●
● Intercostal muscle

Inferior suprarenal artery;
right suprarenal vein ●
Kidney

(Accessory renal artery) ●
Ureter

Inferior vena cava ●
● ● Testicular artery; vein

Renal artery; vein ● ●
Rib XI

Kidney, Perinephric fat
● Subcostal nerve

Ureter
● ● Lumbar artery; vein I

External oblique ●
● Iliohypogastric nerve

Internal oblique ●
● Inferior mesenteric artery

Transversus abdominis ●
● Ilio-inguinal nerve

Testicular vein; artery ● ●
● Quadratus lumborum

Psoas major ●
Iliolumbar ligament

Sigmoid arteries ●
● Left colic artery

(Psoas minor) ●
● Lateral cutaneous nerve of thigh

Common iliac ● ●
arteries; veins
● Iliacus

Genito-femoral nerve {
Femoral branch ●
Genital branch ●
● ● Iliolumbar artery; vein, iliac branches

Internal iliac artery; ● ●
vein
● Femoral nerve

Sigmoid mesocolon
Femoral branch ●
Genital branch ●
} Genito-femoral nerve

Recto-vesical pouch
● Internal iliac artery

Medial umbilical fold
● Superior rectal artery

Urinary bladder
● ● Inferior epigastric artery; vein

Rectus abdominis ●
● ● Median sacral artery; vein

Median umbilical fold
Sigmoid colon

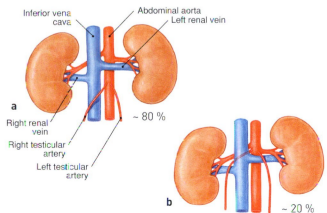

Inferior vena cava
Abdominal aorta
Left renal vein

a
~ 80 %

Right renal vein
Right testicular artery
Left testicular artery

b
~ 20 %

Fig. 886 Position of the retroperitoneal structures of the male.
Whereas the left testicular vein opens into the left renal vein, the right testicular vein drains directly into the inferior vena cava. The same applies to the ovarian veins.

Fig. 887 a, b Variability of the course of the testicular arteries.
a "Textbook case"
b Both testicular arteries branch off cranially to the renal veins; the right artery passes posterior to the inferior vena cava and the left artery passes anterior to the left renal vein.

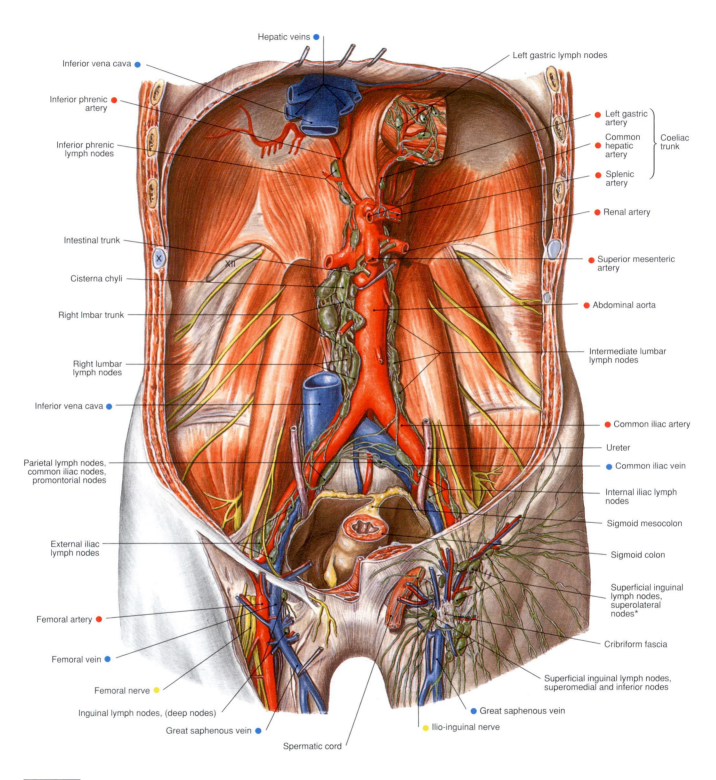

Hepatic veins ●

Inferior vena cava ●

Inferior phrenic artery ●

Inferior phrenic lymph nodes

Intestinal trunk

Cisterna chyli

Right lmbar trunk

Right lumbar lymph nodes

Inferior vena cava ●

Parietal lymph nodes, common iliac nodes, promontorial nodes

External iliac lymph nodes

Femoral artery ●

Femoral vein ●

Femoral nerve ●

Inguinal lymph nodes, (deep nodes)

Great saphenous vein ●

Spermatic cord

Left gastric lymph nodes

● Left gastric artery
● Common hepatic artery } Coeliac trunk
● Splenic artery

● Renal artery

● Superior mesenteric artery

● Abdominal aorta

Intermediate lumbar lymph nodes

● Common iliac artery

Ureter

● Common iliac vein

Internal iliac lymph nodes

Sigmoid mesocolon

Sigmoid colon

Superficial inguinal lymph nodes, superolateral nodes*

Cribriform fascia

Superficial inguinal lymph nodes, superomedial and inferior nodes

● Great saphenous vein

● Ilio-inguinal nerve

→ 1121

Fig. 888 Lymph nodes and lymphatics of the posterior abdominal wall and the inguinal region; ventral view.

The numbers X and XII indicate the respective ribs.

* Clinical term: „horizontal chain", draining the lower abdominal wall, the gluteal region, the perineum and the external genital

Lymphatics of the retroperitoneal space, radiography

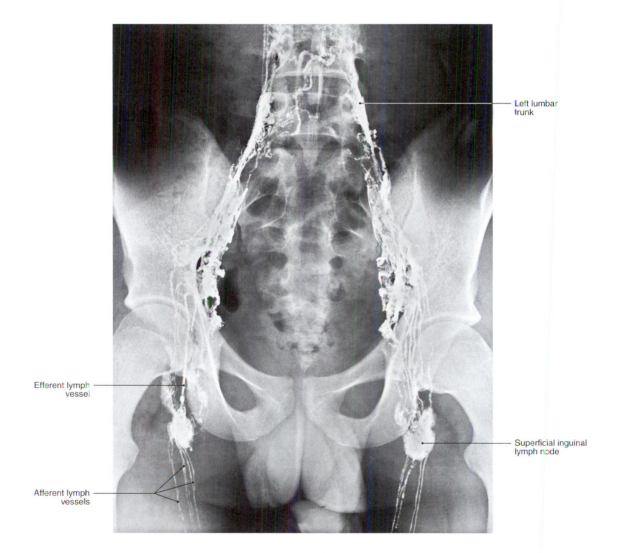

Left lumbar trunk

Efferent lymph vessel

Superficial inguinal lymph node

Afferent lymph vessels

Fig. 889 Lymphatics and lymph nodes of the inguinal, the pelvic and the lumbar region;
AP-radiograph after bilateral injection of a contrast medium into lymphatics of the foot (lymphography).
This formerly applied technique visualizes the position and size of lymphatics and lymph nodes.

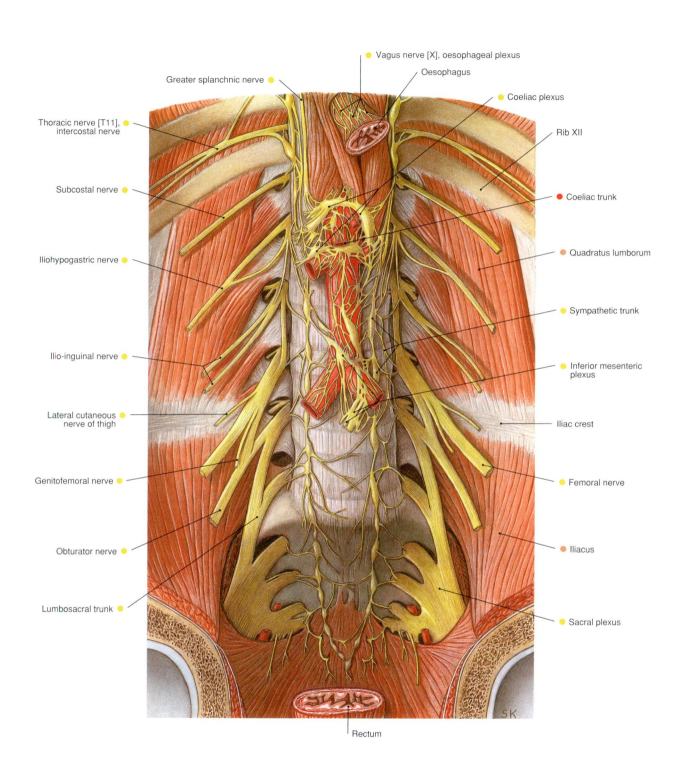

Vagus nerve [X], oesophageal plexus

Greater splanchnic nerve

Oesophagus

Coeliac plexus

Thoracic nerve [T11], intercostal nerve

Rib XII

Subcostal nerve

Coeliac trunk

Quadratus lumborum

Iliohypogastric nerve

Sympathetic trunk

Ilio-inguinal nerve

Inferior mesenteric plexus

Iliac crest

Lateral cutaneous nerve of thigh

Femoral nerve

Genitofemoral nerve

Iliacus

Obturator nerve

Lumbosacral trunk

Sacral plexus

Rectum

→ 47, 49, 50

Fig. 890 Nerves of the posterior abdominal wall, the lumbosacral plexus and the abdominal part of the autonomous nervous system; ventral view.

Vessels and nerves of the retroperitoneal space

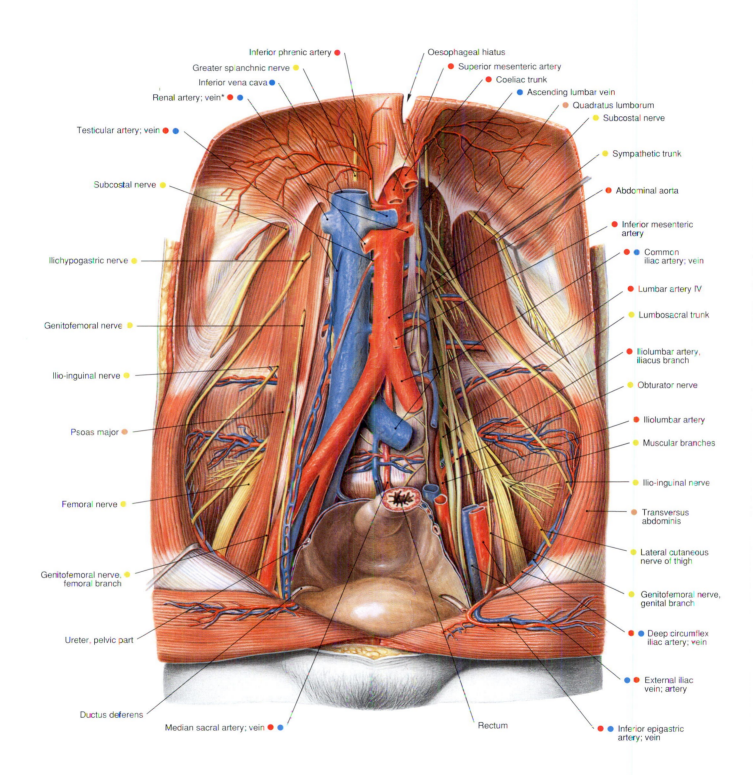

Inferior phrenic artery ●
Greater splanchnic nerve ●
Inferior vena cava ●
Renal artery; vein* ● ●
Testicular artery; vein ● ●
Subcostal nerve ●
Ilichypogastric nerve ●
Genitofemoral nerve ●
Ilio-inguinal nerve ●
Psoas major ●
Femoral nerve ●
Genitofemoral nerve, femoral branch ●
Ureter, pelvic part
Ductus deferens
Median sacral artery; vein ● ●

Oesophageal hiatus
Superior mesenteric artery ●
Coeliac trunk ●
Ascending lumbar vein ●
Quadratus lumborum ●
Subcostal nerve ●
Sympathetic trunk ●
Abdominal aorta ●
Inferior mesenteric artery ●
● ● Common iliac artery; vein
Lumbar artery IV ●
Lumbosacral trunk ●
Iliolumbar artery, iliacus branch ●
Obturator nerve ●
Iliolumbar artery ●
Muscular branches ●
Ilio-inguinal nerve ●
Transversus abdominis ●
Lateral cutaneous nerve of thigh ●
Genitofemoral nerve, genital branch ●
● ● Deep circumflex iliac artery; vein
● ● External iliac vein; artery
Rectum
● ● Inferior epigastric artery; vein

Fig. 891 Vessels and nerves of the posterior abdominal wall of the male.

* In ~10% the left renal vein passes posterior to the aorta.

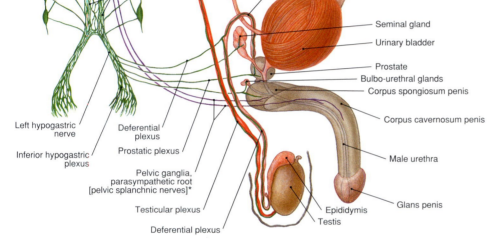

Fig. 892 Male genitalia;
diagram demonstrating the autonomous innervation of the left side;
ventral and lateral view, respectively.
Green = sympathetic nervous system
Purple = parasympathetic nervous system

* Also: erigent nerves

Surgical removal of paraaortic lymph nodes or operations at the abdominal aorta and the large arteries of the pelvis can cause damage to the sympathetic nerves with the consequence of ejaculatory impotency (Impotentia generandi). Prostate operations, in turn, may damage the parasympathetic fibres innervating the penis, thus leading to erectile impotency (Impotentia coeundi).

Innervation of the male genitalia

	Origin	Course	Organ	Function
Parasympathetic	Sacral part of the spinal cord (S2 – S4)	Pelvic ganglia, parasympathetic root (pelvic splanchnic nerves)	Penis Corpus cavernosum	Vasodilatation Erection
Sympathetic	Thoracic part of the spinal cord (T10 – T12)	Superior and inferior mesenteric plexus ↓ Sympathetic trunk ↓ Testicular plexus ↓	Testis	Regulation of blood flow
	Lumbar part of the spinal cord (L1 – L2)	Superior hypogastric plexus ↓ Hypogastric nerve ↓		
		Inferior hypogastric plexus	Bulbo-urethral glands	Expulsion of its fluid
			Ductus (vas) deferens	Contraction, transport of the sperms into the urethra
			Vesicular gland Prostata	Expulsion of its content into the urethra
Somatomotor, somatosensory	Sacral part of the spinal cord (S2 – S4)	Pudendal nerve	(Sphincter vesicae)	Closure of the urinary bladder to prevent retrograde ejaculation
			Ischiocavernosus Bulbospongiosus	Expulsion of the ejaculate out of the urethra
		Posterior scrotal nerves Dorsal nerve of penis	Scrotal skin Penile skin	

Innervation of the female genitalia

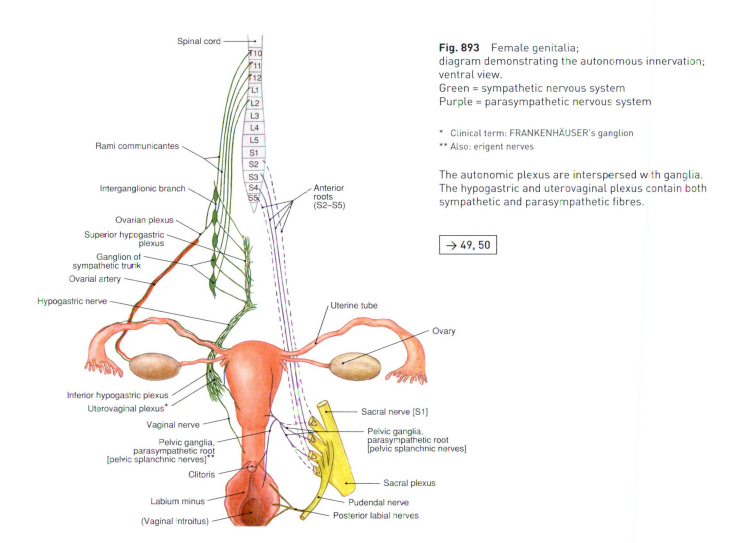

Fig. 893 Female genitalia;
diagram demonstrating the autonomous innervation;
ventral view.
Green = sympathetic nervous system
Purple = parasympathetic nervous system

* Clinical term: FRANKENHÄUSER's ganglion
** Also: erigent nerves

The autonomic plexus are interspersed with ganglia.
The hypogastric and uterovaginal plexus contain both
sympathetic and parasympathetic fibres.

→ 49, 50

Innervation of the female genitalia

	Origin	Course		Organ	Function
Parasympathetic	Sacral part of the spinal cord [S2 – S4]	Pelvic ganglia, parasympathetic root (pelvic splanchnic nerves) ↓		Uterine tube Uterus	Vasodilatation Vasodilatation
		Cavernous nerves of clitoris		Vagina Clitoris	Transsudation Erection
Sympathetic	Thoracic part of the spinal cord (T10 – T12)	Superior mesenteric plexus ↘ Ovarian plexus ↗ Renal plexus		Ovary	Vasoconstriction
		Sympathetic trunk ↓			
	Lumbar part of the spinal cord (L1 – L2)	Superior hypogastric plexus ↓ Hypogastric nerve Inferior hypogastric plexus ↓		-	
		Uterovaginal plexus (FRANKENHÄUSER's ganglion)		Uteri Uterus Vagina	Contraction
Somatomotor, somatosensory	Sacral part of the spinal cord [S2 – S4]	Pudendal nerve	↗ Dorsal nerve of clitoris	Clitoris	
			↘ Posterior labial nerves	Labia majora Ischiocavernosus Bulbospongiosus	Contraction

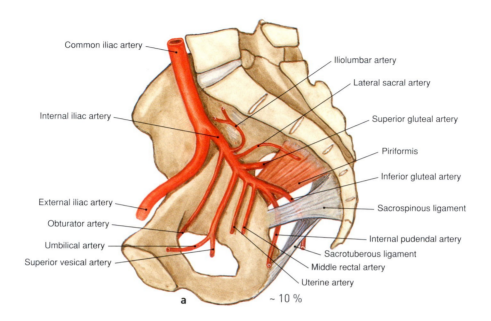

Common iliac artery

Iliolumbar artery

Lateral sacral artery

Internal iliac artery

Superior gluteal artery

Piriformis

Inferior gluteal artery

External iliac artery

Sacrospinous ligament

Obturator artery

Internal pudendal artery

Umbilical artery

Sacrotuberous ligament

Superior vesical artery

Middle rectal artery

Uterine artery

a   ~ 10 %

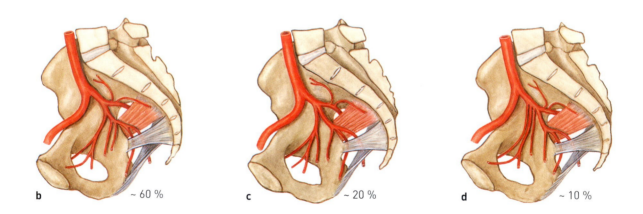

b   ~ 60 %

c   ~ 20 %

d   ~ 10 %

Fig. 894 a–d   Variability of the branching pattern of the internal iliac artery; viewed from the left.
a   All branches arise from the same stem.
b   The internal iliac artery divides into two major branches („textbook case").
c   The internal iliac artery divides into three major branches.
d   The internal iliac artery divides into more than three major branches.

Vessels and nerves of the pelvic wall

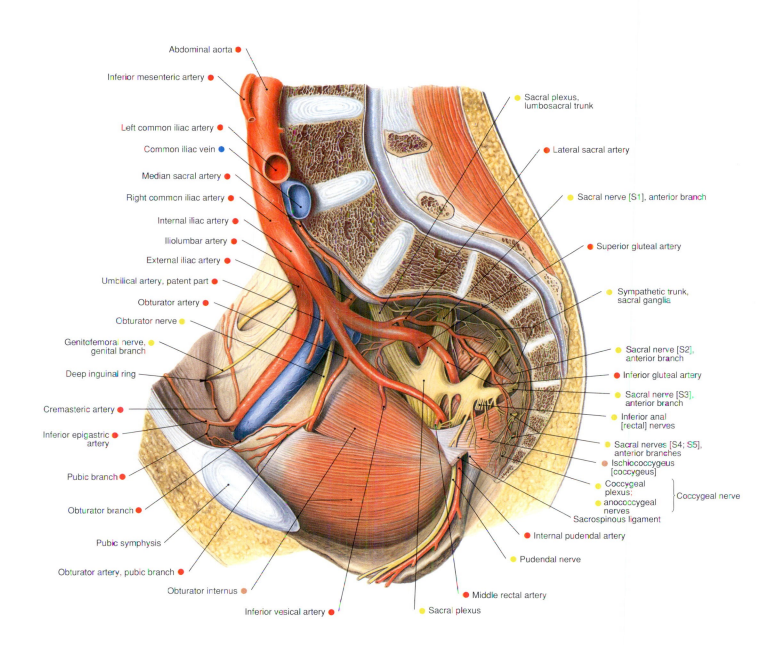

Abdominal aorta ●

Inferior mesenteric artery ●

Left common iliac artery ●

Common iliac vein ●

Median sacral artery ●

Right common iliac artery ●

Internal iliac artery ●

Iliolumbar artery ●

External iliac artery ●

Umbilical artery, patent part ●

Obturator artery ●

Obturator nerve ●

Genitofemoral nerve, genital branch ●

Deep inguinal ring

Cremasteric artery ●

Inferior epigastric artery ●

Pubic branch ●

Obturator branch ●

Pubic symphysis

Obturator artery, pubic branch ●

Obturator internus ●

Inferior vesical artery ●

Sacral plexus, lumbosacral trunk ●

● Lateral sacral artery

● Sacral nerve [S1], anterior branch

● Superior gluteal artery

● Sympathetic trunk, sacral ganglia

● Sacral nerve [S2], anterior branch

● Inferior gluteal artery

● Sacral nerve [S3], anterior branch

● Inferior anal [rectal] nerves

● Sacral nerves [S4; S5], anterior branches

● Ischiococcygeus [coccygeus]

● Coccygeal plexus; ● anococcygeal nerves } Coccygeal nerve

Sacrospinous ligament

● Internal pudendal artery

● Pudendal nerve

● Middle rectal artery

● Sacral plexus

Fig. 895 Internal iliac artery and sacral plexus; viewed from the left.

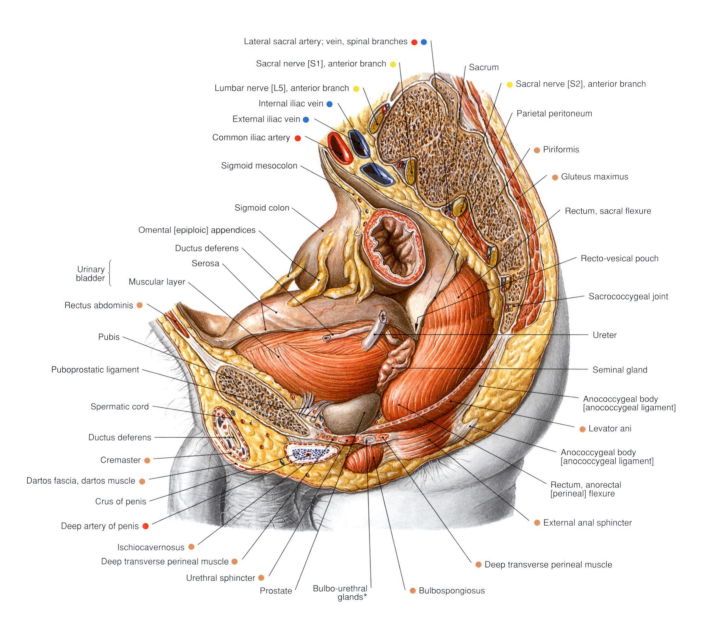

Lateral sacral artery; vein, spinal branches ● ●

Sacral nerve [S1], anterior branch ●

Sacrum

Sacral nerve [S2], anterior branch ●

Lumbar nerve [L5], anterior branch ●

Internal iliac vein ●

Parietal peritoneum

External iliac vein ●

Piriformis ●

Common iliac artery ●

Gluteus maximus ●

Sigmoid mesocolon

Rectum, sacral flexure

Sigmoid colon

Recto-vesical pouch

Omental [epiploic] appendices

Ductus deferens

Sacrococcygeal joint

Urinary bladder { Serosa

Muscular layer

Ureter

Rectus abdominis ●

Seminal gland

Pubis

Anococcygeal body [anococcygeal ligament]

Puboprostatic ligament

Levator ani ●

Spermatic cord

Anococcygeal body [anococcygeal ligament]

Ductus deferens

Rectum, anorectal [perineal] flexure

Cremaster ●

Dartos fascia, dartos muscle ●

External anal sphincter ●

Crus of penis

Deep artery of penis ●

Ischiocavernosus ●

Deep transverse perineal muscle ●

Deep transverse perineal muscle ●

Urethral sphincter ●

Prostate

Bulbo-urethral glands*

Bulbospongiosus ●

Fig. 896   Organs of the male pelvis.

* Clinical term: COWPER's gland

Vessels of the male pelvis

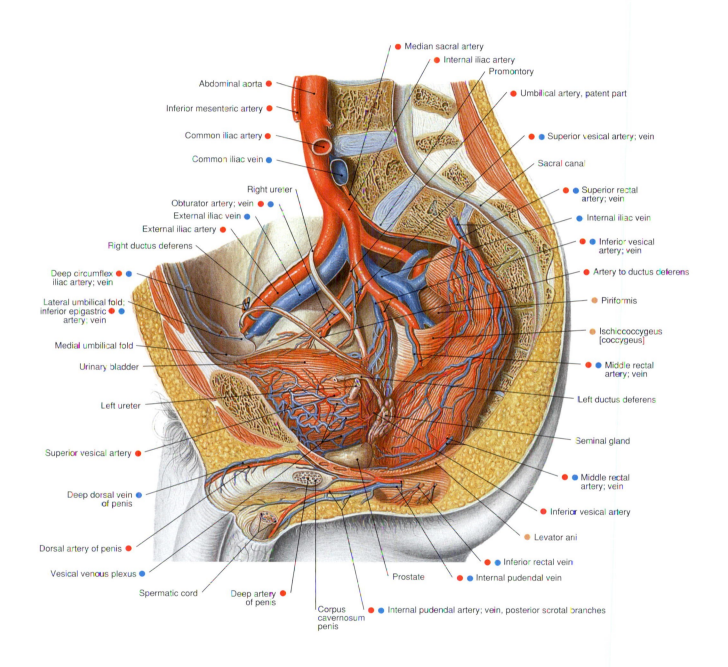

- Median sacral artery
- Internal iliac artery
Promontory
Abdominal aorta ●
Inferior mesenteric artery ●
Common iliac artery ●
Common iliac vein ●
Right ureter
Obturator artery; vein ● ●
External iliac vein ●
External iliac artery ●
Right ductus deferens
Deep circumflex ● ●
iliac artery; vein
Lateral umbilical fold;
inferior epigastric ● ●
artery; vein
Medial umbilical fold
Urinary bladder
Left ureter
Superior vesical artery ●
Deep dorsal vein ●
of penis
Dorsal artery of penis ●
Vesical venous plexus ●
Spermatic cord
Deep artery ●
of penis
Corpus
cavernosum
penis

- Umbilical artery, patent part
● ● Superior vesical artery; vein
Sacral canal
● ● Superior rectal
artery; vein
● Internal iliac vein
● ● Inferior vesical
artery; vein
● Artery to ductus deferens
● Piriformis
● Ischiococcygeus
[coccygeus]
● ● Middle rectal
artery; vein
Left ductus deferens
Seminal gland
● ● Middle rectal
artery; vein
● Inferior vesical artery
● Levator ani
● ● Inferior rectal vein
● ● Internal pudendal vein
Prostate
● ● Internal pudendal artery; vein, posterior scrotal branches

Fig. 897 Blood supply of the male pelvis.

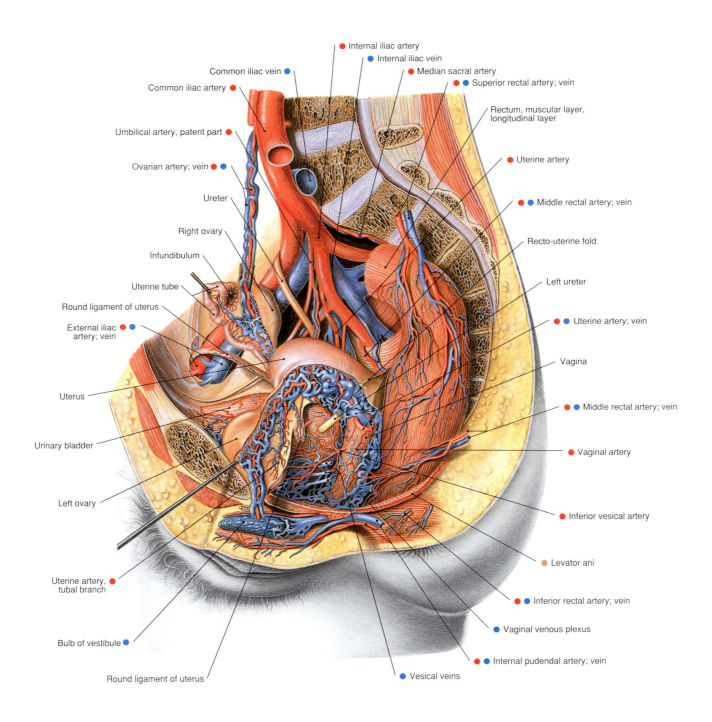

Internal iliac artery

Internal iliac vein

Common iliac vein

Median sacral artery

Common iliac artery

Superior rectal artery; vein

Rectum, muscular layer, longitudinal layer

Umbilical artery, patent part

Uterine artery

Ovarian artery; vein

Middle rectal artery; vein

Ureter

Right ovary

Recto-uterine fold

Infundibulum

Left ureter

Uterine tube

Round ligament of uterus

Uterine artery; vein

External iliac artery; vein

Vagina

Uterus

Middle rectal artery; vein

Urinary bladder

Vaginal artery

Left ovary

Inferior vesical artery

Levator ani

Uterine artery, tubal branch

Inferior rectal artery; vein

Vaginal venous plexus

Bulb of vestibule

Internal pudendal artery; vein

Round ligament of uterus

Vesical veins

Fig. 898   Blood supply of the female pelvis.

Vessels of the female pelvis

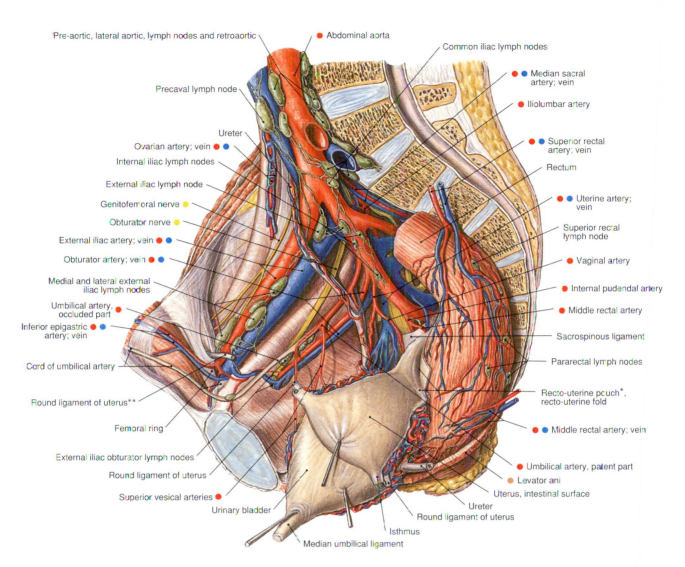

Pre-aortic, lateral aortic, lymph nodes and retroaortic

Abdominal aorta

Common iliac lymph nodes

Precaval lymph node

Median sacral artery; vein

Iliolumbar artery

Ureter

Ovarian artery; vein

Superior rectal artery; vein

Internal iliac lymph nodes

Rectum

External iliac lymph node

Uterine artery; vein

Genitofemoral nerve

Obturator nerve

Superior rectal lymph node

External iliac artery; vein

Vaginal artery

Obturator artery; vein

Internal pudendal artery

Medial and lateral external iliac lymph nodes

Middle rectal artery

Umbilical artery, occluded part

Inferior epigastric artery; vein

Sacrospinous ligament

Cord of umbilical artery

Pararectal lymph nodes

Recto-uterine pouch*, recto-uterine fold

Round ligament of uterus**

Middle rectal artery; vein

Femoral ring

External iliac obturator lymph nodes

Umbilical artery, patent part

Round ligament of uterus

Levator ani

Uterus, intestinal surface

Superior vesical arteries

Ureter

Urinary bladder

Round ligament of uterus

Isthmus

Median umbilical ligament

Fig. 899 Lymphatics and lymph nodes of the pelvic wall of the female.

The lymph nodes are frequently much smaller than illustrated but they are always present. Tumour cells from the uterus can reach the superficial inguinal lymph nodes via lymphatics of the round ligament of uterus.

* Clinical term: pouch of DOUGLAS
** Clinical term: round ligament

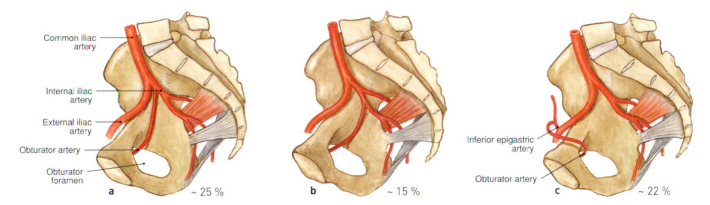

Common iliac artery

Internal iliac artery

External iliac artery

Obturator artery

Obturator foramen

Inferior epigastric artery

Obturator artery

a ~ 25 %   **b** ~ 15 %   **c** ~ 22 %

Fig. 900 a–c Variability of the origin of the obturator artery; medial view.
a Origin from the anterior branch of the internal iliac artery („textbook case")

b Origin as an independent branch from the internal iliac artery
c Origin from the external iliac artery
Only in 75% of the cases, the obturator artery originates from the trunk of the internal iliac artery

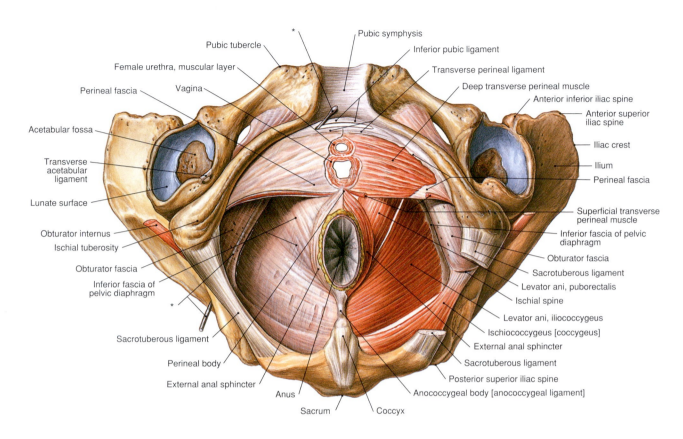

Fig. 901 Perineal muscles and the pelvic diaphragm of the female; inferior view.

* Probe in the pudendal canal (ALCOCK's canal)

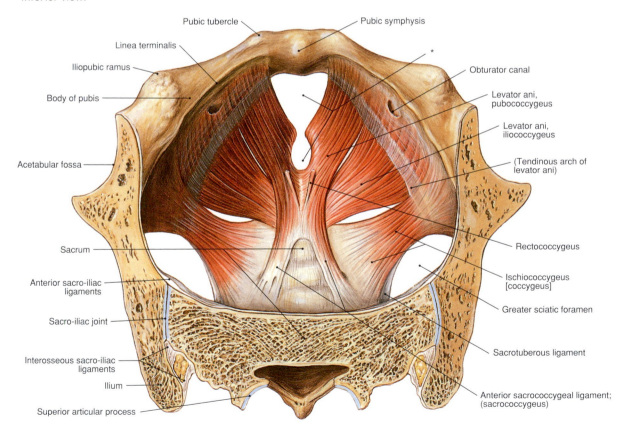

Fig. 902 Pelvic diaphragm of the female; superior view.

* Clinical term: levator hiatus

Female pelvic diaphragm

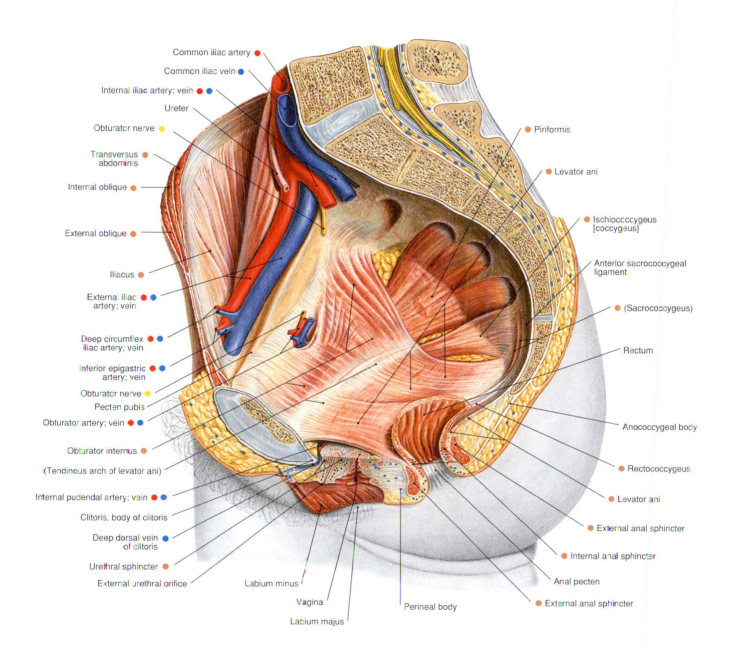

Common iliac artery ●
Common iliac vein ●
Internal iliac artery; vein ● ●
Ureter
Obturator nerve ●
Transversus abdominis ●
Internal oblique ●
External oblique ●
Iliacus ●
External iliac artery; vein ● ●
Deep circumflex iliac artery; vein ● ●
Inferior epigastric artery; vein ● ●
Obturator nerve ●
Pecten pubis
Obturator artery; vein ● ●
Obturator internus ●
(Tendinous arch of levator ani)
Internal pudendal artery; vein ● ●
Clitoris, body of clitoris
Deep dorsal vein of clitoris ●
Urethral sphincter ●
External urethral orifice

Labium minus
Vagina
Labium majus
Perineal body

Piriformis ●
Levator ani ●
Ischiococcygeus [coccygeus] ●
Anterior sacrococcygeal ligament
(Sacrococcygeus) ●
Rectum
Anococcygeal body
Rectococcygeus ●
Levator ani ●
External anal sphincter ●
Internal anal sphincter ●
Anal pecten
External anal sphincter ●

Fig. 903 Muscles of the pelvic diaphragm of the female.

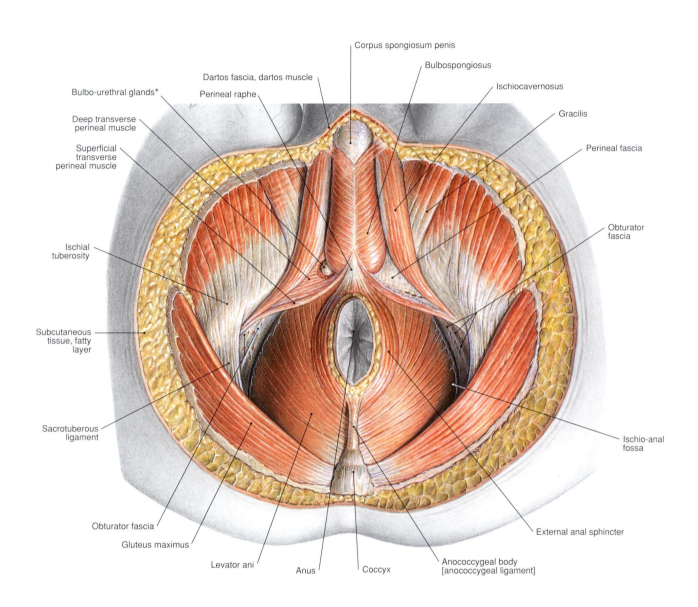

Corpus spongiosum penis

Bulbospongiosus

Dartos fascia, dartos muscle

Ischiocavernosus

Bulbo-urethral glands*

Perineal raphe

Gracilis

Deep transverse
perineal muscle

Perineal fascia

Superficial
transverse
perineal muscle

Obturator
fascia

Ischial
tuberosity

Subcutaneous
tissue, fatty
layer

Ischio-anal
fossa

Sacrotuberous
ligament

External anal sphincter

Obturator fascia

Gluteus maximus

Anococcygeal body
[anococcygeal ligament]

Levator ani

Anus

Coccyx

→ T 22

Fig. 904 Perineum and pelvic diaphragm of the male;
inferior view.

* Clinical term: COWPER's gland

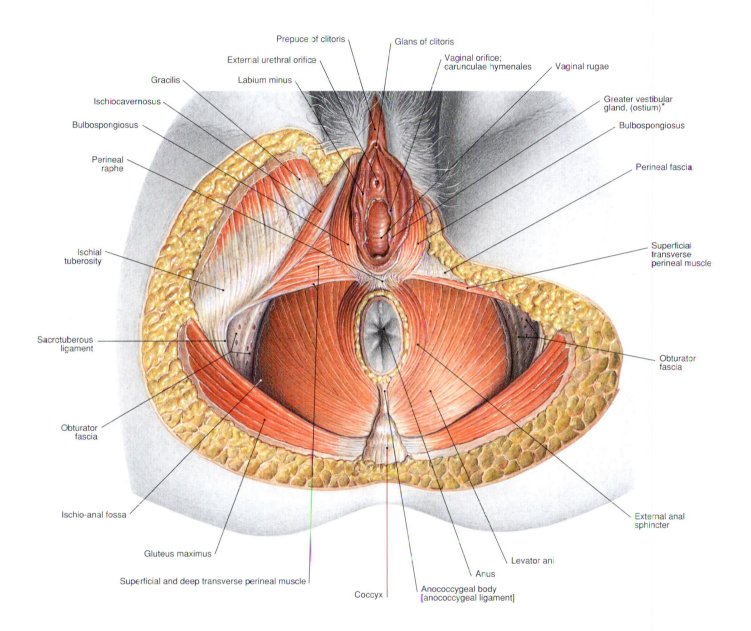

Prepuce of clitoris
Glans of clitoris
External urethral orifice
Vaginal orifice; carunculae hymenales
Vaginal rugae
Gracilis
Labium minus
Greater vestibular gland, (ostium)*
Ischiocavernosus
Bulbospongiosus
Bulbospongiosus
Perineal raphe
Perineal fascia
Ischial tuberosity
Superficial transverse perineal muscle
Sacrotuberous ligament
Obturator fascia
Obturator fascia
External anal sphincter
Ischio-anal fossa
Gluteus maximus
Levator ani
Superficial and deep transverse perineal muscle
Anus
Coccyx
Anococcygeal body [anococcygeal ligament]

Fig. 905 Perineum; pelvic diaphragm and female external genitalia; inferior view.

* Clinical term: BARTHOLIN's gland

→ T 22

The vaginal and the anal orifices are located in close proximity. During delivery the skin and muscles of the perineum can rupture up to the sphincter muscles of the anus (I. – III. degree perineal lacerations). These can be prevented by surgical incisions directed either laterally or in the median plane (perineal incision = lateral or medial episiotomy).

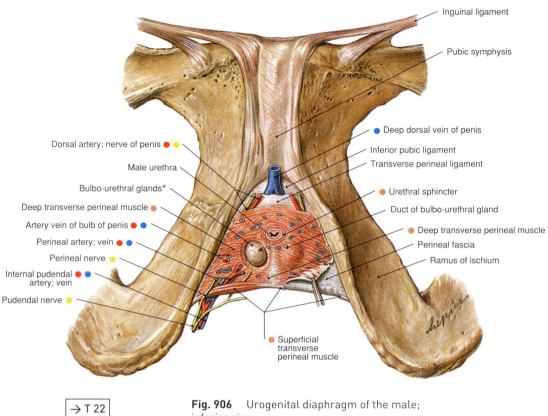

Inguinal ligament

Pubic symphysis

Deep dorsal vein of penis ●

Dorsal artery; nerve of penis ● ●

Inferior pubic ligament

Transverse perineal ligament

Male urethra

Urethral sphincter ●

Bulbo-urethral glands*

Deep transverse perineal muscle ●

Duct of bulbo-urethral gland

Artery vein of bulb of penis ● ●

Deep transverse perineal muscle ●

Perineal artery; vein ● ●

Perineal fascia

Perineal nerve ●

Ramus of ischium

Internal pudendal artery; vein ● ●

Pudendal nerve ●

Superficial transverse perineal muscle ●

→ T 22

Fig. 906 Urogenital diaphragm of the male; inferior view.

* Clinical term: COWPER's gland

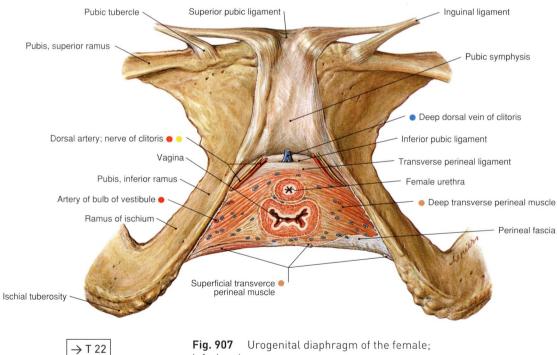

Pubic tubercle

Superior pubic ligament

Inguinal ligament

Pubis, superior ramus

Pubic symphysis

Deep dorsal vein of clitoris ●

Dorsal artery; nerve of clitoris ● ●

Inferior pubic ligament

Vagina

Transverse perineal ligament

Pubis, inferior ramus

Female urethra

Artery of bulb of vestibule ●

Deep transverse perineal muscle ●

Ramus of ischium

Perineal fascia

Ischial tuberosity

Superficial transverce perineal muscle ●

→ T 22

Fig. 907 Urogenital diaphragm of the female; inferior view.

Female external genitalia

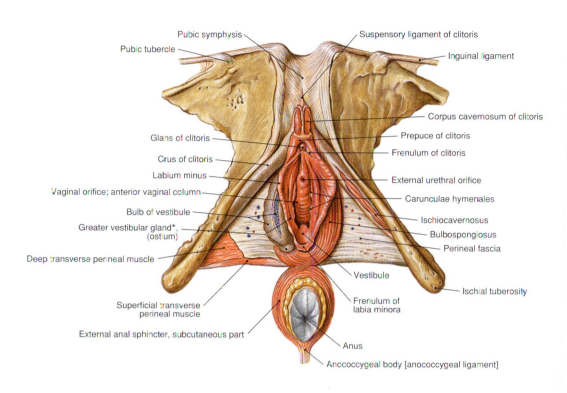

Pubic symphysis
Pubic tubercle
Suspensory ligament of clitoris
Inguinal ligament
Corpus cavernosum of clitoris
Glans of clitoris
Prepuce of clitoris
Crus of clitoris
Frenulum of clitoris
Labium minus
External urethral orifice
Vaginal orifice; anterior vaginal column
Carunculae hymenales
Bulb of vestibule
Ischiocavernosus
Greater vestibular gland*, (ostium)
Bulbospongiosus
Deep transverse perineal muscle
Perineal fascia
Vestibule
Superficial transverse perineal muscle
Ischial tuberosity
Frenulum of labia minora
External anal sphincter, subcutaneous part
Anus
Anococcygeal body [anococcygeal ligament]

Fig. 908 Female external genitalia; ventroinferior view.

* Clinical term: BARTHOLIN's gland

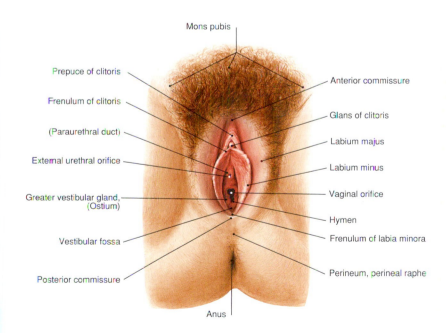

Mons pubis
Prepuce of clitoris
Anterior commissure
Frenulum of clitoris
Glans of clitoris
(Paraurethral duct)
Labium majus
External urethral orifice
Labium minus
Greater vestibular gland, (Ostium)
Vaginal orifice
Vestibular fossa
Hymen
Frenulum of labia minora
Posterior commissure
Perineum, perineal raphe
Anus

Fig. 909 Female external genitalia; inferior view.

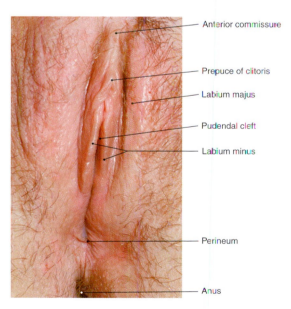

Anterior commissure
Prepuce of clitoris
Labium majus
Pudendal cleft
Labium minus
Perineum
Anus

Fig. 910 Female external genitalia; inferior view.

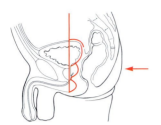

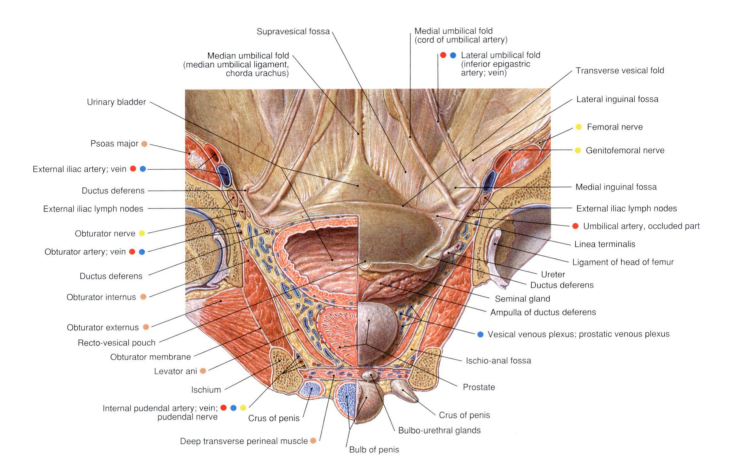

Fig. 911 Pelvic diaphragm;
pelvic organs and anterior abdominal wall of the male;
frontal section through the head of the femur
and the urinary bladder on the left;
dorsal view.

Female pelvic organs and retroperitoneal space

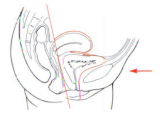

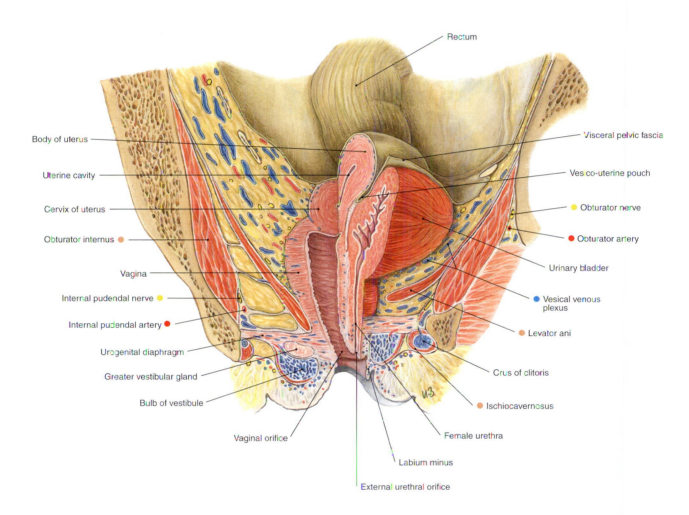

Rectum

Body of uterus

Uterine cavity

Cervix of uterus

Obturator internus ●

Vagina

Internal pudendal nerve ●

Internal pudendal artery ●

Urogenital diaphragm

Greater vestibular gland

Bulb of vestibule

Vaginal orifice

External urethral orifice

Labium minus

Female urethra

Ischiocavernosus ●

Crus of clitoris

Levator ani ●

Vesical venous plexus ●

Urinary bladder

Obturator artery ●

Obturator nerve ●

Vesico-uterine pouch

Visceral pelvic fascia

Fig. 912 Pelvic diaphragm and pelvic organs of the female; frontal section (on the right) combined with a median section; ventral view.

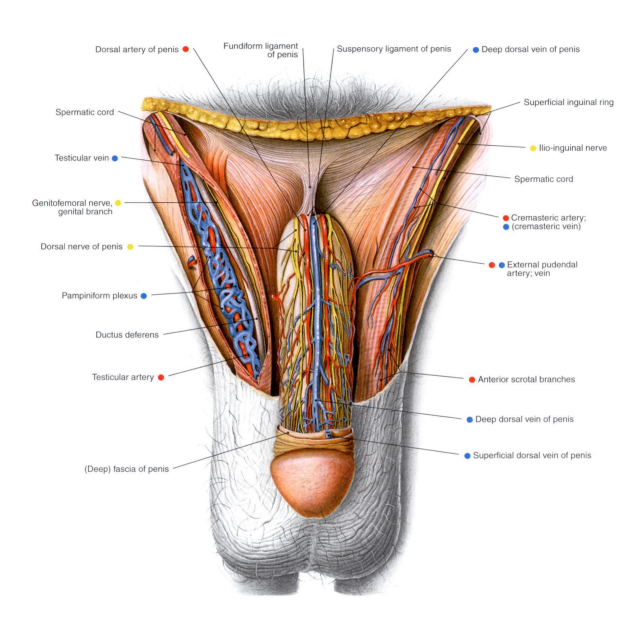

Dorsal artery of penis ●
Fundiform ligament of penis
Suspensory ligament of penis
● Deep dorsal vein of penis

Spermatic cord

Testicular vein ●

Genitofemoral nerve, genital branch ●

Dorsal nerve of penis ●

Pampiniform plexus ●

Ductus deferens

Testicular artery ●

(Deep) fascia of penis

Superficial inguinal ring

● Ilio-inguinal nerve

Spermatic cord

● Cremasteric artery;
● (cremasteric vein)

● ● External pudendal artery; vein

● Anterior scrotal branches

● Deep dorsal vein of penis

● Superficial dorsal vein of penis

Fig. 913   Male external genitalia.

Male external genitalia

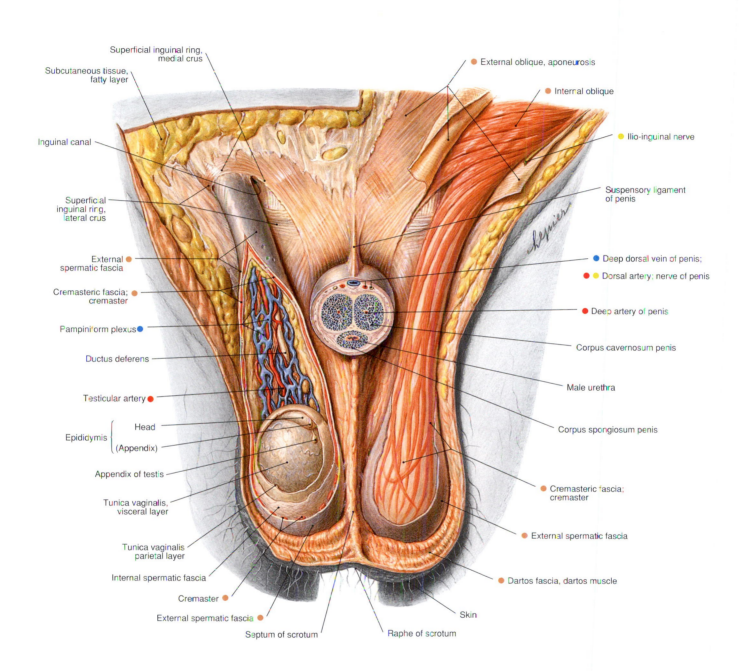

Superficial inguinal ring, medial crus

Subcutaneous tissue, fatty layer

Inguinal canal

Superficial inguinal ring, lateral crus

External spermatic fascia

Cremasteric fascia; cremaster

Pampiniform plexus

Ductus deferens

Testicular artery

Epididymis { Head / (Appendix) }

Appendix of testis

Tunica vaginalis, visceral layer

Tunica vaginalis parietal layer

Internal spermatic fascia

Cremaster

External spermatic fascia

Septum of scrotum

External oblique, aponeurosis

Internal oblique

Ilio-inguinal nerve

Suspensory ligament of penis

Deep dorsal vein of penis;

Dorsal artery; nerve of penis

Deep artery of penis

Corpus cavernosum penis

Male urethra

Corpus spongiosum penis

Cremasteric fascia; cremaster

External spermatic fascia

Dartos fascia, dartos muscle

Skin

Raphe of scrotum

Fig. 914   Male genitalia.   → 837, 849

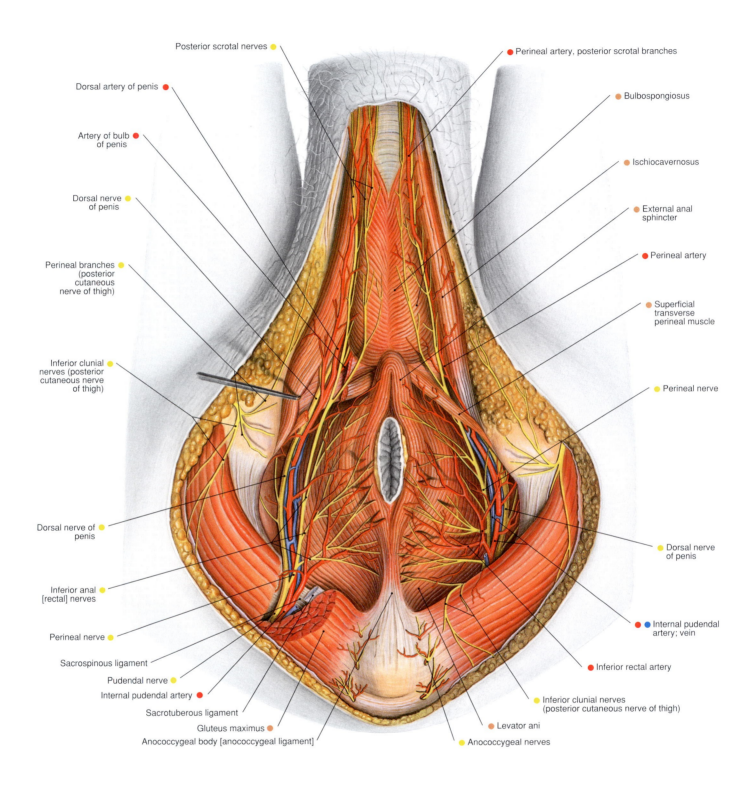

Posterior scrotal nerves ●

Dorsal artery of penis ●

Artery of bulb of penis ●

Dorsal nerve of penis ●

Perineal branches (posterior cutaneous nerve of thigh) ●

Inferior clunial nerves (posterior cutaneous nerve of thigh) ●

Dorsal nerve of penis ●

Inferior anal [rectal] nerves ●

Perineal nerve ●

Sacrospinous ligament

Pudendal nerve ●

Internal pudendal artery ●

Sacrotuberous ligament

Gluteus maximus ●

Anococcygeal body [anococcygeal ligament]

● Perineal artery, posterior scrotal branches

● Bulbospongiosus

● Ischiocavernosus

● External anal sphincter

● Perineal artery

● Superficial transverse perineal muscle

● Perineal nerve

● Dorsal nerve of penis

●● Internal pudendal artery; vein

● Inferior rectal artery

● Inferior clunial nerves (posterior cutaneous nerve of thigh)

● Levator ani

Anococcygeal nerves

Fig. 915   Vessels and nerves of the perineum and the male external genitalia.

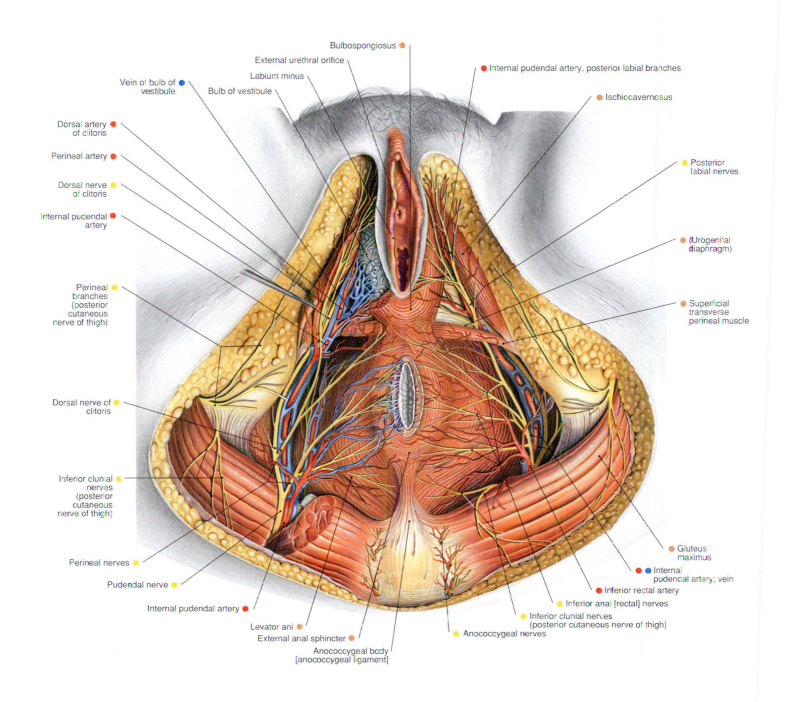

Bulbospongiosus
External urethral orifice
Labium minus
Vein of bulb of vestibule
Bulb of vestibule

Internal pudendal artery, posterior labial branches

Ischiocavernosus

Dorsal artery of clitoris

Perineal artery

Dorsal nerve of clitoris

Internal pudendal artery

Posterior labial nerves

(Urogenital diaphragm)

Superficial transverse perineal muscle

Perineal branches (posterior cutaneous nerve of thigh)

Dorsal nerve of clitoris

Inferior clunial nerves (posterior cutaneous nerve of thigh)

Gluteus maximus

Internal pudendal artery; vein

Inferior rectal artery

Perineal nerves

Pudendal nerve

Internal pudendal artery

Inferior anal [rectal] nerves

Inferior clunial nerves (posterior cutaneous nerve of thigh)

Levator ani

External anal sphincter

Anococcygeal nerves

Anococcygeal body [anococcygeal ligament]

Fig. 916   Vessels and nerves of the perineum and the female external genitalia.

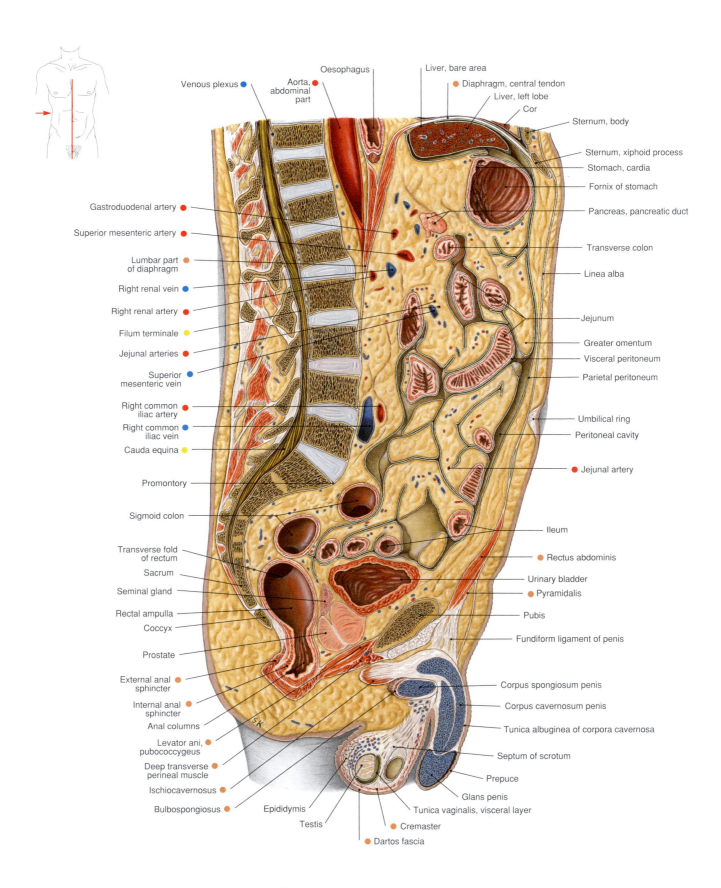

Venous plexus ●
Aorta, abdominal part ●
Oesophagus
Liver, bare area
● Diaphragm, central tendon
Liver, left lobe
Cor
Sternum, body
Sternum, xiphoid process
Stomach, cardia
Fornix of stomach
Pancreas, pancreatic duct
Transverse colon
Linea alba
Jejunum
Greater omentum
Visceral peritoneum
Parietal peritoneum
Umbilical ring
Peritoneal cavity
● Jejunal artery
Ileum
● Rectus abdominis
Urinary bladder
● Pyramidalis
Pubis
Fundiform ligament of penis
Corpus spongiosum penis
Corpus cavernosum penis
Tunica albuginea of corpora cavernosa
Septum of scrotum
Prepuce
Glans penis
Tunica vaginalis, visceral layer
● Cremaster
● Dartos fascia

Gastroduodenal artery ●
Superior mesenteric artery ●
Lumbar part of diaphragm ●
Right renal vein ●
Right renal artery ●
Filum terminale ●
Jejunal arteries ●
Superior mesenteric vein ●
Right common iliac artery ●
Right common iliac vein ●
Cauda equina ●
Promontory
Sigmoid colon
Transverse fold of rectum
Sacrum
Seminal gland
Rectal ampulla
Coccyx
Prostate
External anal sphincter ●
Internal anal sphincter ●
Anal columns
Levator ani, pubococcygeus ●
Deep transverse perineal muscle ●
Ischiocavernosus ●
Bulbospongiosus ●
Epididymis
Testis
Fig. 917 Abdomen and pelvis of the male; median section.

Abdomen, sagittal section

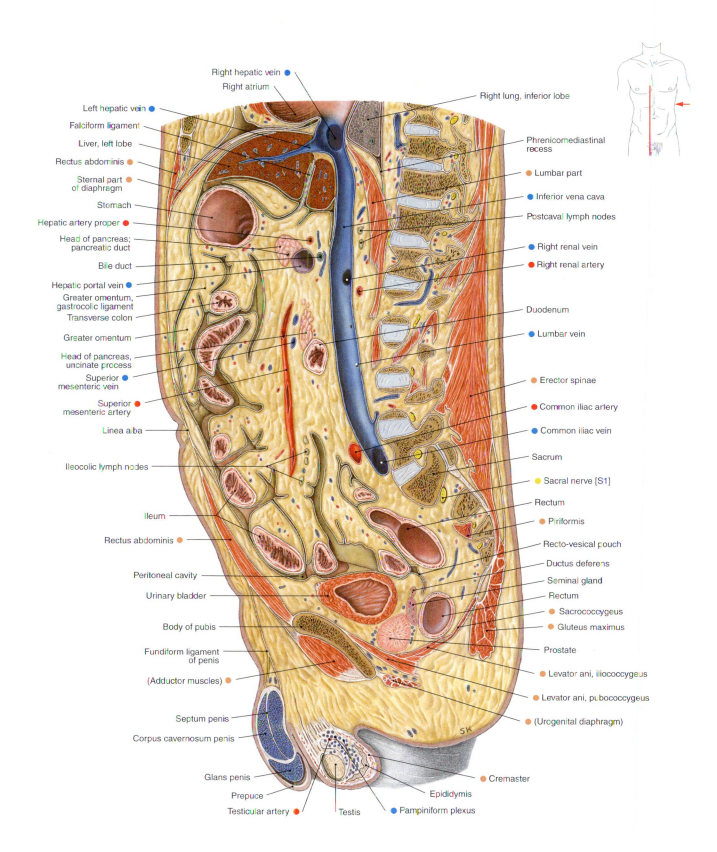

Right hepatic vein ●
Right atrium
Left hepatic vein ●
Falciform ligament
Liver, left lobe
Rectus abdominis ●
Sternal part
of diaphragm
Stomach
Hepatic artery proper ●
Head of pancreas;
pancreatic duct
Bile duct
Hepatic portal vein ●
Greater omentum,
gastrocolic ligament
Transverse colon
Greater omentum
Head of pancreas,
uncinate process
Superior ●
mesenteric vein
Superior ●
mesenteric artery
Linea alba
Ileocolic lymph nodes
Ileum
Rectus abdominis ●
Peritoneal cavity
Urinary bladder
Body of pubis
Fundiform ligament
of penis
(Adductor muscles) ●
Septum penis
Corpus cavernosum penis
Glans penis
Prepuce
Testicular artery ●

Right lung, inferior lobe
Phrenicomediastinal
recess
● Lumbar part
● Inferior vena cava
Postcaval lymph nodes
● Right renal vein
● Right renal artery
Duodenum
● Lumbar vein
● Erector spinae
● Common iliac artery
● Common iliac vein
Sacrum
● Sacral nerve [S1]
Rectum
● Piriformis
Recto-vesical pouch
Ductus deferens
Seminal gland
Rectum
● Sacrococcygeus
● Gluteus maximus
Prostate
● Levator ani, iliococcygeus
● Levator ani, pubococcygeus
● (Urogenital diaphragm)
● Cremaster
Epididymis
Testis ● Pampiniform plexus

Fig. 918 Abdomen and pelvis of the male;
sagittal section to the right of the median plane.

Inferior vena cava

Liver, caudate lobe

Right atrium

Left hepatic vein

Right ventricle

Hepatic portal vein

Left triangular ligament

Hepatic portal vein, right branch

Stomach, cardiac orifice

Hepatic artery proper

Left gastric artery; vein

Duodenum, superior part

Transverse colon

Liver, right lobe

Tail of pancreas

Transverse colon

Gastroduodenal artery

Head of pancreas

Splenic vein

Ascending colon

Duodenum, duodenojejunal flexure

Superior mesenteric artery

Superior mesenteric artery; vein

Jejunal arteries

Ascending colon

Jejunum

Ileum

Peritoneal cavity

Ilium

Descending colon

Sartorius

Tensor fasciae latae

Iliacus

Femoral nerve

Femoral artery

Sigmoid colon

Rectus femoris

Pubis

Femoral vein

Pubic symphysis

Pectineus

Fundiform ligament of penis

Adductor brevis

Dorsal artery of penis

Adductor longus

Male urethra

Penis, tunica albuginea

Deep artery of penis

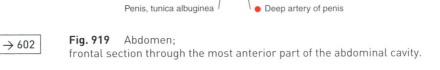

→ 602

Fig. 919   Abdomen;
frontal section through the most anterior part of the abdominal cavity.

Upper abdomen, frontal section

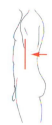

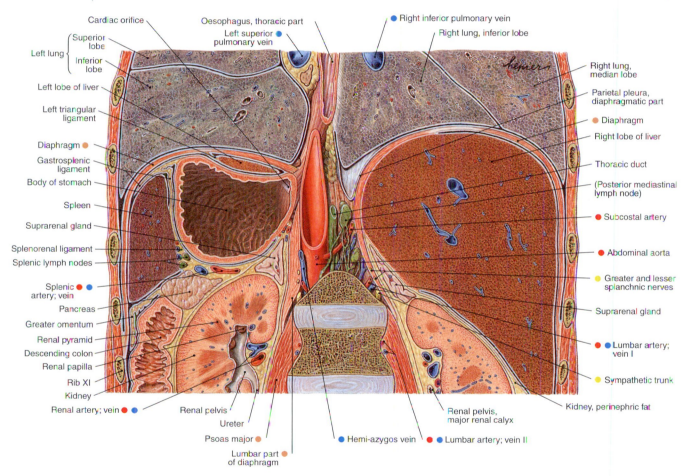

Cardiac orifice
Oesophagus, thoracic part
● Right inferior pulmonary vein
Left superior ●
pulmonary vein
Right lung, inferior lobe

Superior
lobe
Left lung
Inferior
lobe

Left lobe of liver

Right lung,
median lobe

Left triangular
ligament

Parietal pleura,
diaphragmatic part

Diaphragm ●

● Diaphragm

Gastrosplenic
ligament

Right lobe of liver

Body of stomach

Thoracic duct

Spleen

(Posterior mediastinal
lymph node)

Suprarenal gland

● Subcostal artery

Splenorenal ligament
Splenic lymph nodes

● Abdominal aorta

Splenic ● ●
artery; vein

● Greater and lesser
splanchnic nerves

Pancreas

Suprarenal gland

Greater omentum
Renal pyramid

● ● Lumbar artery;
vein I

Descending colon
Renal papilla

● Sympathetic trunk

Rib XI
Kidney

Kidney, perinephric fat

Renal artery; vein ● ●

Renal pelvis
Ureter

Renal pelvis,
major renal calyx

Psoas major ●

● Hemi-azygos vein ● ● Lumbar artery; vein II

Lumbar part ●
of diaphragm

Fig. 920 Abdomen;
frontal section demonstrating the diaphragm,
the organs of the upper abdomen and the kidneys;
dorsal view.

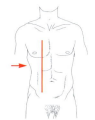

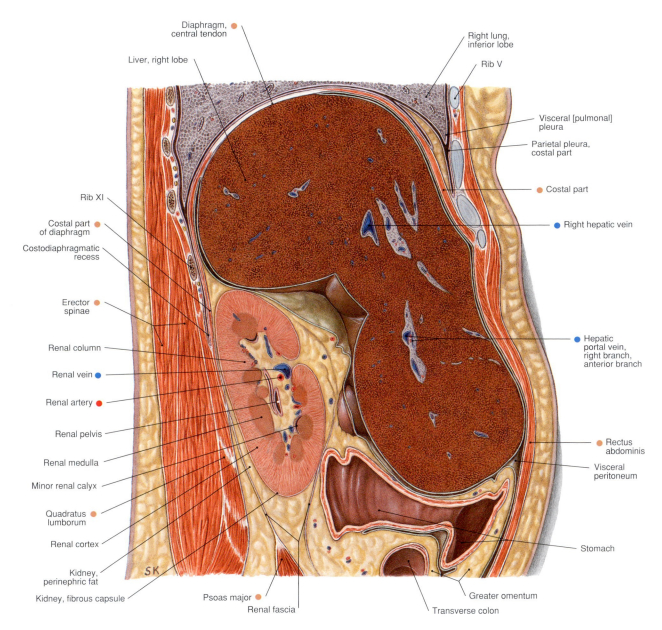

Diaphragm, central tendon

Liver, right lobe

Right lung, inferior lobe

Rib V

Visceral [pulmonal] pleura

Parietal pleura, costal part

Rib XI

Costal part of diaphragm

Costodiaphragmatic recess

Costal part

Right hepatic vein

Erector spinae

Renal column

Renal vein

Renal artery

Renal pelvis

Renal medulla

Minor renal calyx

Quadratus lumborum

Renal cortex

Hepatic portal vein, right branch, anterior branch

Rectus abdominis

Visceral peritoneum

Kidney, perinephric fat

Kidney, fibrous capsule

Psoas major

Renal fascia

Stomach

Greater omentum

Transverse colon

SK

Fig. 921 Abdomen; sagittal section through the upper abdomen at the level of the right kidney; viewed from the right.

Upper abdomen, sagittal section

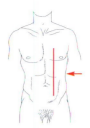

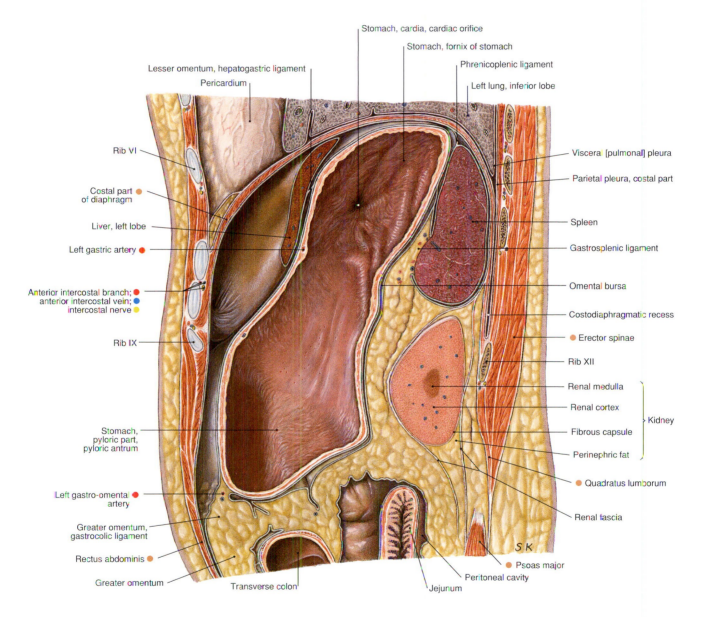

Stomach, cardia, cardiac orifice

Stomach, fornix of stomach

Phrenicoplenic ligament

Lesser omentum, hepatogastric ligament

Left lung, inferior lobe

Pericardium

Rib VI

Visceral [pulmonal] pleura

Costal part
of diaphragm

Parietal pleura, costal part

Liver, left lobe

Spleen

Left gastric artery ●

Gastrosplenic ligament

Anterior intercostal branch; ●
anterior intercostal vein; ●
intercostal nerve ●

Omental bursa

Costodiaphragmatic recess

Rib IX

● Erector spinae

Rib XII

Renal medulla

Renal cortex

Kidney

Stomach,
pyloric part,
pyloric antrum

Fibrous capsule

Perinephric fat

● Quadratus lumborum

Left gastro-omental ●
artery

Renal fascia

Greater omentum,
gastrocolic ligament

S K

Rectus abdominis ●

● Psoas major

Peritoneal cavity

Greater omentum

Transverse colon

Jejunum

Fig. 922 Abdomen;
sagittal section through the upper abdomen at the level of the spleen;
viewed from the left.

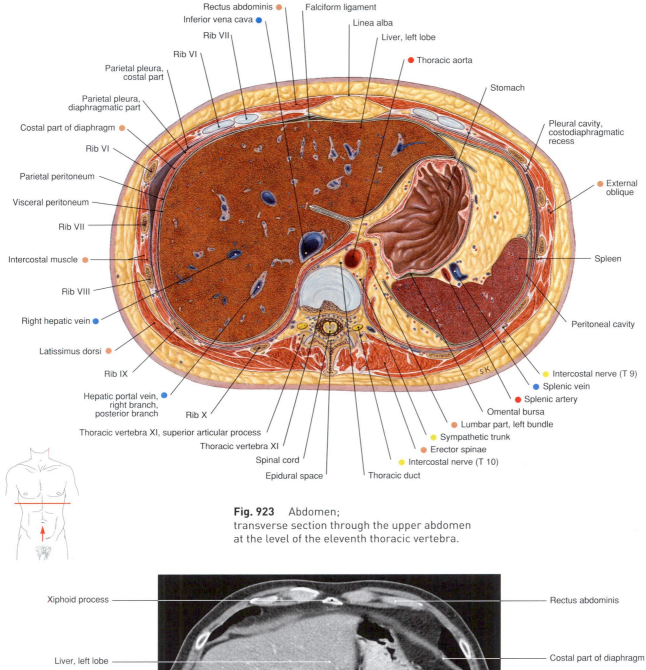

Fig. 923 Abdomen; transverse section through the upper abdomen at the level of the eleventh thoracic vertebra.

Fig. 924 Abdomen; computed tomographic cross-section (CT) at the level of the tenth thoracic vertebra; inferior view.

Upper abdomen, transverse sections

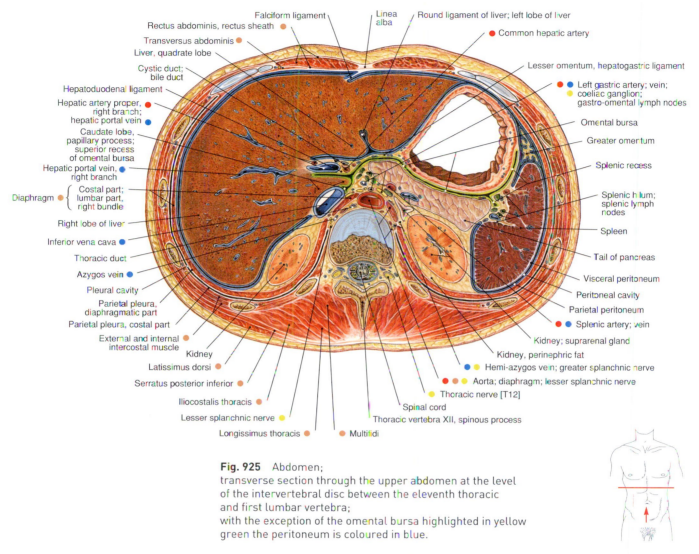

Falciform ligament
Rectus abdominis, rectus sheath ●
Transversus abdominis ●
Liver, quadrate lobe
Cystic duct; bile duct
Hepatoduodenal ligament
Hepatic artery proper, right branch; ●
hepatic portal vein ●
Caudate lobe, papillary process; superior recess of omental bursa
Hepatic portal vein, ● right branch
Diaphragm ● { Costal part; lumbar part, right bundle
Right lobe of liver
Inferior vena cava ●
Thoracic duct
Azygos vein ●
Pleural cavity
Parietal pleura, diaphragmatic part
Parietal pleura, costal part
External and internal ● intercostal muscle
Kidney
Latissimus dorsi ●
Serratus posterior inferior ●
Iliocostalis thoracis ●
Lesser splanchnic nerve ●
Longissimus thoracis ●   ● Multifidi

Linea alba
Round ligament of liver; left lobe of liver
● Common hepatic artery
Lesser omentum, hepatogastric ligament
● ● Left gastric artery; vein;
● coeliac ganglion; gastro-omental lymph nodes
Omental bursa
Greater omentum
Splenic recess
Splenic hilum; splenic lymph nodes
Spleen
Tail of pancreas
Visceral peritoneum
Peritoneal cavity
Parietal peritoneum
● ● Splenic artery; vein
Kidney; suprarenal gland
Kidney, perinephric fat
● ● Hemi-azygos vein; greater splanchnic nerve
● ● ● Aorta; diaphragm; lesser splanchnic nerve
● Thoracic nerve [T12]
Spinal cord
Thoracic vertebra XII, spinous process

Fig. 925 Abdomen;
transverse section through the upper abdomen at the level of the intervertebral disc between the eleventh thoracic and first lumbar vertebra;
with the exception of the omental bursa highlighted in yellow green the peritoneum is coloured in blue.

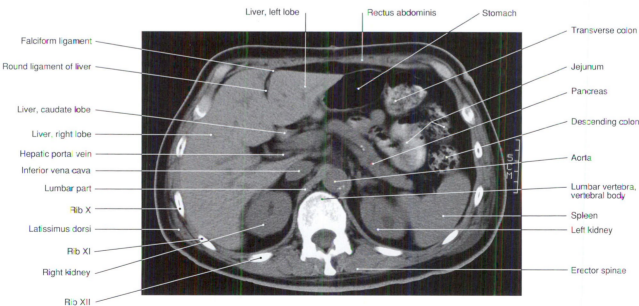

Liver, left lobe
Rectus abdominis
Stomach
Falciform ligament
Round ligament of liver
Liver, caudate lobe
Liver, right lobe
Hepatic portal vein
Inferior vena cava
Lumbar part
Rib X
Latissimus dorsi
Rib XI
Right kidney
Rib XII

Transverse colon
Jejunum
Pancreas
Descending colon
Aorta
Lumbar vertebra, vertebral body
Spleen
Left kidney
Erector spinae

5 C M

Fig. 926 Abdomen;
computed tomographic section (CT)
at the level of the first lumbar vertebra.
The intestine is partially filled with a contrast medium.

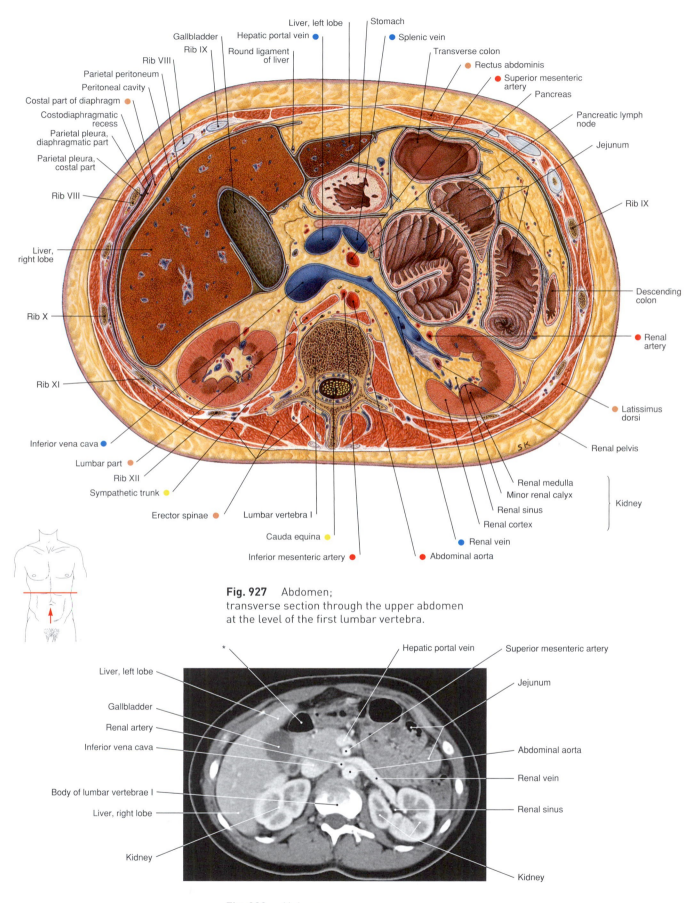

Fig. 927 Abdomen;
transverse section through the upper abdomen
at the level of the first lumbar vertebra.

Fig. 928 Abdomen;
computed tomographic section (CT)
at the level of the first lumbar vertebra;
inferior view.

* Intestinal gas

Lower abdomen, transverse sections

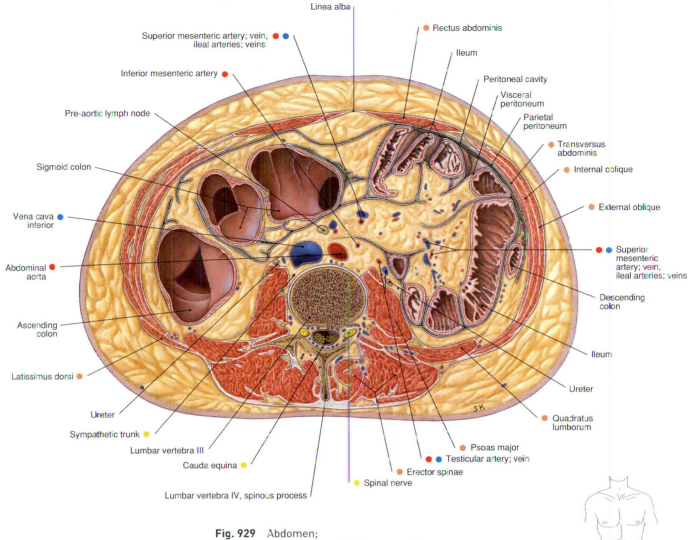

Linea alba

Superior mesenteric artery; vein, ● ●
ileal arteries; veins

Inferior mesenteric artery ●

Pre-aortic lymph node

Sigmoid colon

Vena cava ●
inferior

Abdominal ●
aorta

Ascending
colon

Latissimus dorsi ●

Ureter

Sympathetic trunk ●

Lumbar vertebra III

Cauda equina ●

Lumbar vertebra IV, spinous process

Rectus abdominis ●

Ileum

Peritoneal cavity

Visceral
peritoneum

Parietal
peritoneum

Transversus ●
abdominis

Internal oblique ●

External oblique ●

● ● Superior
mesenteric
artery; vein,
ileal arteries; veins

Descending
colon

Ileum

Ureter

Quadratus ●
lumborum

Psoas major ●

● ● Testicular artery; vein

Erector spinae ●

Spinal nerve ●

Fig. 929   Abdomen;
transverse section through the lower abdomen
at the level of the third lumbar vertebra.

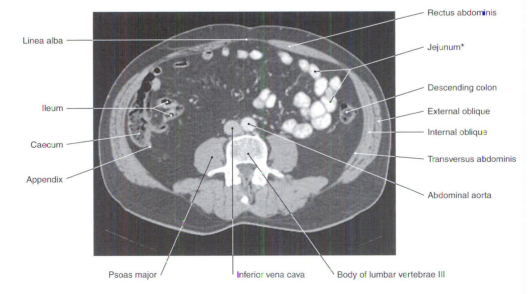

Linea alba

Ileum

Caecum

Appendix

Rectus abdominis

Jejunum*

Descending colon

External oblique

Internal oblique

Transversus abdominis

Abdominal aorta

Psoas major

Inferior vena cava

Body of lumbar vertebrae III

Fig. 930   Abdomen;
computed tomographic section (CT)
at the level of the third lumbar vertebra;
inferior view.

*   Jejunum filled with a contrast medium

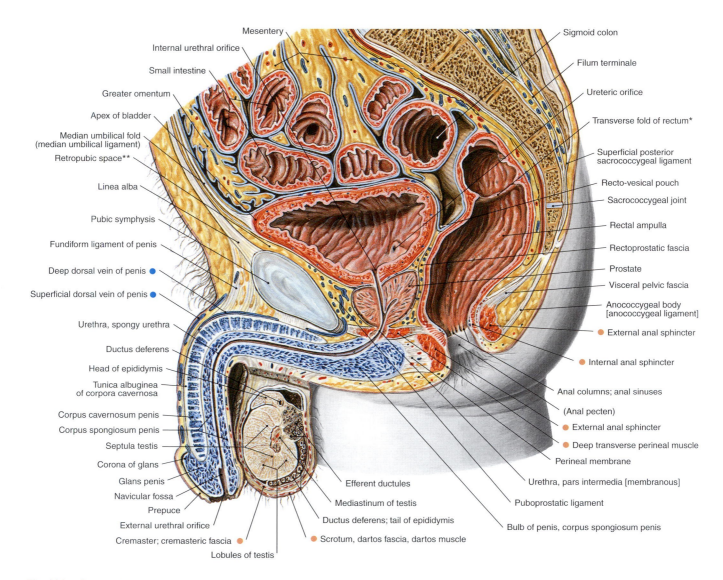

Mesentery
Internal urethral orifice
Small intestine
Greater omentum
Apex of bladder
Median umbilical fold (median umbilical ligament)
Retropubic space**
Linea alba
Pubic symphysis
Fundiform ligament of penis
Deep dorsal vein of penis
Superficial dorsal vein of penis
Urethra, spongy urethra
Ductus deferens
Head of epididymis
Tunica albuginea of corpora cavernosa
Corpus cavernosum penis
Corpus spongiosum penis
Septula testis
Corona of glans
Glans penis
Navicular fossa
Prepuce
External urethral orifice
Cremaster; cremasteric fascia
Lobules of testis

Sigmoid colon
Filum terminale
Ureteric orifice
Transverse fold of rectum*
Superficial posterior sacrococcygeal ligament
Recto-vesical pouch
Sacrococcygeal joint
Rectal ampulla
Rectoprostatic fascia
Prostate
Visceral pelvic fascia
Anococcygeal body [anococcygeal ligament]
External anal sphincter
Internal anal sphincter
Anal columns; anal sinuses
(Anal pecten)
External anal sphincter
Deep transverse perineal muscle
Perineal membrane
Urethra, pars intermedia [membranous]
Puboprostatic ligament
Bulb of penis, corpus spongiosum penis

Efferent ductules
Mediastinum of testis
Ductus deferens; tail of epididymis
Scrotum, dartos fascia, dartos muscle

Fig. 931 Pelvis of the male; median section; viewed from the left.

* Clinical term: KOHLRAUSCH's fold
** Clinical term: cave of RETZIUS

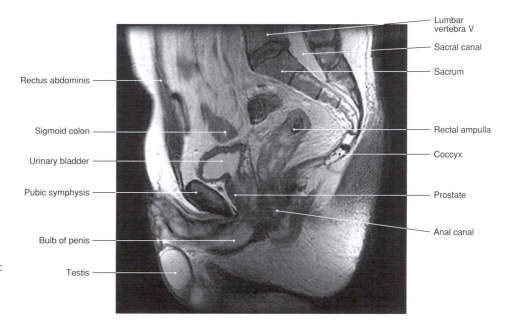

Rectus abdominis
Sigmoid colon
Urinary bladder
Pubic symphysis
Bulb of penis
Testis

Lumbar vertebra V
Sacral canal
Sacrum
Rectal ampulla
Coccyx
Prostate
Anal canal

Fig. 932 Pelvis of the male; magnetic resonance tomographic image (MRI); paramedian section; viewed from the left.

Female pelvis, median sections

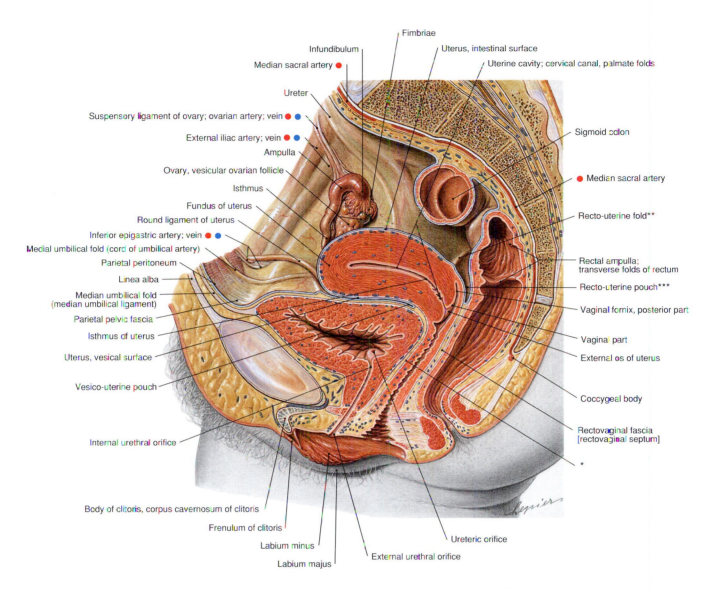

Fimbriae

Infundibulum

Median sacral artery ●

Ureter

Suspensory ligament of ovary; ovarian artery; vein ● ●

External iliac artery; vein ● ●

Ampulla

Ovary, vesicular ovarian follicle

Isthmus

Fundus of uterus

Round ligament of uterus

Inferior epigastric artery; vein ● ●

Medial umbilical fold (cord of umbilical artery)

Parietal peritoneum

Linea alba

Median umbilical fold (median umbilical ligament)

Parietal pelvic fascia

Isthmus of uterus

Uterus, vesical surface

Vesico-uterine pouch

Internal urethral orifice

Body of clitoris, corpus cavernosum of clitoris

Frenulum of clitoris

Labium minus

Labium majus

Uterus, intestinal surface

Uterine cavity; cervical canal, palmate folds

Sigmoid colon

● Median sacral artery

Recto-uterine fold**

Rectal ampulla; transverse folds of rectum

Recto-uterine pouch***

Vaginal fornix, posterior part

Vaginal part

External os of uterus

Coccygeal body

Rectovaginal fascia [rectovaginal septum]

*

Ureteric orifice

External urethral orifice

Fig. 933 Pelvis of the female; median section; the intestine has been almost completely removed with some remnants of the sigmoid and rectum; viewed from the left.

*   Clinical term: vesicovaginal septum
** Clinical term: sacrouterine ligament
*** Clinical term: pouch of DOUGLAS

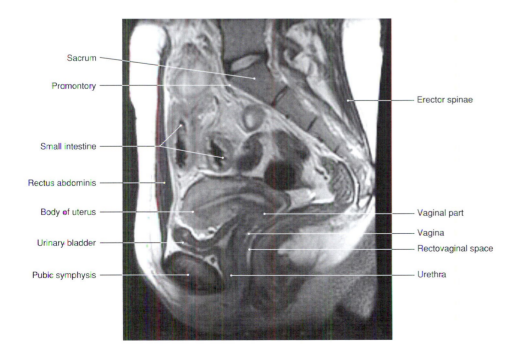

Sacrum

Promontory

Small intestine

Rectus abdominis

Body of uterus

Urinary bladder

Pubic symphysis

Erector spinae

Vaginal part

Vagina

Rectovaginal space

Urethra

Fig. 934 Pelvis of the female; magnetic resonance tomographic image (MRI); paramedian section; viewed from the left.

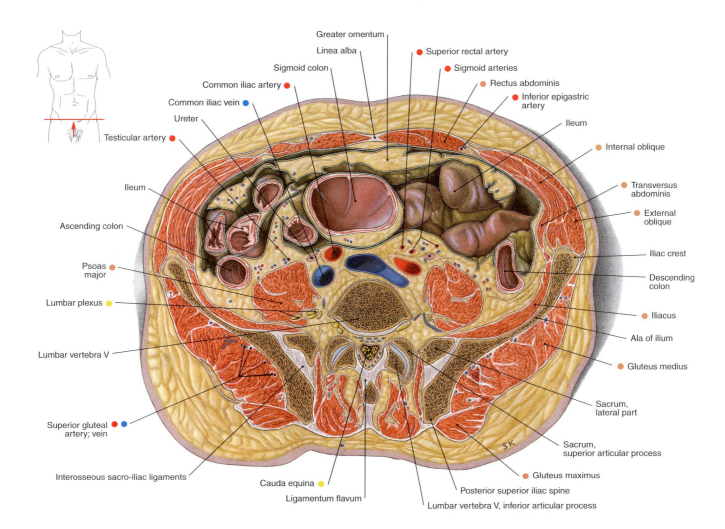

Fig. 935 Pelvis;
transverse section at the level of the fifth lumbar vertebra. This male specimen is different from Fig. 923, 925, 927 and 929.

As the sigmoid reaches far into the upper abdomen the figure also displays the dome of colonic flexure. The thickness of the adipose tissue layer on the gluteus medius muscle must be taken into consideration when injecting intramuscularly.

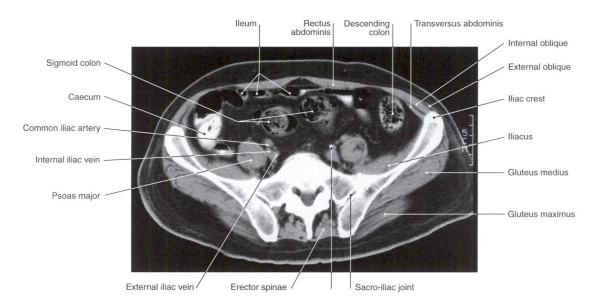

Fig. 936 Pelvis;
computed tomographic cross-section (CT) at the level of the first sacral vertebra after administration

of a contrast medium into the colon; supine position; inferior view.

* Calcification in the wall of the iliac artery.

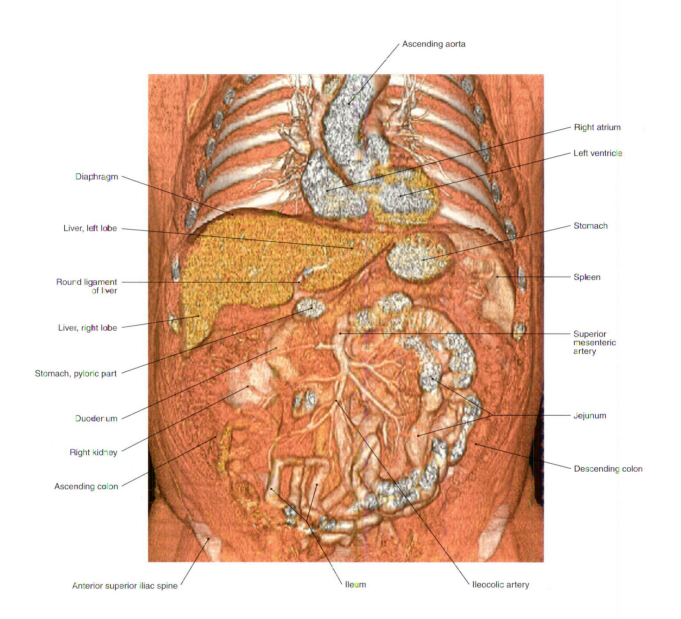

Ascending aorta

Right atrium

Left ventricle

Diaphragm

Liver, left lobe

Stomach

Round ligament
of liver

Spleen

Liver, right lobe

Superior
mesenteric
artery

Stomach, pyloric part

Duodenum

Jejunum

Right kidney

Descending colon

Ascending colon

Anterior superior iliac spine

Ileum

Ileocolic artery

Fig. 937 Abdomen;
volume-guided reconstruction in the frontal plane
based on horizontal computed tomographic sections (CT).
The section planes of organs such as the heart,
the stomach, the liver and parts of the small intestine,
appear granulate

→ 802, 919

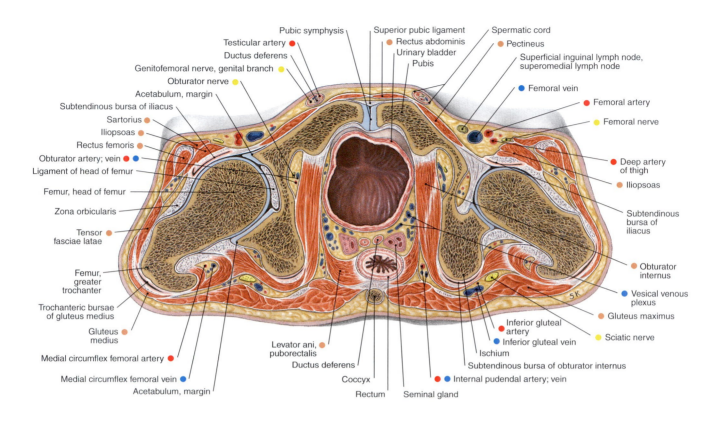

Pubic symphysis
Testicular artery ●
Ductus deferens
Genitofemoral nerve, genital branch ●
Obturator nerve ●
Acetabulum, margin
Subtendinous bursa of iliacus
Sartorius ●
Iliopsoas ●
Rectus femoris ●
Obturator artery; vein ● ●
Ligament of head of femur
Femur, head of femur
Zona orbicularis
Tensor fasciae latae ●
Femur, greater trochanter
Trochanteric bursae of gluteus medius
Gluteus medius ●
Medial circumflex femoral artery ●
Medial circumflex femoral vein ●
Acetabulum, margin

Superior pubic ligament
Rectus abdominis ●
Urinary bladder
Pubis
Spermatic cord
Pectineus ●
Superficial inguinal lymph node, superomedial lymph node
Femoral vein ●
Femoral artery ●
Femoral nerve ●
Deep artery of thigh ●
Iliopsoas ●
Subtendinous bursa of iliacus
Obturator internus ●
Vesical venous plexus ●
Gluteus maximus ●
Sciatic nerve ●
Inferior gluteal artery ●
Inferior gluteal vein ●
Ischium
Subtendinous bursa of obturator internus
Internal pudendal artery; vein ● ●

Levator ani, puborectalis ●
Ductus deferens
Coccyx
Rectum
Seminal gland

Fig. 938 Pelvis of the male;
transverse section through the lesser pelvis.

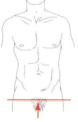

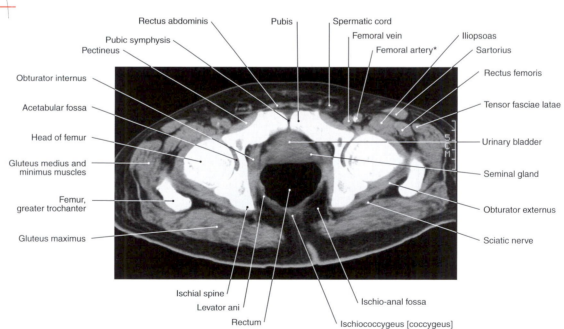

Rectus abdominis
Pubic symphysis
Pectineus
Obturator internus
Acetabular fossa
Head of femur
Gluteus medius and minimus muscles
Femur, greater trochanter
Gluteus maximus

Pubis
Spermatic cord
Femoral vein
Femoral artery*
Iliopsoas
Sartorius
Rectus femoris
Tensor fasciae latae
Urinary bladder
Seminal gland
Obturator externus
Sciatic nerve

Ischial spine
Levator ani
Rectum
Ischiococcygeus [coccygeus]
Ischio-anal fossa

Fig. 939 Pelvis of the male;
computed tomographic cross-section (CT) through
the lesser pelvis with the subject in supine position.

* Calcification in the medial part of the femoral artery

Female pelvis, transverse sections

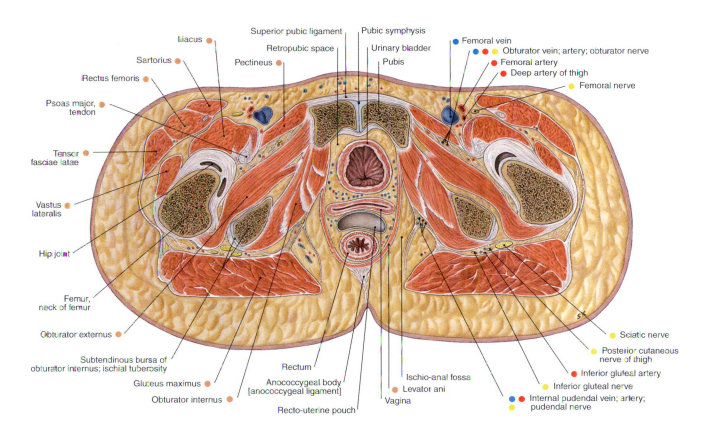

Superior pubic ligament
Iliacus
Pubic symphysis
Sartorius
Retropubic space
Urinary bladder
Pectineus
Pubis
Rectus femoris
Femoral vein
Obturator vein; artery; obturator nerve
Psoas major, tendon
Femoral artery
Deep artery of thigh
Femoral nerve
Tensor fasciae latae
Vastus lateralis
Hip joint
Femur, neck of femur
Obturator externus
Sciatic nerve
Posterior cutaneous nerve of thigh
Subtendinous bursa of obturator internus; ischial tuberosity
Inferior gluteal artery
Rectum
Inferior gluteal nerve
Gluteus maximus
Anococcygeal body [anococcygeal ligament]
Ischio-anal fossa
Internal pudendal vein; artery; pudendal nerve
Obturator internus
Levator ani
Recto-uterine pouch
Vagina

Fig. 940 Pelvis of the female;
transverse section through the lesser pelvis
at the level of the symphysis.

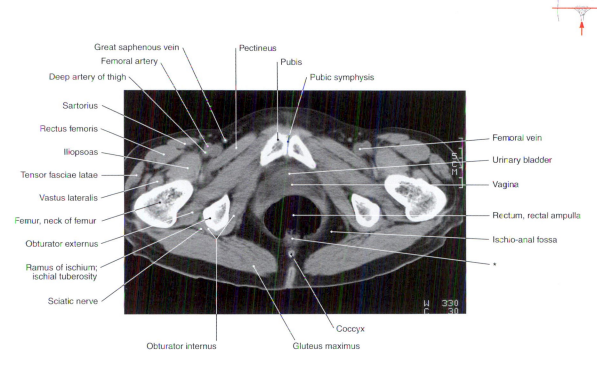

Great saphenous vein
Pectineus
Femoral artery
Pubis
Deep artery of thigh
Pubic symphysis
Sartorius
Rectus femoris
Iliopsoas
Femoral vein
Tensor fasciae latae
Urinary bladder
Vastus lateralis
Vagina
Femur, neck of femur
Rectum, rectal ampulla
Obturator externus
Ischio-anal fossa
Ramus of ischium; ischial tuberosity
*
Sciatic nerve
Coccyx
Obturator internus
Gluteus maximus

Fig. 941 Pelvis of the female;
computed tomographic cross-section (CT) through
the lesser pelvis with the subject in supine position.

* Remnants of contrasting intestinal contents

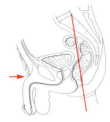

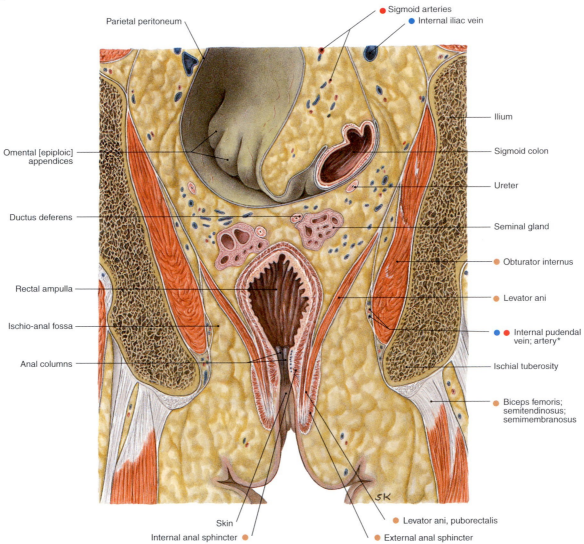

Parietal peritoneum

● Sigmoid arteries
● Internal iliac vein

Omental [epiploic] appendices

Ductus deferens

Rectal ampulla

Ischio-anal fossa

Anal columns

Ilium

Sigmoid colon

Ureter

Seminal gland

● Obturator internus

● Levator ani

● ● Internal pudendal vein; artery*

Ischial tuberosity

● Biceps femoris; semitendinosus; semimembranosus

Skin

Internal anal sphincter ●

● Levator ani, puborectalis

● External anal sphincter

Fig. 942   Pelvis of the male;
oblique frontal section through the lesser pelvis.

*   Clinical term: ALCOCK's canal

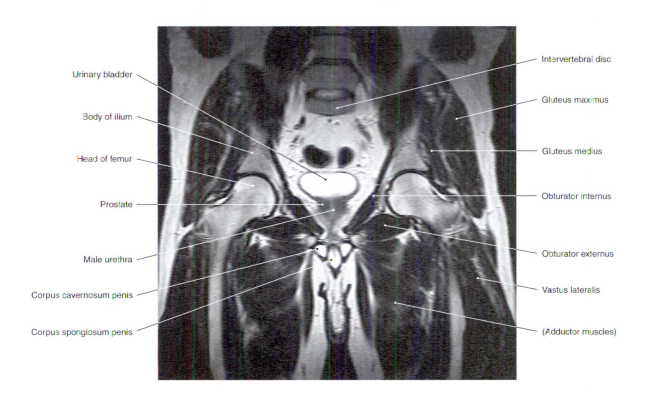

Fig. 943 Pelvis of the male;
magnetic resonance tomographic image (MRI);
frontal section at the level of the hip joints;
ventral view.

Urinary bladder
Body of ilium
Head of femur
Prostate
Male urethra
Corpus cavernosum penis
Corpus spongiosum penis

Intervertebral disc
Gluteus maximus
Gluteus medius
Obturator internus
Obturator externus
Vastus lateralis
(Adductor muscles)

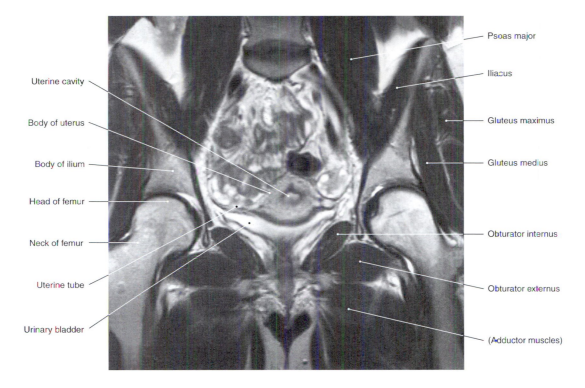

Fig. 944 Pelvis of the female;
magnetic resonance tomographic image (MRI);
frontal section at the level of the hip joints;
ventral view.

Uterine cavity
Body of uterus
Body of ilium
Head of femur
Neck of femur
Uterine tube
Urinary bladder

Psoas major
Iliacus
Gluteus maximus
Gluteus medius
Obturator internus
Obturator externus
(Adductor muscles)

When the urinary bladder is empty, the uterus lies on the apex
of the bladder due to its anteflexion.

Male pelvis diaphragm, angled-frontal section

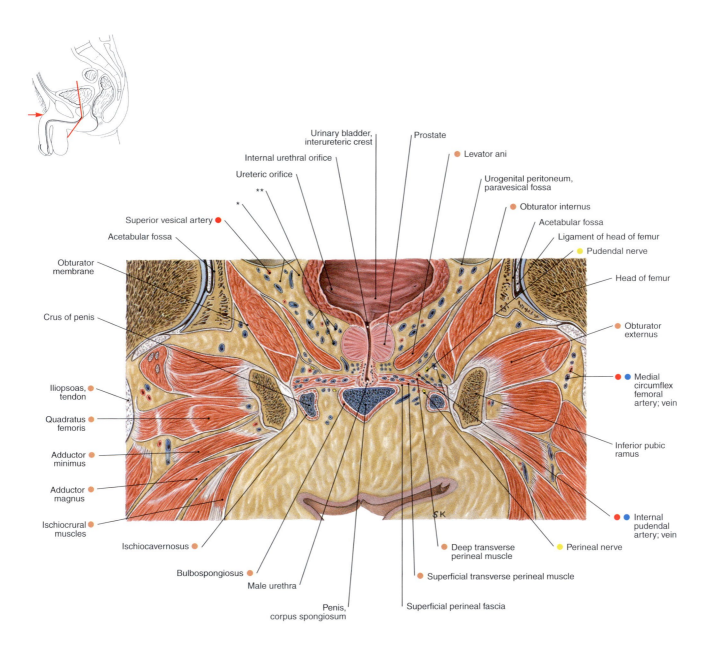

Urinary bladder, interureteric crest

Prostate

Internal urethral orifice

Levator ani

Ureteric orifice

Urogenital peritoneum, paravesical fossa

**

*

Obturator internus

Superior vesical artery ●

Acetabular fossa

Acetabular fossa

Ligament of head of femur

● Pudendal nerve

Obturator membrane

Head of femur

Crus of penis

● Obturator externus

Iliopsoas, tendon ●

● ● Medial circumflex femoral artery; vein

Quadratus femoris ●

Inferior pubic ramus

Adductor minimus ●

Adductor magnus

Ischiocrural muscles ●

● ● Internal pudendal artery; vein

Ischiocavernosus ●

Deep transverse perineal muscle ●

● Perineal nerve

Bulbospongiosus ●

● Superficial transverse perineal muscle

Male urethra

Penis, corpus spongiosum

Superficial perineal fascia

Fig. 945 Pelvis of the male; angled-frontal section through the urinary bladder.

* Clinical term: paracystium
** Clinical term: prostatic venous plexus

Female pelvic diaphragm, angled-frontal section

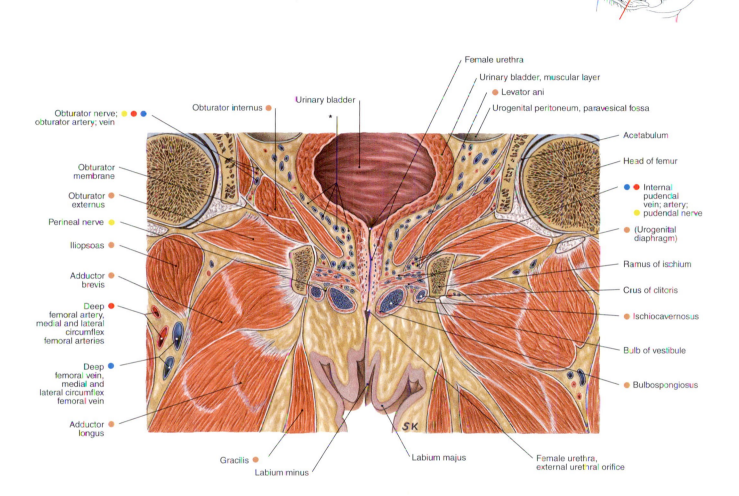

Obturator nerve;
obturator artery; vein

Obturator
membrane

Obturator
externus

Perineal nerve

Iliopsoas

Adductor
brevis

Deep
femoral artery,
medial and lateral
circumflex
femoral arteries

Deep
femoral vein,
medial and
lateral circumflex
femoral vein

Adductor
longus

Gracilis

Labium minus

Obturator internus

Urinary bladder

*

Female urethra

Urinary bladder, muscular layer

Levator ani

Urogenital peritoneum, paravesical fossa

Acetabulum

Head of femur

Internal
pudendal
vein; artery;
pudendal nerve

(Urogenital
diaphragm)

Ramus of ischium

Crus of clitoris

Ischiocavernosus

Bulb of vestibule

Bulbospongiosus

Labium majus

Female urethra,
external urethral orifice

S K

Fig. 946 Pelvis of the female;
angled-frontal section through the urinary bladder.

* Paracystium with venous plexus

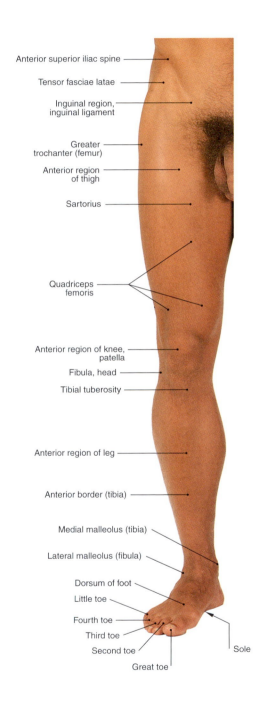

Anterior superior iliac spine

Tensor fasciae latae

Inguinal region, inguinal ligament

Greater trochanter (femur)

Anterior region of thigh

Sartorius

Quadriceps femoris

Anterior region of knee, patella

Fibula, head

Tibial tuberosity

Anterior region of leg

Anterior border (tibia)

Medial malleolus (tibia)

Lateral malleolus (fibula)

Dorsum of foot

Little toe

Fourth toe

Third toe

Second toe

Great toe

Sole

Fig. 947   Lower limb.

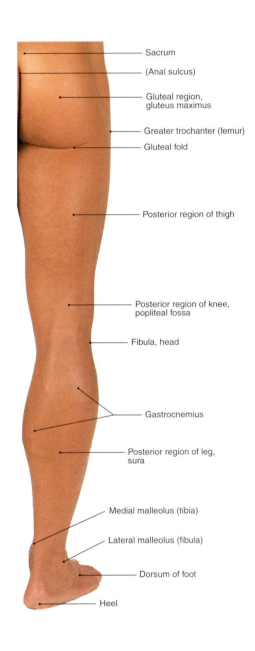

Sacrum

(Anal sulcus)

Gluteal region, gluteus maximus

Greater trochanter (femur)

Gluteal fold

Posterior region of thigh

Posterior region of knee, popliteal fossa

Fibula, head

Gastrocnemius

Posterior region of leg, sura

Medial malleolus (tibia)

Lateral malleolus (fibula)

Dorsum of foot

Heel

Fig. 948   Lower limb.

Skeleton of the lower limb, overview

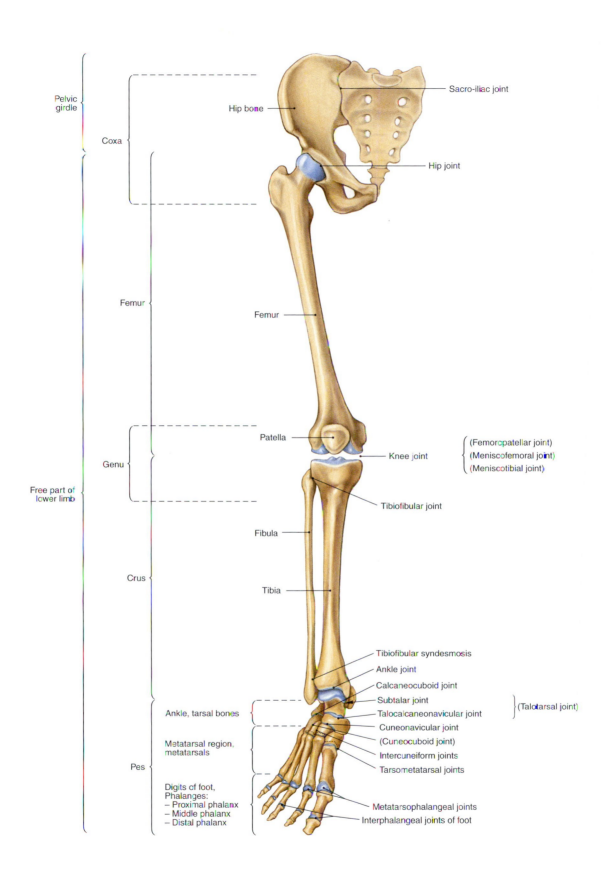

Pelvic girdle

Coxa

Femur

Genu

Free part of lower limb

Crus

Pes

Ankle, tarsal bones

Metatarsal region, metatarsals

Digits of foot,
Phalanges:
– Proximal phalanx
– Middle phalanx
– Distal phalanx

Hip bone

Femur

Patella

Fibula

Tibia

Sacro-iliac joint

Hip joint

Knee joint

(Femoropatellar joint)
(Meniscofemoral joint)
(Meniscotibial joint)

Tibiofibular joint

Tibiofibular syndesmosis
Ankle joint
Calcaneocuboid joint
Subtalar joint
Talocalcaneonavicular joint
Cuneonavicular joint
(Cuneocuboid joint)
Intercuneiform joints
Tarsometatarsal joints
Metatarsophalangeal joints
Interphalangeal joints of foot

(Talotarsal joint)

Fig. 949 Lower limb;
skeleton and joints.

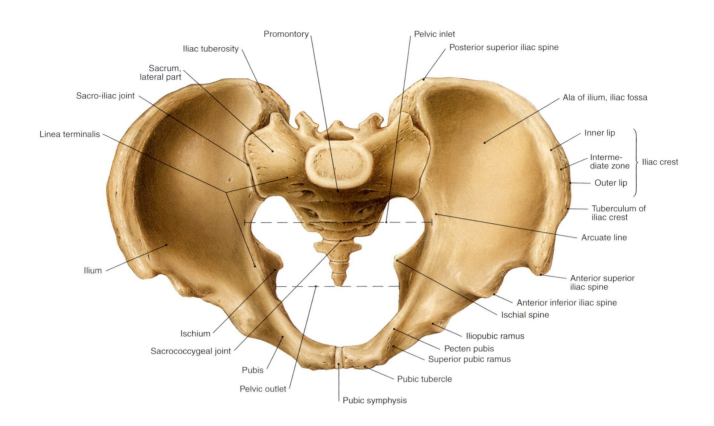

Fig. 950 Sacrum and pelvic girdle.
The region cranial to the linea terminalis is referred to as the greater pelvis and the region caudal to it is known as lesser pelvis.

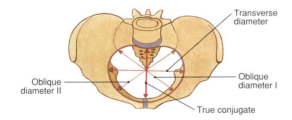

Fig. 951 Pelvis;
shape and dimensions of the pelvic inlet of the female.

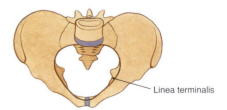

Fig. 952 Pelvis;
shape of the pelvic inlet of the male.

k – k = Pelvic axis
a – b = Anatomical conjugate
a – e = Diagonal conjugate
          12.5–13 cm
a – c = True conjugate
          10.4–11 cm

h – d = Sagittal diameter of the
          pelvic brim 12–12.5 cm
e – g = Sagittal diameter of the
          pelvic constriction
          11–11.5 cm
e – f = Sagittal diameter of the
          pelvic outlet
          (= pubococcygeal distance)
          9–10 cm

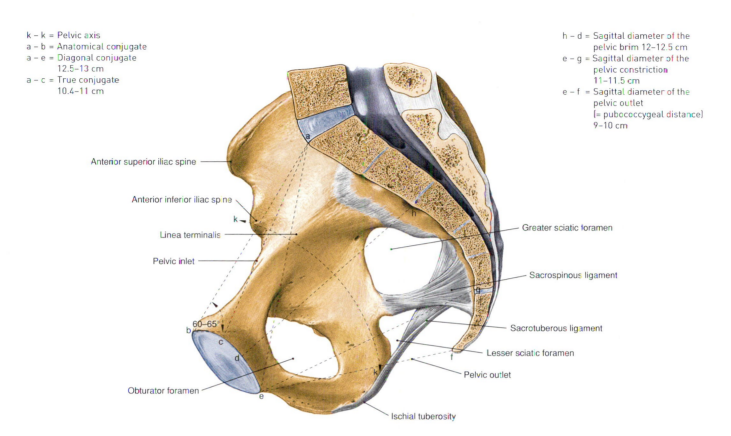

Anterior superior iliac spine
Anterior inferior iliac spine
Linea terminalis
Pelvic inlet

60–65°

Obturator foramen
Ischial tuberosity

Greater sciatic foramen
Sacrospinous ligament
Sacrotuberous ligament
Lesser sciatic foramen
Pelvic outlet

Fig. 953 Pelvis;
dimensions in the female;
median section.

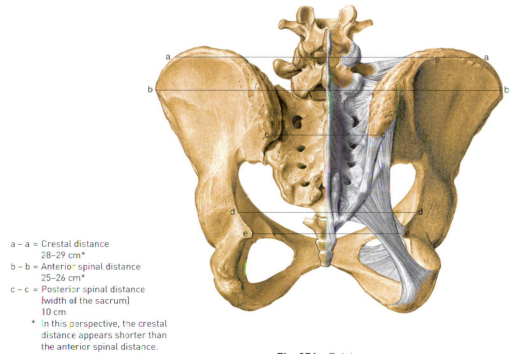

a – a = Crestal distance
          28–29 cm*
b – b = Anterior spinal distance
          25–26 cm*
c – c = Posterior spinal distance
          (width of the sacrum)
          10 cm
      * In this perspective, the crestal
          distance appears shorter than
          the anterior spinal distance.

d – d = Transverse diameter
          of the pelvic brim
          (= interacetabular line)
          12–12.5 cm
e – e = Transverse diameter of
          the pelvic constriction
          (= interspinal line)
          10.5 cm
f – f = Transverse diameter of
          the pelvic outlet
          (= tuberal diameter)
          11–12 cm

Fig. 954 Pelvis;
dimensions in the female.

Hip bone

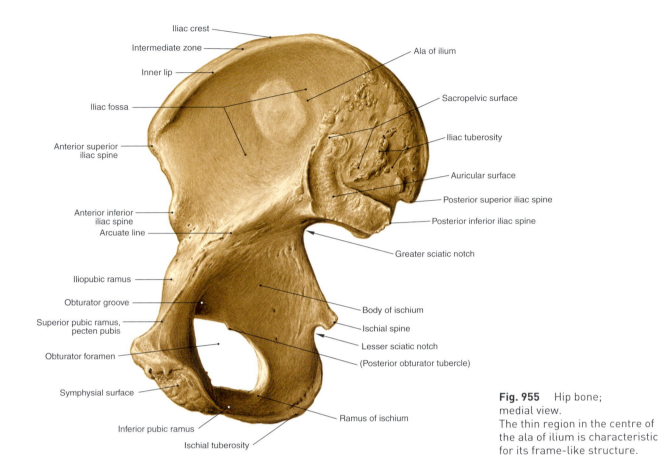

Iliac crest
Intermediate zone
Inner lip
Iliac fossa
Anterior superior iliac spine
Anterior inferior iliac spine
Arcuate line
Iliopubic ramus
Obturator groove
Superior pubic ramus, pecten pubis
Obturator foramen
Symphysial surface
Inferior pubic ramus
Ischial tuberosity

Ala of ilium
Sacropelvic surface
Iliac tuberosity
Auricular surface
Posterior superior iliac spine
Posterior inferior iliac spine
Greater sciatic notch
Body of ischium
Ischial spine
Lesser sciatic notch
(Posterior obturator tubercle)
Ramus of ischium

Fig. 955 Hip bone; medial view.
The thin region in the centre of the ala of ilium is characteristic for its frame-like structure.

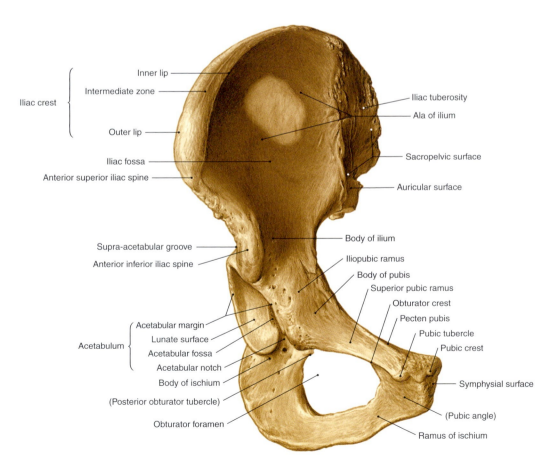

Iliac crest {
Inner lip
Intermediate zone
Outer lip
Iliac fossa
Anterior superior iliac spine

Supra-acetabular groove
Anterior inferior iliac spine

Acetabulum {
Acetabular margin
Lunate surface
Acetabular fossa
Acetabular notch
Body of ischium
(Posterior obturator tubercle)
Obturator foramen

Iliac tuberosity
Ala of ilium
Sacropelvic surface
Auricular surface
Body of ilium
Iliopubic ramus
Body of pubis
Superior pubic ramus
Obturator crest
Pecten pubis
Pubic tubercle
Pubic crest
Symphysial surface
(Pubic angle)
Ramus of ischium

Fig. 956 Hip bone; ventral view.

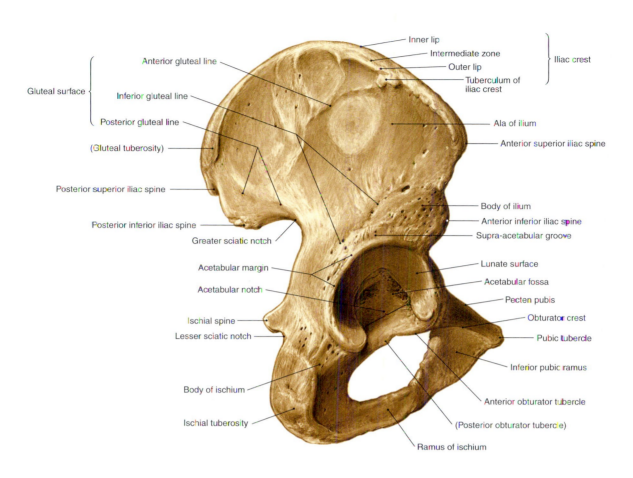

Inner lip
Intermediate zone
Outer lip
Iliac crest
Tuberculum of iliac crest

Anterior gluteal line
Gluteal surface
Inferior gluteal line
Posterior gluteal line
(Gluteal tuberosity)
Posterior superior iliac spine
Posterior inferior iliac spine
Greater sciatic notch
Acetabular margin
Acetabular notch
Ischial spine
Lesser sciatic notch
Body of ischium
Ischial tuberosity

Ala of ilium
Anterior superior iliac spine
Body of ilium
Anterior inferior iliac spine
Supra-acetabular groove
Lunate surface
Acetabular fossa
Pecten pubis
Obturator crest
Pubic tubercle
Inferior pubic ramus
Anterior obturator tubercle
(Posterior obturator tubercle)
Ramus of ischium

Fig. 957 Hip bone; dorsolateral view.

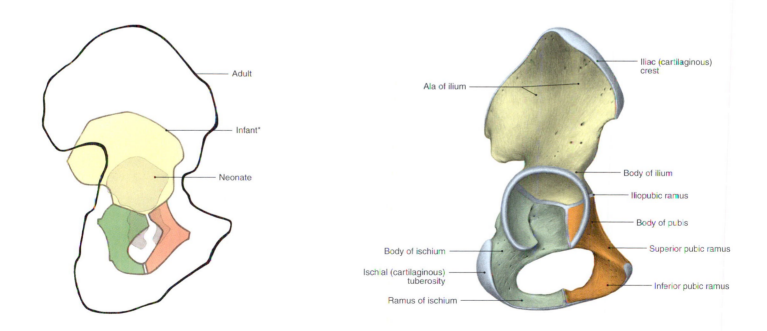

Adult
Infant*
Neonate

Fig. 958 Hip bone; development.

* Approximately sixth year of life

Iliac (cartilaginous) crest
Ala of ilium
Body of ilium
Iliopubic ramus
Body of pubis
Body of ischium
Superior pubic ramus
Ischial (cartilaginous) tuberosity
Inferior pubic ramus
Ramus of ischium

Fig. 959 Hip bone;
stage of development in a 6-year-old child.
In the acetabulum, the three parts of the hip bone are fused to a Y-shaped cartilaginous junction. This junction ossifies at the age of 13–18 years.

Joints of the pelvic girdle

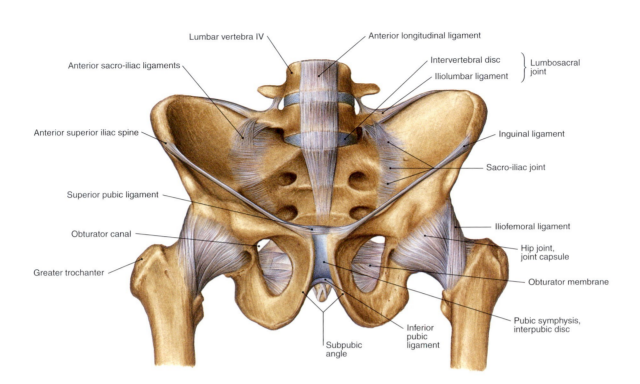

Lumbar vertebra IV

Anterior longitudinal ligament

Anterior sacro-iliac ligaments

Intervertebral disc ⎫ Lumbosacral
Iliolumbar ligament ⎬ joint

Anterior superior iliac spine

Inguinal ligament

Sacro-iliac joint

Superior pubic ligament

Obturator canal

Iliofemoral ligament

Greater trochanter

Hip joint, joint capsule

Obturator membrane

Pubic symphysis, interpubic disc

Subpubic angle

Inferior pubic ligament

Fig. 960 Joints of the pelvic girdle and the lumbosacral joint of the male.

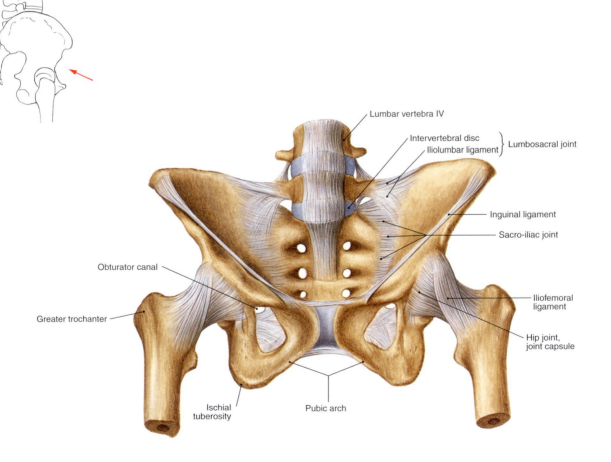

Lumbar vertebra IV

Intervertebral disc ⎫ Lumbosacral
Iliolumbar ligament ⎬ joint

Inguinal ligament

Sacro-iliac joint

Obturator canal

Iliofemoral ligament

Greater trochanter

Hip joint, joint capsule

Ischial tuberosity

Pubic arch

Fig. 961 Joints of the pelvic girdle and the lumbosacral joint of the female.

Joints of the pelvic girdle

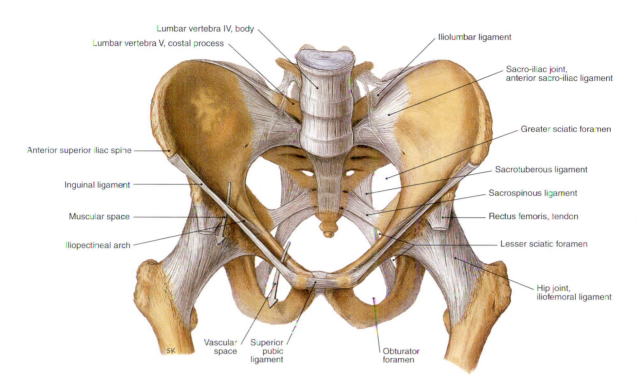

Lumbar vertebra IV, body
Lumbar vertebra V, costal process
Iliolumbar ligament
Sacro-iliac joint, anterior sacro-iliac ligament
Anterior superior iliac spine
Greater sciatic foramen
Inguinal ligament
Sacrotuberous ligament
Muscular space
Sacrospinous ligament
Iliopectineal arch
Rectus femoris, tendon
Lesser sciatic foramen
Hip joint, iliofemoral ligament
Vascular space
Superior pubic ligament
Obturator foramen

Fig. 962   Joints of the pelvic girdle and the lumbosacral joint of the male.

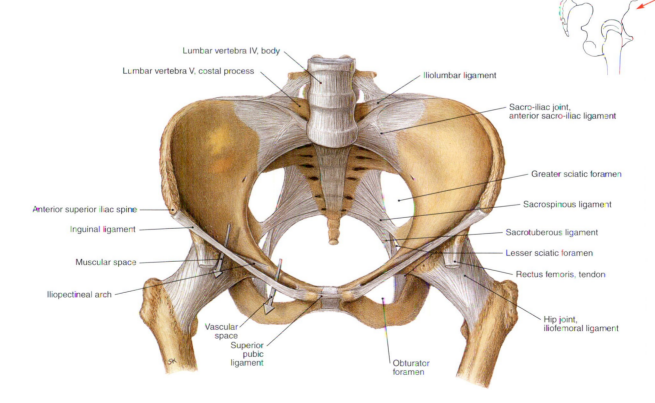

Lumbar vertebra IV, body
Lumbar vertebra V, costal process
Iliolumbar ligament
Sacro-iliac joint, anterior sacro-iliac ligament
Anterior superior iliac spine
Greater sciatic foramen
Inguinal ligament
Sacrospinous ligament
Muscular space
Sacrotuberous ligament
Iliopectineal arch
Lesser sciatic foramen
Rectus femoris, tendon
Vascular space
Hip joint, iliofemoral ligament
Superior pubic ligament
Obturator foramen

Fig. 963   Joints of the pelvic girdle and the lumbosacral joint of the female.

Joints of the pelvic girdle

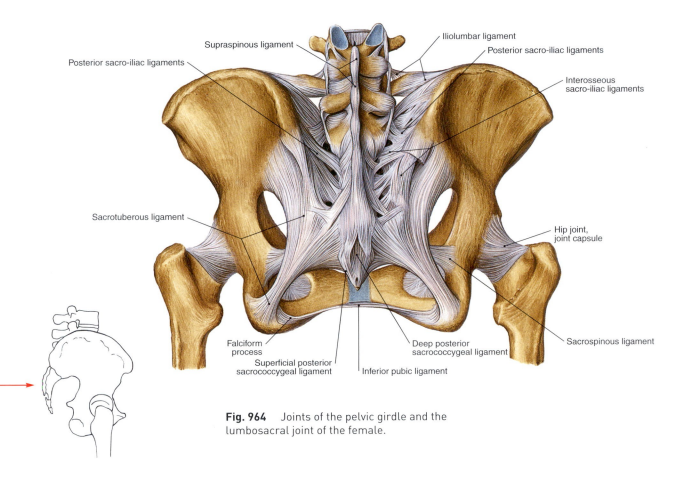

Supraspinous ligament

Posterior sacro-iliac ligaments

Iliolumbar ligament

Posterior sacro-iliac ligaments

Interosseous sacro-iliac ligaments

Sacrotuberous ligament

Hip joint, joint capsule

Falciform process

Deep posterior sacrococcygeal ligament

Superficial posterior sacrococcygeal ligament

Inferior pubic ligament

Sacrospinous ligament

Fig. 964   Joints of the pelvic girdle and the lumbosacral joint of the female.

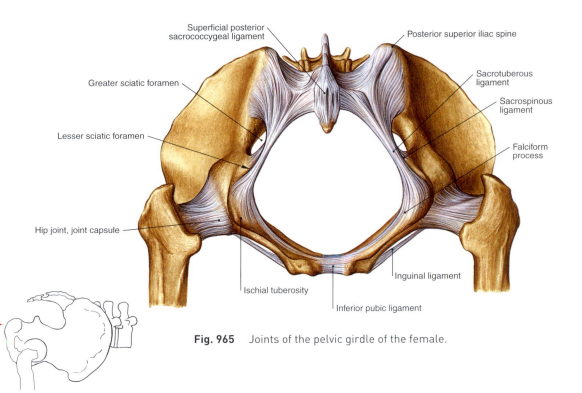

Superficial posterior sacrococcygeal ligament

Posterior superior iliac spine

Greater sciatic foramen

Sacrotuberous ligament

Sacrospinous ligament

Lesser sciatic foramen

Falciform process

Hip joint, joint capsule

Inguinal ligament

Ischial tuberosity

Inferior pubic ligament

Fig. 965   Joints of the pelvic girdle of the female.

Joints of the pelvic girdle

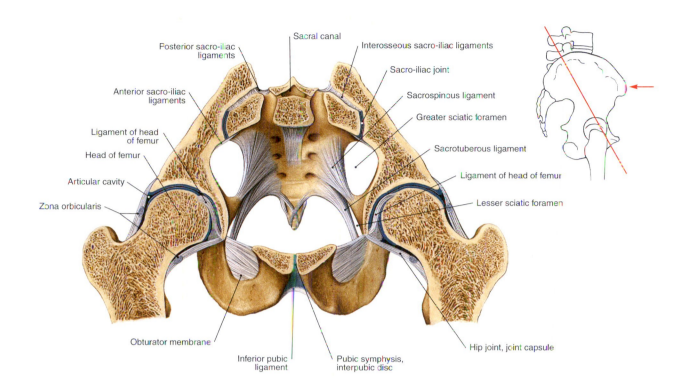

Fig. 966 Joints of the pelvic girdle
of the female.

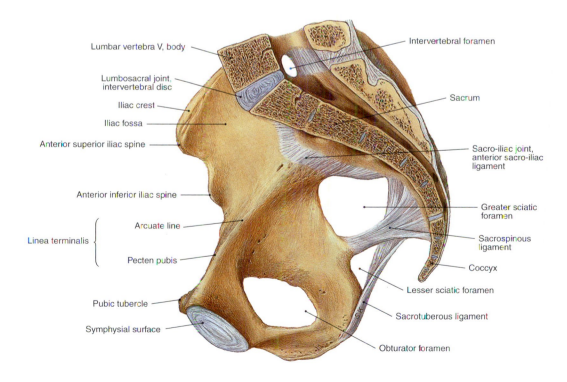

Fig. 967 Joints of the pelvic girdle and the
lumbosacral joint of the female;
median section.

Normally, the anterior border of the lowest intervertebral disc
forms the furthest projecting point of the posterior circumference
of the pelvic inlet. Radiographically, the most anterior part of the
sacrum is referred to as promontory.

Joints of the pelvic girdle

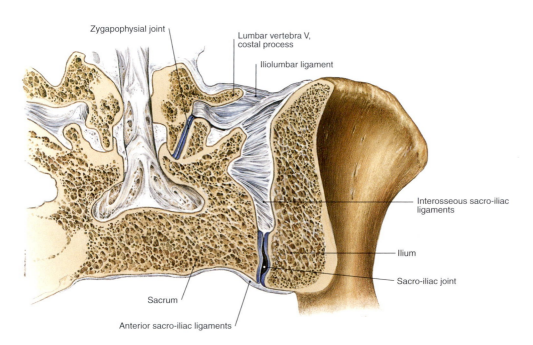

Fig. 968 Sacroiliac joint;
frontal section.

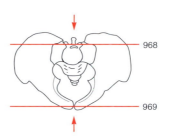

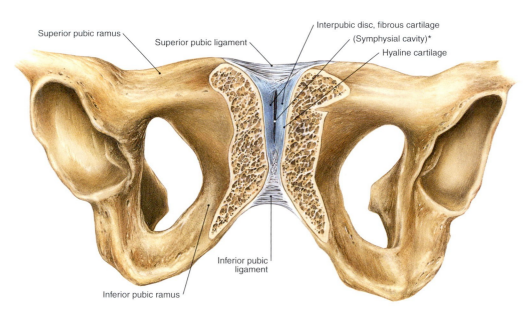

Fig. 969 Pubic symphysis;
oblique section in the direction of the longitudinal
axis of the symphysis.
The interpubic disc consists of fibrous cartilage, with
the exception of the articular symphysial surfaces of
both pubic bones that are covered with hyaline
cartilage. A longitudinal flat cleft occurs after the
first decade of life (*).

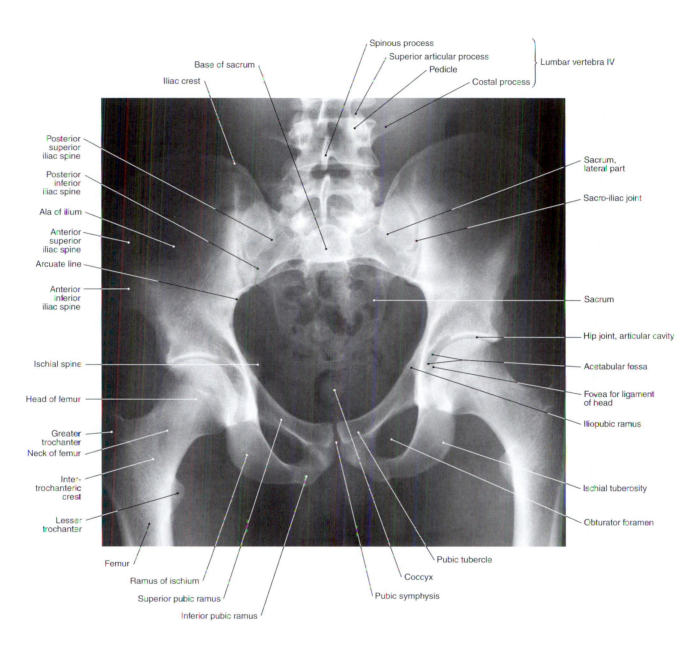

Spinous process

Superior articular process

Base of sacrum

Pedicle

Lumbar vertebra IV

Iliac crest

Costal process

Posterior superior iliac spine

Sacrum, lateral part

Posterior inferior iliac spine

Sacro-iliac joint

Ala of ilium

Anterior superior iliac spine

Arcuate line

Anterior inferior iliac spine

Sacrum

Hip joint, articular cavity

Ischial spine

Acetabular fossa

Head of femur

Fovea for ligament of head

Greater trochanter

Iliopubic ramus

Neck of femur

Inter-trochanteric crest

Ischial tuberosity

Lesser trochanter

Obturator foramen

Femur

Ramus of ischium

Pubic tubercle

Superior pubic ramus

Coccyx

Inferior pubic ramus

Pubic symphysis

Fig. 970   Pelvis of the male;
AP-radiograph with the central beam directed
onto the third sacral segment; upright position.

Pelvis, development

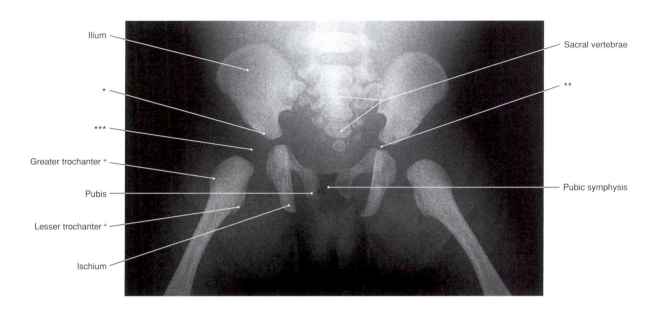

Fig. 971 Pelvis and femur;
AP-radiograph of a female, premature baby
(eighth month of pregnancy).

* Osseous roof of the acetabulum
** Y-shaped junction in the acetabular fossa
*** The ossification centre in the head of the femur does not appear
before the third to fifth month of life.
+ At this age, both greater trochanters only become apparent as small
protuberances of the bone of the diaphysis.

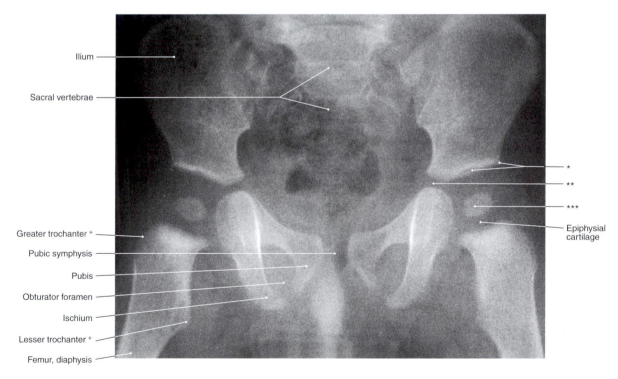

Fig. 972 Pelvis and femur;
AP-radiograph of a 12-month-old boy.

* Osseous roof of the acetabulum
** Y-shaped junction in the acetabular fossa
*** Ossification centre in the epiphysis of the head of the femur
+ At this age, both greater trochanters only become apparent as small
protuberances of the bone of the diaphysis.

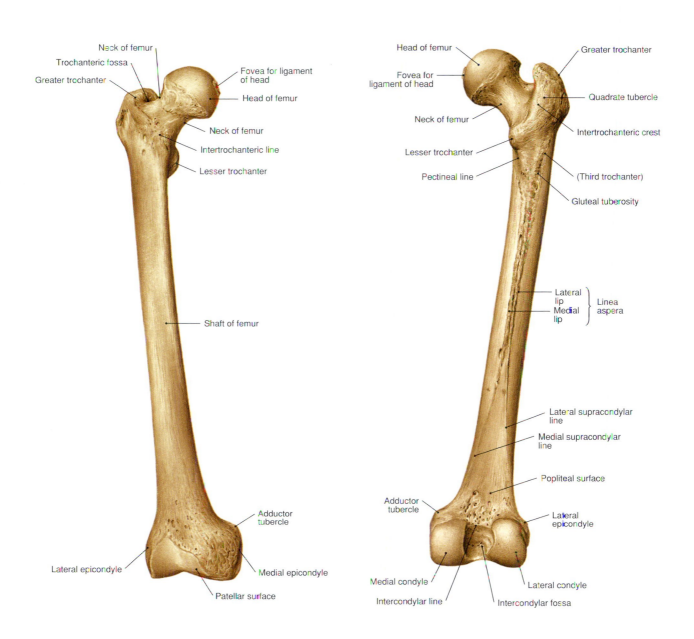

Fig. 973 Femur; ventral view.

Fig. 974 Femur; dorsal view.

Femur

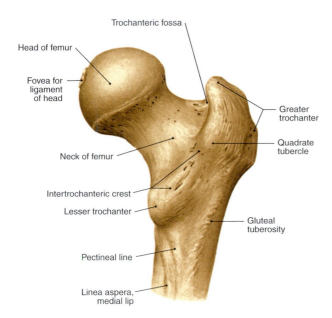

Fig. 975   Femur;
proximal extremity;
dorsal view.

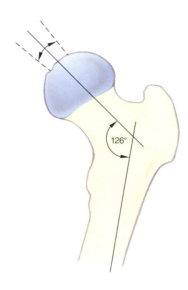

Fig. 976   Femur;
variability of the angle of the neck of the femur;
dorsal view.
The angle between the neck and the shaft of the femur is
referred to as neck-shaft angle. It is 150° in infants and about
126° in the adult.

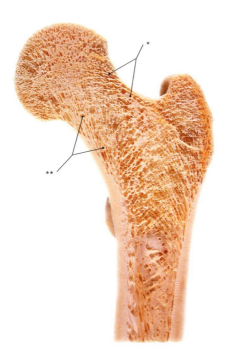

Fig. 977   Femur;
trabecular structure of the femoral bone with a large
neck-shaft angle; section in the plane of the angle of
anterior torsion (60%).
The lateral plates of the trabecular bone* („tensile system")
are only poorly developed, whereas the medial plates**
(„compressive system") are much stronger.

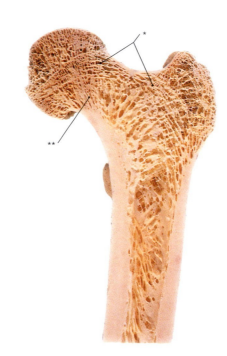

Fig. 978   Femur;
trabecular structure of the femoral bone with a small
neck-shaft angle (coxa vara); section in the plane of the
angle of anterior torsion (60%).
The lateral plates of the trabecular bone * („tensile system") are well developed, while the medial plates **
(„compressive system") are developed less strong. As a
result of the high demand of flexion, the cortex on the
inner side of the femoral neck is particularly thick.

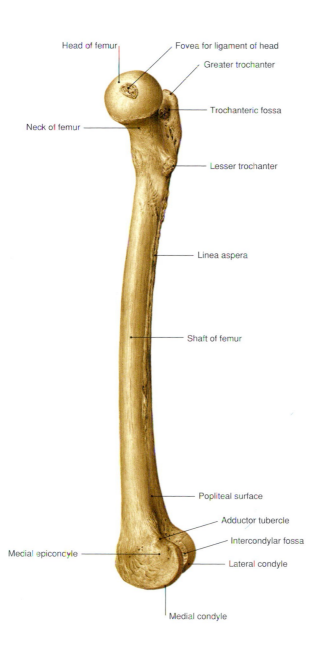

Head of femur

Fovea for ligament of head

Greater trochanter

Trochanteric fossa

Neck of femur

Lesser trochanter

Linea aspera

Shaft of femur

Popliteal surface

Adductor tubercle

Intercondylar fossa

Medial epiconcyle

Lateral condyle

Medial condyle

Fig. 979 Femur;
medial view.

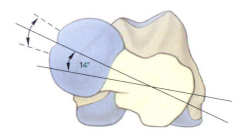

Fig. 980 Femur;
variability of the angle of anterior torsion; the proximal
end of the femur has been projected over the distal end;
proximal view.
The angle of anterior torsion is about 30° in infants
and about 14° in adults.

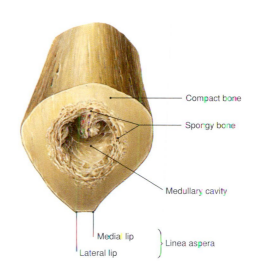

Compact bone

Sporgy bone

Medullary cavity

Medial lip } Linea aspera
Lateral lip

Fig. 981 Femur;
cross-section through the middle of the shaft;
distal view.

Hip joint

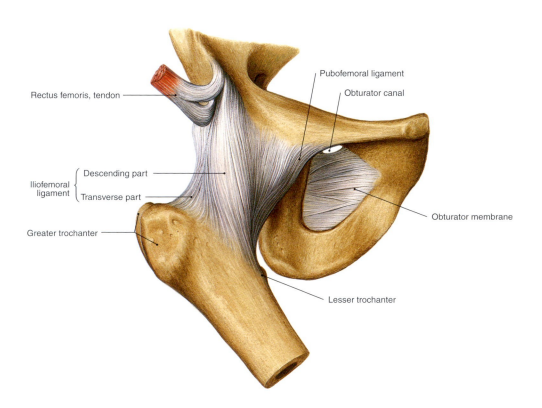

Rectus femoris, tendon

Pubofemoral ligament

Obturator canal

Iliofemoral ligament
- Descending part
- Transverse part

Greater trochanter

Obturator membrane

Lesser trochanter

Fig. 982   Hip joint;
ventrodistal view.

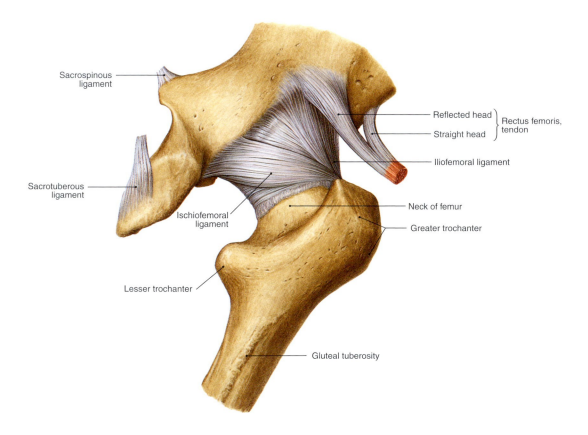

Sacrospinous ligament

Reflected head
Straight head
} Rectus femoris, tendon

Iliofemoral ligament

Sacrotuberous ligament

Ischiofemoral ligament

Neck of femur

Greater trochanter

Lesser trochanter

Gluteal tuberosity

Fig. 983   Hip joint;
dorsal view.

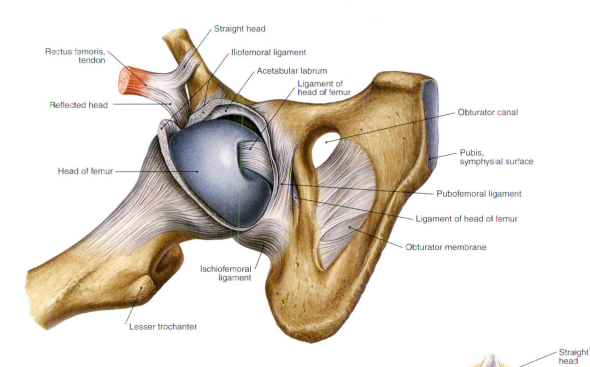

Fig. 984 Hip joint;
the articular capsule has been opened and the
head of the femur has been partly exarticulated;
laterodistal view.

Fig. 985 Hip joint;
aspect of the acetabulum after removal of the articular
capsule and exarticulation of the head of the femur;
laterodistal view.

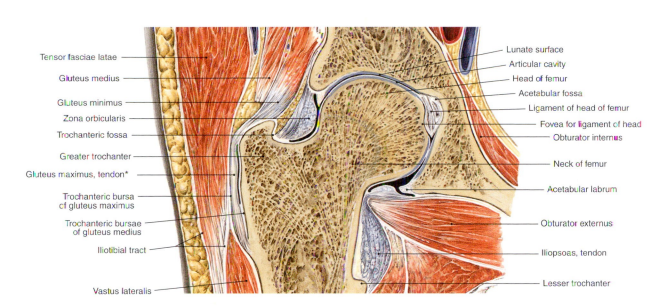

Fig. 986 Hip joint;
vertical section at the plane of the angle of antetorsion.

* Radiations into the iliotibial tract

Hip joint, radiography

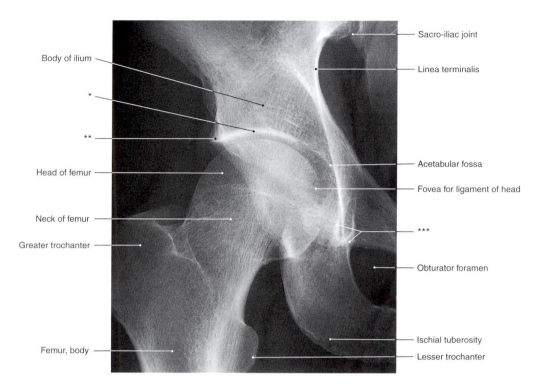

Body of ilium

*

**

Head of femur

Neck of femur

Greater trochanter

Femur, body

Sacro-iliac joint

Linea terminalis

Acetabular fossa

Fovea for ligament of head

***

Obturator foramen

Ischial tuberosity

Lesser trochanter

Fig. 987   Hip joint;
AP-radiograph; upright position on both legs.

*   Clinical term: acetabular roof = tangential projection of the lunate surface
**   Clinical term: edge of the acetabular roof = the most lateral projection
      of the acetabulum
*** Clinical term: KÖHLER's teardrop = projection of the acetabular fossa

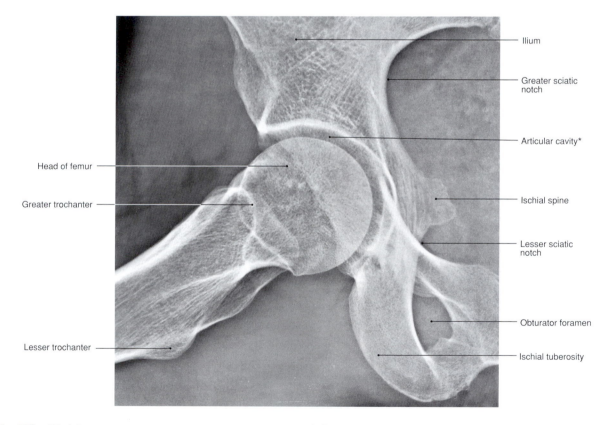

Head of femur

Greater trochanter

Lesser trochanter

Ilium

Greater sciatic
notch

Articular cavity*

Ischial spine

Lesser sciatic
notch

Obturator foramen

Ischial tuberosity

Fig. 988   Hip joint;
AP-radiograph; supine position with the thigh abducted
and flexed (so-called LAUENSTEIN projection).

*   Due to minimal absorption of X-rays by cartilage, the articular cleft
    appears abnormally broad.

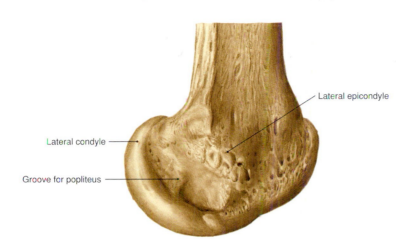

Fig. 989 Femur;
distal extremity;
lateral view.

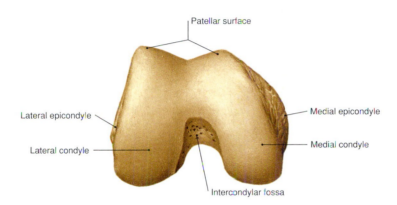

Fig. 990 Femur;
distal extremity;
distal view.

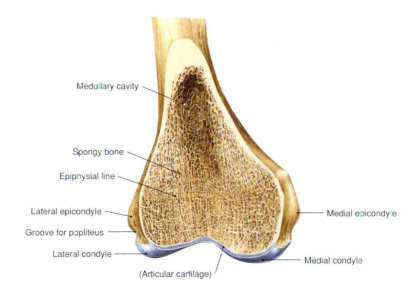

Fig. 991 Femur;
frontal section through the distal part;
ventral view.

Tibia

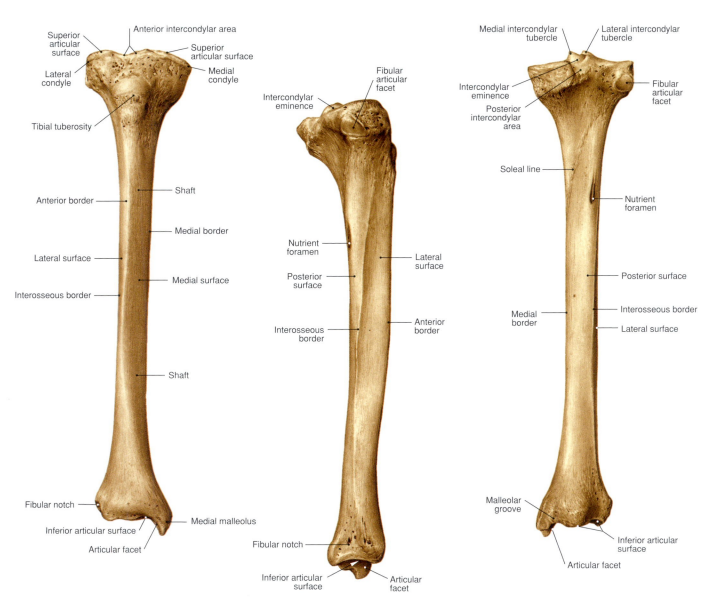

Fig. 992 Tibia;
ventral view.

Fig. 993 Tibia;
lateral view.

Fig. 994 Tibia;
dorsal view.

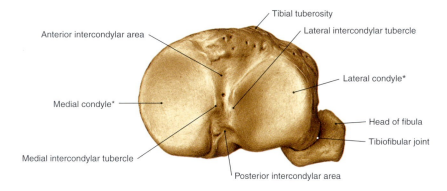

Fig. 995 Tibia and fibula;
proximal view.

* The articular surfaces of the condyles together are referred to as
superior articular surface.

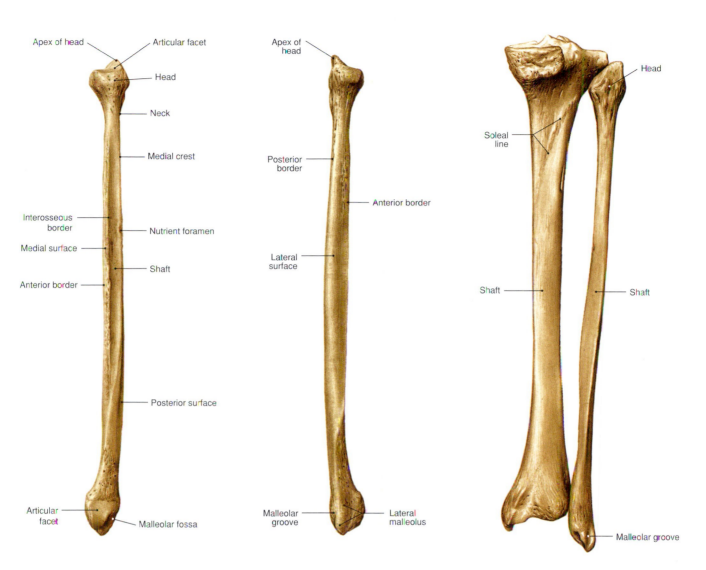

Fig. 996 Fibula;
medial view.

Fig. 997 Fibula;
lateral view.

Fig. 998 Tibia, and fibula;
dorsal view.

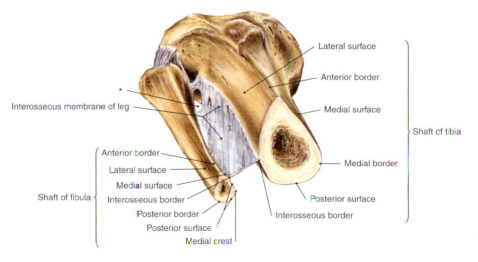

Fig. 999 Tibia and fibula;
cross-section with the interosseous membrane of leg;
distal view.

* Opening for the anterior tibial artery

Patella and knee joint

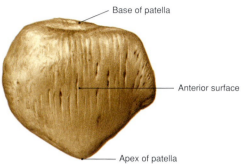

Base of patella

Anterior surface

Apex of patella

Fig. 1000 Patella;
ventral view.

Base of patella

Articular surface

Apex of patella

Fig. 1001 Patella;
dorsal view.

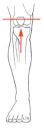

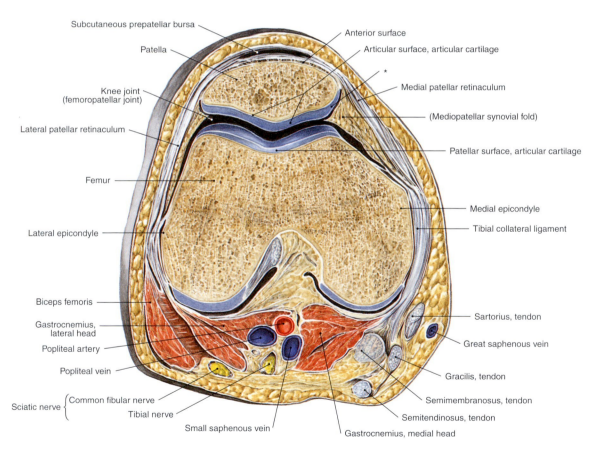

Subcutaneous prepatellar bursa

Patella

Knee joint
(femoropatellar joint)

Lateral patellar retinaculum

Femur

Lateral epicondyle

Biceps femoris

Gastrocnemius,
lateral head

Popliteal artery

Popliteal vein

Sciatic nerve { Common fibular nerve

Tibial nerve

Small saphenous vein

Anterior surface

Articular surface, articular cartilage

*

Medial patellar retinaculum

(Mediopatellar synovial fold)

Patellar surface, articular cartilage

Medial epicondyle

Tibial collateral ligament

Sartorius, tendon

Great saphenous vein

Gracilis, tendon

Semimembranosus, tendon

Semitendinosus, tendon

Gastrocnemius, medial head

Fig. 1002 Knee joint;
cross-section.

* Medial border facet

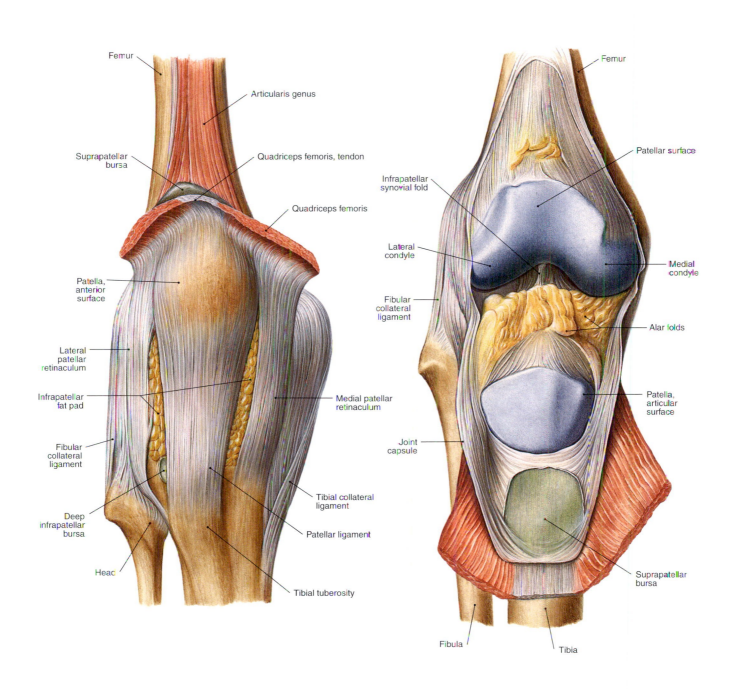

Fig. 1003 Knee joint;
intact articular capsule;
ventral view.

Fig. 1004 Knee joint;
the anterior part of the articular capsule has
been reflected downwards after dissection of
the quadriceps muscle;
the suprapatellar bursa has been opened;
ventral view.

Knee joint

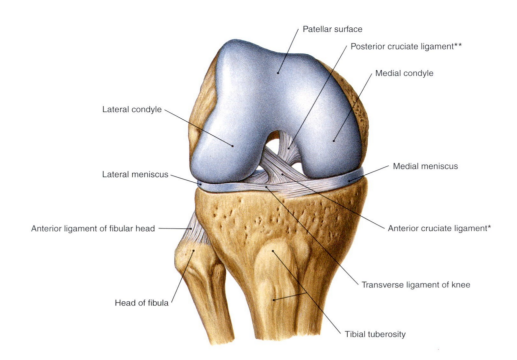

Fig. 1005 Knee joint;
in 90° flexion; the articular capsule and the lateral
ligaments have been removed;
ventral view.

* Clinical term: ACL (= anterior cruciate ligament)
** Clinical term: PCL (= posterior cruciate ligament)

Labels for Fig. 1005:
- Patellar surface
- Posterior cruciate ligament**
- Medial condyle
- Lateral condyle
- Lateral meniscus
- Medial meniscus
- Anterior ligament of fibular head
- Anterior cruciate ligament*
- Head of fibula
- Transverse ligament of knee
- Tibial tuberosity

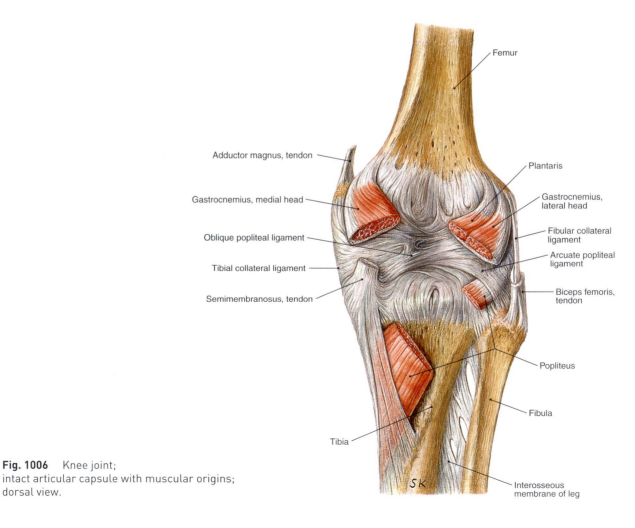

Fig. 1006 Knee joint;
intact articular capsule with muscular origins;
dorsal view.

Labels for Fig. 1006:
- Femur
- Adductor magnus, tendon
- Plantaris
- Gastrocnemius, medial head
- Gastrocnemius, lateral head
- Oblique popliteal ligament
- Fibular collateral ligament
- Tibial collateral ligament
- Arcuate popliteal ligament
- Semimembranosus, tendon
- Biceps femoris, tendon
- Popliteus
- Fibula
- Tibia
- Interosseous membrane of leg

SK

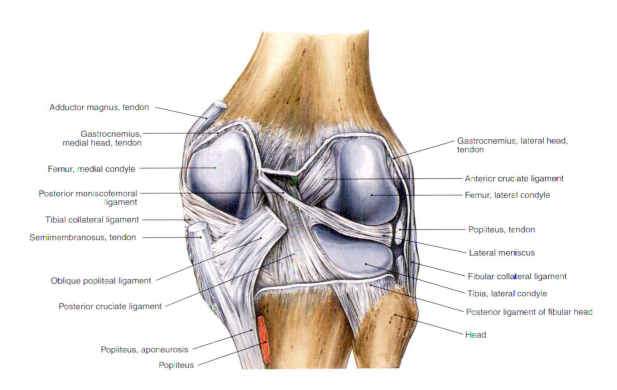

Adductor magnus, tendon
Gastrocnemius, medial head, tendon
Femur, medial condyle
Posterior meniscofemoral ligament
Tibial collateral ligament
Semimembranosus, tendon
Oblique popliteal ligament
Posterior cruciate ligament
Popliteus, aponeurosis
Popliteus

Gastrocnemius, lateral head, tendon
Anterior cruciate ligament
Femur, lateral condyle
Popliteus, tendon
Lateral meniscus
Fibular collateral ligament
Tibia, lateral condyle
Posterior ligament of fibular head
Head

Fig. 1007 Knee joint;
exposure of the cruciate ligaments and the menisci;
dorsal view.

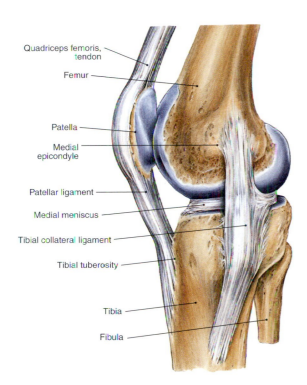

Quadriceps femoris, tendon
Femur
Patella
Medial epicondyle
Patellar ligament
Medial meniscus
Tibial collateral ligament
Tibial tuberosity
Tibia
Fibula

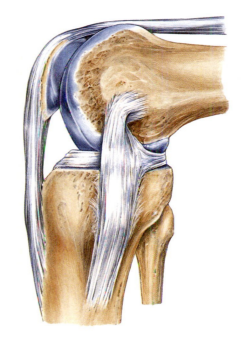

Fig. 1008 Tibial collateral ligament;
knee in extended position;
medial view.
Only the posterior fibres of the tibial collateral ligament are
attached to the medial meniscus.

Fig. 1009 Tibial collateral ligament;
knee in flexed position (90°);
medial view.
In the course of flexion, the posterior and proximal fibres of the
tibial collateral ligament become twisted, thereby stabilizing
the medial meniscus.

Knee joint

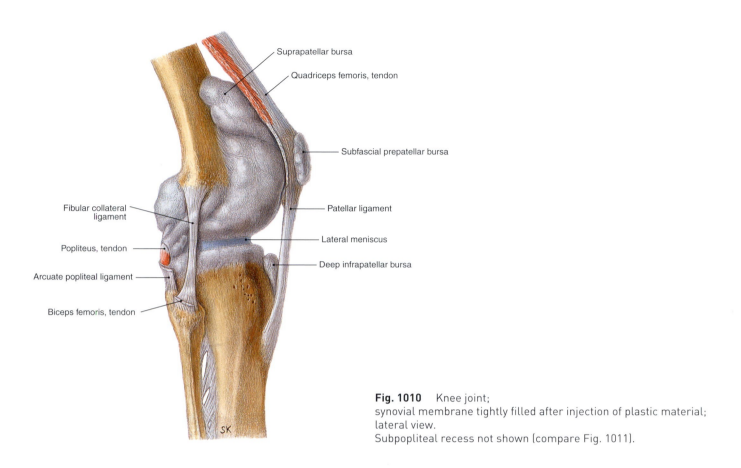

Fig. 1010   Knee joint;
synovial membrane tightly filled after injection of plastic material;
lateral view.
Subpopliteal recess not shown (compare Fig. 1011).

Labels for Fig. 1010:
- Suprapatellar bursa
- Quadriceps femoris, tendon
- Subfascial prepatellar bursa
- Patellar ligament
- Lateral meniscus
- Deep infrapatellar bursa
- Fibular collateral ligament
- Popliteus, tendon
- Arcuate popliteal ligament
- Biceps femoris, tendon

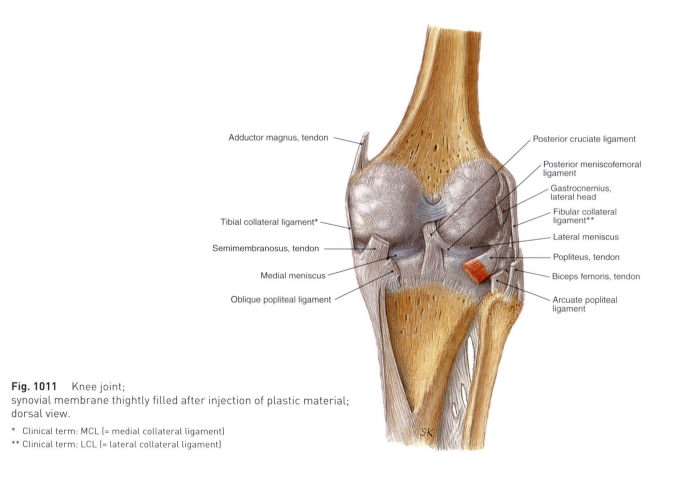

Labels for Fig. 1011:
- Adductor magnus, tendon
- Posterior cruciate ligament
- Posterior meniscofemoral ligament
- Gastrocnemius, lateral head
- Fibular collateral ligament**
- Lateral meniscus
- Tibial collateral ligament*
- Popliteus, tendon
- Semimembranosus, tendon
- Biceps femoris, tendon
- Medial meniscus
- Arcuate popliteal ligament
- Oblique popliteal ligament

Fig. 1011   Knee joint;
synovial membrane thightly filled after injection of plastic material;
dorsal view.

*   Clinical term: MCL (= medial collateral ligament)
** Clinical term: LCL (= lateral collateral ligament)

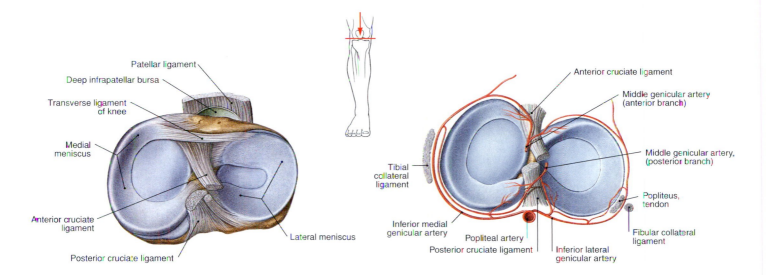

Fig. 1012 Menisci of the knee joint
and cruciate ligaments;
proximal view.

Fig. 1013 Menisci of the knee joint;
arterial supply;
proximal view.

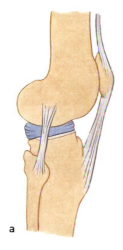

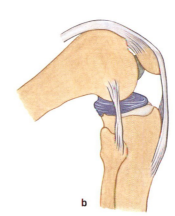

Fig. 1014 a, b Displacement of the menisci during flexion;
lateral view.

a Extended position
b Flexed position

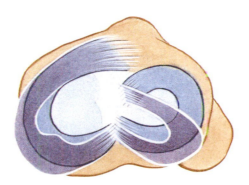

Fig. 1015 Displacement of the menisci during flexion;
proximal view.
In flexion, both menisci are displaced posteriorly over the
edges of the tibial condyles. The greater mobility of the lateral
meniscus accounts for its lesser risk of damage.

Knee joint, sections

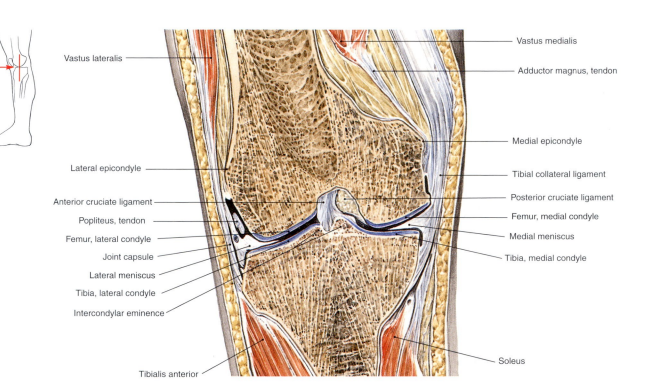

Vastus lateralis

Vastus medialis

Adductor magnus, tendon

Medial epicondyle

Lateral epicondyle

Tibial collateral ligament

Anterior cruciate ligament

Posterior cruciate ligament

Popliteus, tendon

Femur, medial condyle

Femur, lateral condyle

Medial meniscus

Joint capsule

Tibia, medial condyle

Lateral meniscus

Tibia, lateral condyle

Intercondylar eminence

Soleus

Tibialis anterior

Fig. 1016   Knee joint;
frontal section.

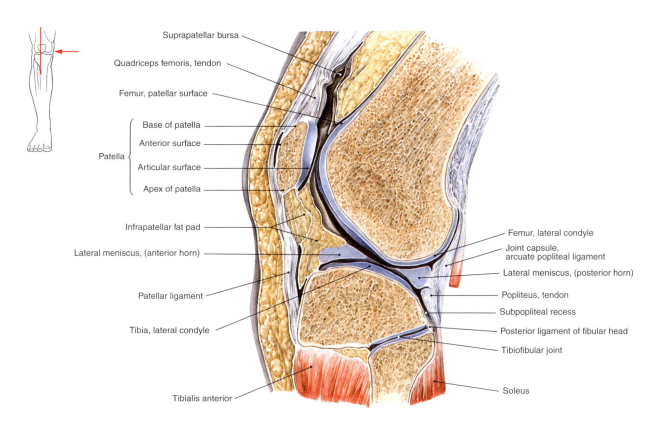

Suprapatellar bursa

Quadriceps femoris, tendon

Femur, patellar surface

Base of patella

Anterior surface

Patella {

Articular surface

Apex of patella

Infrapatellar fat pad

Femur, lateral condyle

Lateral meniscus, (anterior horn)

Joint capsule,
arcuate popliteal ligament

Lateral meniscus, (posterior horn)

Popliteus, tendon

Patellar ligament

Subpopliteal recess

Posterior ligament of fibular head

Tibia, lateral condyle

Tibiofibular joint

Soleus

Tibialis anterior

Fig. 1017   Knee joint;
sagittal section through the lateral part of the joint.

Knee joint, radiography

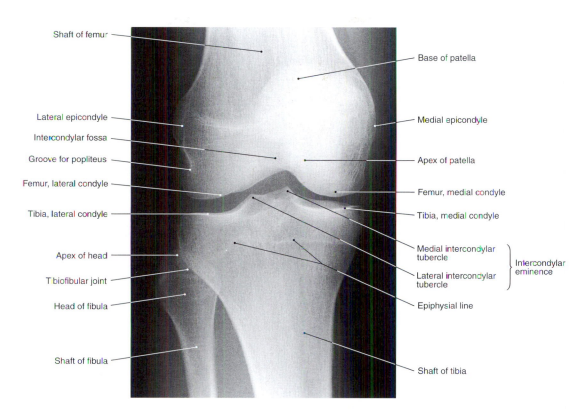

Shaft of femur

Base of patella

Lateral epicondyle

Medial epicondyle

Intercondylar fossa

Groove for popliteus

Apex of patella

Femur, lateral condyle

Tibia, lateral condyle

Femur, medial condyle

Tibia, medial condyle

Apex of head

Medial intercondylar tubercle

Tibiofibular joint

Lateral intercondylar tubercle

Intercondylar eminence

Head of fibula

Epiphysial line

Shaft of fibula

Shaft of tibia

Fig. 1018 Knee joint;
AP-radiograph with the central beam directed onto
the middle of the joint; subject reclined.

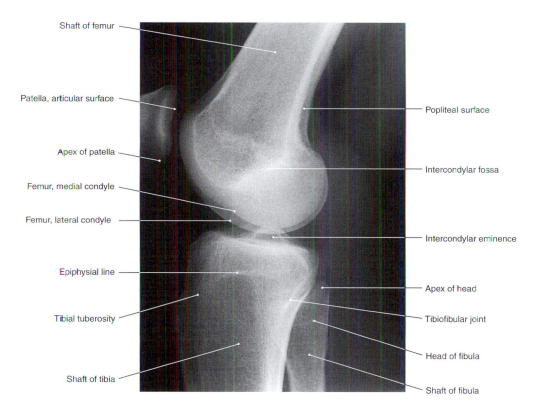

Shaft of femur

Patella, articular surface

Popliteal surface

Apex of patella

Intercondylar fossa

Femur, medial condyle

Femur, lateral condyle

Intercondylar eminence

Epiphysial line

Apex of head

Tibial tuberosity

Tibiofibular joint

Head of fibula

Shaft of tibia

Shaft of fibula

Fig. 1019 Knee joint;
lateral radiograph with the central beam directed onto
the middle of the joint; subject reclined.

Knee joint, arthroscopy

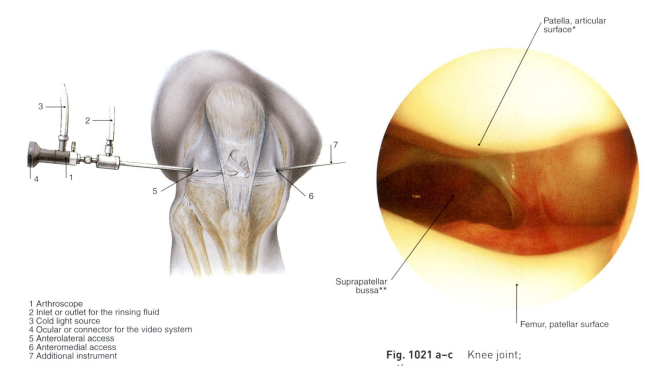

1 Arthroscope
2 Inlet or outlet for the rinsing fluid
3 Cold light source
4 Ocular or connector for the video system
5 Anterolateral access
6 Anteromedial access
7 Additional instrument

Fig. 1020   Accesses for arthroscopy.

Fig. 1021 a–c   Knee joint; arthroscopy.

a   Distal view into the femoropatellar joint

* Patellar roof ridge: ridge between the medial and lateral articular surfaces

** Clinical term: suprapatellar recess

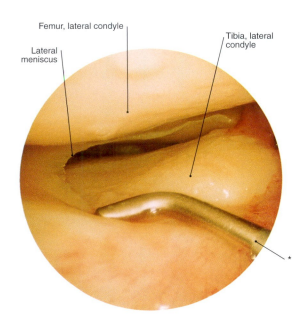

b   Medial view of the free inner edge of the lateral meniscus;
retractor (*) slightly depressing the anterior part of the meniscus

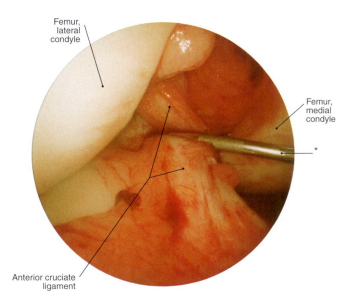

c   Anterolateral view of the distal part of the anterior cruciate ligament.
The ligament is covered by a richly vascularized synovial membrane. It is drawn medially by a retractor (*).

Knee joint, imaging

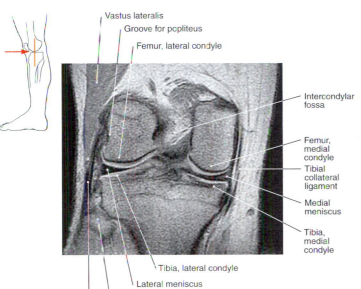

Vastus lateralis
Groove for popliteus
Femur, lateral condyle

Intercondylar fossa

Femur, medial condyle

Tibial collateral ligament

Medial meniscus

Tibia, medial condyle

Tibia, lateral condyle
Lateral meniscus
Head of fibula
Fibular collateral ligament

Fig. 1022 Knee joint;
magnetic resonance tomographic image (MRI);
frontal section;
knee in the extended position.
In this imaging technique, compact bone appears black.

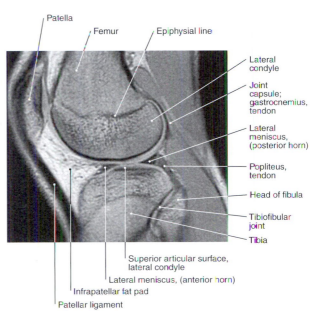

Patella
Femur
Epiphysial line

Lateral condyle

Joint capsule; gastrocnemius, tendon

Lateral meniscus, (posterior horn)

Popliteus, tendon

Head of fibula

Tibiofibular joint

Tibia

Superior articular surface, lateral condyle
Lateral meniscus, (anterior horn)
Infrapatellar fat pad
Patellar ligament

Fig. 1023 Knee joint;
magnetic resonance tomographic image (MRI);
sagittal section through the lateral part of the joint;
knee in the extended position.

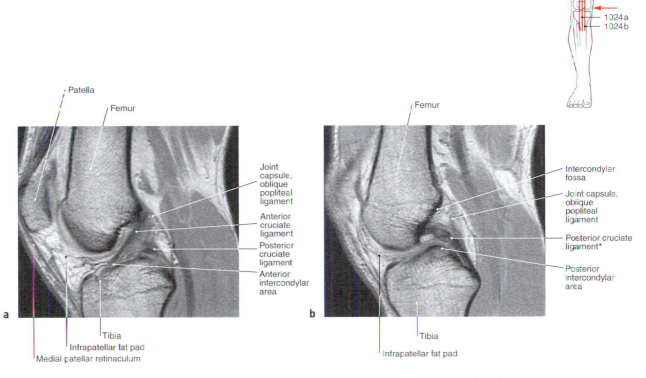

Patella
Femur

Joint capsule, oblique popliteal ligament

Anterior cruciate ligament

Posterior cruciate ligament

Anterior intercondylar area

a

Tibia
Infrapatellar fat pad
Medial patellar retinaculum

Femur

Intercondylar fossa

Joint capsule, oblique popliteal ligament

Posterior cruciate ligament*

Posterior intercondylar area

b

Tibia
Infrapatellar fat pad

Fig. 1024 a, b Knee joint;
magnetic resonance tomographic image (MRI);
sagittal sections to demonstrate the cruciate ligaments;
knee in the extended position.

a Anterior cruciate ligament (ACL)
b Posterior cruciate ligament (PCL)

* The inhomogeneity is due to oblique sectioning of the fibre bundles.

Joints of the bones of the leg

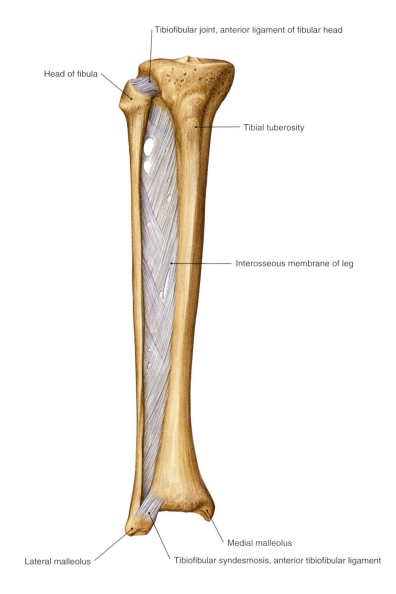

Tibiofibular joint, anterior ligament of fibular head

Head of fibula

Tibial tuberosity

Interosseous membrane of leg

Medial malleolus

Lateral malleolus

Tibiofibular syndesmosis, anterior tibiofibular ligament

Fig. 1025   Joints of the bones of the leg; ventral view.

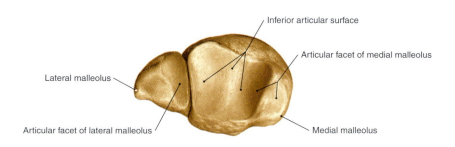

Inferior articular surface

Articular facet of medial malleolus

Lateral malleolus

Medial malleolus

Articular facet of lateral malleolus

Fig. 1026   Tibia and fibula; distal view.

Skeleton of the foot

Fig. 1027 Skeleton of the foot; proximal view.

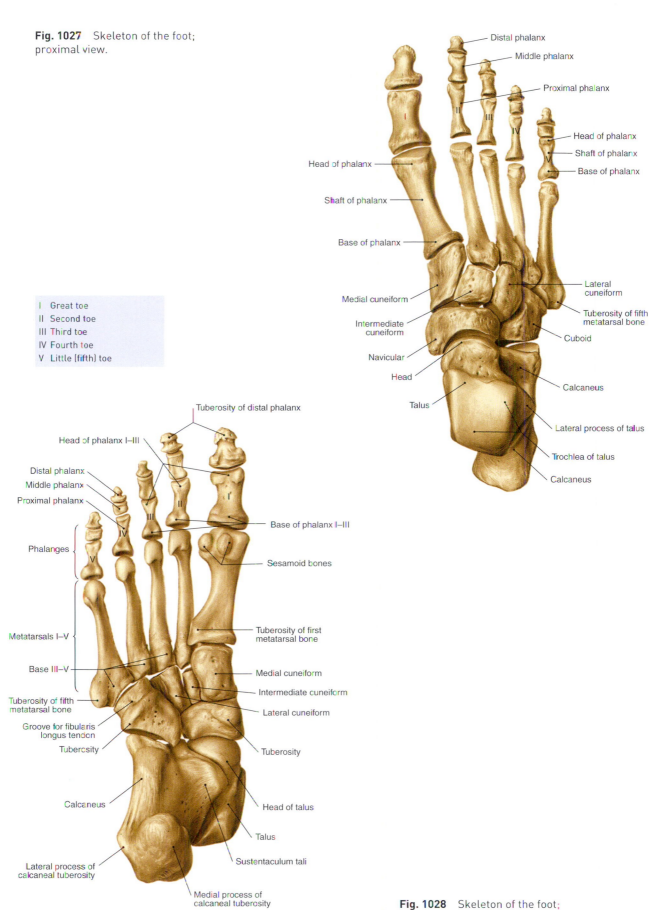

Distal phalanx
Middle phalanx
Proximal phalanx
Head of phalanx
Shaft of phalanx
Base of phalanx
Head of phalanx
Shaft of phalanx
Base of phalanx
Lateral cuneiform
Medial cuneiform
Intermediate cuneiform
Tuberosity of fifth metatarsal bone
Cuboid
Navicular
Head
Calcaneus
Talus
Lateral process of talus
Trochlea of talus
Calcaneus

I Great toe
II Second toe
III Third toe
IV Fourth toe
V Little (fifth) toe

Tuberosity of distal phalanx
Head of phalanx I–III
Distal phalanx
Middle phalanx
Proximal phalanx
Phalanges
Base of phalanx I–III
Sesamoid bones
Metatarsals I–V
Tuberosity of first metatarsal bone
Base III–V
Medial cuneiform
Tuberosity of fifth metatarsal bone
Intermediate cuneiform
Groove for fibularis longus tendon
Lateral cuneiform
Tuberosity
Tuberosity
Head of talus
Calcaneus
Talus
Sustentaculum tali
Lateral process of calcaneal tuberosity
Medial process of calcaneal tuberosity

Fig. 1028 Skeleton of the foot; plantar view.

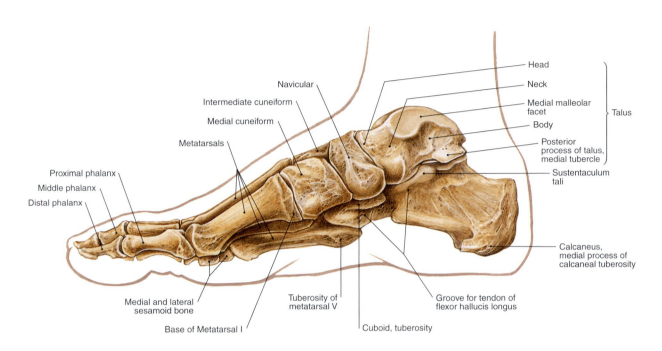

Fig. 1029   Skeleton of the foot;
medial view.

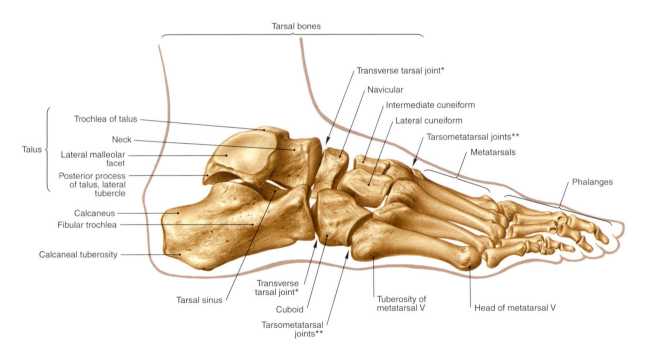

Fig. 1030   Skeleton of the foot;
lateral view.

*   Also: CHOPART´s joint
** Also: LISFRANC´s joint

Tatus and calcaneus

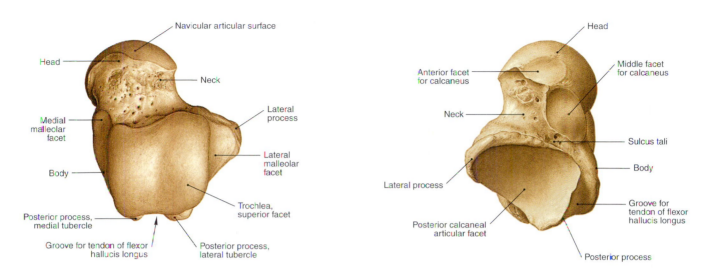

Navicular articular surface

Head

Neck

Medial malleolar facet

Body

Lateral process

Lateral malleolar facet

Posterior process, medial tubercle

Trochlea, superior facet

Groove for tendon of flexor hallucis longus

Posterior process, lateral tubercle

Fig. 1031   Talus;
proximal view.

Head

Anterior facet for calcaneus

Middle facet for calcaneus

Neck

Sulcus tali

Body

Lateral process

Groove for tendon of flexor hallucis longus

Posterior calcaneal articular facet

Posterior process

Fig. 1032   Talus;
plantar view.

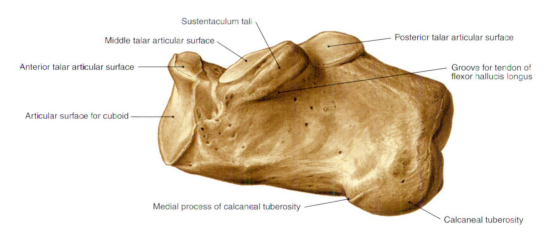

Sustentaculum tali

Middle talar articular surface

Posterior talar articular surface

Anterior talar articular surface

Groove for tendon of flexor hallucis longus

Articular surface for cuboid

Medial process of calcaneal tuberosity

Calcaneal tuberosity

Fig. 1033   Calcaneus;
medial view.

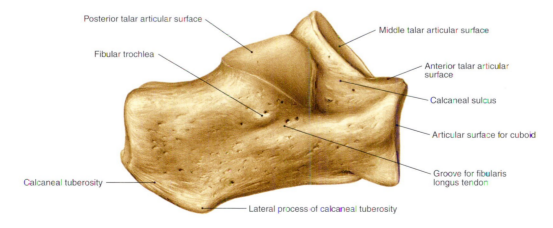

Posterior talar articular surface

Middle talar articular surface

Fibular trochlea

Anterior talar articular surface

Calcaneal sulcus

Articular surface for cuboid

Groove for fibularis longus tendon

Calcaneal tuberosity

Lateral process of calcaneal tuberosity

Fig. 1034   Calcaneus;
lateral view.

Tarsal bones

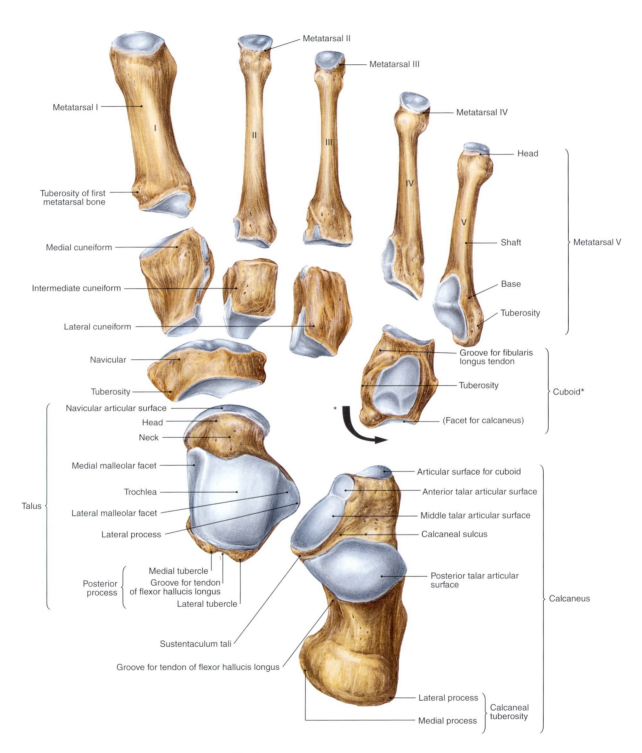

Fig. 1035 Tarsal bones and metatarsal bones; proximal view.

* The cuboid bone is shown in a medial view.

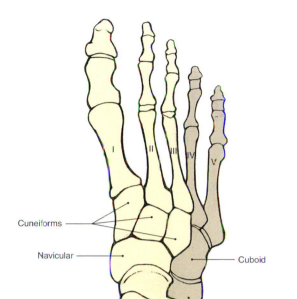

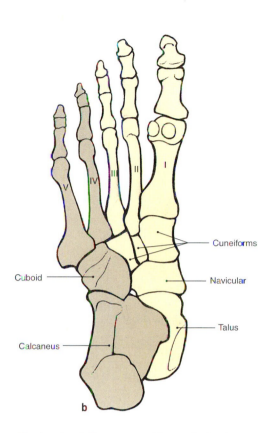

Fig. 1036 a, b Skeleton of the foot; structural organisation.
a Proximal view
b Plantar view

The heads of all metatarsal bones lie in the plantar plane. The cuneiform bones, the navicular bone and the talus rest upon the lateral parts of the skeleton, especially in the posterior part of the foot. The talus is therefore situated above the calcaneus and the longitudinal arch is formed.
The wedge-shaped cross-section of the cuneiform bones and the bases of the metatarsal bones contribute to the formation of the transverse vault.

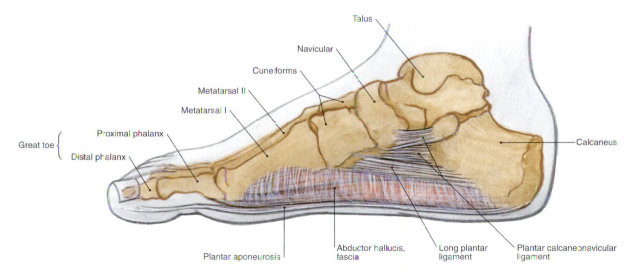

Fig. 1037 Supporting structures of the medial arch of the longitudinal vault of the foot; medial view.

The ligaments shown in this illustration are mostly directed in the longitudinal axis of the foot and support passively the longitudinal vault of the foot. The short muscles of the foot primarily support this construction.

Joints of the foot

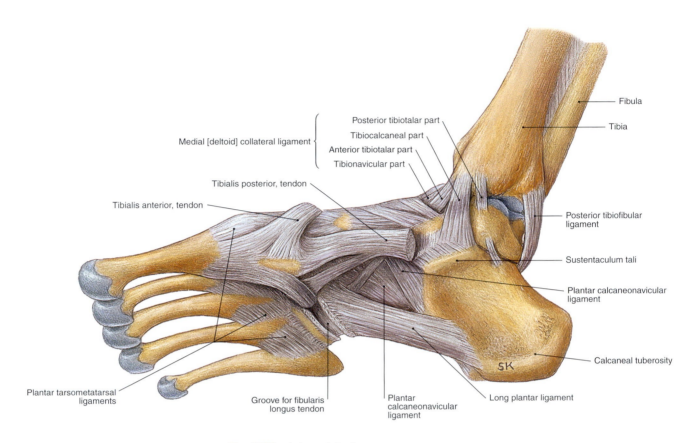

Medial [deltoid] collateral ligament {

Posterior tibiotalar part
Tibiocalcaneal part
Anterior tibiotalar part
Tibionavicular part

Tibialis posterior, tendon

Tibialis anterior, tendon

Fibula

Tibia

Posterior tibiofibular ligament

Sustentaculum tali

Plantar calcaneonavicular ligament

Calcaneal tuberosity

Plantar tarsometatarsal ligaments

Groove for fibularis longus tendon

Plantar calcaneonavicular ligament

Long plantar ligament

SK

Fig. 1038   Joints of the foot; ligaments and tendons; medial view.

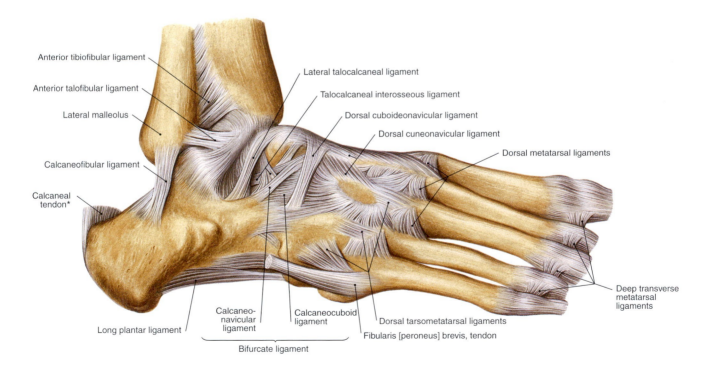

Anterior tibiofibular ligament

Anterior talofibular ligament

Lateral malleolus

Calcaneofibular ligament

Calcaneal tendon*

Long plantar ligament

Calcaneo-navicular ligament

Calcaneocuboid ligament

Bifurcate ligament

Lateral talocalcaneal ligament

Talocalcaneal interosseous ligament

Dorsal cuboideonavicular ligament

Dorsal cuneonavicular ligament

Dorsal metatarsal ligaments

Deep transverse metatarsal ligaments

Dorsal tarsometatarsal ligaments

Fibularis [peroneus] brevis, tendon

Fig. 1039   Joints of the foot; ligaments and tendons; lateral view.

*   Also: Achilles tendon

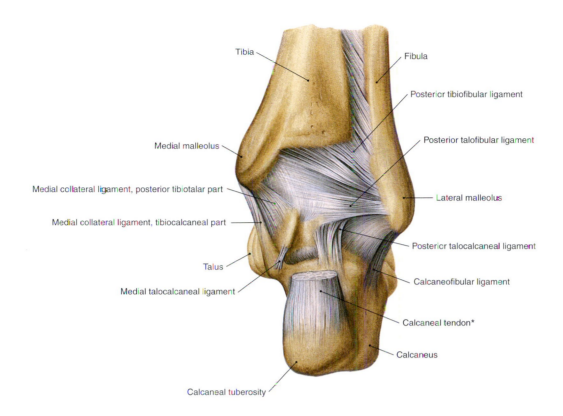

Fig. 1040 Joints of the foot;
ligaments and tendons of the posterior part of the foot.

* Also: Achilles tendon

Labels (Fig. 1040):
- Tibia
- Fibula
- Posterior tibiofibular ligament
- Posterior talofibular ligament
- Medial malleolus
- Lateral malleolus
- Medial collateral ligament, posterior tibiotalar part
- Medial collateral ligament, tibiocalcaneal part
- Posterior talocalcaneal ligament
- Talus
- Calcaneofibular ligament
- Medial talocalcaneal ligament
- Calcaneal tendon*
- Calcaneus
- Calcaneal tuberosity

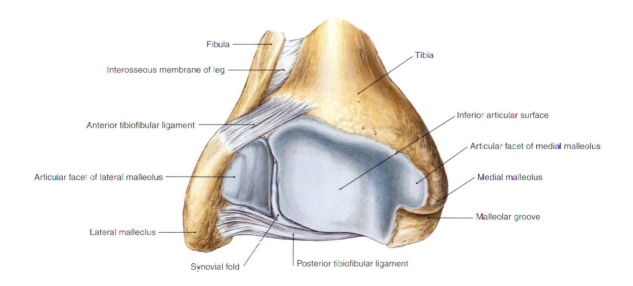

Fig. 1041 Ankle joint;
proximal articular surfaces;
distal view.

Labels (Fig. 1041):
- Fibula
- Tibia
- Interosseous membrane of leg
- Inferior articular surface
- Anterior tibiofibular ligament
- Articular facet of medial malleolus
- Articular facet of lateral malleolus
- Medial malleolus
- Malleolar groove
- Lateral malleolus
- Synovial fold
- Posterior tibiofibular ligament

Joints of the foot

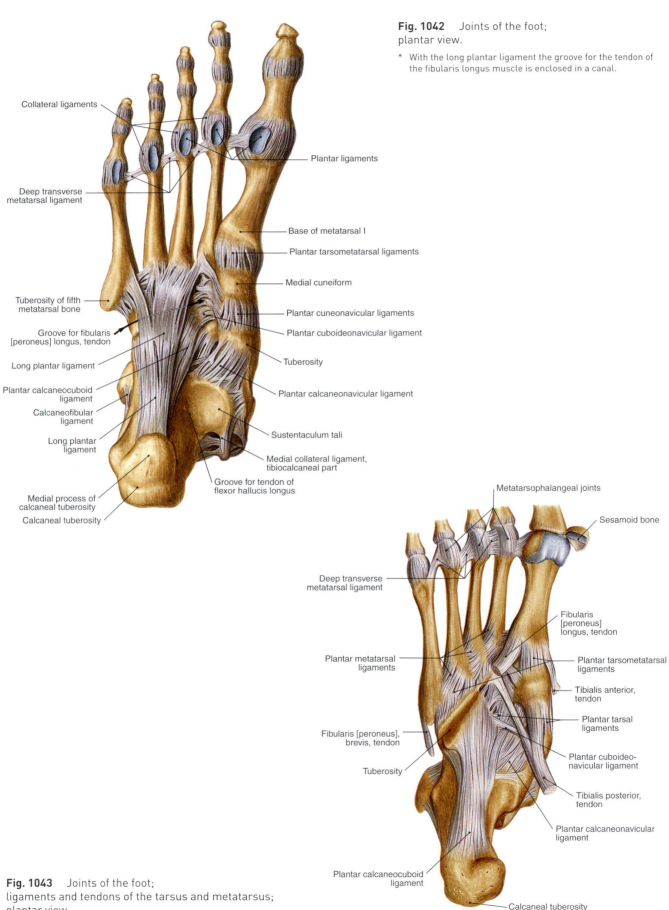

Collateral ligaments

Plantar ligaments

Deep transverse
metatarsal ligament

Base of metatarsal I

Plantar tarsometatarsal ligaments

Medial cuneiform

Tuberosity of fifth
metatarsal bone

Plantar cuneonavicular ligaments

Groove for fibularis
[peroneus] longus, tendon

Plantar cuboideonavicular ligament

Long plantar ligament

Tuberosity

Plantar calcaneocuboid
ligament

Plantar calcaneonavicular ligament

Calcaneofibular
ligament

Long plantar
ligament

Sustentaculum tali

Medial collateral ligament,
tibiocalcaneal part

Medial process of
calcaneal tuberosity

Groove for tendon of
flexor hallucis longus

Calcaneal tuberosity

Fig. 1042 Joints of the foot;
plantar view.

* With the long plantar ligament the groove for the tendon of
the fibularis longus muscle is enclosed in a canal.

Metatarsophalangeal joints

Sesamoid bone

Deep transverse
metatarsal ligament

Fibularis
[peroneus]
longus, tendon

Plantar metatarsal
ligaments

Plantar tarsometatarsal
ligaments

Tibialis anterior,
tendon

Plantar tarsal
ligaments

Fibularis [peroneus],
brevis, tendon

Plantar cuboideo-
navicular ligament

Tuberosity

Tibialis posterior,
tendon

Plantar calcaneonavicular
ligament

Plantar calcaneocuboid
ligament

Calcaneal tuberosity

Fig. 1043 Joints of the foot;
ligaments and tendons of the tarsus and metatarsus;
plantar view.

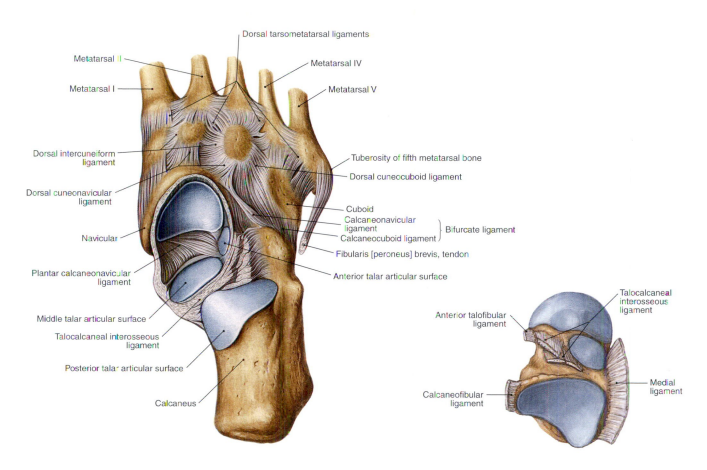

Dorsal tarsometatarsal ligaments

Metatarsal II

Metatarsal I

Dorsal intercuneiform ligament

Dorsal cuneonavicular ligament

Navicular

Plantar calcaneonavicular ligament

Middle talar articular surface

Talocalcaneal interosseous ligament

Posterior talar articular surface

Calcaneus

Metatarsal IV

Metatarsal V

Tuberosity of fifth metatarsal bone

Dorsal cuneocuboid ligament

Cuboid

Calcaneonavicular ligament
Calcaneocuboid ligament } Bifurcate ligament

Fibularis [peroneus] brevis, tendon

Anterior talar articular surface

Anterior talofibular ligament

Talocalcaneal interosseous ligament

Calcaneofibular ligament

Medial ligament

Fig. 1044 Talotarsal joint; distal articular surfaces; proximal view.

Fig. 1045 Talotarsal joint; proximal articular surfaces; distal view.

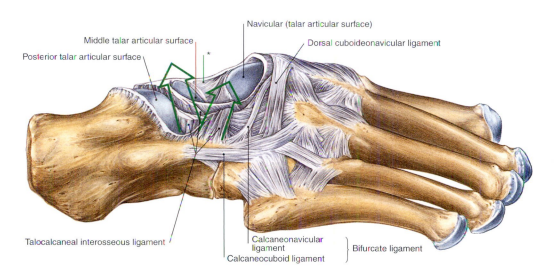

Navicular (talar articular surface)

Middle talar articular surface

Posterior talar articular surface

Dorsal cuboideonavicular ligament

Talocalcaneal interosseous ligament

Calcaneonavicular ligament
Calcaneocuboid ligament } Bifurcate ligament

Fig. 1046 Talotarsal joint;
the talus and the lateral ligaments have been removed; lateral view.
The two arrows point out the helical distorsion of the talocalcaneal interosseous ligament.

* Tight connective tissue layer between the plantar calcaneonavicular ligament and the tibionavicular part of the deltoid ligament limiting a medially directed gliding of the head of the talus; slackening of this layer results in flattening of the longitudinal vault (flat-foot, pes valgus)

Ankle and talotarsal joint, sections

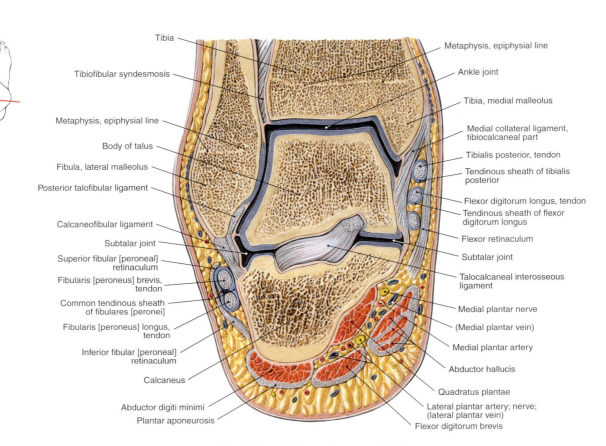

Tibia

Tibiofibular syndesmosis

Metaphysis, epiphysial line

Body of talus

Fibula, lateral malleolus

Posterior talofibular ligament

Calcaneofibular ligament

Subtalar joint

Superior fibular [peroneal] retinaculum

Fibularis [peroneus] brevis, tendon

Common tendinous sheath of fibulares [peronei]

Fibularis [peroneus] longus, tendon

Inferior fibular [peroneal] retinaculum

Calcaneus

Abductor digiti minimi

Plantar aponeurosis

Metaphysis, epiphysial line

Ankle joint

Tibia, medial malleolus

Medial collateral ligament, tibiocalcaneal part

Tibialis posterior, tendon

Tendinous sheath of tibialis posterior

Flexor digitorum longus, tendon

Tendinous sheath of flexor digitorum longus

Flexor retinaculum

Subtalar joint

Talocalcaneal interosseous ligament

Medial plantar nerve

(Medial plantar vein)

Medial plantar artery

Abductor hallucis

Quadratus plantae

Lateral plantar artery; nerve; (lateral plantar vein)

Flexor digitorum brevis

Fig. 1047 Ankle and talotarsal joint; frontal section.

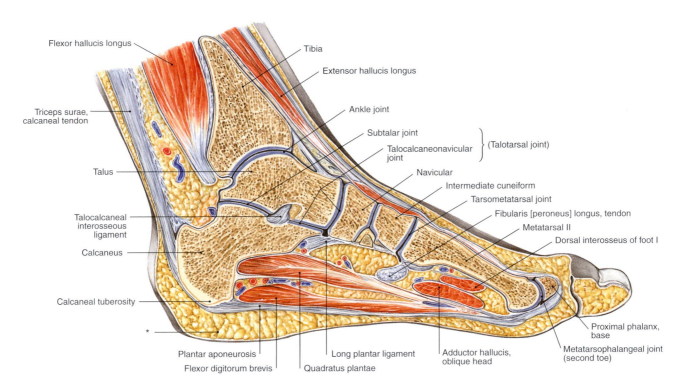

Flexor hallucis longus

Triceps surae, calcaneal tendon

Talus

Talocalcaneal interosseous ligament

Calcaneus

Calcaneal tuberosity

*

Plantar aponeurosis

Flexor digitorum brevis

Quadratus plantae

Long plantar ligament

Tibia

Extensor hallucis longus

Ankle joint

Subtalar joint

Talocalcaneonavicular joint

} (Talotarsal joint)

Navicular

Intermediate cuneiform

Tarsometatarsal joint

Fibularis [peroneus] longus, tendon

Metatarsal II

Dorsal interosseus of foot I

Proximal phalanx, base

Metatarsophalangeal joint (second toe)

Adductor hallucis, oblique head

Fig. 1048 Ankle and talotarsal joint; sagittal section.

* Fat pad of the heel

Ankle and talotarsal joint, radiography

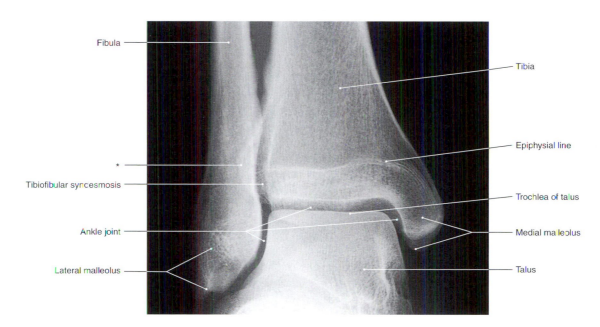

Fibula

Tibia

Epiphysial line

*

Tibiofibular syndesmosis

Trochlea of talus

Ankle joint

Medial malleolus

Lateral malleolus

Talus

Fig. 1049 Ankle joint;
AP-radiograph with the subject reclined and the central beam directed tangentially onto the trochlea of talus.

* Clinically, the posterior border of the fibular notch is also referred to as the third malleolus.

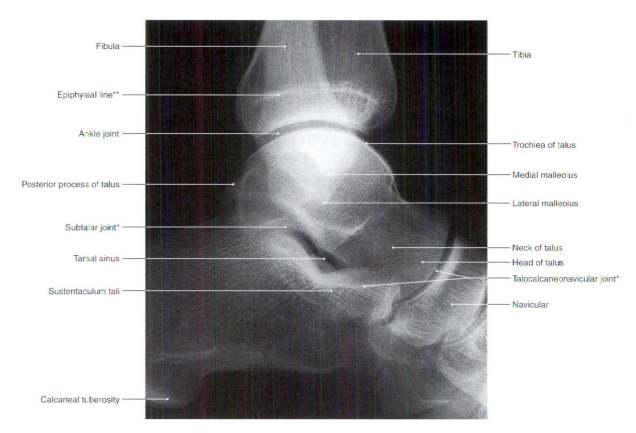

Fibula

Tibia

Epiphysial line**

Ankle joint

Trochlea of talus

Medial malleolus

Lateral malleolus

Posterior process of talus

Subtalar joint*

Neck of talus

Tarsal sinus

Head of talus

Talocalcaneonavicular joint*

Sustentaculum tali

Navicular

Calcaneal tuberosity

Fig. 1050 Ankle and talotarsal joint;
AP-radiograph with the subject reclined and the central beam directed tangentially onto the apex of the trochlea of talus.

* Due to their helical distorsion, the joint clefts are not displayed orthogonally.

** Overlapping epiphyseal lines of the tibia and fibula

→ 1160, 1162

Fasciae of the lower limb

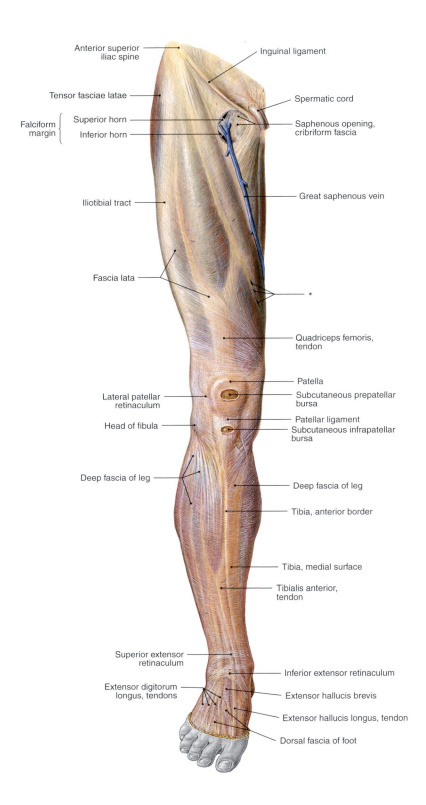

Fig. 1051 Fascia lata and deep fascia of leg.
The transition zone between the aponeurosis of the external
oblique abdominal muscle and the fascia lata is known as
inguinal ligament. This ligament extends laterally from the
anterior superior iliac spine to its attachment on the pubic
tubercle medially.

* Openings in the fascia for the perforator veins (DODD's veins)

Fasciae of the lower limb

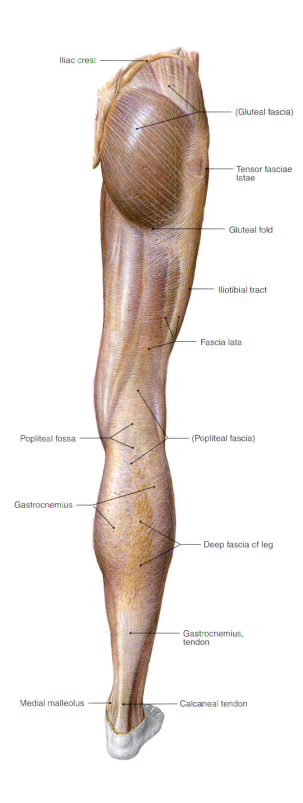

Iliac crest

(Gluteal fascia)

Tensor fasciae latae

Gluteal fold

Iliotibial tract

Fascia lata

Popliteal fossa

(Popliteal fascia)

Gastrocnemius

Deep fascia of leg

Gastrocnemius, tendon

Medial malleolus

Calcaneal tendon

Fig. 1052   Fascia lata and deep fascia of leg.

Muscles of the lower limb, overview

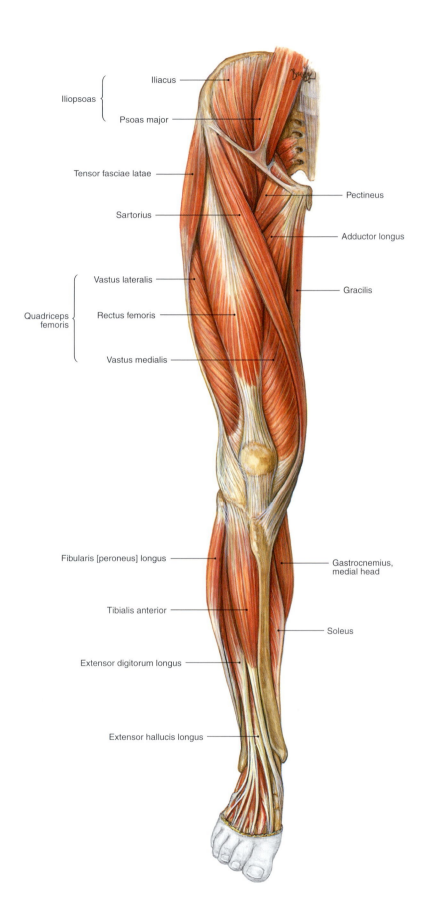

Iliopsoas { Iliacus

Psoas major

Tensor fasciae latae

Sartorius

Pectineus

Adductor longus

Quadriceps femoris { Vastus lateralis

Rectus femoris

Vastus medialis

Gracilis

Fibularis [peroneus] longus

Tibialis anterior

Extensor digitorum longus

Extensor hallucis longus

Gastrocnemius, medial head

Soleus

→ T 42, T 44, T 45, T 47, T 48

Fig. 1053   Muscles of the lower limb; overview.

Muscles of the lower limb, overview

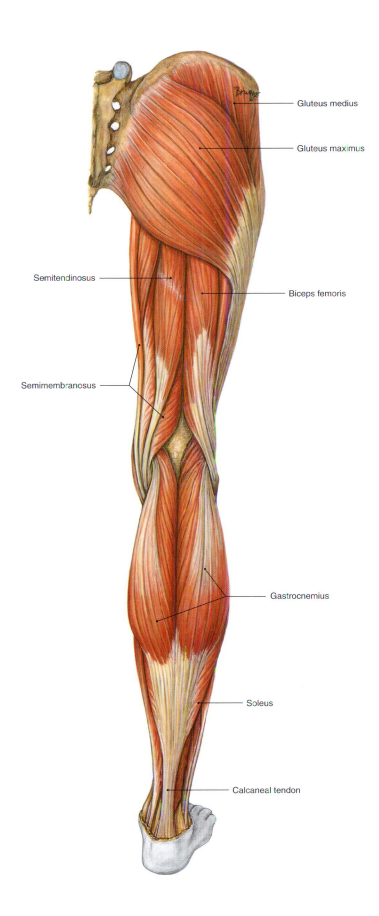

Gluteus medius

Gluteus maximus

Semitendinosus

Biceps femoris

Semimembranosus

Gastrocnemius

Soleus

Calcaneal tendon

Fig. 1054   Muscles of the lower limb;
overview.

→ T 43, T 46, T 49

Origins and insertions of the muscles of the hip, the thigh and the leg

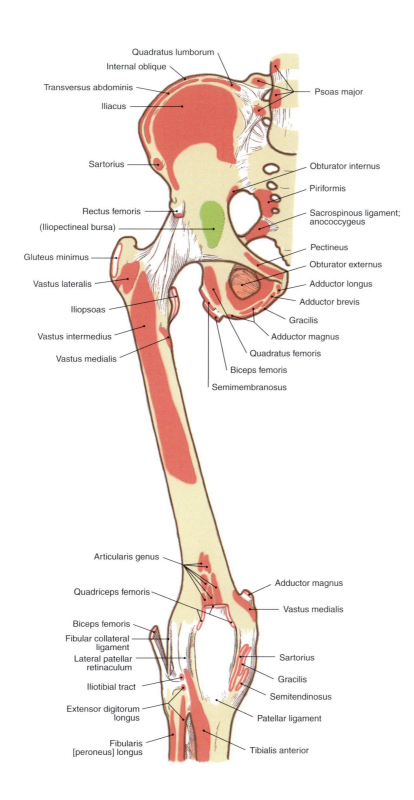

Quadratus lumborum

Internal oblique

Transversus abdominis

Iliacus

Psoas major

Sartorius

Obturator internus

Piriformis

Rectus femoris

Sacrospinous ligament;
anococcygeus

(Iliopectineal bursa)

Pectineus

Gluteus minimus

Obturator externus

Vastus lateralis

Adductor longus

Iliopsoas

Adductor brevis

Vastus intermedius

Gracilis

Vastus medialis

Adductor magnus

Quadratus femoris

Biceps femoris

Semimembranosus

Articularis genus

Quadriceps femoris

Adductor magnus

Vastus medialis

Biceps femoris

Fibular collateral
ligament

Lateral patellar
retinaculum

Sartorius

Iliotibial tract

Gracilis

Extensor digitorum
longus

Semitendinosus

Patellar ligament

Fibularis
[peroneus] longus

Tibialis anterior

→ T 42–T 48

Fig. 1055 Origins and insertions of the muscles at the
lower lumbar vertebrae, the pelvic bones, the femur and
the proximal extremities of the bones of the leg;
ventral view.

Origins and insertions of the muscles of the hip, the thigh and the leg

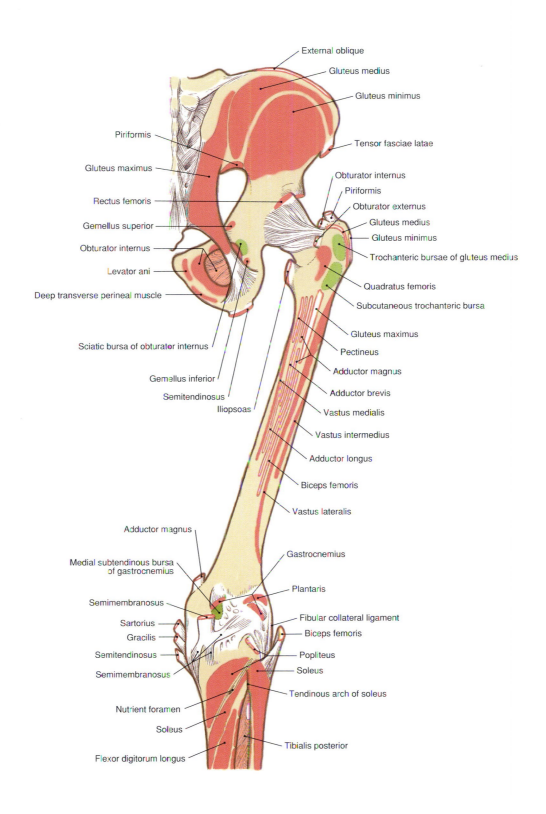

External oblique
Gluteus medius
Gluteus minimus
Piriformis
Tensor fasciae latae
Gluteus maximus
Obturator internus
Piriformis
Rectus femoris
Obturator externus
Gemellus superior
Gluteus medius
Obturator internus
Gluteus minimus
Levator ani
Trochanteric bursae of gluteus medius
Deep transverse perineal muscle
Quadratus femoris
Subcutaneous trochanteric bursa
Gluteus maximus
Pectineus
Sciatic bursa of obturator internus
Adductor magnus
Gemellus inferior
Adductor brevis
Semitendinosus
Vastus medialis
Iliopsoas
Vastus intermedius
Adductor longus
Biceps femoris
Vastus lateralis
Adductor magnus
Gastrocnemius
Medial subtendinous bursa
of gastrocnemius
Plantaris
Semimembranosus
Sartorius
Fibular collateral ligament
Gracilis
Biceps femoris
Semitendinosus
Popliteus
Semimembranosus
Soleus
Tendinous arch of soleus
Nutrient foramen
Soleus
Tibialis posterior
Flexor digitorum longus

Fig. 1056 Origins and insertions of the muscles at
the pelvic bones, the femur and the proximal extremities
of the bones of the leg;
dorsal view.

→ T 43–T 46, T 49, T 50

Muscles of the thigh

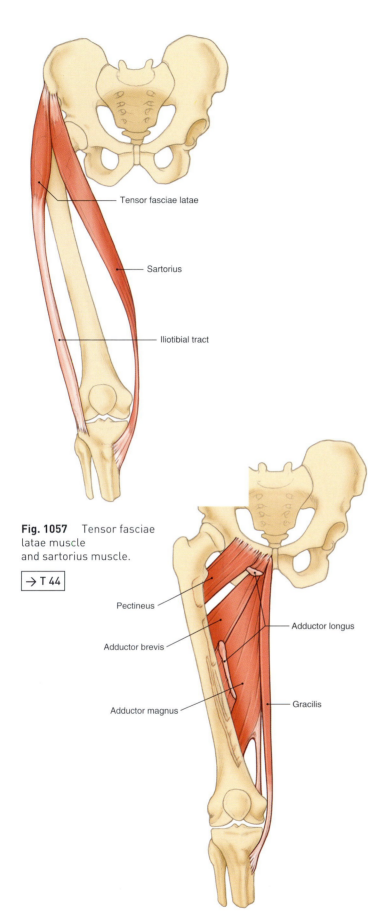

Tensor fasciae latae

Sartorius

Iliotibial tract

Fig. 1057 Tensor fasciae latae muscle and sartorius muscle.

→ T 44

Pectineus

Adductor brevis

Adductor magnus

Adductor longus

Gracilis

Fig. 1059 Adductor muscles.

→ T 45

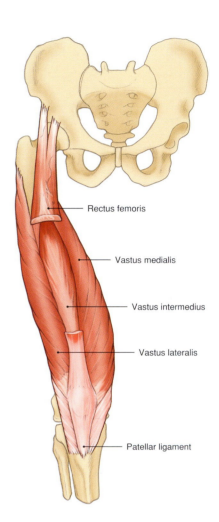

Rectus femoris

Vastus medialis

Vastus intermedius

Vastus lateralis

Patellar ligament

Fig. 1058 Quadriceps femoris muscle.

→ T 44

Psoas major

Iliacus

Fig. 1060 Iliopsoas muscle.

→ T 42

Muscles of the thigh

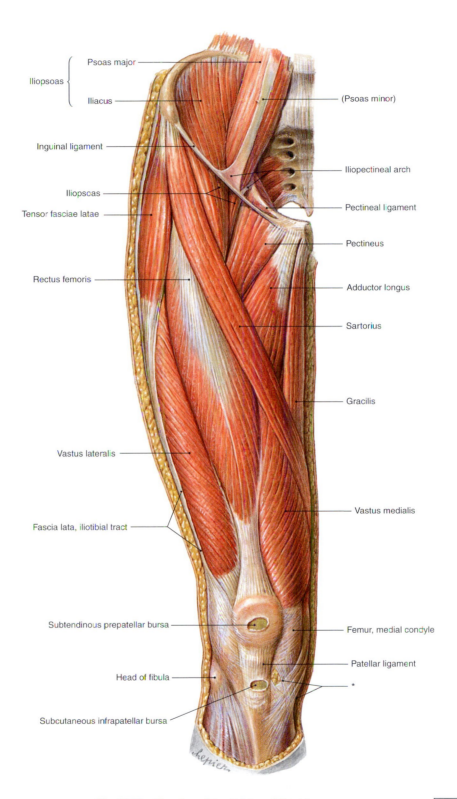

Psoas major

Iliopsoas

Iliacus

(Psoas minor)

Inguinal ligament

Iliopectineal arch

Iliopscas

Pectineal ligament

Tensor fasciae latae

Pectineus

Rectus femoris

Adductor longus

Sartorius

Gracilis

Vastus lateralis

Vastus medialis

Fascia lata, iliotibial tract

Subtendinous prepatellar bursa

Femur, medial condyle

Patellar ligament

Head of fibula

*

Subcutaneous infrapatellar bursa

Fig. 1061   Muscles of the thigh and the hip;
after removal of the fascia lata except for the iliotibial tract.

→ T 42, T 44, T 45

*   Common insertion of the sartorius, gracilis and semitendinosus muscles just
below the medial condyle of the tibia (formerly known as the superficial pes
anserinus

Muscles of the thigh

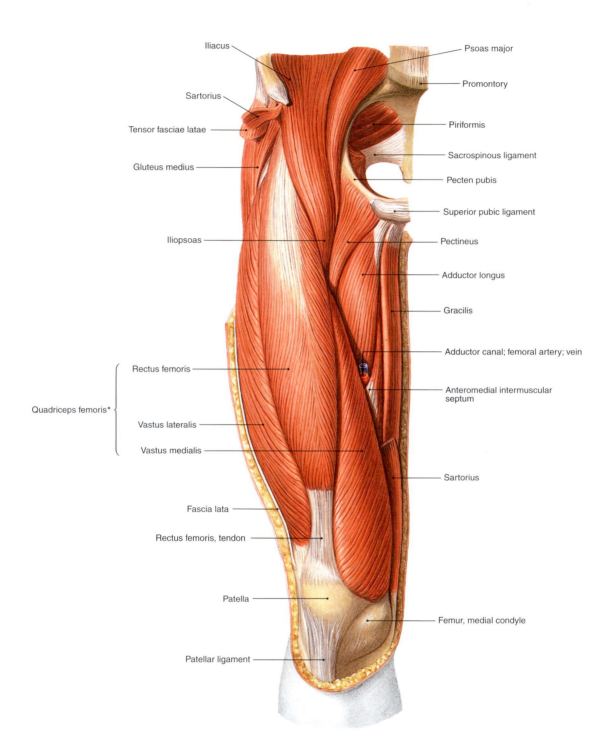

Iliacus

Sartorius

Tensor fasciae latae

Gluteus medius

Iliopsoas

Quadriceps femoris*

Rectus femoris

Vastus lateralis

Vastus medialis

Fascia lata

Rectus femoris, tendon

Patella

Patellar ligament

Psoas major

Promontory

Piriformis

Sacrospinous ligament

Pecten pubis

Superior pubic ligament

Pectineus

Adductor longus

Gracilis

Adductor canal; femoral artery; vein

Anteromedial intermuscular septum

Sartorius

Femur, medial condyle

→ T 42, T 44, T 45

Fig. 1062   Muscles of the thigh and the hip;
after removal of the fascia lata, the tensor fasciae latae
muscle and the sartorius muscle.

* The fourth head of the quadriceps muscle, the vastus intermedius muscle, is
   covered by the rectus femoris muscle.

Muscles of the thigh

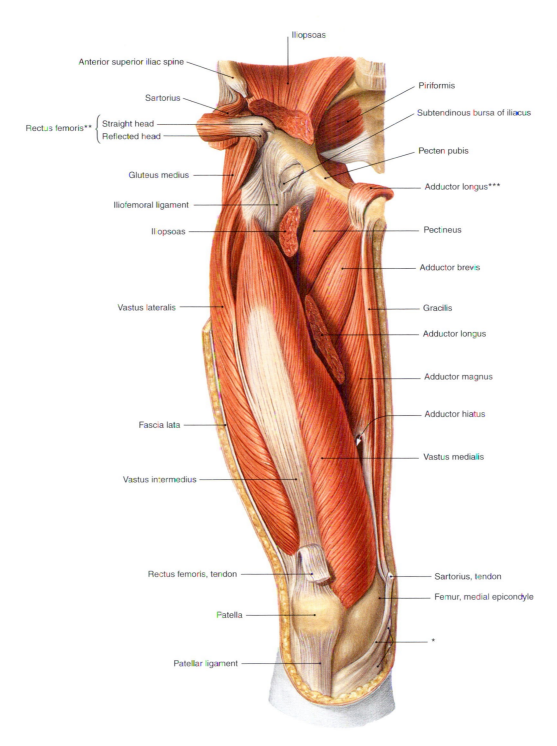

Iliopsoas

Anterior superior iliac spine

Piriformis

Sartorius

Subtendinous bursa of iliacus

Rectus femoris** { Straight head / Reflected head }

Pecten pubis

Gluteus medius

Adductor longus***

Iliofemoral ligament

Pectineus

Iliopsoas

Adductor brevis

Vastus lateralis

Gracilis

Adductor longus

Adductor magnus

Adductor hiatus

Fascia lata

Vastus medialis

Vastus intermedius

Rectus femoris, tendon

Sartorius, tendon

Femur, medial epicondyle

Patella

*

Patellar ligament

Fig. 1063 Muscles of the thigh and the hip;
deep layer after removal of the sartorius, the rectus femoris
and the adductor longus muscles as well as parts of the
iliopsoas muscle in the joint region.

* Common insertion of the sartorius, gracilis and semitendinosus muscles just
below the medial condyle of the tibia
** The origin of the rectus femoris muscle has been flapped laterally upwards.
*** A part of the adductor longus muscle has been flapped upwards.

→ T 42, T 44, T 45

Muscles of the thigh

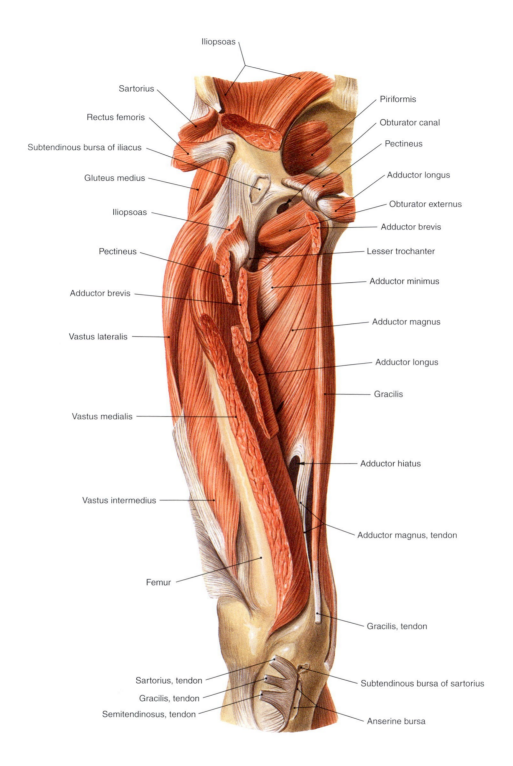

Iliopsoas

Sartorius

Rectus femoris

Subtendinous bursa of iliacus

Gluteus medius

Iliopsoas

Pectineus

Adductor brevis

Vastus lateralis

Vastus medialis

Vastus intermedius

Femur

Piriformis

Obturator canal

Pectineus

Adductor longus

Obturator externus

Adductor brevis

Lesser trochanter

Adductor minimus

Adductor magnus

Adductor longus

Gracilis

Adductor hiatus

Adductor magnus, tendon

Gracilis, tendon

Sartorius, tendon

Gracilis, tendon

Semitendinosus, tendon

Subtendinous bursa of sartorius

Anserine bursa

→ T 42, T 44, T 45

Fig. 1064   Muscles of the thigh and the hip;
after almost complete removal of superficial and
several deeper muscles;
ventral view.

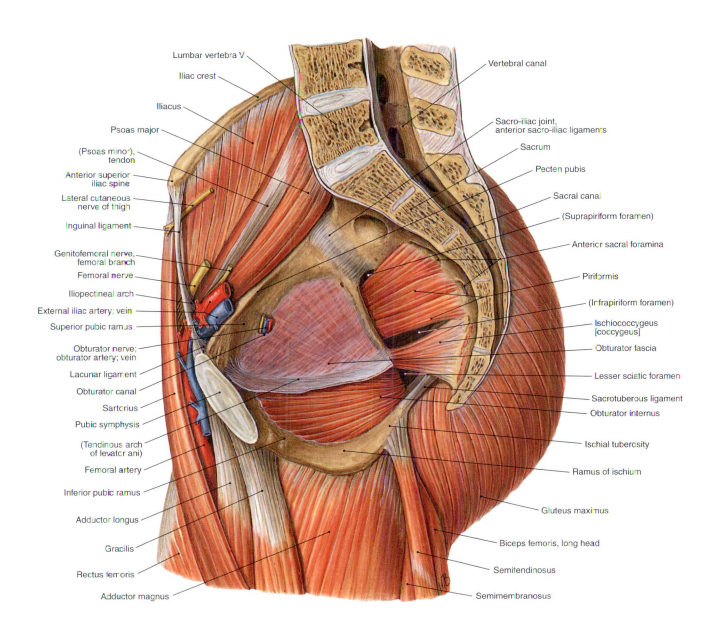

Lumbar vertebra V

Iliac crest

Iliacus

Psoas major

(Psoas minor), tendon

Anterior superior iliac spine

Lateral cutaneous nerve of thigh

Inguinal ligament

Genitofemoral nerve, femoral branch

Femoral nerve

Iliopectineal arch

External iliac artery; vein

Superior pubic ramus

Obturator nerve; obturator artery; vein

Lacunar ligament

Obturator canal

Sartorius

Pubic symphysis

(Tendinous arch of levator ani)

Femoral artery

Inferior pubic ramus

Adductor longus

Gracilis

Rectus femoris

Adductor magnus

Vertebral canal

Sacro-iliac joint, anterior sacro-iliac ligaments

Sacrum

Pecten pubis

Sacral canal

(Suprapiriform foramen)

Anterior sacral foramina

Piriformis

(Infrapiriform foramen)

Ischiococcygeus [coccygeus]

Obturator fascia

Lesser sciatic foramen

Sacrotuberous ligament

Obturator internus

Ischial tuberosity

Ramus of ischium

Gluteus maximus

Biceps femoris, long head

Semitendinosus

Semimembranosus

Fig. 1065 Muscles of the thigh and the hip; medial view.

→ T 22 a, T 42–T 46

Muscles of the thigh and the hip

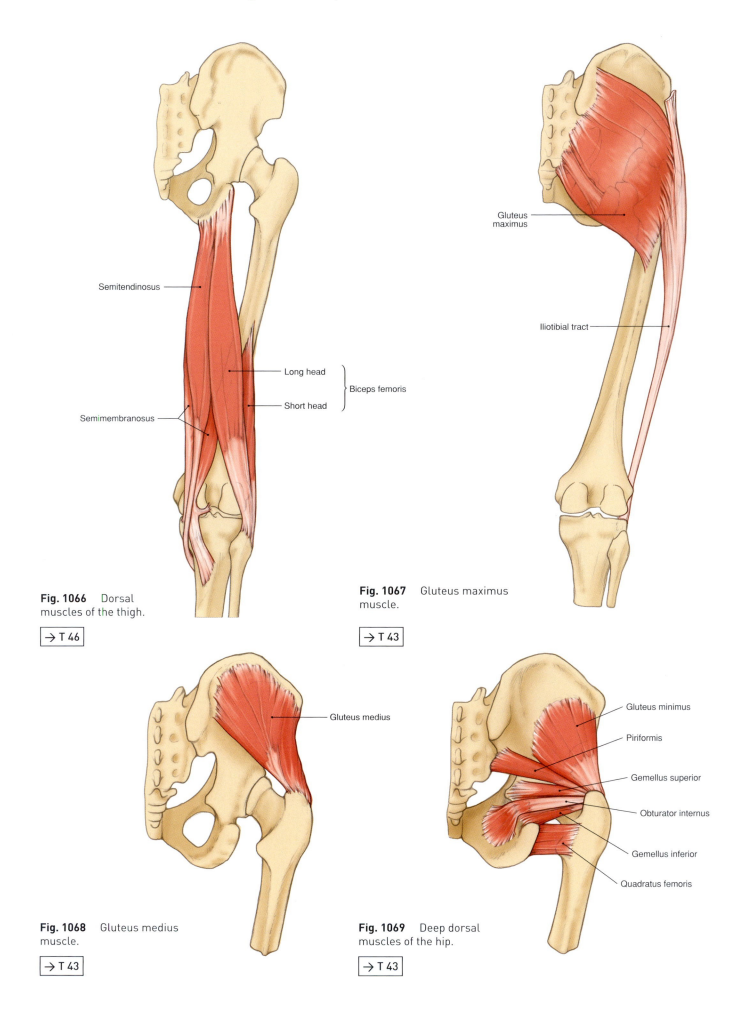

Fig. 1066   Dorsal muscles of the thigh.

→ T 46

Semitendinosus

Long head
} Biceps femoris
Short head

Semimembranosus

Fig. 1067   Gluteus maximus muscle.

→ T 43

Gluteus maximus

Iliotibial tract

Fig. 1068   Gluteus medius muscle.

→ T 43

Gluteus medius

Fig. 1069   Deep dorsal muscles of the hip.

→ T 43

Gluteus minimus

Piriformis

Gemellus superior

Obturator internus

Gemellus inferior

Quadratus femoris

Muscles of the thigh and the hip

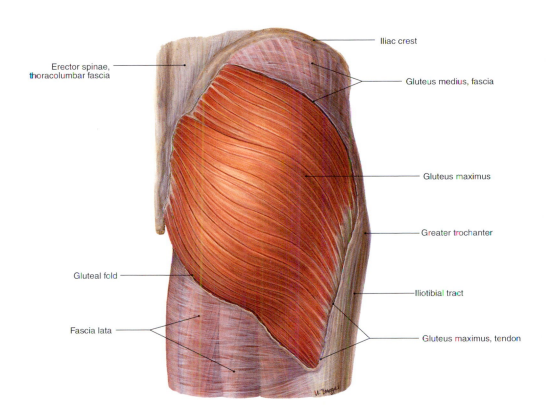

Erector spinae, thoracolumbar fascia

Iliac crest

Gluteus medius, fascia

Gluteus maximus

Greater trochanter

Gluteal fold

Iliotibial tract

Fascia lata

Gluteus maximus, tendon

Fig. 1070 Muscles of the thigh and the hip.

→ T 43

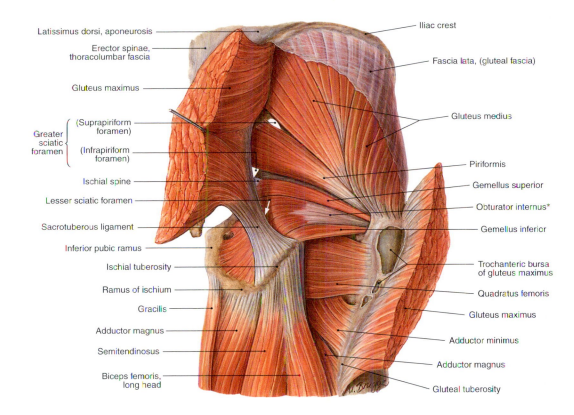

Latissimus dorsi, aponeurosis

Erector spinae, thoracolumbar fascia

Gluteus maximus

Greater sciatic foramen { (Suprapiriform foramen) / (Infrapiriform foramen)

Ischial spine

Lesser sciatic foramen

Sacrotuberous ligament

Inferior pubic ramus

Ischial tuberosity

Ramus of ischium

Gracilis

Adductor magnus

Semitendinosus

Biceps femoris, long head

Iliac crest

Fascia lata, (gluteal fascia)

Gluteus medius

Piriformis

Gemellus superior

Obturator internus*

Gemellus inferior

Trochanteric bursa of gluteus maximus

Quadratus femoris

Gluteus maximus

Adductor minimus

Adductor magnus

Gluteal tuberosity

Fig. 1071 Muscles of the thigh and the hip; the gluteus maximus muscle has been sectioned; dorsal view.

* The part of the obturator internus muscle between the curved edge of the lesser sciatic notch and the insertion in the trochanteric fossa frequently consists of tendinous bands.

→ T 43, T 45, T 46

Muscles of the thigh and the hip

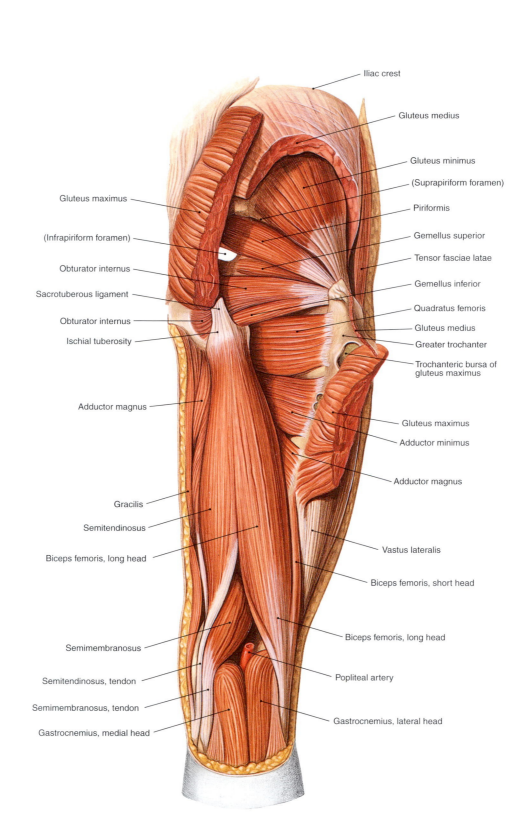

Iliac crest

Gluteus medius

Gluteus minimus

(Suprapiriform foramen)

Piriformis

Gluteus maximus

Gemellus superior

(Infrapiriform foramen)

Tensor fasciae latae

Obturator internus

Gemellus inferior

Sacrotuberous ligament

Quadratus femoris

Obturator internus

Gluteus medius

Ischial tuberosity

Greater trochanter

Trochanteric bursa of gluteus maximus

Adductor magnus

Gluteus maximus

Adductor minimus

Adductor magnus

Gracilis

Semitendinosus

Biceps femoris, long head

Vastus lateralis

Biceps femoris, short head

Semimembranosus

Biceps femoris, long head

Semitendinosus, tendon

Popliteal artery

Semimembranosus, tendon

Gastrocnemius, medial head

Gastrocnemius, lateral head

→ T 43, T 45, T 46

Fig. 1072   Muscles of the thigh and the hip;
the gluteus maximus and medius muscles have
been partially removed;
dorsal view.

Muscles of the thigh and the hip

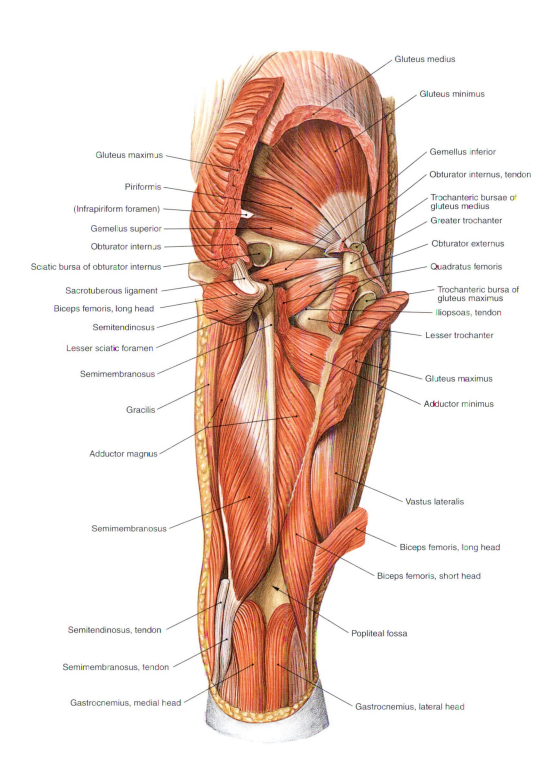

Gluteus medius

Gluteus minimus

Gluteus maximus

Piriformis

(Infrapiriform foramen)

Gemellus superior

Obturator internus

Sciatic bursa of obturator internus

Sacrotuberous ligament

Biceps femoris, long head

Semitendinosus

Lesser sciatic foramen

Semimembranosus

Gracilis

Adductor magnus

Semimembranosus

Semitendinosus, tendon

Semimembranosus, tendon

Gastrocnemius, medial head

Gemellus inferior

Obturator internus, tendon

Trochanteric bursae of gluteus medius

Greater trochanter

Obturator externus

Quadratus femoris

Trochanteric bursa of gluteus maximus

Iliopsoas, tendon

Lesser trochanter

Gluteus maximus

Adductor minimus

Vastus lateralis

Biceps femoris, long head

Biceps femoris, short head

Popliteal fossa

Gastrocnemius, lateral head

Fig. 1073   Muscles of the thigh and the hip;
deep layer after almost complete removal of the
superficial gluteal and the ischiocrural muscles;
dorsal view.

→ T 43, T 45, T 46

Muscles of the thigh and the hip

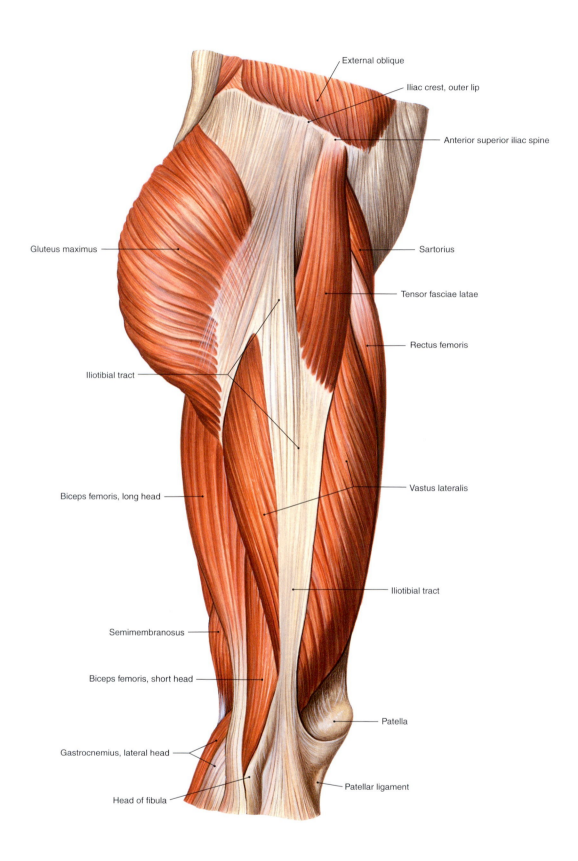

External oblique

Iliac crest, outer lip

Anterior superior iliac spine

Gluteus maximus

Sartorius

Tensor fasciae latae

Rectus femoris

Iliotibial tract

Biceps femoris, long head

Vastus lateralis

Iliotibial tract

Semimembranosus

Biceps femoris, short head

Patella

Gastrocnemius, lateral head

Head of fibula

Patellar ligament

→ T 43, T 44, T 46

Fig. 1074   Muscles of the thigh and the hip;
after removal of the fascia lata except for the iliotibial tract.

Muscles of the thigh

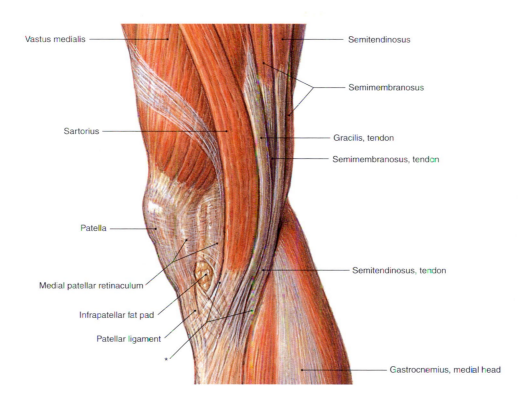

Vastus medialis
Semitendinosus
Semimembranosus
Sartorius
Gracilis, tendon
Semimembranosus, tendon
Patella
Semitendinosus, tendon
Medial patellar retinaculum
Infrapatellar fat pad
Patellar ligament
Gastrocnemius, medial head

Fig. 1075 Muscles in the region of the knee joint; medial view. → T 44–T 46, T 49

* Common insertion just below the medial condyle of the tibia (formerly known as superficial pes anserinus)

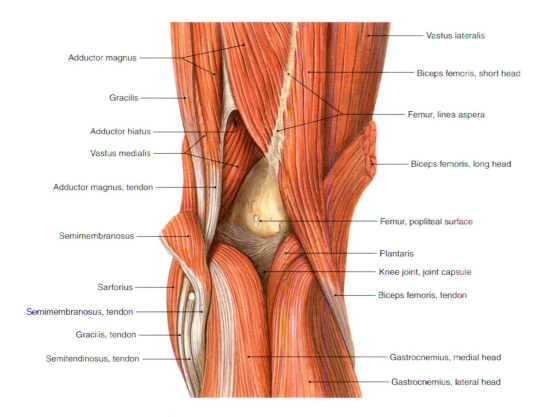

Adductor magnus
Vastus lateralis
Biceps femoris, short head
Gracilis
Adductor hiatus
Femur, linea aspera
Vastus medialis
Adductor magnus, tendon
Biceps femoris, long head
Femur, popliteal surface
Semimembranosus
Plantaris
Knee joint, joint capsule
Sartorius
Biceps femoris, tendon
Semimembranosus, tendon
Gracilis, tendon
Semitendinosus, tendon
Gastrocnemius, medial head
Gastrocnemius, lateral head

Fig. 1076 Muscles in the region of the knee joint; after almost complete removal of the ischiocrural muscles; dorsal view. → T 44–T 46, T 49

Origins and insertions of the muscles of the thigh and the ventral part of the leg

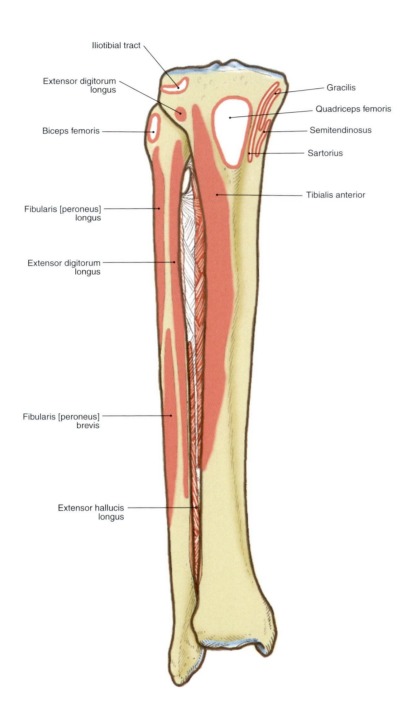

Iliotibial tract

Extensor digitorum longus

Biceps femoris

Fibularis [peroneus] longus

Extensor digitorum longus

Fibularis [peroneus] brevis

Extensor hallucis longus

Gracilis

Quadriceps femoris

Semitendinosus

Sartorius

Tibialis anterior

→ T 44–T 47

Fig. 1077 Origins and insertions of the muscles at the bones of the leg; ventral view.

Origins and insertions of the muscles of the thigh and the dorsal part of the leg

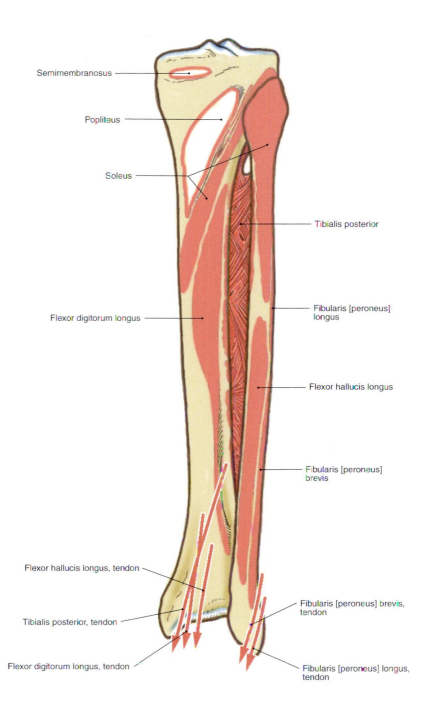

Semimembranosus

Popliteus

Soleus

Tibialis posterior

Flexor digitorum longus

Fibularis [peroneus] longus

Flexor hallucis longus

Fibularis [peroneus] brevis

Flexor hallucis longus, tendon

Tibialis posterior, tendon

Fibularis [peroneus] brevis, tendon

Flexor digitorum longus, tendon

Fibularis [peroneus] longus, tendon

Fig. 1078 Origins and insertions of the muscles at the bones of the leg; dorsal view.

→ T 46, T 48–T 50

Muscles of the leg

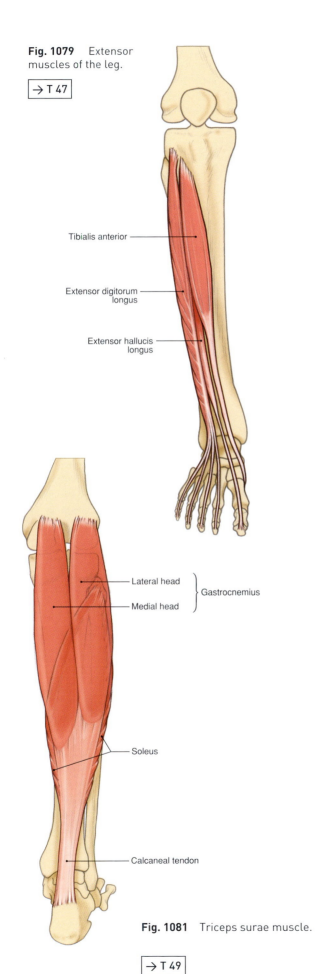

Fig. 1079   Extensor muscles of the leg.

→ T 47

Tibialis anterior

Extensor digitorum longus

Extensor hallucis longus

Lateral head ⎫ Gastrocnemius
Medial head ⎭

Soleus

Calcaneal tendon

Fig. 1081   Triceps surae muscle.

→ T 49

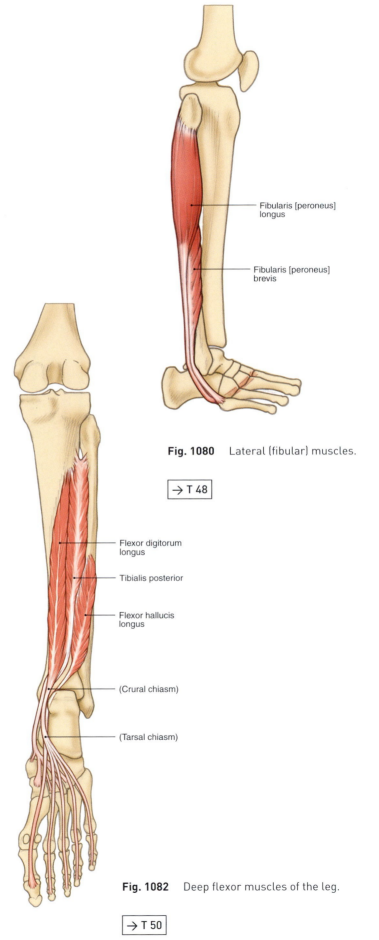

Fibularis [peroneus] longus

Fibularis [peroneus] brevis

Fig. 1080   Lateral (fibular) muscles.

→ T 48

Flexor digitorum longus

Tibialis posterior

Flexor hallucis longus

(Crural chiasm)

(Tarsal chiasm)

Fig. 1082   Deep flexor muscles of the leg.

→ T 50

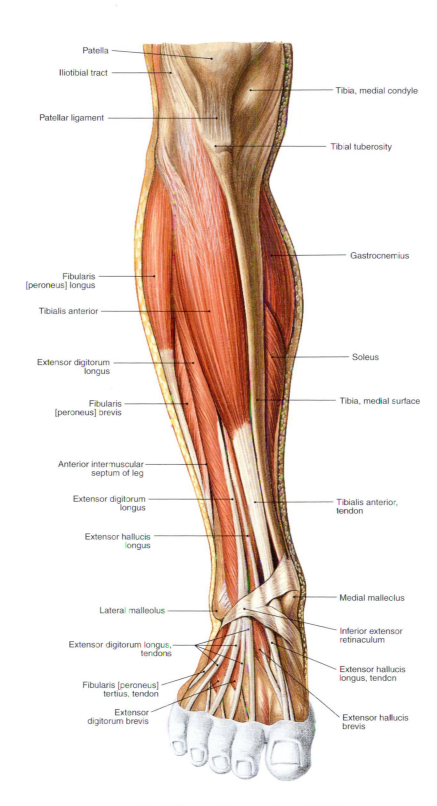

Patella

Iliotibial tract

Patellar ligament

Tibia, medial condyle

Tibial tuberosity

Gastrocnemius

Fibularis [peroneus] longus

Tibialis anterior

Extensor digitorum longus

Soleus

Fibularis [peroneus] brevis

Tibia, medial surface

Anterior intermuscular septum of leg

Extensor digitorum longus

Tibialis anterior, tendon

Extensor hallucis longus

Medial malleolus

Lateral malleolus

Inferior extensor retinaculum

Extensor digitorum longus, tendons

Extensor hallucis longus, tendon

Fibularis [peroneus] tertius, tendon

Extensor digitorum brevis

Extensor hallucis brevis

Fig. 1083   Muscles of the leg and the foot.

→ T 47, T 48

Muscles of the leg

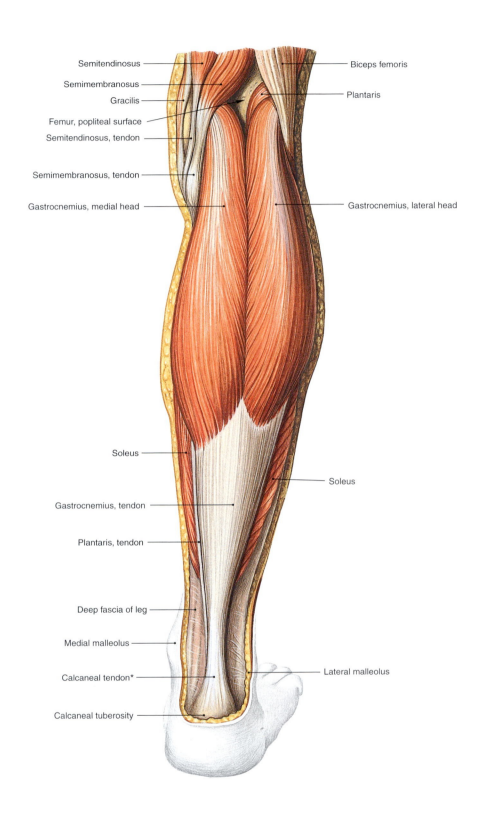

Semitendinosus

Semimembranosus

Gracilis

Femur, popliteal surface

Semitendinosus, tendon

Semimembranosus, tendon

Gastrocnemius, medial head

Biceps femoris

Plantaris

Gastrocnemius, lateral head

Soleus

Soleus

Gastrocnemius, tendon

Plantaris, tendon

Deep fascia of leg

Medial malleolus

Calcaneal tendon*

Calcaneal tuberosity

Lateral malleolus

→ T 49

Fig. 1084 Muscles of the leg; superficial layer.

* Also: Achilles tendon

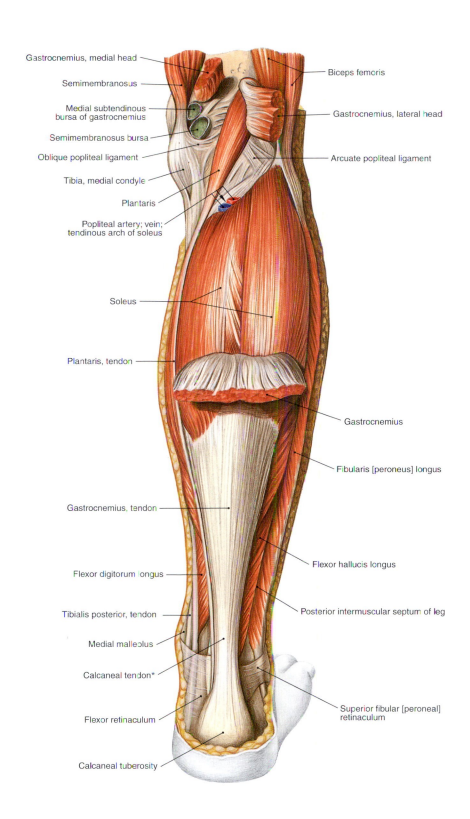

Gastrocnemius, medial head

Semimembranosus

Medial subtendinous
bursa of gastrocnemius

Semimembranosus bursa

Oblique popliteal ligament

Tibia, medial condyle

Plantaris

Popliteal artery; vein;
tendinous arch of soleus

Soleus

Plantaris, tendon

Gastrocnemius, tendon

Flexor digitorum longus

Tibialis posterior, tendon

Medial malleolus

Calcaneal tendon*

Flexor retinaculum

Calcaneal tuberosity

Biceps femoris

Gastrocnemius, lateral head

Arcuate popliteal ligament

Gastrocnemius

Fibularis [peroneus] longus

Flexor hallucis longus

Posterior intermuscular septum of leg

Superior fibular [peroneal]
retinaculum

Fig. 1085   Muscles of the leg;
superficial layer after partial removal
of the gastrocnemius muscle.

* Also: Achilles tendon

→ T 49

Muscles of the leg

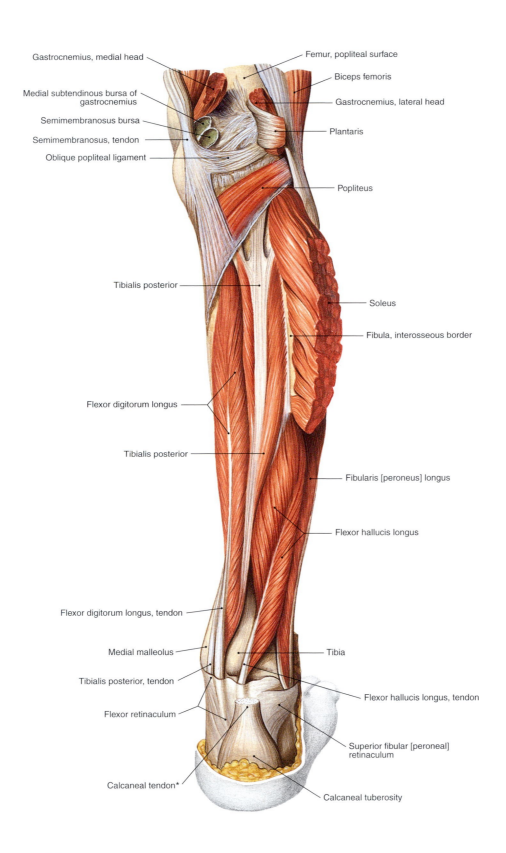

Gastrocnemius, medial head

Medial subtendinous bursa of
gastrocnemius

Semimembranosus bursa

Semimembranosus, tendon

Oblique popliteal ligament

Tibialis posterior

Flexor digitorum longus

Tibialis posterior

Flexor digitorum longus, tendon

Medial malleolus

Tibialis posterior, tendon

Flexor retinaculum

Calcaneal tendon*

Femur, popliteal surface

Biceps femoris

Gastrocnemius, lateral head

Plantaris

Popliteus

Soleus

Fibula, interosseous border

Fibularis [peroneus] longus

Flexor hallucis longus

Tibia

Flexor hallucis longus, tendon

Superior fibular [peroneal]
retinaculum

Calcaneal tuberosity

→ T 50

Fig. 1086 Muscles of the leg;
deep layer.

* Also: Achilles tendon

Muscles of the leg

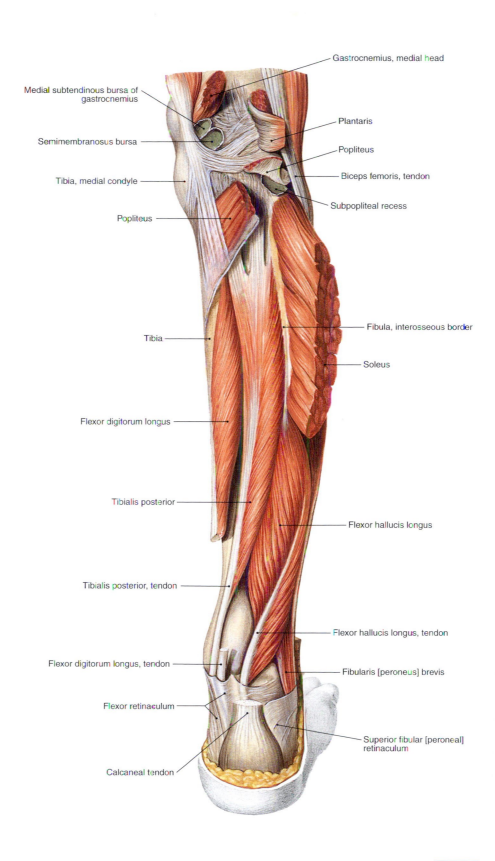

Gastrocnemius, medial head

Medial subtendinous bursa of gastrocnemius

Plantaris

Semimembranosus bursa

Popliteus

Tibia, medial condyle

Biceps femoris, tendon

Popliteus

Subpopliteal recess

Fibula, interosseous border

Tibia

Soleus

Flexor digitorum longus

Tibialis posterior

Flexor hallucis longus

Tibialis posterior, tendon

Flexor hallucis longus, tendon

Flexor digitorum longus, tendon

Fibularis [peroneus] brevis

Flexor retinaculum

Superior fibular [peroneal] retinaculum

Calcaneal tendon

Fig. 1087 Muscles of the leg; deepest layer.

→ T 50

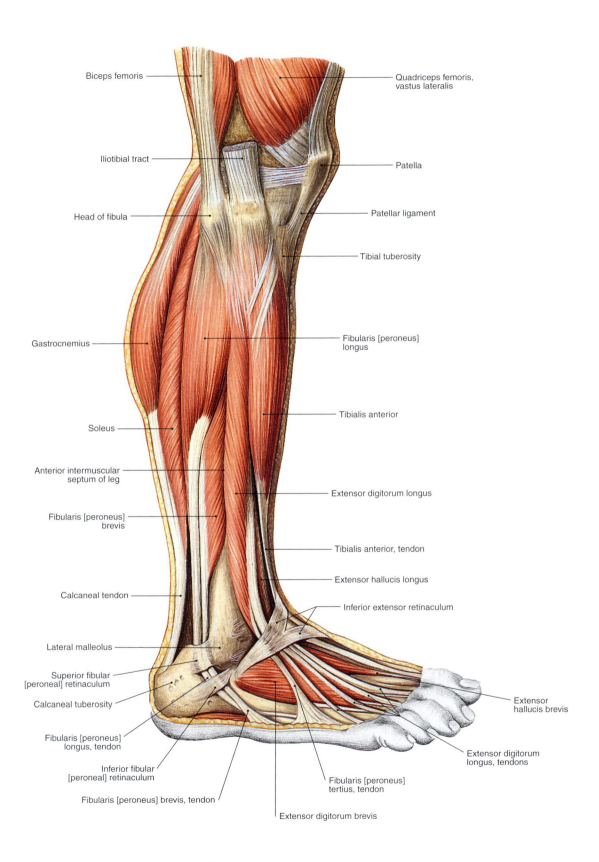

Biceps femoris

Quadriceps femoris, vastus lateralis

Iliotibial tract

Patella

Head of fibula

Patellar ligament

Tibial tuberosity

Gastrocnemius

Fibularis [peroneus] longus

Tibialis anterior

Soleus

Anterior intermuscular septum of leg

Extensor digitorum longus

Fibularis [peroneus] brevis

Tibialis anterior, tendon

Extensor hallucis longus

Calcaneal tendon

Inferior extensor retinaculum

Lateral malleolus

Superior fibular [peroneal] retinaculum

Calcaneal tuberosity

Extensor hallucis brevis

Fibularis [peroneus] longus, tendon

Inferior fibular [peroneal] retinaculum

Extensor digitorum longus, tendons

Fibularis [peroneus] brevis, tendon

Fibularis [peroneus] tertius, tendon

Extensor digitorum brevis

→ T 47–T49, T 51

Fig. 1088   Muscles of the leg and the foot.

Origins and insertions of the muscles of the foot and the leg

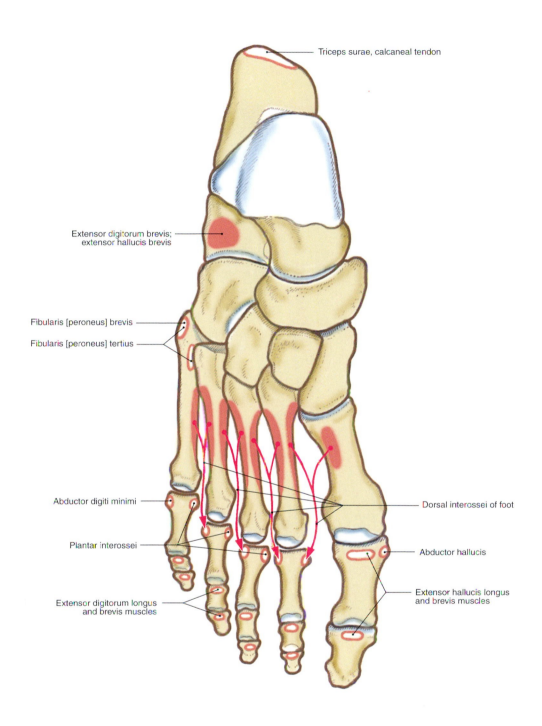

Triceps surae, calcaneal tendon

Extensor digitorum brevis; extensor hallucis brevis

Fibularis [peroneus] brevis

Fibularis [peroneus] tertius

Abductor digiti minimi

Plantar interossei

Extensor digitorum longus and brevis muscles

Dorsal interossei of foot

Abductor hallucis

Extensor hallucis longus and brevis muscles

Fig. 1089 Origins and insertions of the muscles at the bones of the foot; dorsal view.

→ T 47, T 48, T 51, T 53, T 54

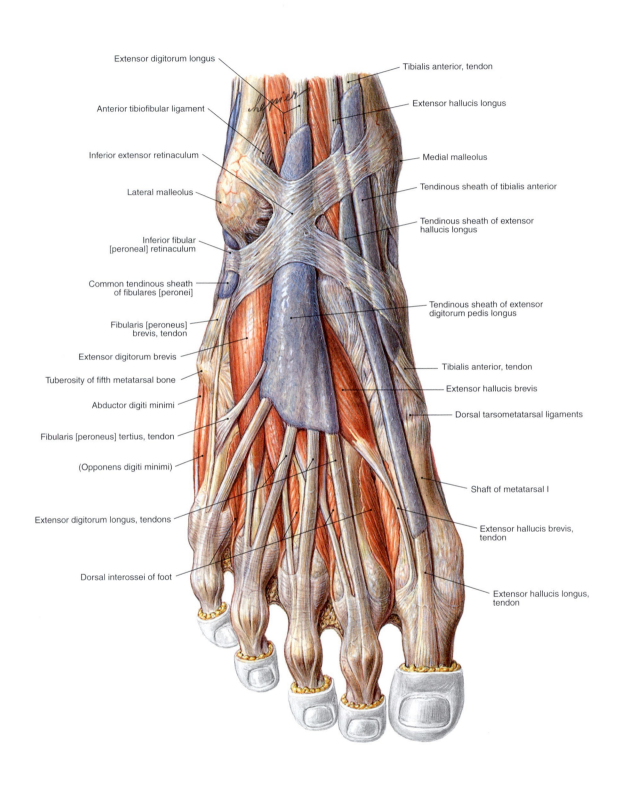

Extensor digitorum longus

Anterior tibiofibular ligament

Inferior extensor retinaculum

Lateral malleolus

Inferior fibular
[peroneal] retinaculum

Common tendinous sheath
of fibulares [peronei]

Fibularis [peroneus]
brevis, tendon

Extensor digitorum brevis

Tuberosity of fifth metatarsal bone

Abductor digiti minimi

Fibularis [peroneus] tertius, tendon

(Opponens digiti minimi)

Extensor digitorum longus, tendons

Dorsal interossei of foot

Tibialis anterior, tendon

Extensor hallucis longus

Medial malleolus

Tendinous sheath of tibialis anterior

Tendinous sheath of extensor
hallucis longus

Tendinous sheath of extensor
digitorum pedis longus

Tibialis anterior, tendon

Extensor hallucis brevis

Dorsal tarsometatarsal ligaments

Shaft of metatarsal I

Extensor hallucis brevis,
tendon

Extensor hallucis longus,
tendon

Fig. 1090   Tendon sheaths of the foot.

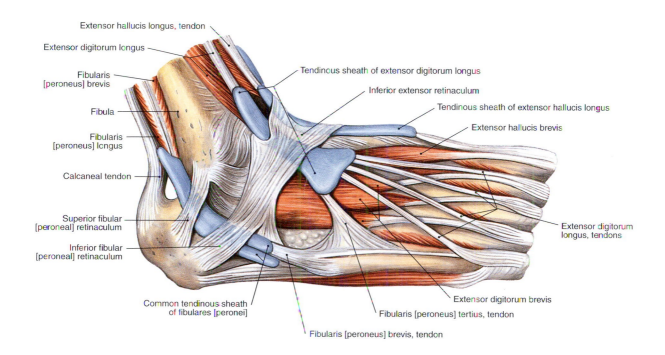

Extensor hallucis longus, tendon

Extensor digitorum longus

Fibularis [peroneus] brevis

Fibula

Fibularis [peroneus] longus

Calcaneal tendon

Superior fibular [peroneal] retinaculum

Inferior fibular [peroneal] retinaculum

Tendinous sheath of extensor digitorum longus

Inferior extensor retinaculum

Tendinous sheath of extensor hallucis longus

Extensor hallucis brevis

Extensor digitorum longus, tendons

Extensor digitorum brevis

Common tendinous sheath of fibulares [peronei]

Fibularis [peroneus] tertius, tendon

Fibularis [peroneus] brevis, tendon

Fig. 1091   Tendon sheaths of the foot.

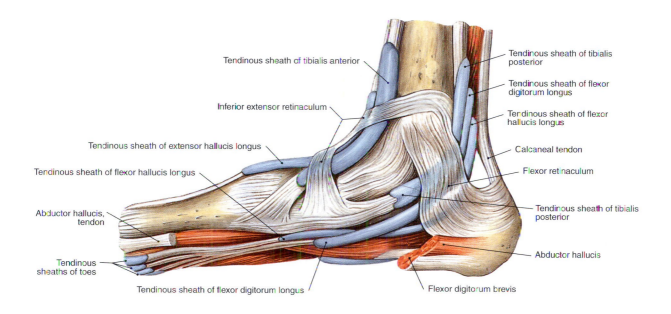

Tendinous sheath of tibialis anterior

Tendinous sheath of tibialis posterior

Tendinous sheath of flexor digitorum longus

Inferior extensor retinaculum

Tendinous sheath of flexor hallucis longus

Tendinous sheath of extensor hallucis longus

Calcaneal tendon

Tendinous sheath of flexor hallucis longus

Flexor retinaculum

Abductor hallucis, tendon

Tendinous sheath of tibialis posterior

Tendinous sheaths of toes

Abductor hallucis

Tendinous sheath of flexor digitorum longus

Flexor digitorum brevis

Fig. 1092   Tendon sheaths of the foot.

Muscles of the foot

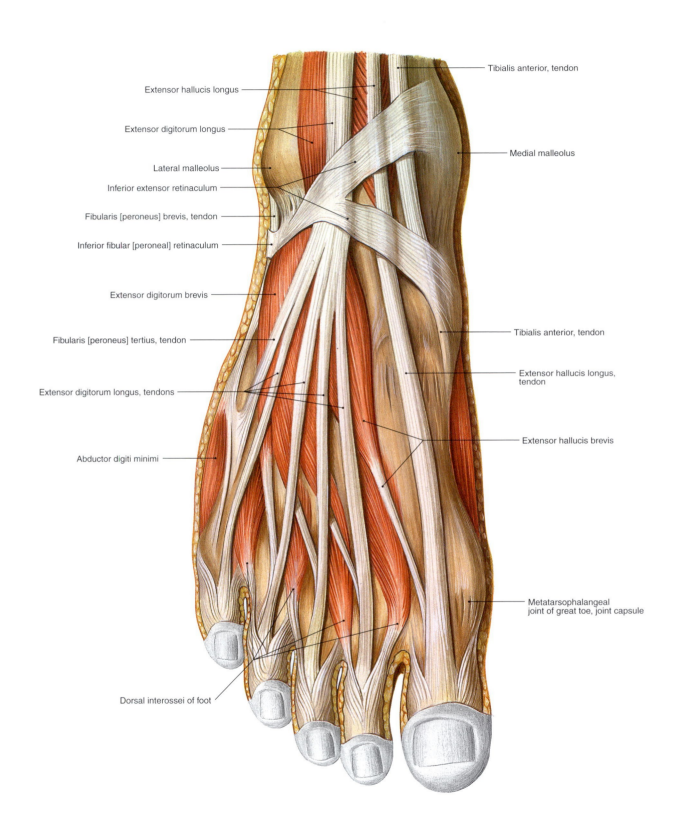

Extensor hallucis longus

Extensor digitorum longus

Lateral malleolus

Inferior extensor retinaculum

Fibularis [peroneus] brevis, tendon

Inferior fibular [peroneal] retinaculum

Extensor digitorum brevis

Fibularis [peroneus] tertius, tendon

Extensor digitorum longus, tendons

Abductor digiti minimi

Dorsal interossei of foot

Tibialis anterior, tendon

Medial malleolus

Tibialis anterior, tendon

Extensor hallucis longus, tendon

Extensor hallucis brevis

Metatarsophalangeal joint of great toe, joint capsule

→ T 47, T 51, T 53

Fig. 1093   Muscles of the foot; after removal of the tendon sheaths.

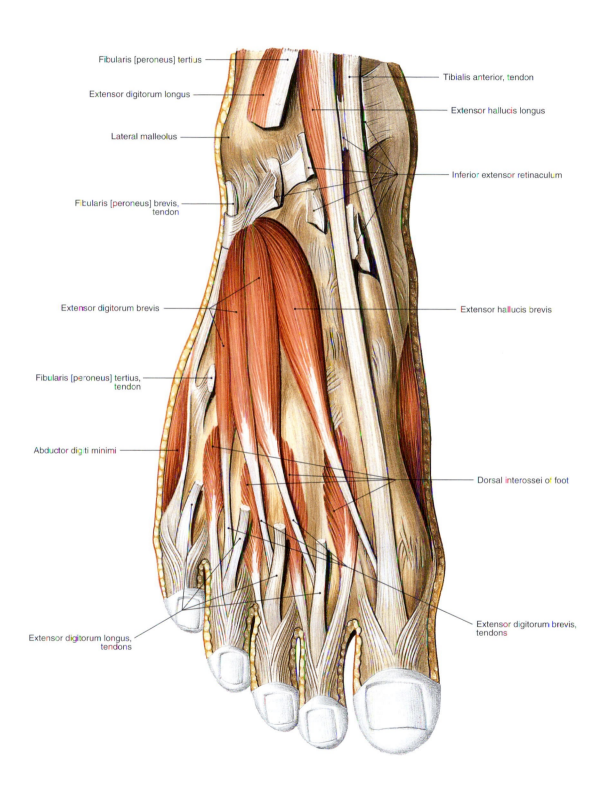

Fibularis [peroneus] tertius

Extensor digitorum longus

Lateral malleolus

Fibularis [peroneus] brevis, tendon

Extensor digitorum brevis

Fibularis [peroneus] tertius, tendon

Abductor digiti minimi

Extensor digitorum longus, tendons

Tibialis anterior, tendon

Extensor hallucis longus

Inferior extensor retinaculum

Extensor hallucis brevis

Dorsal interossei of foot

Extensor digitorum brevis, tendons

Fig. 1094   Muscles of the foot; after section of the inferior extensor retinaculum.

→ T 47, T 51, T 53

Muscles of the foot

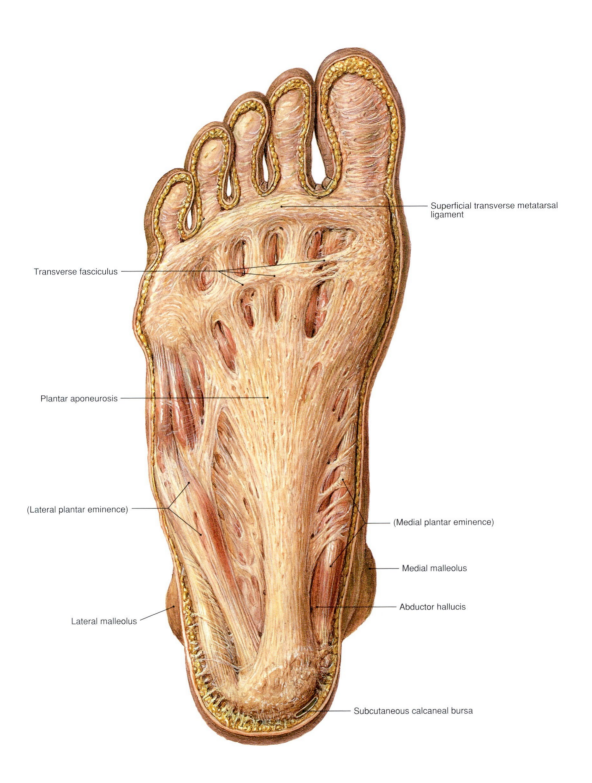

Superficial transverse metatarsal ligament

Transverse fasciculus

Plantar aponeurosis

(Lateral plantar eminence)

(Medial plantar eminence)

Medial malleolus

Abductor hallucis

Lateral malleolus

Subcutaneous calcaneal bursa

Fig. 1095   Muscles of the foot;
plantar aponeurosis.

Origins and insertions of the muscles of the foot and the leg

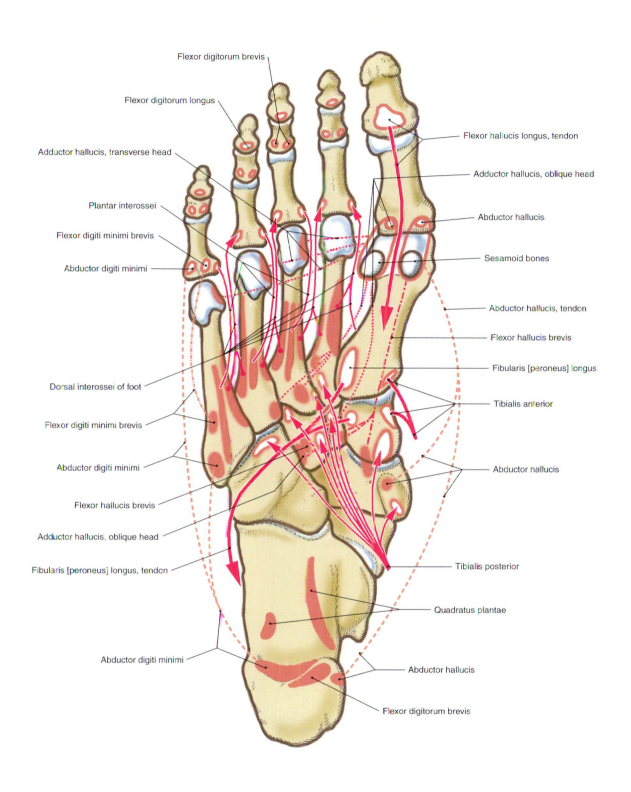

Fig. 1096 Origins and insertions of the muscles at the bones of the foot; plantar view.

→ T 42, T 48, T 50, T 52–T 54

Muscles of the foot

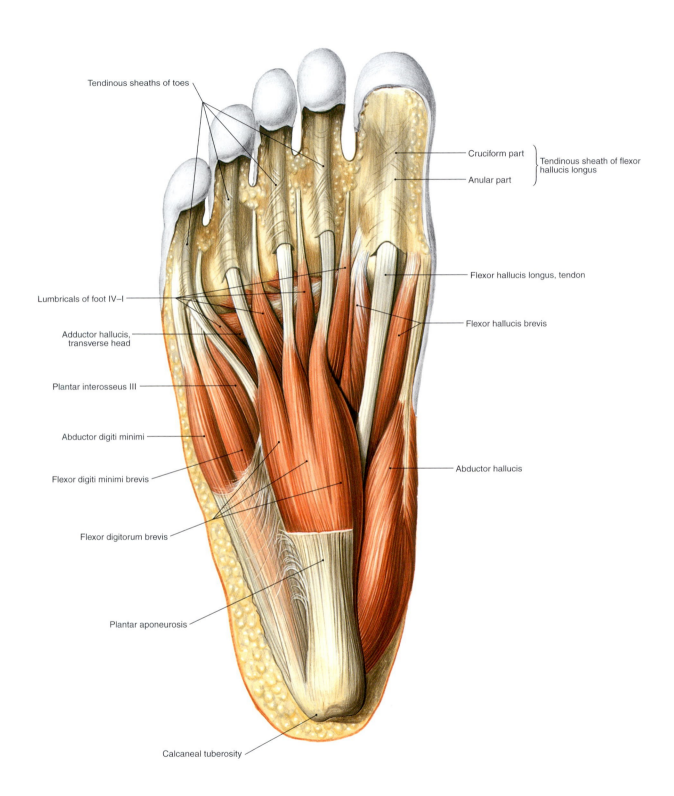

Tendinous sheaths of toes

Cruciform part ⎫ Tendinous sheath of flexor
                ⎬ hallucis longus
Anular part   ⎭

Flexor hallucis longus, tendon

Lumbricals of foot IV–I

Flexor hallucis brevis

Adductor hallucis, transverse head

Plantar interosseus III

Abductor digiti minimi

Flexor digiti minimi brevis

Abductor hallucis

Flexor digitorum brevis

Plantar aponeurosis

Calcaneal tuberosity

→ T 52–T 54

Fig. 1097 Muscles of the foot; the plantar aponeurosis has been removed.

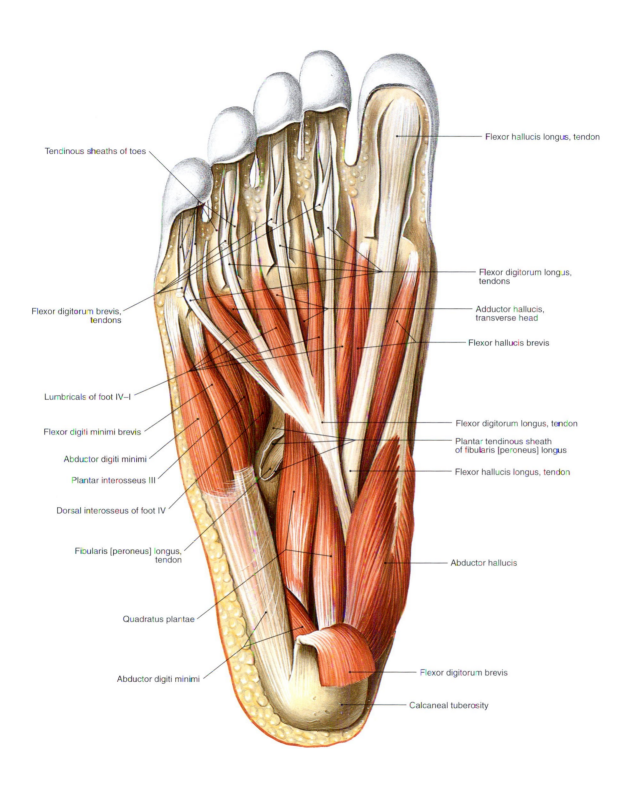

Tendinous sheaths of toes

Flexor digitorum brevis, tendons

Lumbricals of foot IV–I

Flexor digiti minimi brevis

Abductor digiti minimi

Plantar interosseus III

Dorsal interosseus of foot IV

Fibularis [peroneus] longus, tendon

Quadratus plantae

Abductor digiti minimi

Flexor hallucis longus, tendon

Flexor digitorum longus, tendons

Adductor hallucis, transverse head

Flexor hallucis brevis

Flexor digitorum longus, tendon

Plantar tendinous sheath of fibularis [peroneus] longus

Flexor hallucis longus, tendon

Abductor hallucis

Flexor digitorum brevis

Calcaneal tuberosity

Fig. 1098 Muscles of the foot; middle layer after almost complete removal of the flexor digitorum brevis muscle.

→ T 50, T 52–T 54

Muscles of the foot

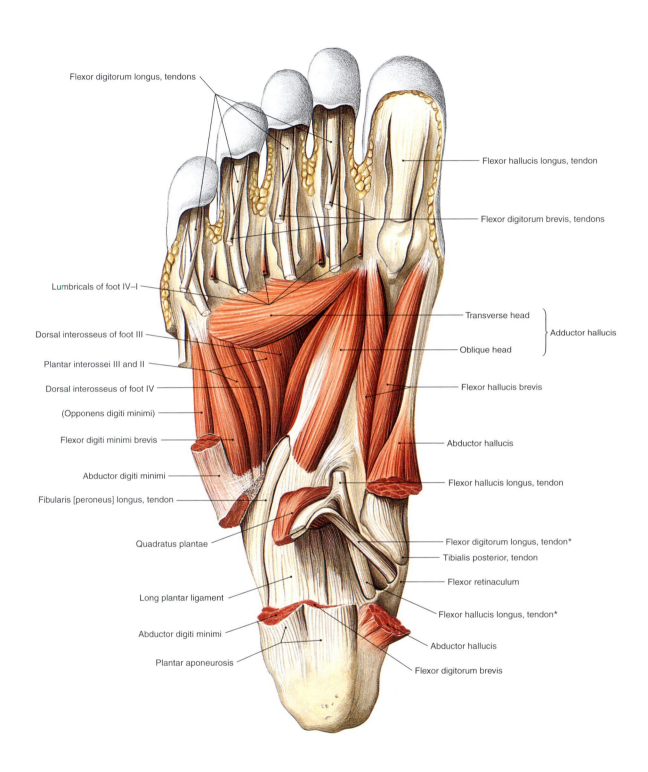

Flexor digitorum longus, tendons

Flexor hallucis longus, tendon

Flexor digitorum brevis, tendons

Lumbricals of foot IV–I

Transverse head
Oblique head ⎫ Adductor hallucis

Dorsal interosseus of foot III

Plantar interossei III and II

Dorsal interosseus of foot IV

Flexor hallucis brevis

(Opponens digiti minimi)

Flexor digiti minimi brevis

Abductor hallucis

Abductor digiti minimi

Flexor hallucis longus, tendon

Fibularis [peroneus] longus, tendon

Flexor digitorum longus, tendon*

Tibialis posterior, tendon

Quadratus plantae

Flexor retinaculum

Long plantar ligament

Flexor hallucis longus, tendon*

Abductor digiti minimi

Abductor hallucis

Plantar aponeurosis

Flexor digitorum brevis

→ T 50, 52–T 54

Fig. 1099 Muscles of the foot;
deep layer.

* The site where the tendon of the flexor digitorum longus muscle
crosses the tendon of the flexor hallucis longus muscle is commonly
referred to as plantar chiasm.

Muscles of the foot

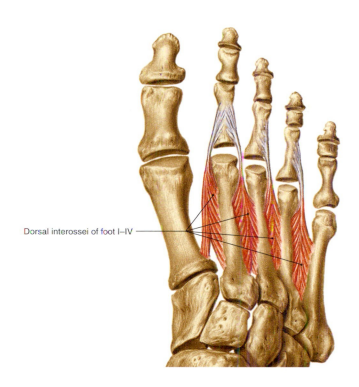

Fig. 1100   Dorsal interossei muscles;
dorsal view.

Dorsal interossei of foot I–IV

→ T 53

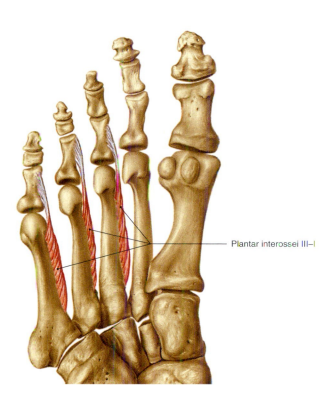

Fig. 1101   Plantar interossei muscles;
plantar view.

Plantar interossei III–I

→ T 53

Lumbosacral plexus

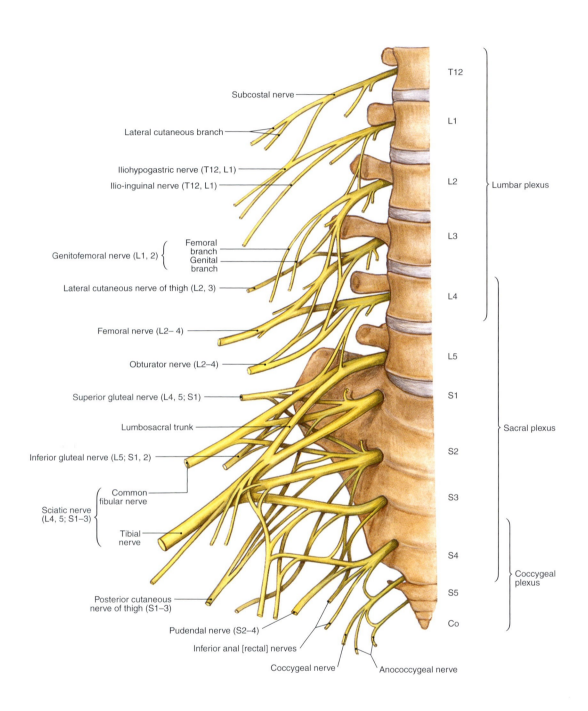

Subcostal nerve

Lateral cutaneous branch

Iliohypogastric nerve (T12, L1)

Ilio-inguinal nerve (T12, L1)

Genitofemoral nerve (L1, 2) {
Femoral branch
Genital branch

Lateral cutaneous nerve of thigh (L2, 3)

Femoral nerve (L2–4)

Obturator nerve (L2–4)

Superior gluteal nerve (L4, 5; S1)

Lumbosacral trunk

Inferior gluteal nerve (L5; S1, 2)

Sciatic nerve (L4, 5; S1–3) {
Common fibular nerve
Tibial nerve

Posterior cutaneous nerve of thigh (S1–3)

Pudendal nerve (S2–4)

Inferior anal [rectal] nerves

Coccygeal nerve

Anococcygeal nerve

T12

L1

L2

L3

L4

L5

S1

S2

S3

S4

S5

Co

Lumbar plexus

Sacral plexus

Coccygeal plexus

→ 595

Fig. 1102 Lumbosacral and coccygeal plexus; segmental organisation of nerves.

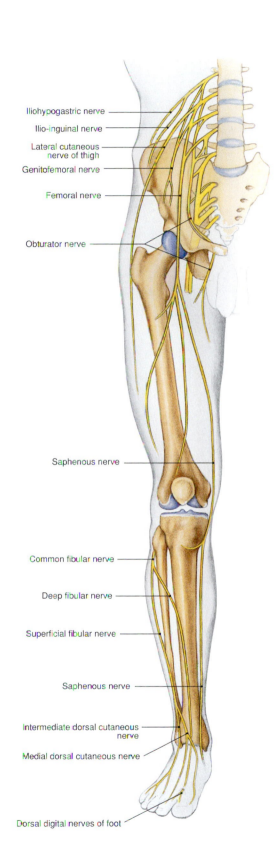

Iliohypogastric nerve

Ilio-inguinal nerve

Lateral cutaneous nerve of thigh

Genitofemoral nerve

Femoral nerve

Obturator nerve

Saphenous nerve

Common fibular nerve

Deep fibular nerve

Superficial fibular nerve

Saphenous nerve

Intermediate dorsal cutaneous nerve

Medial dorsal cutaneous nerve

Dorsal digital nerves of foot

Fig. 1103   Nerves of the lower limb; overview.

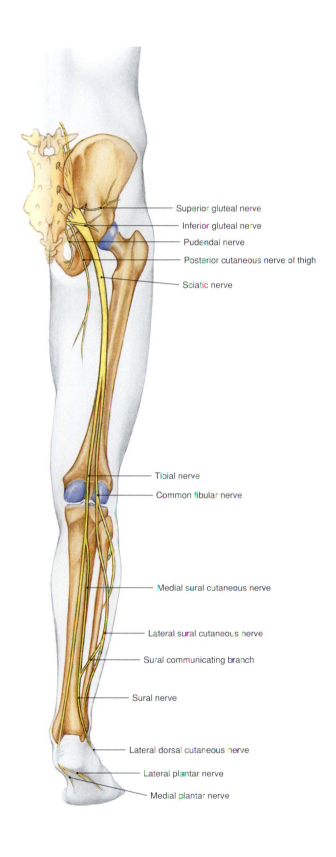

Superior gluteal nerve

Inferior gluteal nerve

Pudendal nerve

Posterior cutaneous nerve of thigh

Sciatic nerve

Tibial nerve

Common fibular nerve

Medial sural cutaneous nerve

Lateral sural cutaneous nerve

Sural communicating branch

Sural nerve

Lateral dorsal cutaneous nerve

Lateral plantar nerve

Medial plantar nerve

Fig. 1104   Nerves of the lower limb; overview.

Cutaneous innervation

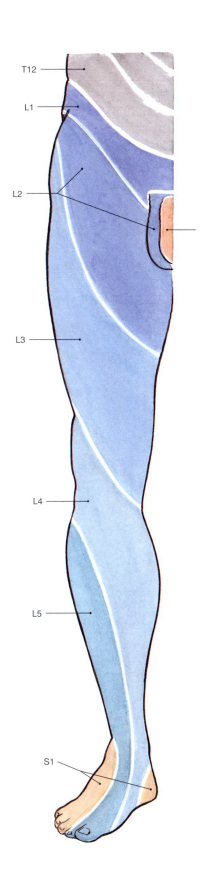

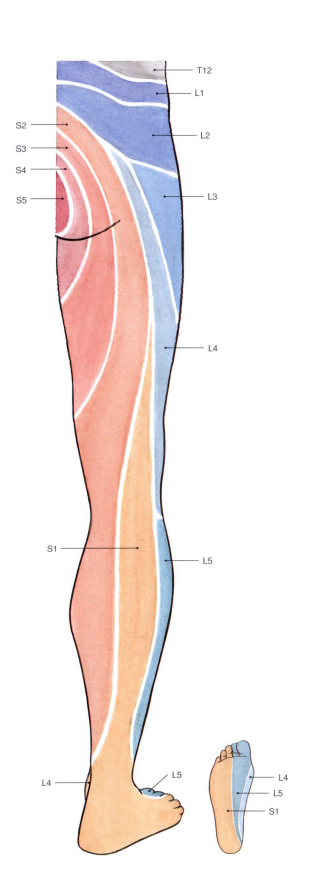

Fig. 1105 Segmental cutaneous innervation (dermatomes) of the lower limb.

Fig. 1106 Segmental cutaneous innervation (dermatomes) of the lower limb.

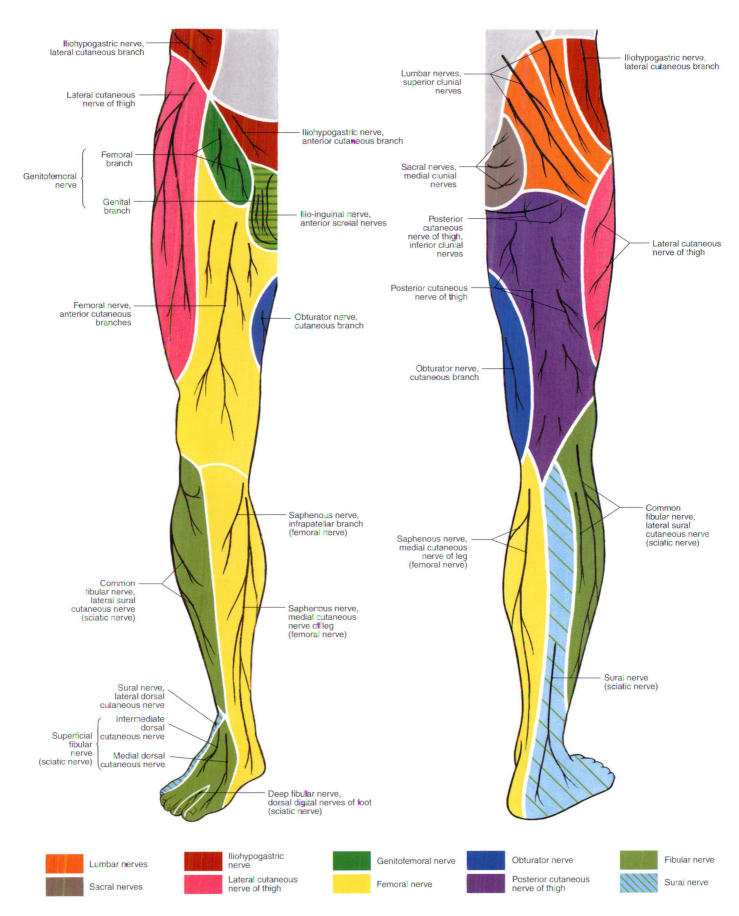

Iliohypogastric nerve, lateral cutaneous branch

Lateral cutaneous nerve of thigh

Genitofemoral nerve — Femoral branch

Genital branch

Iliohypogastric nerve, anterior cutaneous branch

Ilio-inguinal nerve, anterior scrotal nerves

Femoral nerve, anterior cutaneous branches

Obturator nerve, cutaneous branch

Saphenous nerve, infrapatellar branch (femoral nerve)

Common fibular nerve, lateral sural cutaneous nerve (sciatic nerve)

Saphenous nerve, medial cutaneous nerve of leg (femoral nerve)

Sural nerve, lateral dorsal cutaneous nerve

Superficial fibular nerve (sciatic nerve) — Intermediate dorsal cutaneous nerve

Medial dorsal cutaneous nerve

Deep fibular nerve, dorsal digital nerves of foot (sciatic nerve)

Lumbar nerves, superior clunial nerves

Iliohypogastric nerve, lateral cutaneous branch

Sacral nerves, medial clunial nerves

Posterior cutaneous nerve of thigh, inferior clunial nerves

Lateral cutaneous nerve of thigh

Posterior cutaneous nerve of thigh

Obturator nerve, cutaneous branch

Common fibular nerve, lateral sural cutaneous nerve (sciatic nerve)

Saphenous nerve, medial cutaneous nerve of leg (femoral nerve)

Sural nerve (sciatic nerve)

Lumbar nerves

Sacral nerves

Iliohypogastric nerve

Lateral cutaneous nerve of thigh

Genitofemoral nerve

Femoral nerve

Obturator nerve

Posterior cutaneous nerve of thigh

Fibular nerve

Sural nerve

Fig. 1107 Cutaneous nerves of the lower limb.

Fig. 1108 Cutaneous nerves of the lower limb.

Fermoral and obturator nerve

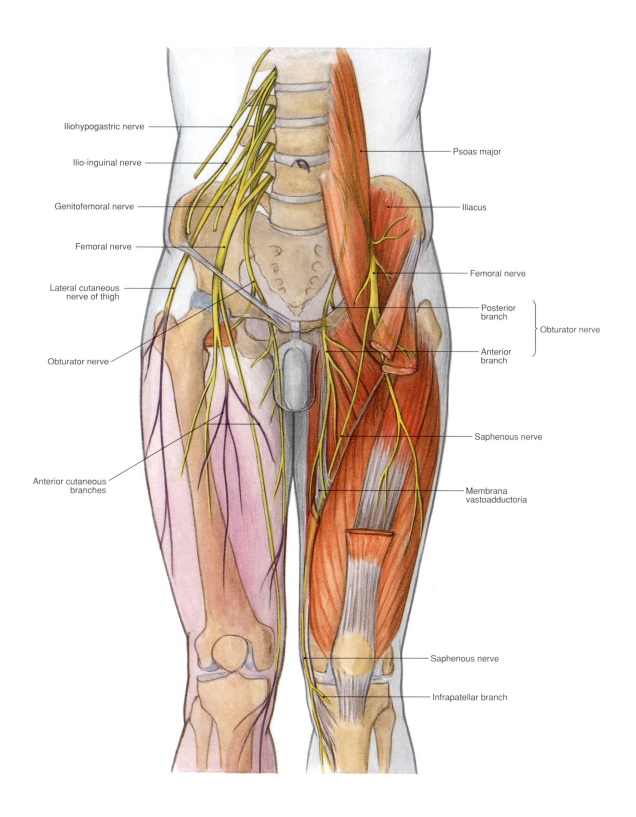

Iliohypogastric nerve

Ilio-inguinal nerve

Genitofemoral nerve

Femoral nerve

Lateral cutaneous nerve of thigh

Obturator nerve

Anterior cutaneous branches

Psoas major

Iliacus

Femoral nerve

Posterior branch

Obturator nerve

Anterior branch

Saphenous nerve

Membrana vastoadductoria

Saphenous nerve

Infrapatellar branch

Fig. 1109 Femoral and obturator nerve;
overview;
cutaneous innervation illustrated with purple.

Gluteal nerves and sciatic nerve

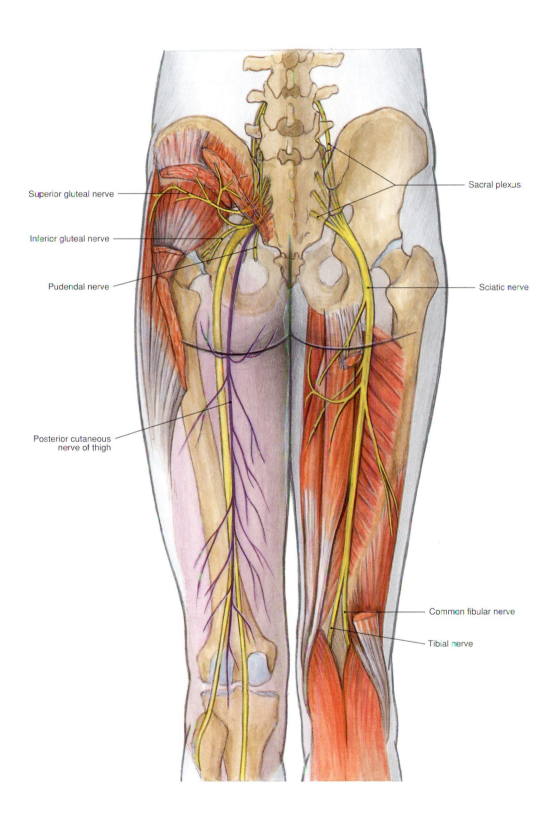

Superior gluteal nerve

Inferior gluteal nerve

Pudendal nerve

Posterior cutaneous nerve of thigh

Sacral plexus

Sciatic nerve

Common fibular nerve

Tibial nerve

Fig. 1110   Gluteal nerves and sciatic nerve;
overview;
cutaneous innervation illustrated with purple.

Tibial and fibular nerve

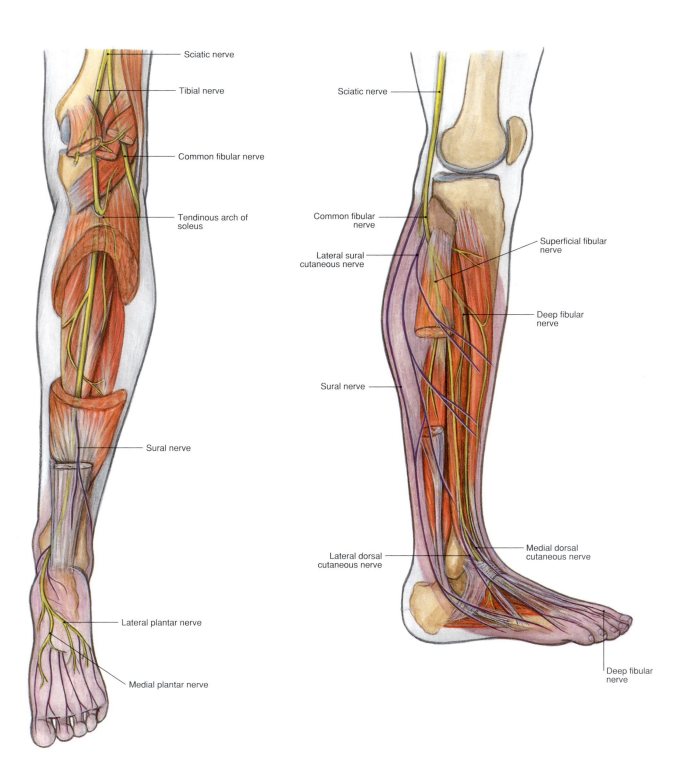

Fig. 1111 Tibial nerve; overview; cutaneous innervation illustrated with purple.

Fig. 1112 Fibular nerve; overview; cutaneous innervation illustrated with purple.

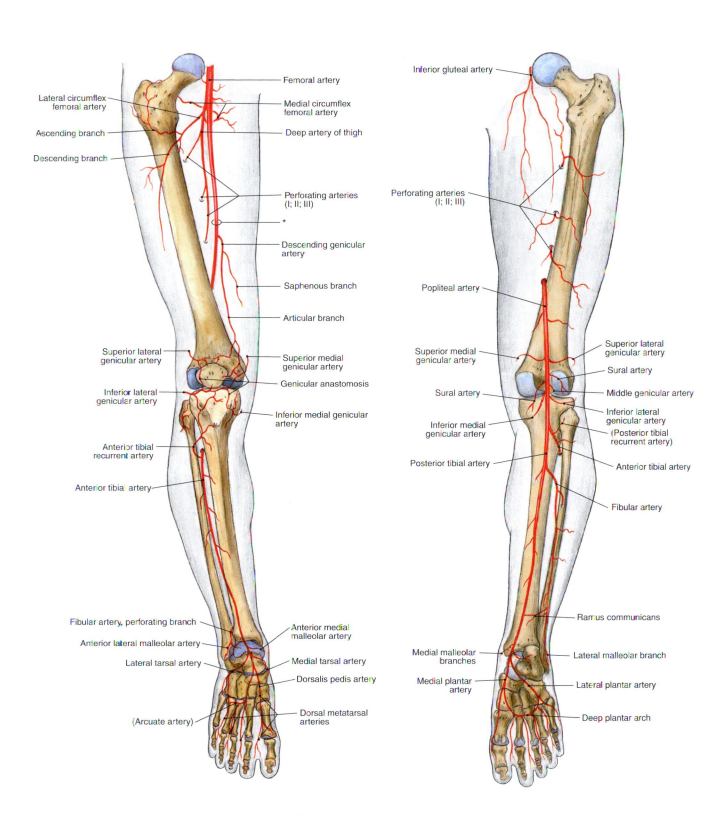

Femoral artery

Lateral circumflex femoral artery

Medial circumflex femoral artery

Ascending branch

Deep artery of thigh

Descending branch

Perforating arteries (I; II; III)

*

Descending genicular artery

Saphenous branch

Articular branch

Superior lateral genicular artery

Superior medial genicular artery

Genicular anastomosis

Inferior lateral genicular artery

Inferior medial genicular artery

Anterior tibial recurrent artery

Anterior tibial artery

Fibular artery, perforating branch

Anterior lateral malleolar artery

Anterior medial malleolar artery

Lateral tarsal artery

Medial tarsal artery

Dorsalis pedis artery

(Arcuate artery)

Dorsal metatarsal arteries

Inferior gluteal artery

Perforating arteries (I; II; III)

Popliteal artery

Superior medial genicular artery

Superior lateral genicular artery

Sural artery

Sural artery

Middle genicular artery

Inferior medial genicular artery

Inferior lateral genicular artery

(Posterior tibial recurrent artery)

Posterior tibial artery

Anterior tibial artery

Fibular artery

Ramus communicans

Medial malleolar branches

Lateral malleolar branch

Medial plantar artery

Lateral plantar artery

Deep plantar arch

Fig. 1113   Arteries of the lower limb;
overview;
ventral view.
The segment of the femoral artery between the point where
the deep artery of thigh branches off and the point of entry
into the adductor canal (*) is known clinically as superficial
femoral artery.

Fig. 1114   Arteries of the lower limb;
overview;
dorsal view.

Veins and lymphatics of the lower limb

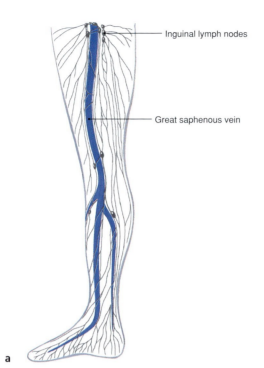

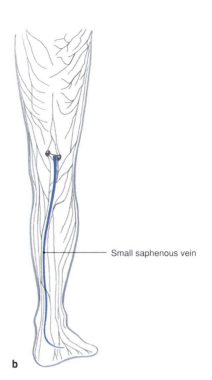

Fig. 1115 a, b Veins and lymphatics of the lower limb; overview.

a Medial view
b Dorsal view

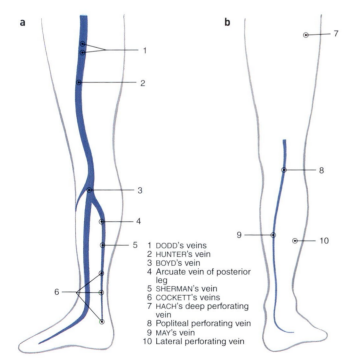

1 DODD's veins
2 HUNTER's vein
3 BOYD's vein
4 Arcuate vein of posterior leg
5 SHERMAN's vein
6 COCKETT's veins
7 HACH's deep perforating vein
8 Popliteal perforating vein
9 MAY's vein
10 Lateral perforating vein

Fig. 1116 a, b Perforating veins; overview (according to HACH, 1986).
a Medial view
b Dorsal view

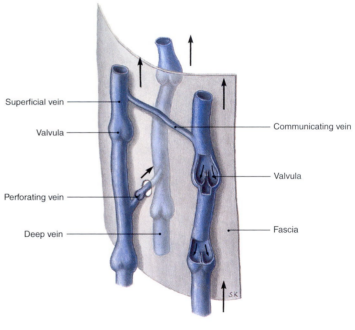

Fig. 1117 Veins of the lower limb; principle of organisation.
Disturbances of the venous flow of the lower limb, especially varicosis, are a common cause of vascular disorders.
If one of the venous systems is entirely occluded, the perforating veins may be of crucial importance to maintain the venous drainage.

Vessels and nerves of the thigh

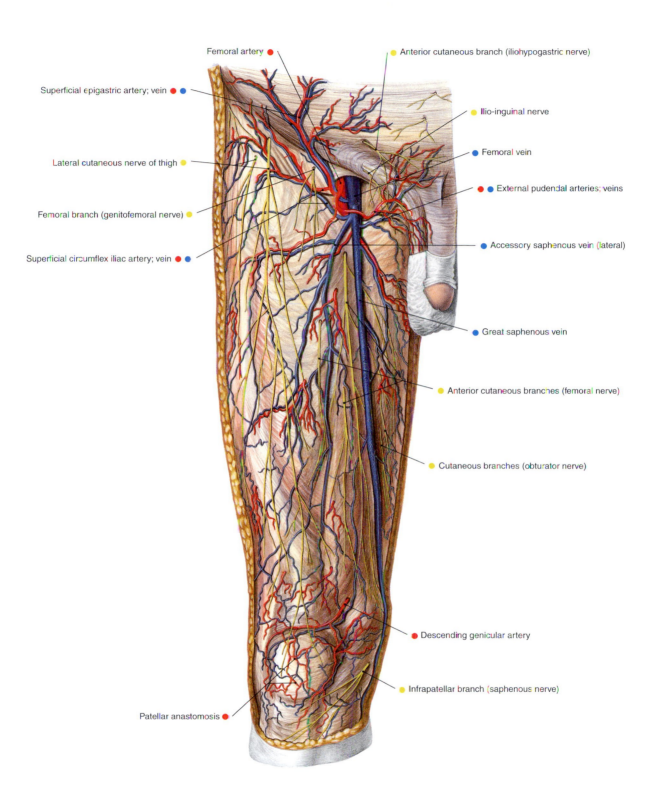

Femoral artery ●

Superficial epigastric artery; vein ● ●

Lateral cutaneous nerve of thigh ●

Femoral branch (genitofemoral nerve) ●

Superficial circumflex iliac artery; vein ● ●

● Anterior cutaneous branch (iliohypogastric nerve)

● Ilio-inguinal nerve

● Femoral vein

● ● External pudendal arteries; veins

● Accessory saphenous vein (lateral)

● Great saphenous vein

● Anterior cutaneous branches (femoral nerve)

● Cutaneous branches (obturator nerve)

● Descending genicular artery

● Infrapatellar branch (saphenous nerve)

Patellar anastomosis ●

Fig. 1118   Epifascial vessels and nerves of the inguinal region, the anterior region of thigh and the anterior region of knee.

592

1123

1135

Lymphatics of the inguinal region

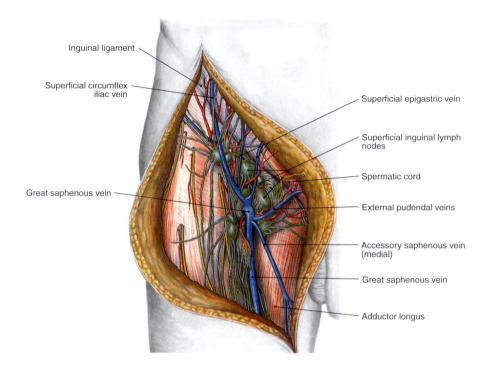

Inguinal ligament

Superficial circumflex iliac vein

Great saphenous vein

Superficial epigastric vein

Superficial inguinal lymph nodes

Spermatic cord

External pudendal veins

Accessory saphenous vein (medial)

Great saphenous vein

Adductor longus

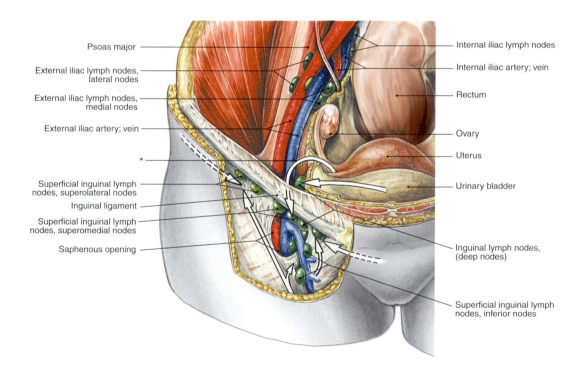

Psoas major

External iliac lymph nodes, lateral nodes

External iliac lymph nodes, medial nodes

External iliac artery; vein

*

Superficial inguinal lymph nodes, superolateral nodes

Inguinal ligament

Superficial inguinal lymph nodes, superomedial nodes

Saphenous opening

Internal iliac lymph nodes

Internal iliac artery; vein

Rectum

Ovary

Uterus

Urinary bladder

Inguinal lymph nodes, (deep nodes)

Superficial inguinal lymph nodes, inferior nodes

Fig. 1120 Draining areas of the lymph nodes in the inguinal region of the female; overview.
The arrows indicate possible directions of the flow of lymph.

* In some rare cases, the medial parts of the uterine tube and the fundus of the uterus may be drained by superficial lymph nodes in the inguinal region via the round ligament of uterus.

Vessels and nerves of the inguinal region

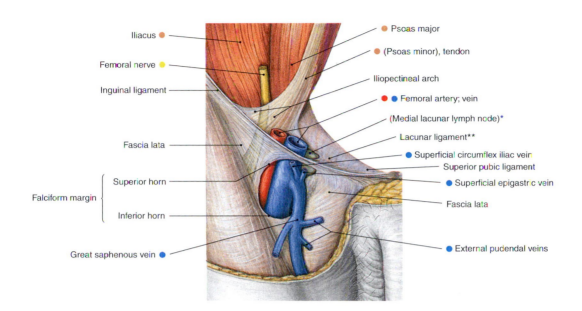

Iliacus ●

Femoral nerve ●

Inguinal ligament

Fascia lata

Falciform margin { Superior horn

Inferior horn

Great saphenous vein ●

● Psoas major

● (Psoas minor), tendon

Iliopectineal arch

● ● Femoral artery; vein

(Medial lacunar lymph node)*

Lacunar ligament**

● Superficial circumflex iliac vein

Superior pubic ligament

● Superficial epigastric vein

Fascia lata

● External pudendal veins

Fig. 1121   Saphenous opening and vascular space; after removal of the anterior abdominal wall and the contents of the abdomen, as well as dissection of the iliac fascia and the femoral septum [CLOQUET].

* Also: ROSENMÜLLER's node
** Also: GIMBERNAT's ligament

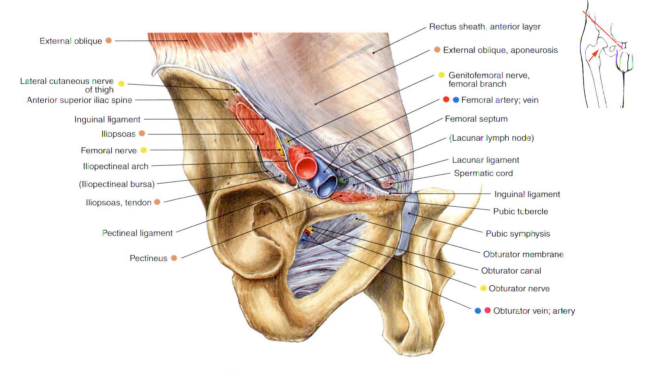

External oblique ●

Lateral cutaneous nerve of thigh ●

Anterior superior iliac spine

Inguinal ligament

Iliopsoas ●

Femoral nerve ●

Iliopectineal arch

(Iliopectineal bursa)

Iliopsoas, tendon ●

Pectineal ligament

Pectineus ●

Rectus sheath, anterior layer

● External oblique, aponeurosis

● Genitofemoral nerve, femoral branch

● ● Femoral artery; vein

Femoral septum

(Lacunar lymph node)

Lacunar ligament

Spermatic cord

Inguinal ligament

Pubic tubercle

Pubic symphysis

Obturator membrane

Obturator canal

● Obturator nerve

● ● Obturator vein; artery

Fig. 1122   Muscular and vascular space; oblique section at the level of the inguinal ligament.

Vessels and nerves of the thigh

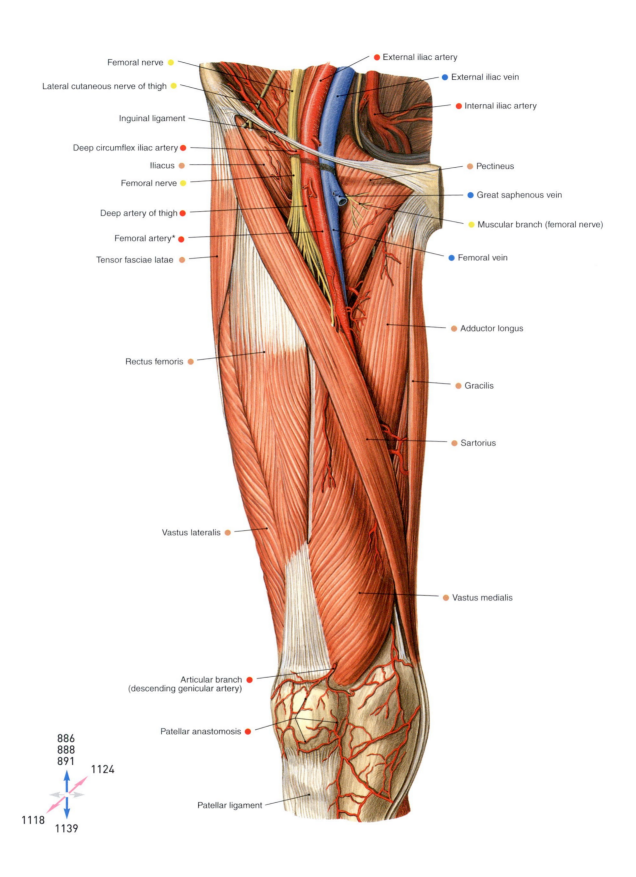

Femoral nerve ●

Lateral cutaneous nerve of thigh ●

Inguinal ligament

Deep circumflex iliac artery ●

Iliacus ●

Femoral nerve ●

Deep artery of thigh ●

Femoral artery* ●

Tensor fasciae latae ●

Rectus femoris ●

Vastus lateralis ●

Articular branch
(descending genicular artery) ●

Patellar anastomosis ●

Patellar ligament

● External iliac artery

● External iliac vein

● Internal iliac artery

● Pectineus

● Great saphenous vein

● Muscular branch (femoral nerve)

● Femoral vein

● Adductor longus

● Gracilis

● Sartorius

● Vastus medialis

886
888
891
1124

1118 1139

Fig. 1123 Vessels and nerves of the anterior region of thigh;
after removal of the fascia lata except for the iliotibial tract.

* Clinically the femoral artery is commonly referred to as superficial
femoral artery to distinguish it from the deep artery of thigh.

Vessels and nerves of the thigh

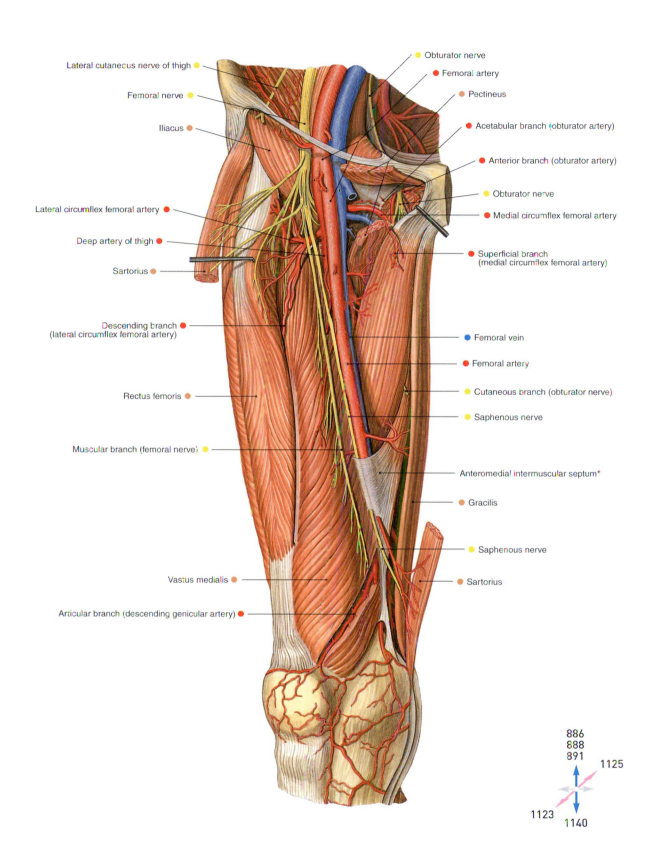

Lateral cutaneous nerve of thigh ●

Femoral nerve ●

Iliacus ●

Lateral circumflex femoral artery ●

Deep artery of thigh ●

Sartorius ●

Descending branch ●
(lateral circumflex femoral artery)

Rectus femoris ●

Muscular branch (femoral nerve) ●

Vastus medialis ●

Articular branch (descending genicular artery) ●

Obturator nerve ●

Femoral artery ●

Pectineus ●

Acetabular branch (obturator artery) ●

Anterior branch (obturator artery) ●

Obturator nerve ●

Medial circumflex femoral artery ●

Superficial branch ●
(medial circumflex femoral artery)

Femoral vein ●

Femoral artery ●

Cutaneous branch (obturator nerve) ●

Saphenous nerve ●

Anteromedial intermuscular septum*

Gracilis ●

Saphenous nerve ●

Sartorius ●

886
888
891
1125
1123
1140

Fig. 1124   Vessels and nerves of the anterior region of thigh;
after partial removal of the sartorius muscle and dissection of
the pectineus muscle.

*   The entrance into the adductor canal is formed by the vastus medialis
and adductor longus muscles as well as by the anteromedial
intermuscular septum spanning between them.

Vessels and nerves of the thigh

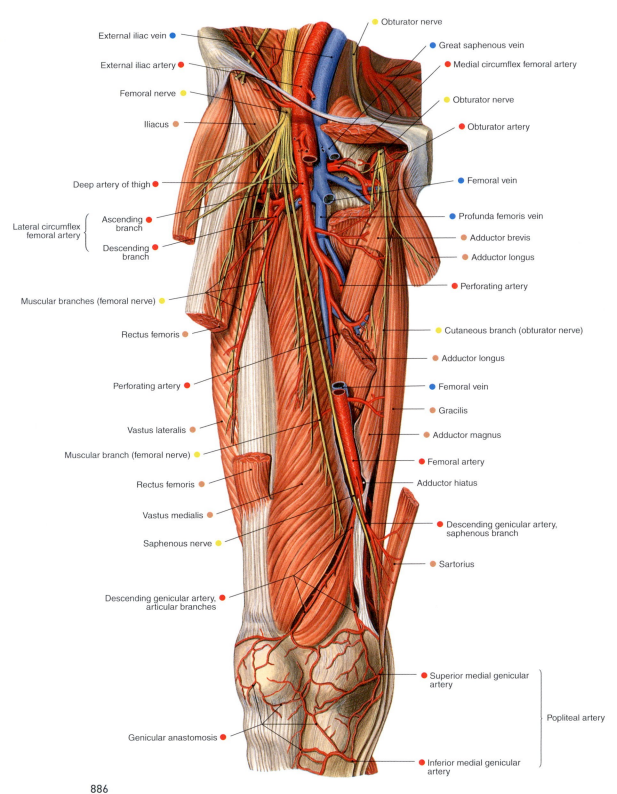

External iliac vein ●
External iliac artery ●
Femoral nerve ●
Iliacus ●
Deep artery of thigh ●
Lateral circumflex femoral artery { Ascending branch ● Descending branch ● }
Muscular branches (femoral nerve) ●
Rectus femoris ●
Perforating artery ●
Vastus lateralis ●
Muscular branch (femoral nerve) ●
Rectus femoris ●
Vastus medialis ●
Saphenous nerve ●
Descending genicular artery, articular branches ●
Genicular anastomosis ●

Obturator nerve ●
● Great saphenous vein
● Medial circumflex femoral artery
● Obturator nerve
● Obturator artery
● Femoral vein
● Profunda femoris vein
● Adductor brevis
● Adductor longus
● Perforating artery
● Cutaneous branch (obturator nerve)
● Adductor longus
● Femoral vein
● Gracilis
● Adductor magnus
● Femoral artery
Adductor hiatus
● Descending genicular artery, saphenous branch
● Sartorius
● Superior medial genicular artery } Popliteal artery
● Inferior medial genicular artery

886
888
891

1124   1140

Fig. 1125 Vessels and nerves of the anterior region of thigh;
deep layer after partial removal of the sartorius and rectus femoris
muscles, the pectineus and adductor longus muscles have been
dissected; the adductor canal is almost entirely opened.

Arteries of the pelvis and the hip

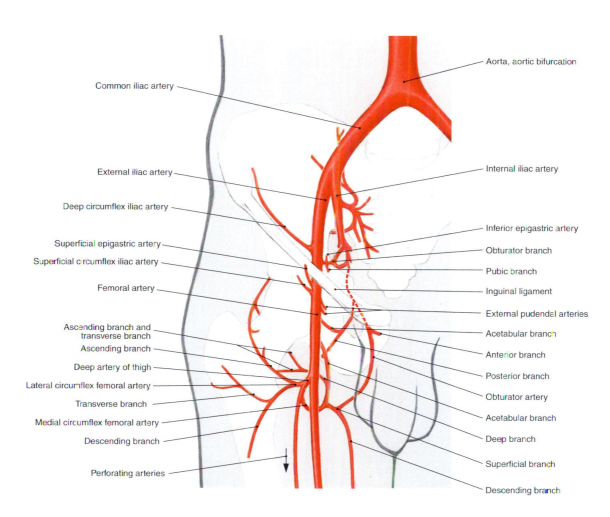

Common iliac artery

External iliac artery

Deep circumflex iliac artery

Superficial epigastric artery

Superficial circumflex iliac artery

Femoral artery

Ascending branch and transverse branch

Ascending branch

Deep artery of thigh

Lateral circumflex femoral artery

Transverse branch

Medial circumflex femoral artery

Descending branch

Perforating arteries

Aorta, aortic bifurcation

Internal iliac artery

Inferior epigastric artery

Obturator branch

Pubic branch

Inguinal ligament

External pudendal arteries

Acetabular branch

Anterior branch

Posterior branch

Obturator artery

Acetabular branch

Deep branch

Superficial branch

Descending branch

Fig. 1126   Arteries of the hip and the thigh; overview.

The branching pattern of these arteries varies considerably. This type of origin and arborisation of the deep artery of thigh occurs in approximately 58% of cases.

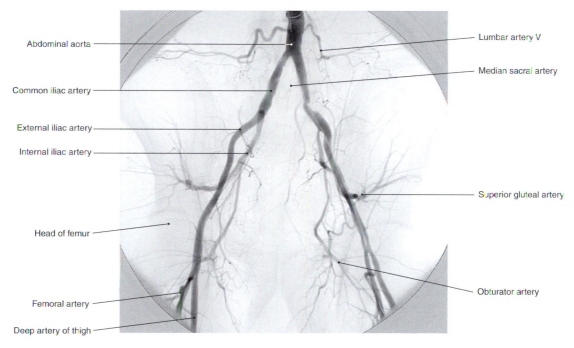

Abdominal aorta

Common iliac artery

External iliac artery

Internal iliac artery

Head of femur

Femoral artery

Deep artery of thigh

Lumbar artery V

Median sacral artery

Superior gluteal artery

Obturator artery

Fig. 1127   Arteries of the pelvis and the thigh; digital subtraction angiography (DSA).

Veins and nerves of the thigh

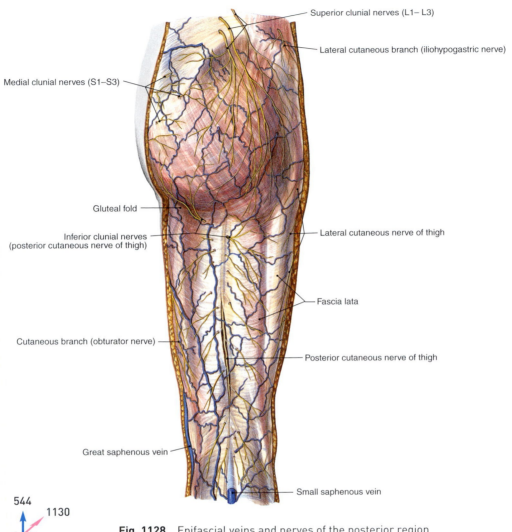

Superior clunial nerves (L1–L3)

Lateral cutaneous branch (iliohypogastric nerve)

Medial clunial nerves (S1–S3)

Gluteal fold

Inferior clunial nerves
(posterior cutaneous nerve of thigh)

Lateral cutaneous nerve of thigh

Fascia lata

Cutaneous branch (obturator nerve)

Posterior cutaneous nerve of thigh

Great saphenous vein

Small saphenous vein

544
1130
1136

Fig. 1128 Epifascial veins and nerves of the posterior region of thigh, the gluteal region and the popliteal fossa.

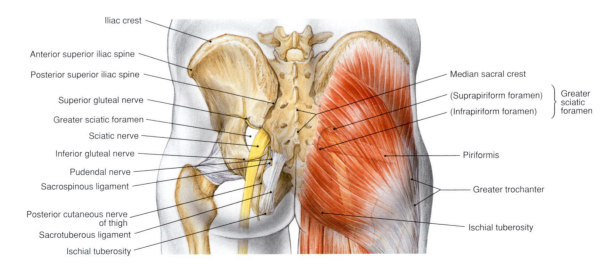

Iliac crest

Anterior superior iliac spine

Posterior superior iliac spine

Superior gluteal nerve

Greater sciatic foramen

Sciatic nerve

Inferior gluteal nerve

Pudendal nerve

Sacrospinous ligament

Posterior cutaneous nerve
of thigh

Sacrotuberous ligament

Ischial tuberosity

Median sacral crest

(Suprapiriform foramen) } Greater
(Infrapiriform foramen) } sciatic
foramen

Piriformis

Greater trochanter

Ischial tuberosity

Fig. 1129 Skeleton contour and sciatic nerve projected onto the surface of the gluteal region.

Vessels and nerves of the thigh

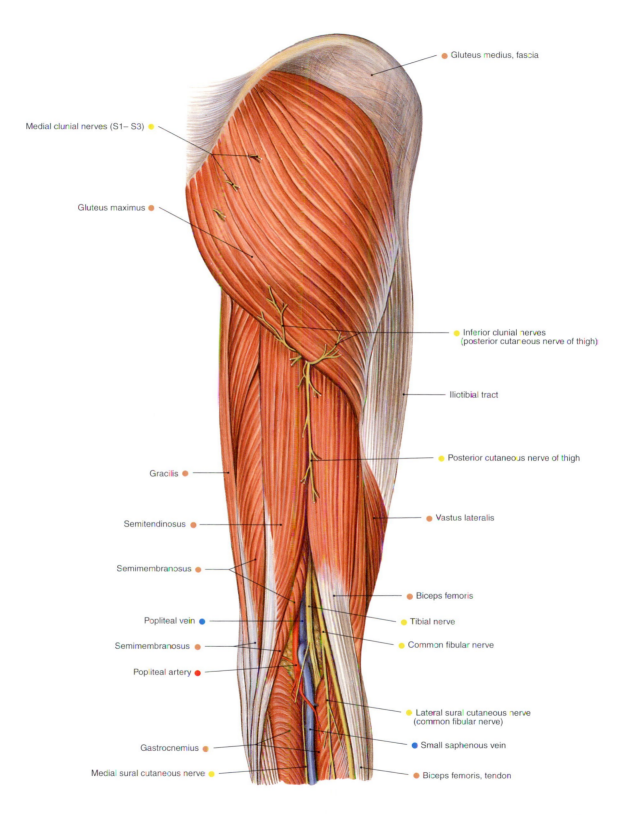

Gluteus medius, fascia

Medial clunial nerves (S1– S3)

Gluteus maximus

Inferior clunial nerves
(posterior cutaneous nerve of thigh)

Iliotibial tract

Posterior cutaneous nerve of thigh

Gracilis

Vastus lateralis

Semitendinosus

Semimembranosus

Biceps femoris

Popliteal vein

Tibial nerve

Semimembranosus

Common fibular nerve

Popliteal artery

Lateral sural cutaneous nerve
(common fibular nerve)

Small saphenous vein

Gastrocnemius

Medial sural cutaneous nerve

Biceps femoris, tendon

Fig. 1130   Vessels and nerves of the gluteal region,
the posterior region of thigh and the popliteal fossa.

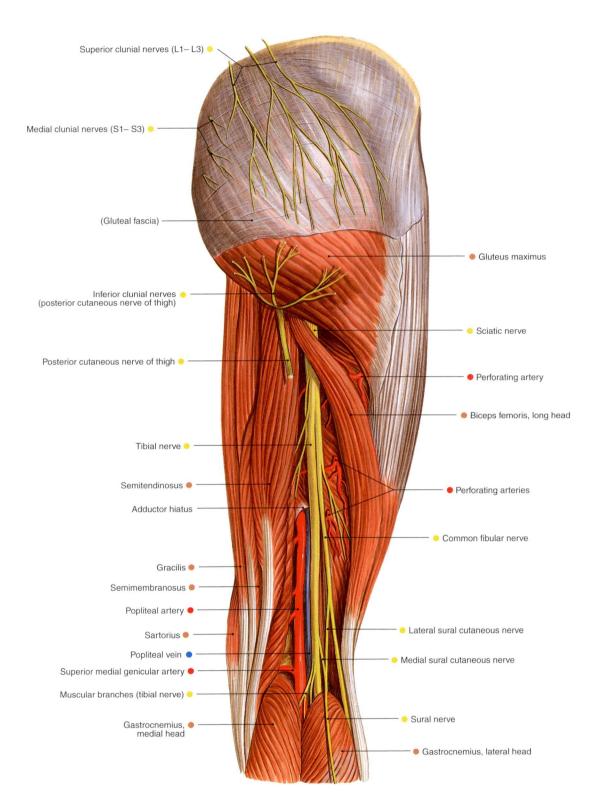

Superior clunial nerves (L1– L3) ●

Medial clunial nerves (S1– S3) ●

(Gluteal fascia)

● Gluteus maximus

Inferior clunial nerves ●
(posterior cutaneous nerve of thigh)

Posterior cutaneous nerve of thigh ●

● Sciatic nerve

● Perforating artery

● Biceps femoris, long head

Tibial nerve ●

Semitendinosus ●

Adductor hiatus

● Perforating arteries

● Common fibular nerve

Gracilis ●

Semimembranosus ●

Popliteal artery ●

Sartorius ●

Popliteal vein ●

Superior medial genicular artery ●

Muscular branches (tibial nerve) ●

Gastrocnemius, ●
medial head

● Lateral sural cutaneous nerve

● Medial sural cutaneous nerve

● Sural nerve

● Gastrocnemius, lateral head

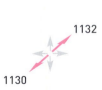

1132

1130

Fig. 1131   Vessels and nerves of the gluteal region,
the posterior region of thigh and the popliteal fossa;
the long head of the biceps femoris muscle has been retracted
laterally. In this specimen, the medial and lateral sural cutaneous
nerves branch off quite far proximally.

Vessels and nerves of the thigh

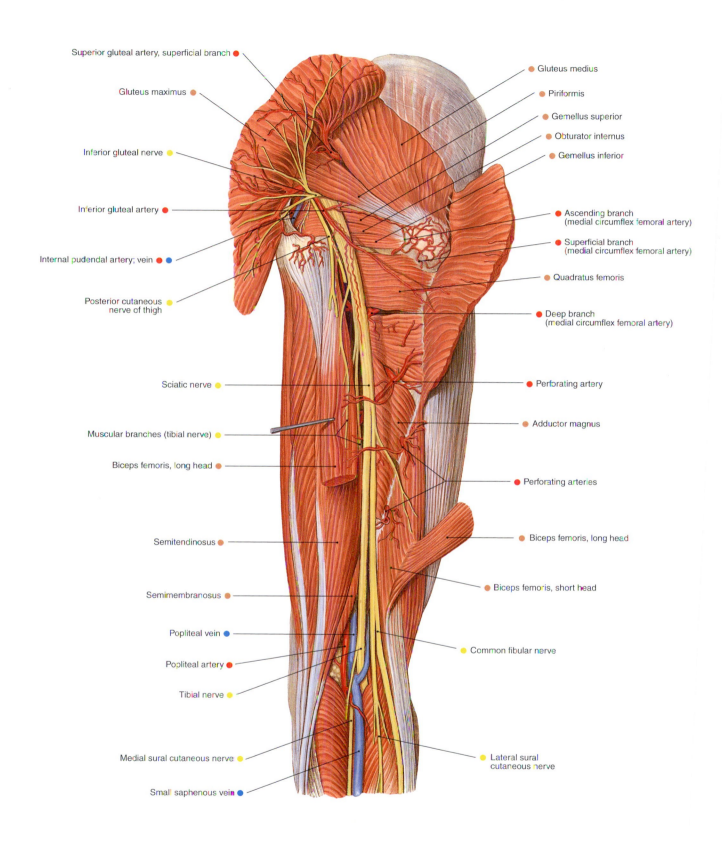

Superior gluteal artery, superficial branch ●

Gluteus maximus ●

Inferior gluteal nerve ●

Inferior gluteal artery ●

Internal pudendal artery; vein ● ●

Posterior cutaneous nerve of thigh ●

Sciatic nerve ●

Muscular branches (tibial nerve) ●

Biceps femoris, long head ●

Semitendinosus ●

Semimembranosus ●

Popliteal vein ●

Popliteal artery ●

Tibial nerve ●

Medial sural cutaneous nerve ●

Small saphenous vein ●

● Gluteus medius

● Piriformis

● Gemellus superior

● Obturator internus

● Gemellus inferior

● Ascending branch (medial circumflex femoral artery)

● Superficial branch (medial circumflex femoral artery)

● Quadratus femoris

● Deep branch (medial circumflex femoral artery)

● Perforating artery

● Adductor magnus

● Perforating arteries

● Biceps femoris, long head

● Biceps femoris, short head

● Common fibular nerve

● Lateral sural cutaneous nerve

Fig. 1132 Vessels and nerves of the gluteal region, the posterior region of thigh and the popliteal fossa; after dissection of the gluteus maximus muscle and the long head of the biceps femoris muscle.

1131

1143
1145
1146

Vessels and nerves of the gluteal region

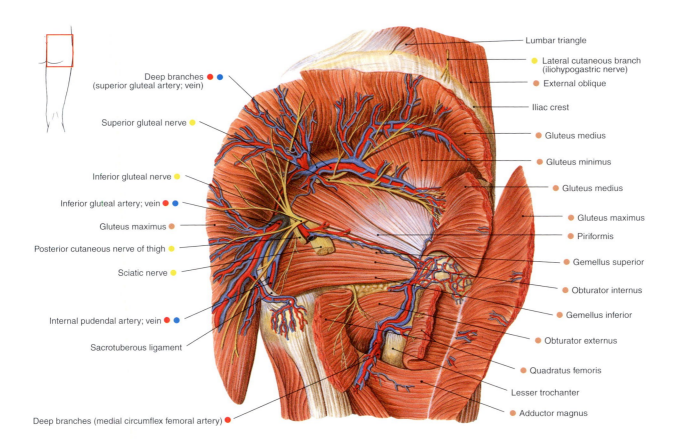

Deep branches 🔴 🔵
(superior gluteal artery; vein)

Superior gluteal nerve 🟡

Inferior gluteal nerve 🟡

Inferior gluteal artery; vein 🔴 🔵

Gluteus maximus 🟤

Posterior cutaneous nerve of thigh 🟡

Sciatic nerve 🟡

Internal pudendal artery; vein 🔴 🔵

Sacrotuberous ligament

Deep branches (medial circumflex femoral artery) 🔴

Lumbar triangle

Lateral cutaneous branch 🟡
(iliohypogastric nerve)

External oblique 🟤

Iliac crest

Gluteus medius 🟤

Gluteus minimus 🟤

Gluteus medius 🟤

Gluteus maximus 🟤

Piriformis 🟤

Gemellus superior 🟤

Obturator internus 🟤

Gemellus inferior 🟤

Obturator externus 🟤

Quadratus femoris 🟤

Lesser trochanter

Adductor magnus 🟤

Fig. 1133 Vessels and nerves of the gluteal region;
after dissection and partial removal of the gluteus maximus and medius muscles;
the sciatic nerve has been removed after its passage through the infrapiriform foramen.

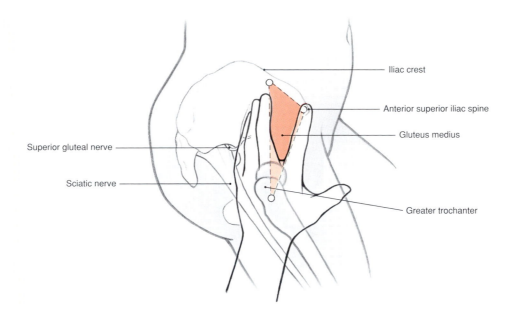

Superior gluteal nerve

Sciatic nerve

Iliac crest

Anterior superior iliac spine

Gluteus medius

Greater trochanter

Fig. 1134 Ventrogluteal injection (according to v. HOCHSTETTER). In order to avoid the superior gluteal nerve and, in particular, the superior gluteal artery the injection is made into the triangular field formed by the two spread fingers and the iliac crest. The index finger – or when using the right hand, the middle finger – is placed on the anterior superior iliac spine and the palm of the hand on the greater trochanter. Since the injected material should be deposited within the belly of the gluteus medius muscle as far away as possible from any vessel, the needle should not cross the lines of the triangle. However, some risk remains for the nerve branch that runs from the superior gluteal nerve to the tensor fasciae latae muscle.

Veins and nerves of the leg

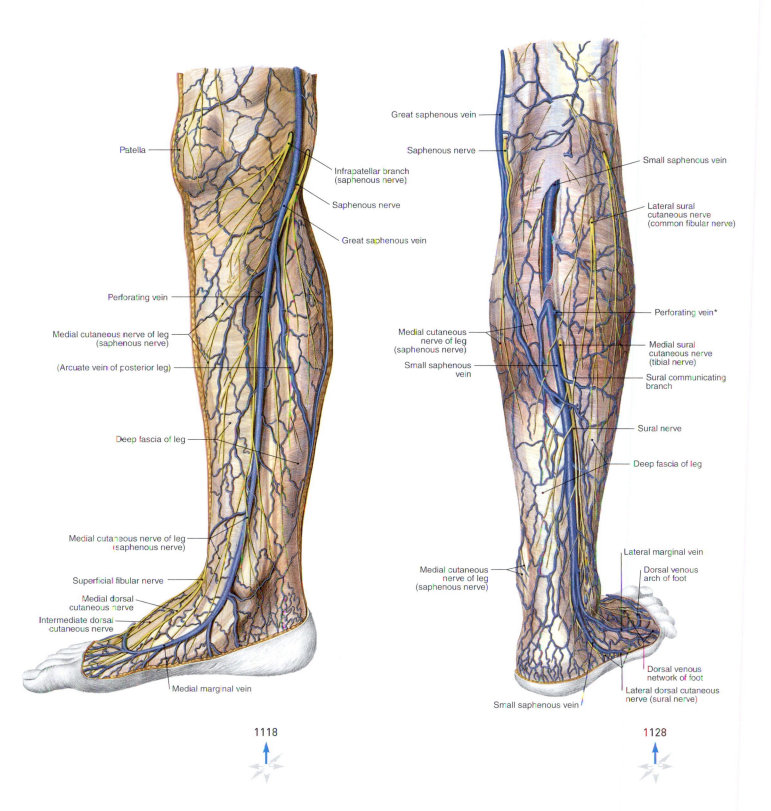

Patella

Infrapatellar branch
(saphenous nerve)

Saphenous nerve

Great saphenous vein

Perforating vein

Medial cutaneous nerve of leg
(saphenous nerve)

(Arcuate vein of posterior leg)

Deep fascia of leg

Medial cutaneous nerve of leg
(saphenous nerve)

Superficial fibular nerve

Medial dorsal
cutaneous nerve

Intermediate dorsal
cutaneous nerve

Medial marginal vein

Great saphenous vein

Saphenous nerve

Small saphenous vein

Lateral sural
cutaneous nerve
(common fibular nerve)

Medial cutaneous
nerve of leg
(saphenous nerve)

Small saphenous
vein

Perforating vein*

Medial sural
cutaneous nerve
(tibial nerve)

Sural communicating
branch

Sural nerve

Deep fascia of leg

Medial cutaneous
nerve of leg
(saphenous nerve)

Lateral marginal vein

Dorsal venous
arch of foot

Dorsal venous
network of foot

Lateral dorsal cutaneous
nerve (sural nerve)

Small saphenous vein

1118

1128

Fig. 1135 Epifascial veins and nerves of the leg
and the foot.

Fig. 1136 Epifascial veins and nerves of the leg
and the foot;
the deep fascia of leg has been dissected
proximally.

* Clinical term: MAY's vein

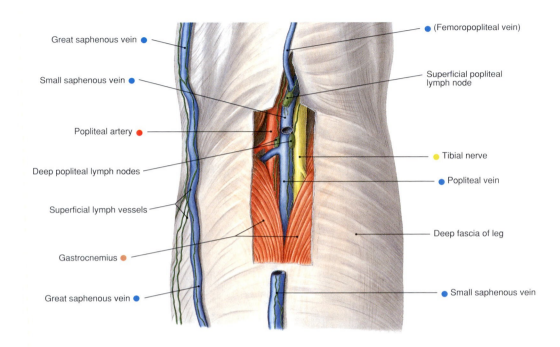

Great saphenous vein ●

Small saphenous vein ●

Popliteal artery ●

Deep popliteal lymph nodes

Superficial lymph vessels

Gastrocnemius ●

Great saphenous vein ●

● (Femoropopliteal vein)

Superficial popliteal lymph node

● Tibial nerve

● Popliteal vein

Deep fascia of leg

● Small saphenous vein

Fig. 1137   Vessels and nerves of the popliteal fossa;
after dissection of the deep fascia of leg and partial removal
of the small saphenous vein.

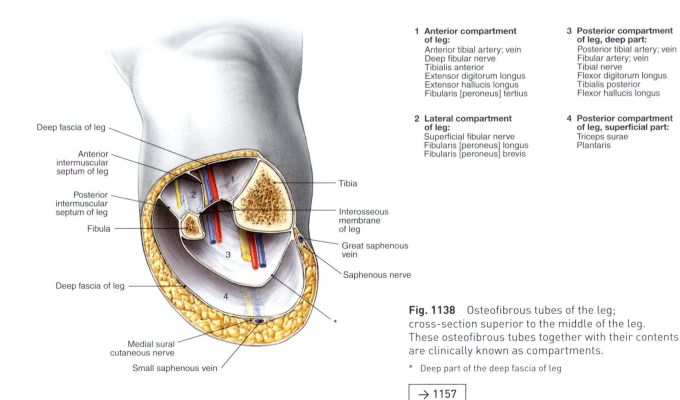

Deep fascia of leg

Anterior
intermuscular
septum of leg

Posterior
intermuscular
septum of leg

Fibula

Deep fascia of leg

Medial sural
cutaneous nerve

Small saphenous vein

Tibia

Interosseous
membrane
of leg

Great saphenous
vein

Saphenous nerve

*

1 **Anterior compartment
   of leg:**
   Anterior tibial artery; vein
   Deep fibular nerve
   Tibialis anterior
   Extensor digitorum longus
   Extensor hallucis longus
   Fibularis [peroneus] tertius

2 **Lateral compartment
   of leg:**
   Superficial fibular nerve
   Fibularis [peroneus] longus
   Fibularis [peroneus] brevis

3 **Posterior compartment
   of leg, deep part:**
   Posterior tibial artery; vein
   Fibular artery; vein
   Tibial nerve
   Flexor digitorum longus
   Tibialis posterior
   Flexor hallucis longus

4 **Posterior compartment
   of leg, superficial part:**
   Triceps surae
   Plantaris

Fig. 1138   Osteofibrous tubes of the leg;
cross-section superior to the middle of the leg.
These osteofibrous tubes together with their contents
are clinically known as compartments.

* Deep part of the deep fascia of leg

→ 1157

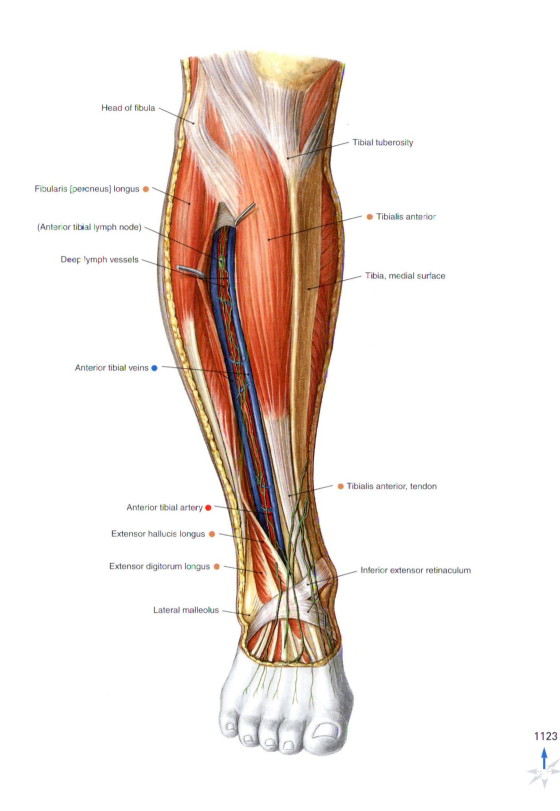

Head of fibula

Tibial tuberosity

Fibularis [peroneus] longus ●

● Tibialis anterior

(Anterior tibial lymph node)

Deep lymph vessels

Tibia, medial surface

Anterior tibial veins ●

Tibialis anterior, tendon ●

Anterior tibial artery ●

Extensor hallucis longus ●

Extensor digitorum longus ●

Inferior extensor retinaculum

Lateral malleolus

1123

Fig. 1139   Vessels of the anterior region of leg; the extensor muscles spread by retractors.

The superficial lymphatics regularly follow the major epifascial veins and converge along the great saphenous vein to the medial side of the leg. The deep lymphatics are found within the connective tissue sheaths of the deep arteries and veins of the leg.

Arteries and nerves of the leg

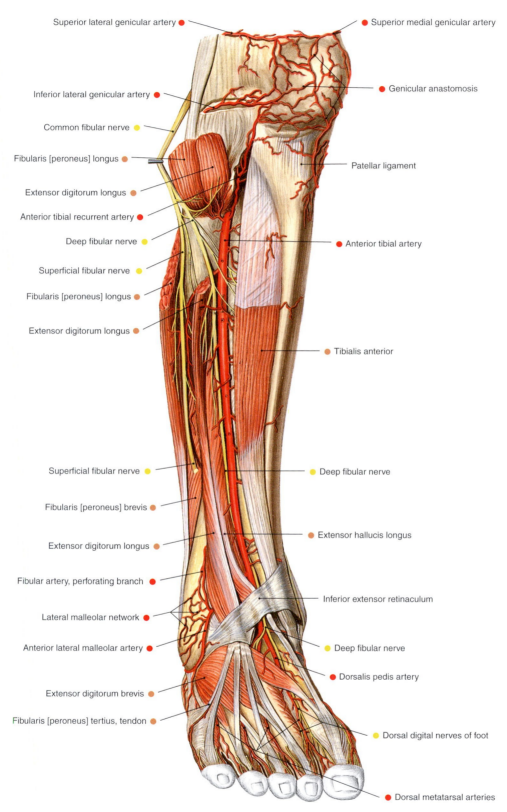

Superior lateral genicular artery ●

Inferior lateral genicular artery ●

Common fibular nerve ●

Fibularis [peroneus] longus ●

Extensor digitorum longus ●

Anterior tibial recurrent artery ●

Deep fibular nerve ●

Superficial fibular nerve ●

Fibularis [peroneus] longus ●

Extensor digitorum longus ●

Superficial fibular nerve ●

Fibularis [peroneus] brevis ●

Extensor digitorum longus ●

Fibular artery, perforating branch ●

Lateral malleolar network ●

Anterior lateral malleolar artery ●

Extensor digitorum brevis ●

Fibularis [peroneus] tertius, tendon ●

● Superior medial genicular artery

● Genicular anastomosis

Patellar ligament

● Anterior tibial artery

● Tibialis anterior

● Deep fibular nerve

● Extensor hallucis longus

Inferior extensor retinaculum

● Deep fibular nerve

● Dorsalis pedis artery

● Dorsal digital nerves of foot

● Dorsal metatarsal arteries

1123
1124
1148
1139

Fig. 1140 Arteries and nerves of the anterior region of leg and the dorsum of foot;
after removal of the deep fascia of leg and dissection of the extensor digitorum longus and fibularis [peroneus] longus muscles.

Arteries and nerves of the popliteal fossa

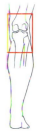

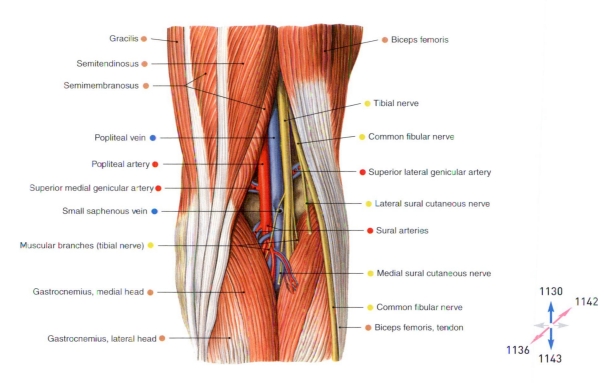

Gracilis ●

Semitendinosus ●

Semimembranosus ●

Popliteal vein ●

Popliteal artery ●

Superior medial genicular artery ●

Small saphenous vein ●

Muscular branches (tibial nerve) ●

Gastrocnemius, medial head ●

Gastrocnemius, lateral head ●

● Biceps femoris

● Tibial nerve

● Common fibular nerve

● Superior lateral genicular artery

● Lateral sural cutaneous nerve

● Sural arteries

● Medial sural cutaneous nerve

● Common fibular nerve

● Biceps femoris, tendon

1130   1142

1136   1143

Fig. 1141 Vessels and nerves of the popliteal fossa;
after removal of the fascia lata and the deep fascia of leg.

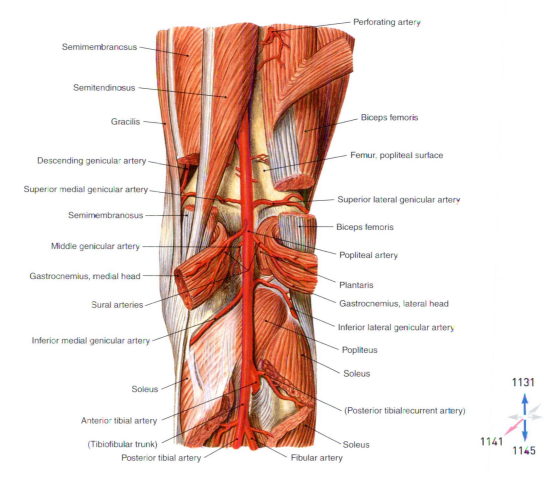

Semimembranosus

Semitendinosus

Gracilis

Descending genicular artery

Superior medial genicular artery

Semimembranosus

Middle genicular artery

Gastrocnemius, medial head

Sural arteries

Inferior medial genicular artery

Soleus

Anterior tibial artery

(Tibiofibular trunk)

Posterior tibial artery

Perforating artery

Biceps femoris

Femur, popliteal surface

Superior lateral genicular artery

Biceps femoris

Popliteal artery

Plantaris

Gastrocnemius, lateral head

Inferior lateral genicular artery

Popliteus

Soleus

(Posterior tibial recurrent artery)

Soleus

Fibular artery

1131

1141   1145

Fig. 1142 Arteries of the popliteal fossa;
demonstration of the arterial supply after partial

removal of the covering muscles.
This branching pattern is found in about 90% of the cases.

Vessels and nerves of the popliteal fossa and the leg

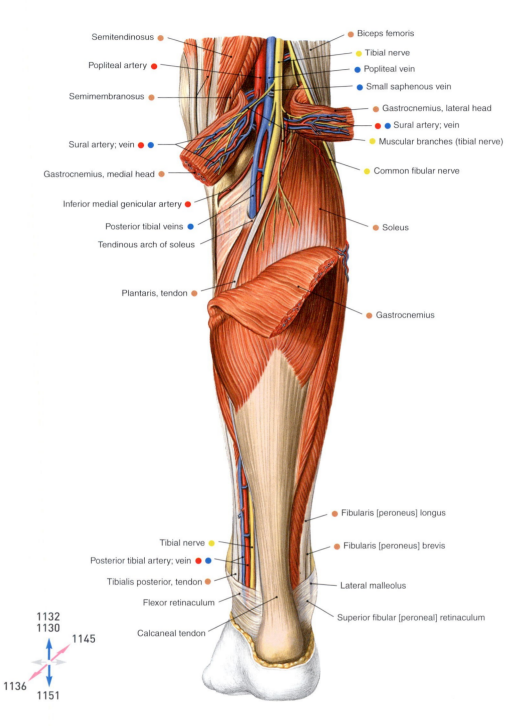

Semitendinosus ●

Popliteal artery ●

Semimembranosus ●

Sural artery; vein ● ●

Gastrocnemius, medial head ●

Inferior medial genicular artery ●

Posterior tibial veins ●

Tendinous arch of soleus

Plantaris, tendon ●

Tibial nerve ●

Posterior tibial artery; vein ● ●

Tibialis posterior, tendon ●

Flexor retinaculum

Calcaneal tendon

● Biceps femoris

● Tibial nerve

● Popliteal vein

● Small saphenous vein

● Gastrocnemius, lateral head

● ● Sural artery; vein

● Muscular branches (tibial nerve)

● Common fibular nerve

● Soleus

● Gastrocnemius

● Fibularis [peroneus] longus

● Fibularis [peroneus] brevis

Lateral malleolus

Superior fibular [peroneal] retinaculum

1132
1130
1145
1136
1151

Fig. 1143 Vessels and nerves of the popliteal fossa and the posterior region of leg; after removal of the deep fascia of leg and dissection of the gastrocnemius muscle.

Fig. 1144 a–d Variations in the branching pattern of the popliteal artery.
a Common trunk of the anterior and posterior tibial artery along with the fibular artery.
b The popliteal artery branches off proximally to the superior border of the popliteal muscle.
c Posterior tibial and fibular artery originate from a common proximal trunk.
d The anterior tibial artery passes ventrally to the popliteal muscle.

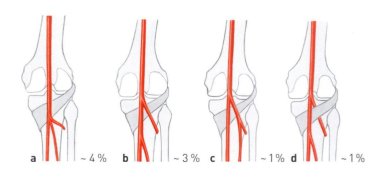

a ~ 4 %   **b** ~ 3 %   **c** ~ 1 %   **d** ~ 1 %

Vessels and nerves of the popliteal fossa and the leg

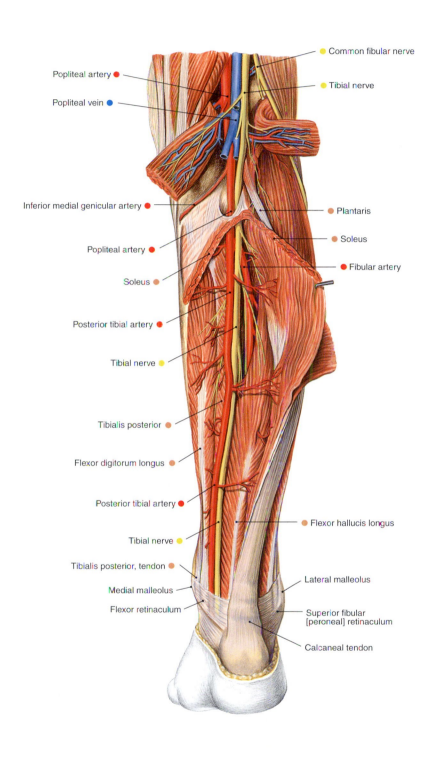

Common fibular nerve

Popliteal artery ●

Popliteal vein ●

Tibial nerve ●

Inferior medial genicular artery ●

Plantaris ●

Popliteal artery ●

Soleus ●

Soleus ●

Fibular artery ●

Posterior tibial artery ●

Tibial nerve ●

Tibialis posterior ●

Flexor digitorum longus ●

Posterior tibial artery ●

Flexor hallucis longus ●

Tibial nerve ●

Tibialis posterior, tendon ●

Lateral malleolus

Medial malleolus

Flexor retinaculum

Superior fibular
[peroneal] retinaculum

Calcaneal tendon

Fig. 1145   Vessels and nerves of the popliteal fossa
and the posterior region of leg;
deep layer.

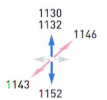

1130
1132
                1146

1143
        1152

Arteries and nerves of the leg

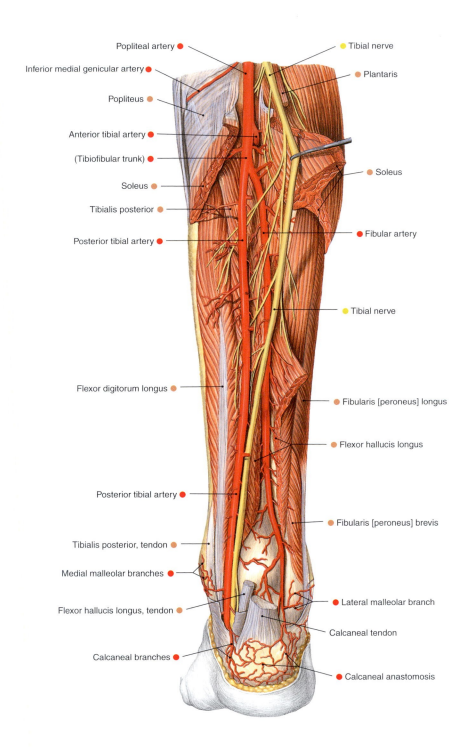

Popliteal artery ●
Inferior medial genicular artery ●
Popliteus ●
Anterior tibial artery ●
(Tibiofibular trunk) ●
Soleus ●
Tibialis posterior ●
Posterior tibial artery ●

● Tibial nerve
● Plantaris
● Soleus
● Fibular artery
● Tibial nerve

Flexor digitorum longus ●

● Fibularis [peroneus] longus
● Flexor hallucis longus

Posterior tibial artery ●

● Fibularis [peroneus] brevis

Tibialis posterior, tendon ●
Medial malleolar branches ●
Flexor hallucis longus, tendon ●
Calcaneal branches ●

● Lateral malleolar branch
Calcaneal tendon
● Calcaneal anastomosis

1130
1132

1145   1153

Fig. 1146 Arteries and nerves of the popliteal fossa
and the posterior region of leg;
deepest layer.

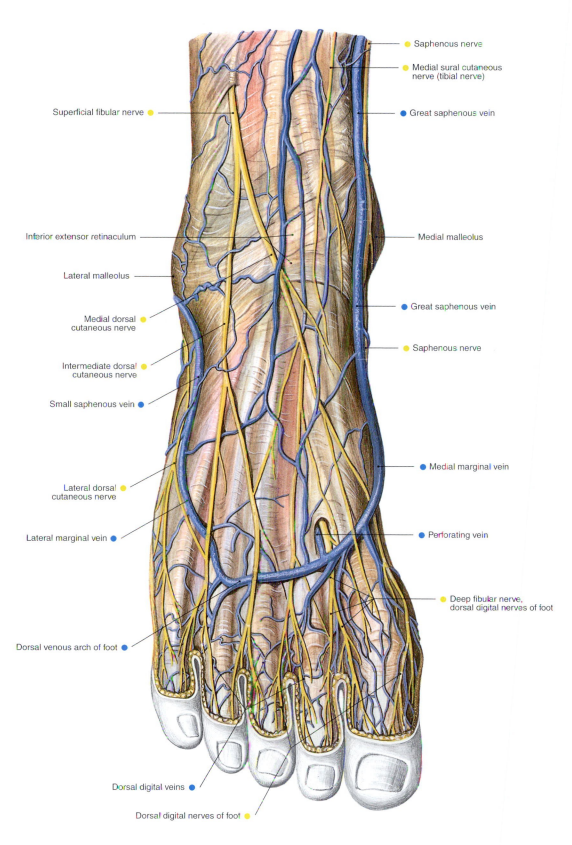

Saphenous nerve

Medial sural cutaneous nerve (tibial nerve)

Great saphenous vein

Superficial fibular nerve

Inferior extensor retinaculum

Medial malleolus

Lateral malleolus

Medial dorsal cutaneous nerve

Great saphenous vein

Intermediate dorsal cutaneous nerve

Saphenous nerve

Small saphenous vein

Lateral dorsal cutaneous nerve

Medial marginal vein

Lateral marginal vein

Perforating vein

Dorsal venous arch of foot

Deep fibular nerve, dorsal digital nerves of foot

Dorsal digital veins

Dorsal digital nerves of foot

1135

1148

Fig. 1147   Epifascial veins and nerves of the dorsum of foot.

Arteries and nerves of the foot

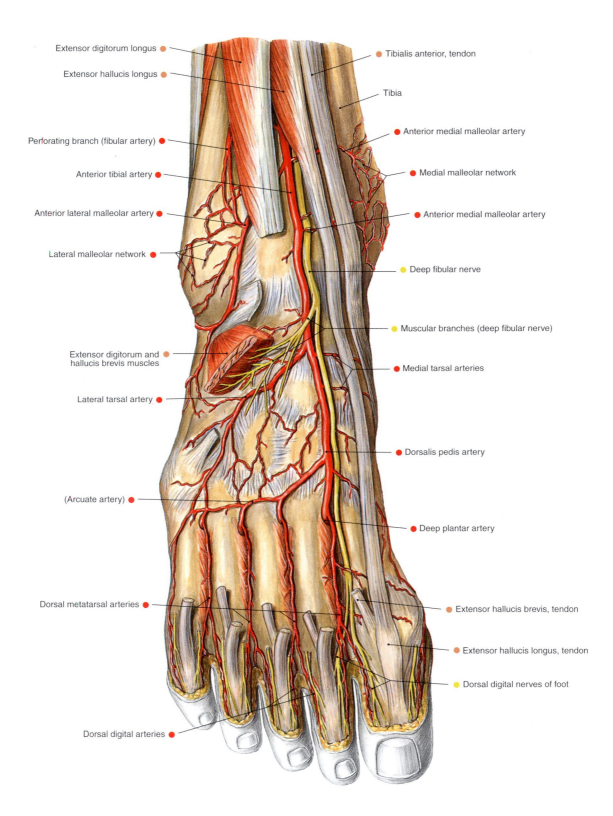

Extensor digitorum longus ●

Extensor hallucis longus ●

Perforating branch (fibular artery) ●

Anterior tibial artery ●

Anterior lateral malleolar artery ●

Lateral malleolar network ●

Extensor digitorum and hallucis brevis muscles ●

Lateral tarsal artery ●

(Arcuate artery) ●

Dorsal metatarsal arteries ●

Dorsal digital arteries ●

● Tibialis anterior, tendon

Tibia

● Anterior medial malleolar artery

● Medial malleolar network

● Anterior medial malleolar artery

● Deep fibular nerve

● Muscular branches (deep fibular nerve)

● Medial tarsal arteries

● Dorsalis pedis artery

● Deep plantar artery

● Extensor hallucis brevis, tendon

● Extensor hallucis longus, tendon

● Dorsal digital nerves of foot

1140

1147

Fig. 1148 Arteries and nerves of the dorsum of foot.

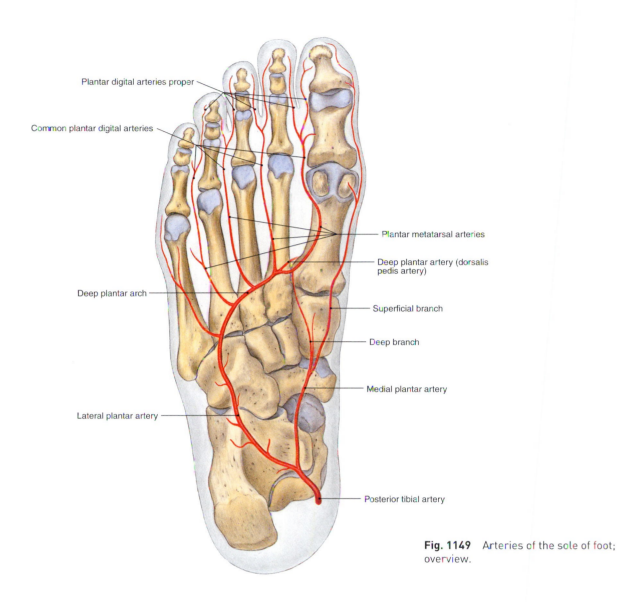

Plantar digital arteries proper

Common plantar digital arteries

Plantar metatarsal arteries

Deep plantar artery (dorsalis pedis artery)

Deep plantar arch

Superficial branch

Deep branch

Medial plantar artery

Lateral plantar artery

Posterior tibial artery

Fig. 1149   Arteries of the sole of foot; overview.

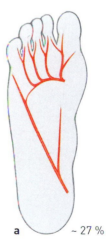

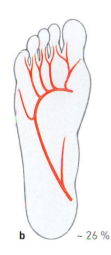

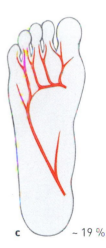

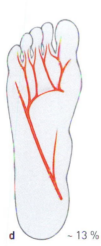

a   ~ 27 %

b   ~ 26 %

c   ~ 19 %

d   ~ 13 %

Fig. 1150 a–d   Variations in the arterial supply of the sole of foot.
a   Dorsalis pedis artery as major supply for the deep plantar arch.
b   Posterior tibial artery as major supply for the deep plantar arch.
c   The fifth toe and lateral parts of the fourth toe are supplied by the posterior tibial artery, whereas the

remaining medially located toes receive their arterial supply through the dorsalis pedis artery.
d   The fifth and fourth toe as well as lateral parts of the third toe are supplied by the posterior tibial artery, whereas all remaining medially located toes receive their arterial supply through the dorsalis pedis artery.

Arteries and nerves of the foot

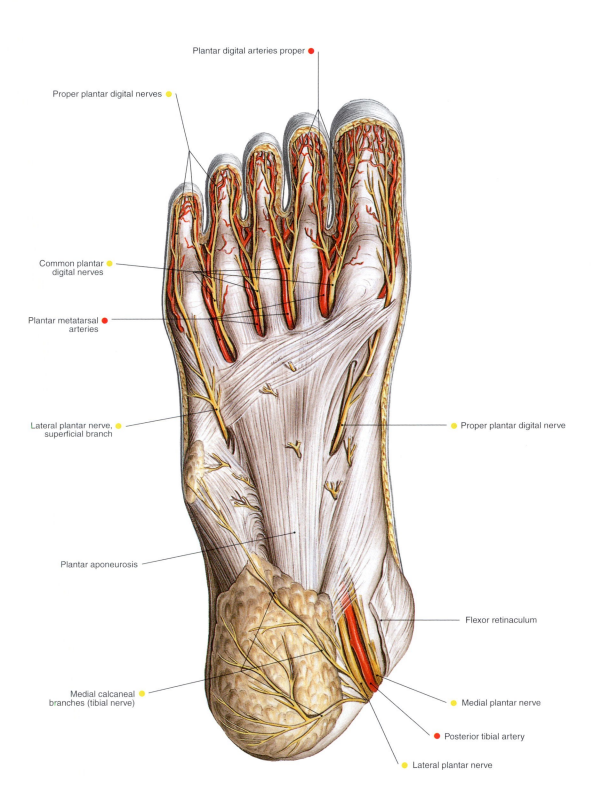

Plantar digital arteries proper ●

Proper plantar digital nerves ●

Common plantar digital nerves ●

Plantar metatarsal arteries ●

Lateral plantar nerve, superficial branch ●

Plantar aponeurosis

Medial calcaneal branches (tibial nerve) ●

● Proper plantar digital nerve

Flexor retinaculum

● Medial plantar nerve

● Posterior tibial artery

● Lateral plantar nerve

1143

1152

Fig. 1151   Arteries and nerves of the sole of foot.

Arteries and nerves of the foot

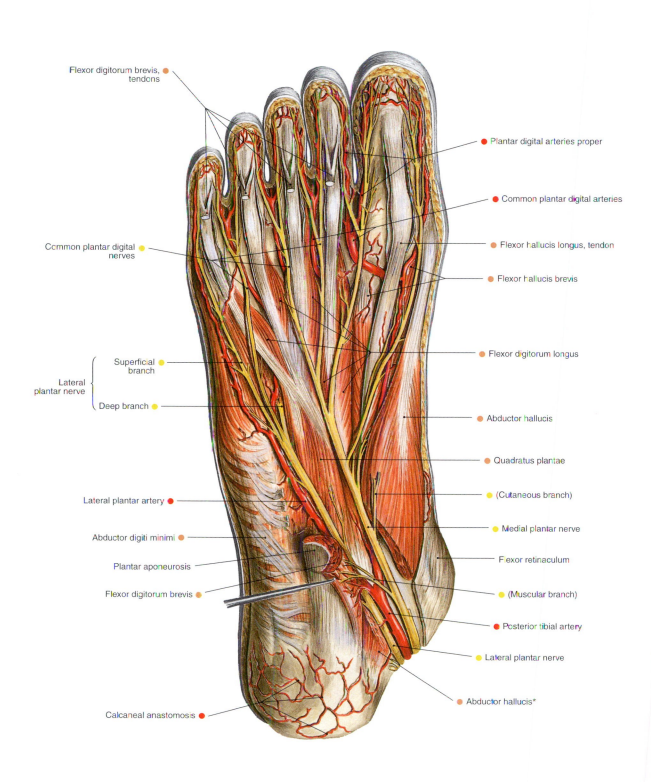

Flexor digitorum brevis, ● tendons

Common plantar digital ● nerves

Superficial ● branch

Lateral plantar nerve

Deep branch ●

Lateral plantar artery ●

Abductor digiti minimi ●

Plantar aponeurosis

Flexor digitorum brevis ●

Calcaneal anastomosis ●

● Plantar digital arteries proper

● Common plantar digital arteries

● Flexor hallucis longus, tendon

● Flexor hallucis brevis

● Flexor digitorum longus

● Abductor hallucis

● Quadratus plantae

● (Cutaneous branch)

● Medial plantar nerve

● Flexor retinaculum

● (Muscular branch)

● Posterior tibial artery

● Lateral plantar nerve

● Abductor hallucis*

Fig. 1152 Arteries and nerves of the sole of foot;
deep layer.

* The distal extension of the medial retromalleolar space
beneath the abductor hallucis muscle is also known as tarsal
tunnel.

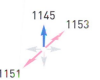

1145

1153

1151

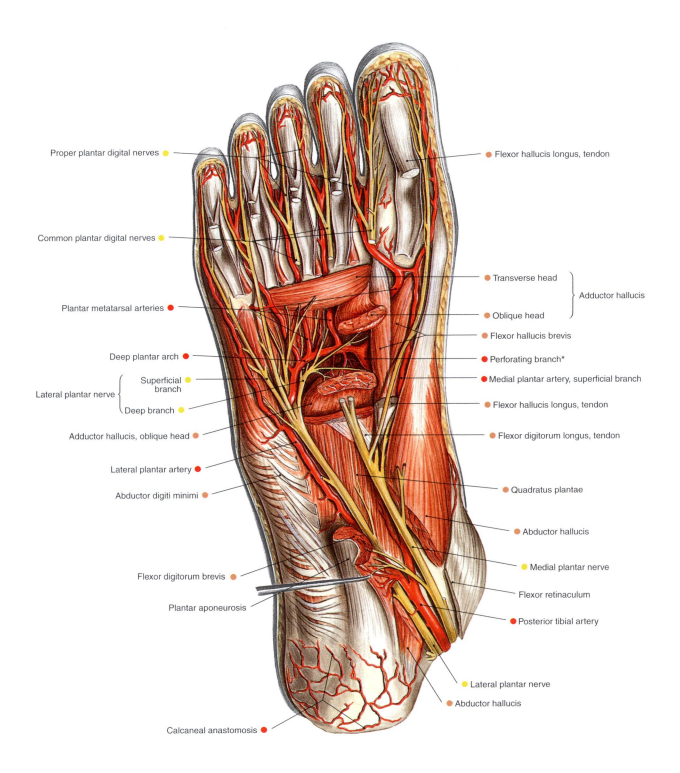

Proper plantar digital nerves ●

Common plantar digital nerves ●

Plantar metatarsal arteries ●

Deep plantar arch ●

Lateral plantar nerve { Superficial branch ●

Deep branch ●

Adductor hallucis, oblique head ●

Lateral plantar artery ●

Abductor digiti minimi ●

Flexor digitorum brevis ●

Plantar aponeurosis

Calcaneal anastomosis ●

● Flexor hallucis longus, tendon

● Transverse head } Adductor hallucis

● Oblique head

● Flexor hallucis brevis

● Perforating branch*

● Medial plantar artery, superficial branch

● Flexor hallucis longus, tendon

● Flexor digitorum longus, tendon

● Quadratus plantae

● Abductor hallucis

● Medial plantar nerve

Flexor retinaculum

● Posterior tibial artery

● Lateral plantar nerve

● Abductor hallucis

1146

1152

Fig. 1153 Arteries and nerves of the sole of foot; deepest layer.

* Anastomosis with the dorsalis pedis artery

Compartments of the foot

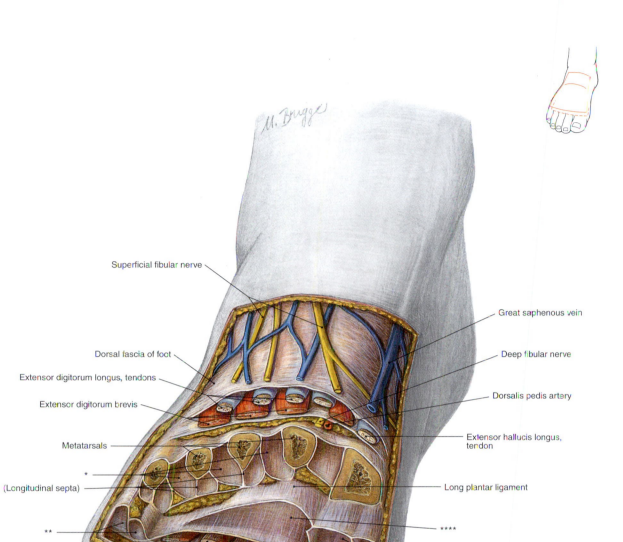

Superficial fibular nerve

Great saphenous vein

Dorsal fascia of foot

Deep fibular nerve

Extensor digitorum longus, tendons

Extensor digitorum brevis

Dorsalis pedis artery

Metatarsals

Extensor hallucis longus, tendon

*

(Longitudinal septa)

Long plantar ligament

**

****

Flexor digitorum muscles, tendons

***

Plantar aponeurosis

Flexor hallucis longus, tendon

Fig. 1154   Compartments of the foot; stepwise section.

*   Space of the interossei muscles
**   Lateral compartment
***   Medial compartment
**** Intermediate compartment

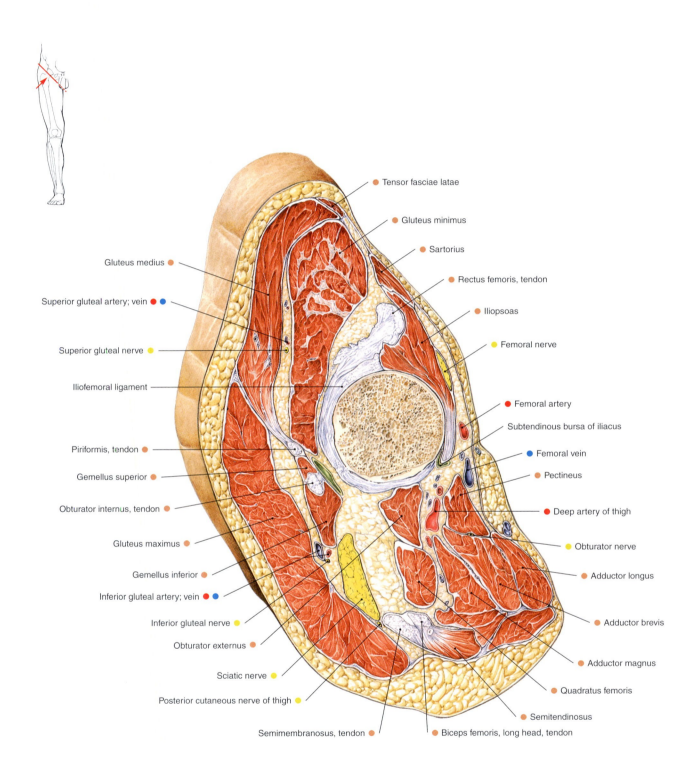

Tensor fasciae latae

Gluteus minimus

Sartorius

Gluteus medius

Rectus femoris, tendon

Superior gluteal artery; vein ● ●

Iliopsoas

Superior gluteal nerve ●

Femoral nerve

Iliofemoral ligament

Femoral artery

Subtendinous bursa of iliacus

Piriformis, tendon ●

Femoral vein

Gemellus superior ●

Pectineus

Obturator internus, tendon ●

Deep artery of thigh

Gluteus maximus ●

Obturator nerve

Gemellus inferior ●

Adductor longus

Inferior gluteal artery; vein ● ●

Adductor brevis

Inferior gluteal nerve ●

Obturator externus ●

Adductor magnus

Sciatic nerve ●

Quadratus femoris

Posterior cutaneous nerve of thigh ●

Semitendinosus

Semimembranosus, tendon ●

Biceps femoris, long head, tendon ●

Fig. 1155 Thigh;
oblique section through the hip joint.

Thigh, cross-sections

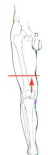

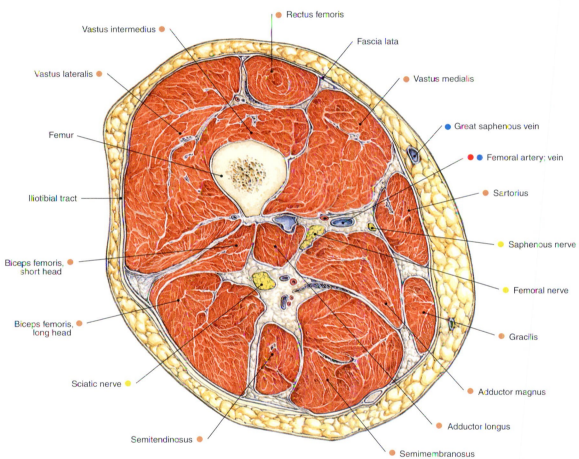

Vastus intermedius ●

Rectus femoris ●

Fascia lata

Vastus lateralis ●

Vastus medialis ●

● Great saphenous vein

Femur

● ● Femoral artery; vein

Iliotibial tract

● Sartorius

● Saphenous nerve

Biceps femoris, ●
short head

● Femoral nerve

Biceps femoris, ●
long head

● Gracilis

Sciatic nerve ●

● Adductor magnus

● Adductor longus

Semitendinosus ●

● Semimembranosus

Fig. 1156   Thigh;
cross-section through the middle of the thigh.

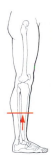

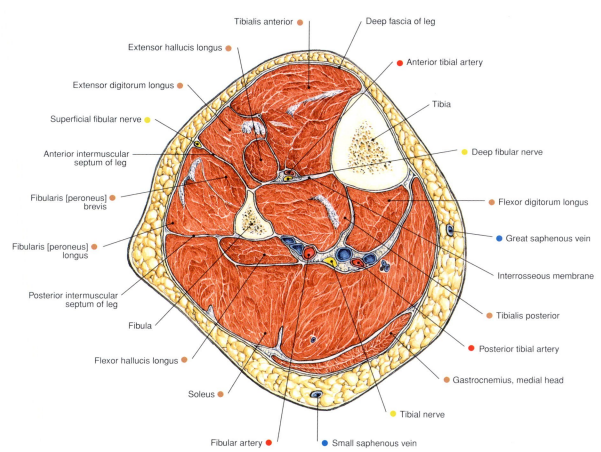

Fig. 1157 Leg;
cross-section through the middle of the leg.

→ 1138

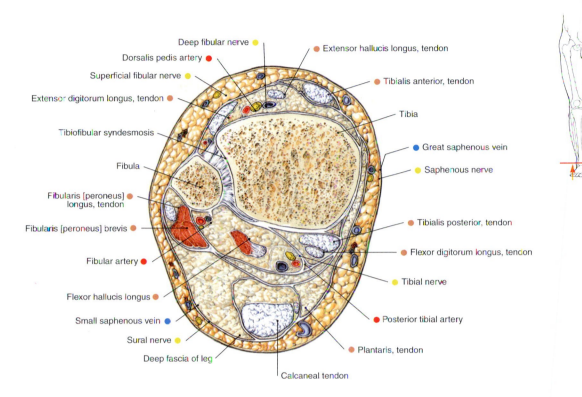

Deep fibular nerve

Dorsalis pedis artery

Superficial fibular nerve

Extensor digitorum longus, tendon

Tibiofibular syndesmosis

Fibula

Fibularis [peroneus] longus, tendon

Fibularis [peroneus] brevis

Fibular artery

Flexor hallucis longus

Small saphenous vein

Sural nerve

Deep fascia of leg

Calcaneal tendon

Extensor hallucis longus, tendon

Tibialis anterior, tendon

Tibia

Great saphenous vein

Saphenous nerve

Tibialis posterior, tendon

Flexor digitorum longus, tendon

Tibial nerve

Posterior tibial artery

Plantaris, tendon

Fig. 1158 Leg;
cross-section just above the ankle joint.

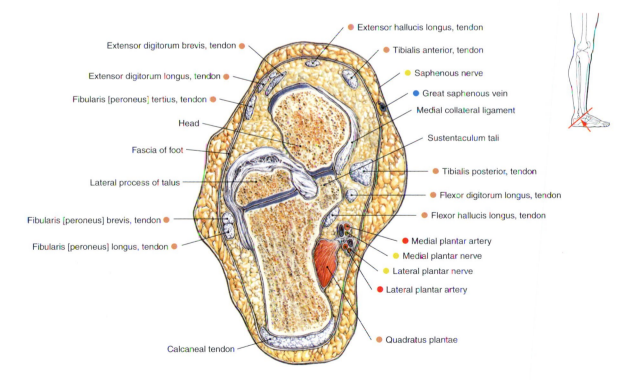

Extensor digitorum brevis, tendon

Extensor digitorum longus, tendon

Fibularis [peroneus] tertius, tendon

Head

Fascia of foot

Lateral process of talus

Fibularis [peroneus] brevis, tendon

Fibularis [peroneus] longus, tendon

Calcaneal tendon

Extensor hallucis longus, tendon

Tibialis anterior, tendon

Saphenous nerve

Great saphenous vein

Medial collateral ligament

Sustentaculum tali

Tibialis posterior, tendon

Flexor digitorum longus, tendon

Flexor hallucis longus, tendon

Medial plantar artery

Medial plantar nerve

Lateral plantar nerve

Lateral plantar artery

Quadratus plantae

Fig. 1159 Foot;
oblique section through the calcaneus and the head of the talus.

Foot, sagittal sections

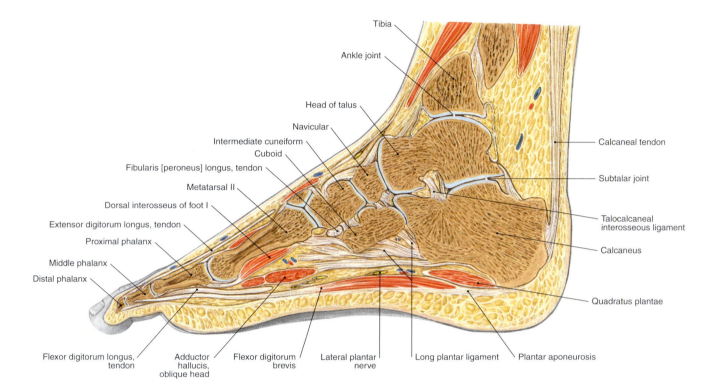

Tibia

Ankle joint

Head of talus

Navicular

Intermediate cuneiform

Cuboid

Fibularis [peroneus] longus, tendon

Metatarsal II

Dorsal interosseus of foot I

Extensor digitorum longus, tendon

Proximal phalanx

Middle phalanx

Distal phalanx

Calcaneal tendon

Subtalar joint

Talocalcaneal interosseous ligament

Calcaneus

Quadratus plantae

Flexor digitorum longus, tendon

Adductor hallucis, oblique head

Flexor digitorum brevis

Lateral plantar nerve

Long plantar ligament

Plantar aponeurosis

→ 1047, 1048

Fig. 1160   Foot;
sagittal section through the second toe.

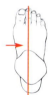

Tibialis anterior, tendon

Tibia

Ankle joint

Talus

(Talonavicular joint)

Navicular

Long plantar ligament

Flexor hallucis longus

Epiphysial line

Triceps surae, calcaneal tendon

Subtalar joint

Talocalcaneal interosseous ligament

Calcaneus

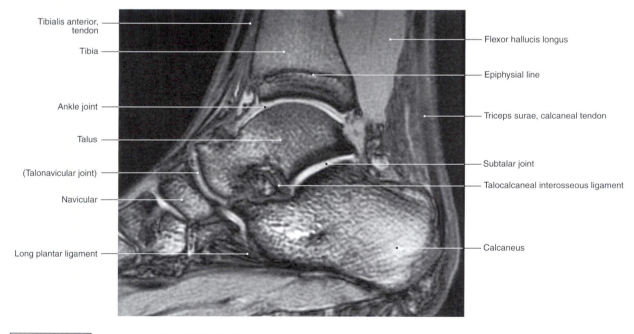

→ 1049, 1050

Fig. 1161   Foot;
magnetic resonance tomography image (MRI); sagittal section.

Foot, cross-section and pedograms

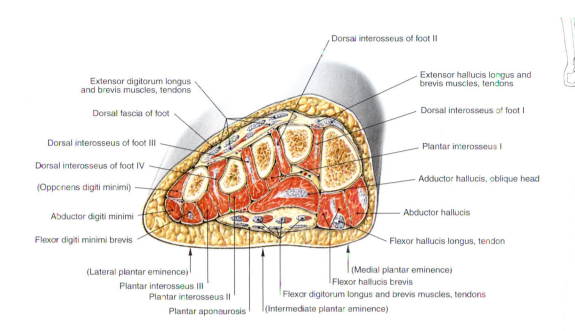

Dorsal interosseus of foot II

Extensor digitorum longus and brevis muscles, tendons

Dorsal fascia of foot

Dorsal interosseus of foot III

Dorsal interosseus of foot IV

(Opponens digiti minimi)

Abductor digiti minimi

Flexor digiti minimi brevis

Extensor hallucis longus and brevis muscles, tendons

Dorsal interosseus of foot I

Plantar interosseus I

Adductor hallucis, oblique head

Abductor hallucis

Flexor hallucis longus, tendon

(Lateral plantar eminence)

Plantar interosseus III

Plantar interosseus II

Plantar aponeurosis

(Medial plantar eminence)

Flexor hallucis brevis

Flexor digitorum longus and brevis muscles, tendons

(Intermediate plantar eminence)

Fig. 1162 Osteofibrous tubes of the foot; frontal section through the metatarsus.

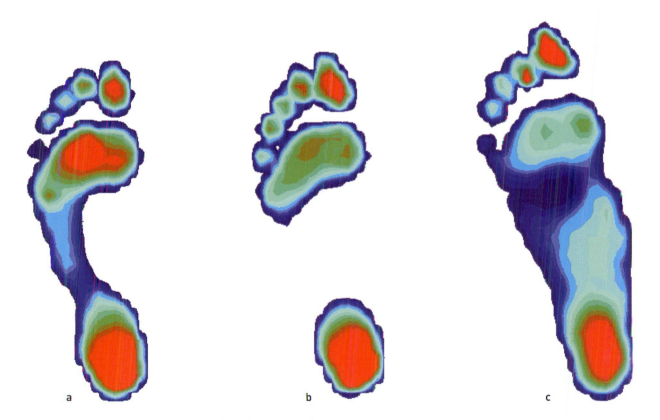

a   b   c

Fig. 1163 Foot prints, pedograms.
a Normal foot
b Pes cavus
c Flat foot

Arteries of the head

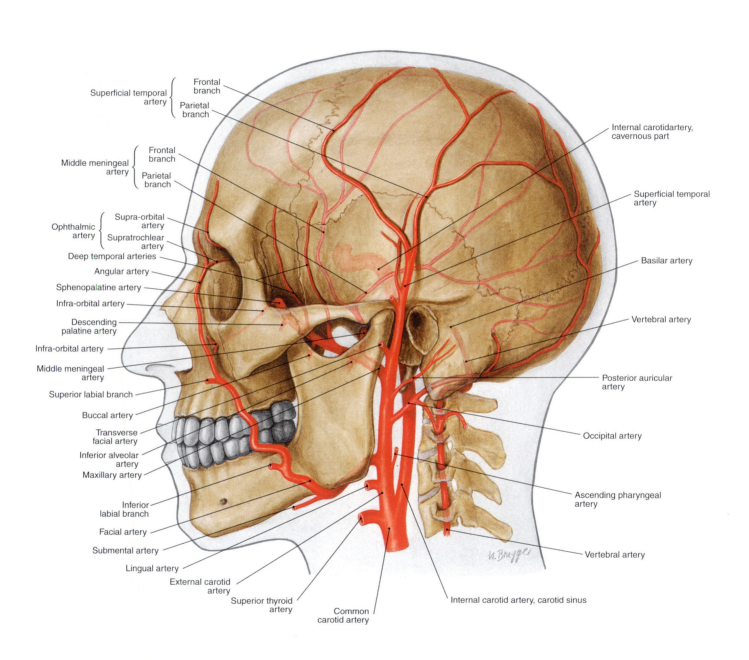

Superficial temporal artery
- Frontal branch
- Parietal branch

Middle meningeal artery
- Frontal branch
- Parietal branch

Ophthalmic artery
- Supra-orbital artery
- Supratrochlear artery

Deep temporal arteries

Angular artery

Sphenopalatine artery

Infra-orbital artery

Descending palatine artery

Infra-orbital artery

Middle meningeal artery

Superior labial branch

Buccal artery

Transverse facial artery

Inferior alveolar artery

Maxillary artery

Inferior labial branch

Facial artery

Submental artery

Lingual artery

External carotid artery

Superior thyroid artery

Common carotid artery

Internal carotid artery, cavernous part

Superficial temporal artery

Basilar artery

Vertebral artery

Posterior auricular artery

Occipital artery

Ascending pharyngeal artery

Vertebral artery

Internal carotid artery, carotid sinus

Fig. 1164 External arteries of the head.

Arteries of the head

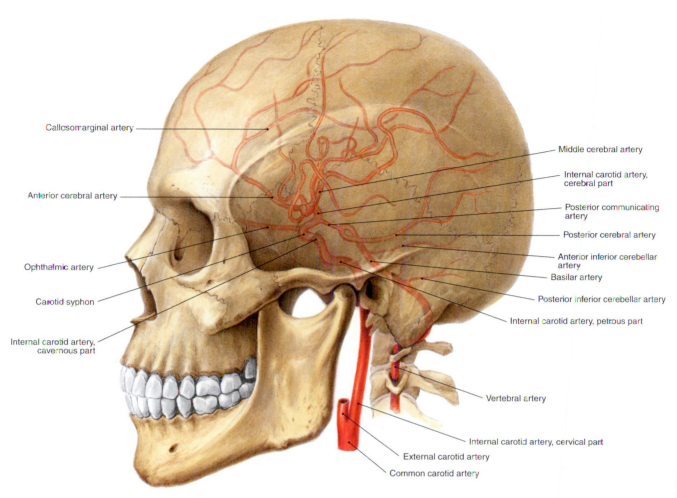

Callosomarginal artery

Middle cerebral artery

Internal carotid artery, cerebral part

Anterior cerebral artery

Posterior communicating artery

Posterior cerebral artery

Anterior inferior cerebellar artery

Ophthalmic artery

Basilar artery

Carotid syphon

Posterior inferior cerebellar artery

Internal carotid artery, petrous part

Internal carotid artery, cavernous part

Vertebral artery

Internal carotid artery, cervical part

External carotid artery

Common carotid artery

Fig. 1165 Internal arteries of the head.

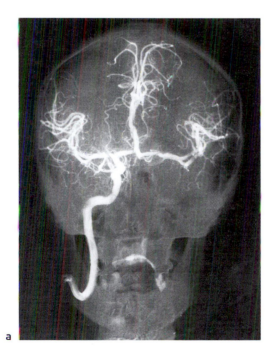

a

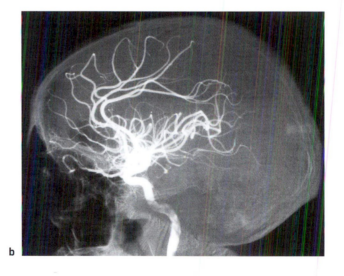

b

Fig. 1166 a, b Internal carotid artery;
radiographs after unilateral injection of a contrast medium
(angiograms).

The contrast medium also distributes to the vessels of the contralateral side via the arterial circle.
a AP-radiograph, digital subtraction angiography (DSA)
b Lateral radiograph, digital subtraction angiography (DSA)

Veins of the head

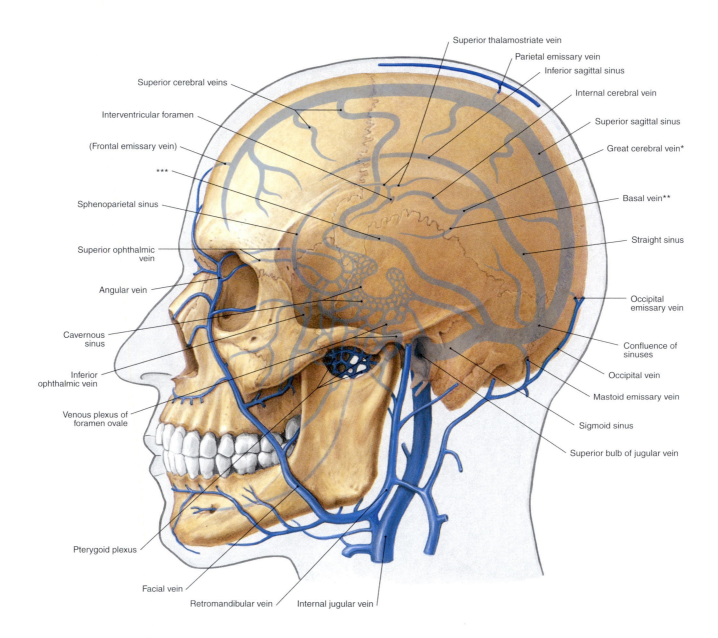

Superior thalamostriate vein
Parietal emissary vein
Inferior sagittal sinus
Superior cerebral veins
Internal cerebral vein
Interventricular foramen
Superior sagittal sinus
(Frontal emissary vein)
Great cerebral vein*
***
Basal vein**
Sphenoparietal sinus
Straight sinus
Superior ophthalmic vein
Angular vein
Occipital emissary vein
Cavernous sinus
Confluence of sinuses
Inferior ophthalmic vein
Occipital vein
Mastoid emissary vein
Venous plexus of foramen ovale
Sigmoid sinus
Superior bulb of jugular vein
Pterygoid plexus
Facial vein
Retromandibular vein
Internal jugular vein

Fig. 1167 Internal and external veins of the head.

*   Vein of GALEN
**   ROSENTHAL's vein
*** Vein of LABBÉ

Emissary veins – Passages through the skull

Parietal emissary vein – parietal foramen
Mastoid emissary vein – mastoid foramen
Occipital emmissary vein – passage in the region of the
   external occipital protuberance
Condylar emmissary vein – condylar canal

Venous plexus of hypoglossal canal – hypoglossal canal
Venous plexus of foramen ovale – foramen ovale
Internal carotid venous plexus – carotid canal

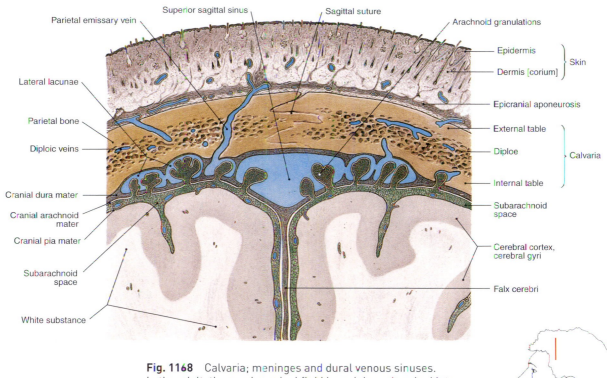

Fig. 1168 Calvaria; meninges and dural venous sinuses.
In the adult, the cerebrospinal fluid is mainly reabsorbed into
the venous system through the arachnoid granulations.
Additionally, reabsorption occurs through the lymphatic
sheaths of small vessels of the cranial pia mater and through
the perineural sheaths of the cranial and the spinal nerves.

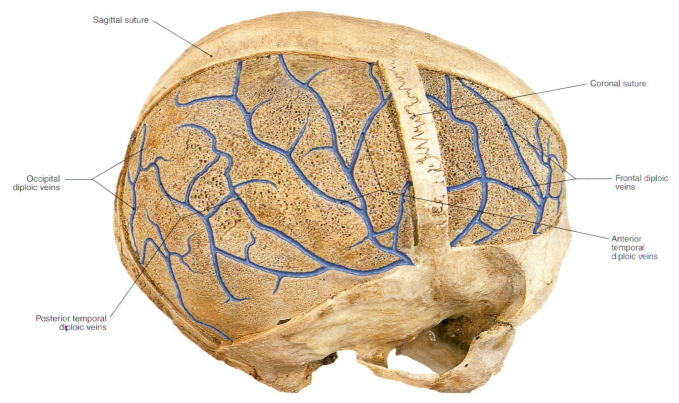

Fig. 1169 Diploic canals and diploic veins
of the calvaria;

the external table of compact bone has been removed from
the calvaria.

Dural venous sinuses

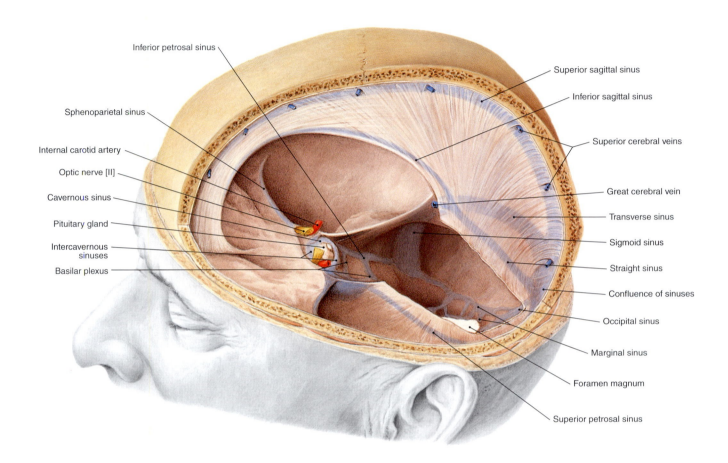

Fig. 1170   Cranial dura mater and dural venous sinuses; after partial removal of the tentorium cerebelli.

Cranial dura mater

The cranial dura mater lines the cranial cavity completely and tightly adheres to the skull bone. The cerebral falx protrudes in the sagittal plane in a sickle-like shape and stretches from the crista galli to the ridge of the tentorium cerebelli, which, in turn, overstretches the posterior cranial fossa and is attached along the transverse sinus and the pyramidal edge. The margins of the tentorial notch envelop the midbrain and taper off into the anterior and posterior clinoid process. The cerebral falx and the tentorium cerebelli divide the cranial cavity into three spaces that are incompletely separated from one another, containing the two cerebral hemispheres and the cerebellum.

Dural venous sinuses

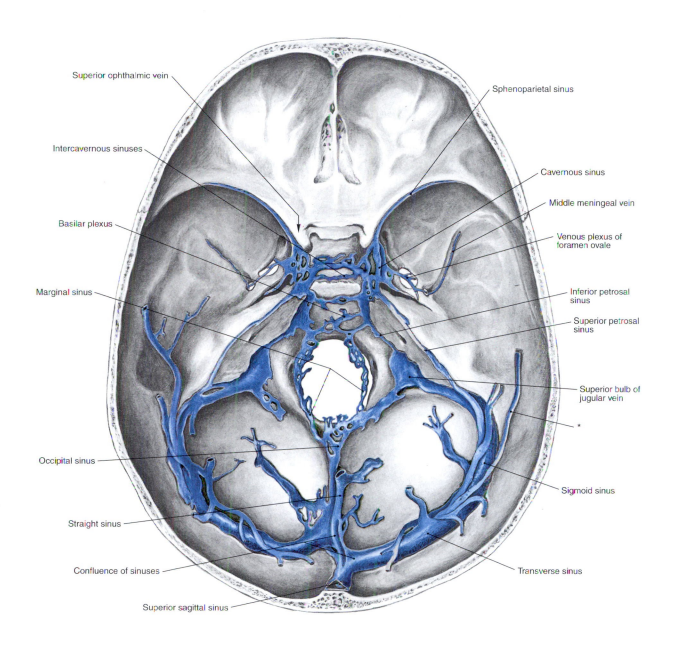

Superior ophthalmic vein

Intercavernous sinuses

Basilar plexus

Marginal sinus

Occipital sinus

Straight sinus

Confluence of sinuses

Superior sagittal sinus

Sphenoparietal sinus

Cavernous sinus

Middle meningeal vein

Venous plexus of
foramen ovale

Inferior petrosal
sinus

Superior petrosal
sinus

Superior bulb of
jugular vein

*

Sigmoid sinus

Transverse sinus

Fig. 1171   Dural venous sinuses;
corrosion cast.
The sinuses contain no valves and feature rigid walls.
*   Vein of LABBÉ to the superficial middle cerebral veins

Dural venous sinuses

The dural venous sinuses are rigid venous channels
without valves draining the venous blood from the brain via
so-called bridging veins.
The main drainage from within the skull occurs via the
sigmoid sinuses into the internal jugular veins. Additionally,
the superior ophthalmic veins and the highly variable emissary veins form a series of smaller, likewise valveless, venous
connections between the intra- and extracranial regions.

The two cavernous sinuses assume a central position by
being situated in the middle cranial fossa to the right
and the left of the sella turcica. They communicate with
each other through the intercavernous sinuses and either
directly or indirectly with most other sinuses and with the
veins of the orbit and the infratemporal fossa.

External surface of the cranial base

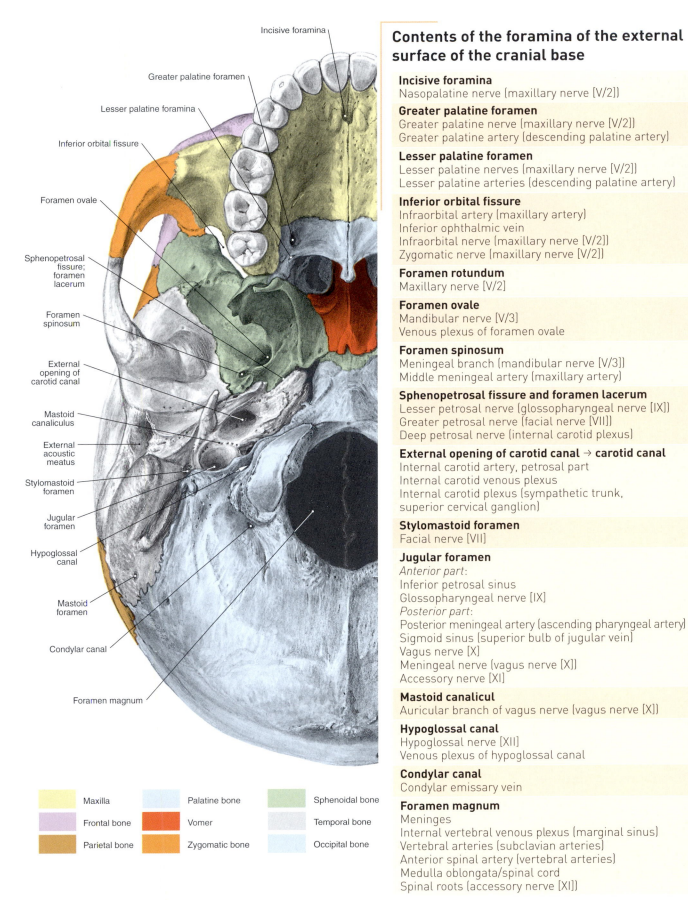

Contents of the foramina of the external surface of the cranial base

Incisive foramina
Nasopalatine nerve (maxillary nerve [V/2])

Greater palatine foramen
Greater palatine nerve (maxillary nerve [V/2])
Greater palatine artery (descending palatine artery)

Lesser palatine foramen
Lesser palatine nerves (maxillary nerve [V/2])
Lesser palatine arteries (descending palatine artery)

Inferior orbital fissure
Infraorbital artery (maxillary artery)
Inferior ophthalmic vein
Infraorbital nerve (maxillary nerve [V/2])
Zygomatic nerve (maxillary nerve [V/2])

Foramen rotundum
Maxillary nerve [V/2]

Foramen ovale
Mandibular nerve [V/3]
Venous plexus of foramen ovale

Foramen spinosum
Meningeal branch (mandibular nerve [V/3])
Middle meningeal artery (maxillary artery)

Sphenopetrosal fissure and foramen lacerum
Lesser petrosal nerve (glossopharyngeal nerve [IX])
Greater petrosal nerve (facial nerve [VII])
Deep petrosal nerve (internal carotid plexus)

External opening of carotid canal → carotid canal
Internal carotid artery, petrosal part
Internal carotid venous plexus
Internal carotid plexus (sympathetic trunk, superior cervical ganglion)

Stylomastoid foramen
Facial nerve [VII]

Jugular foramen
Anterior part:
Inferior petrosal sinus
Glossopharyngeal nerve [IX]
Posterior part:
Posterior meningeal artery (ascending pharyngeal artery)
Sigmoid sinus (superior bulb of jugular vein)
Vagus nerve [X]
Meningeal nerve (vagus nerve [X])
Accessory nerve [XI]

Mastoid canalicul
Auricular branch of vagus nerve (vagus nerve [X])

Hypoglossal canal
Hypoglossal nerve [XII]
Venous plexus of hypoglossal canal

Condylar canal
Condylar emissary vein

Foramen magnum
Meninges
Internal vertebral venous plexus (marginal sinus)
Vertebral arteries (subclavian arteries)
Anterior spinal artery (vertebral arteries)
Medulla oblongata/spinal cord
Spinal roots (accessory nerve [XI])

Incisive foramina
Greater palatine foramen
Lesser palatine foramina
Inferior orbital fissure
Foramen ovale
Sphenopetrosal fissure; foramen lacerum
Foramen spinosum
External opening of carotid canal
Mastoid canaliculus
External acoustic meatus
Stylomastoid foramen
Jugular foramen
Hypoglossal canal
Mastoid foramen
Condylar canal
Foramen magnum

▬ Maxilla	▬ Palatine bone	▬ Sphenoidal bone
▬ Frontal bone	▬ Vomer	▬ Temporal bone
▬ Parietal bone	▬ Zygomatic bone	▬ Occipital bone

Fig. 1172   External surface of the cranial base and foramina.

Contents of the foramina of the internal surface of the cranial base

Lamina cribrosa
Olfactory nerves [I]
Anterior ethmoidal artery (ophthalmic artery)

Optic canal
Optic nerve [II]
Ophthalmic artery (internal carotid artery)
Meninges; sheath of optic nerve

Superior orbital fissure
Medial part:
Nasociliary nerve (ophthalmic nerve [V/1])
Oculomotor nerve [III]
Abducent nerve [VI]
Lateral part:
Trochlear nerve [IV]
Common trunk of the:
– frontal nerve (ophthalmic nerve [V/I])
– lacrimal nerve (ophthalmic nerve [V/I])
Orbital branch (middle meningeal artery)
Superior ophthalmic vein

Foramen rotundum
Maxillary nerve [V/2]

Foramen ovale
Mandibular nerve [V/3]
Venous plexus of foramen ovale

Foramen spinosum
Meningeal branch (mandibular nerve [V/3])
Middle meningeal artery (maxillary artery)

Sphenopetrosal fissure and foramen lacerum
Lesser petrosal nerve (glossopharyngeal nerve [IX])
Greater petrosal nerve (facial nerve [VII])
Deep petrosal nerve (internal carotid plexus)

External opening of carotid canal → carotid canal
Internal carotid artery, petrosal part
Internal carotid venous plexus
Internal carotid plexus (sympathetic trunk, superior cervical ganglion)

Pore → internal acoustic meatus
Facial nerve [VII]
Vestibulocochlear nerve [VIII]
Labyrinthine artery (basilar artery)
Labyrinthine veins

Jugular foramen
Anterior part:
Inferior petrosal sinus
Glossopharyngeal nerve [IX]
Posterior part:
Posterior meningeal artery (ascending pharyngeal artery)
Sigmoid sinus (superior bulb of jugular vein)
Vagus nerve [X]
Accessory nerve [XI]
Meningeal nerve (vagus nerve [X])

Hypoglossal canal
Hypoglossal nerve [XII]
Venous plexus of hypoglossal canal

Condylar canal
Condylar emissary vein

Foramen magnum
Meninges
Internal vertebral venous plexus (marginal sinus)
Vertebral arteries (subclavian arteries)
Anterior spinal artery (vertebral arteries)
Medulla oblongata/spinal cord
Spinal roots (accessory nerve [XI])

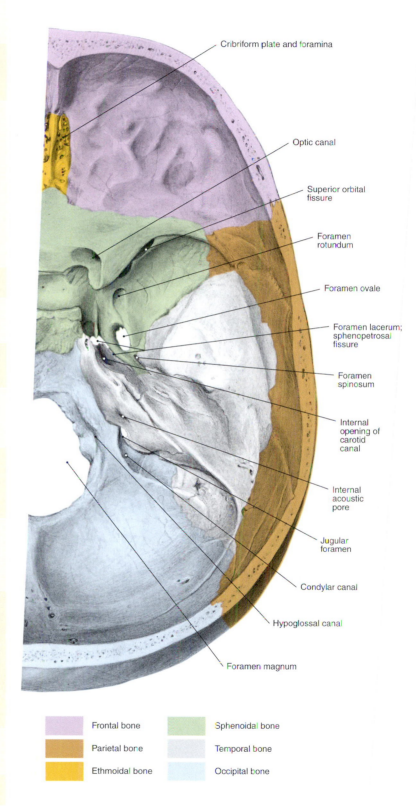

Cribriform plate and foramina

Optic canal

Superior orbital fissure

Foramen rotundum

Foramen ovale

Foramen lacerum; sphenopetrosal fissure

Foramen spinosum

Internal opening of carotid canal

Internal acoustic pore

Jugular foramen

Condylar canal

Hypoglossal canal

Foramen magnum

Frontal bone	Sphenoidal bone
Parietal bone	Temporal bone
Ethmoidal bone	Occipital bone

Fig. 1173 Internal surface of the cranial base and foramina.

Cranial nerves, overview

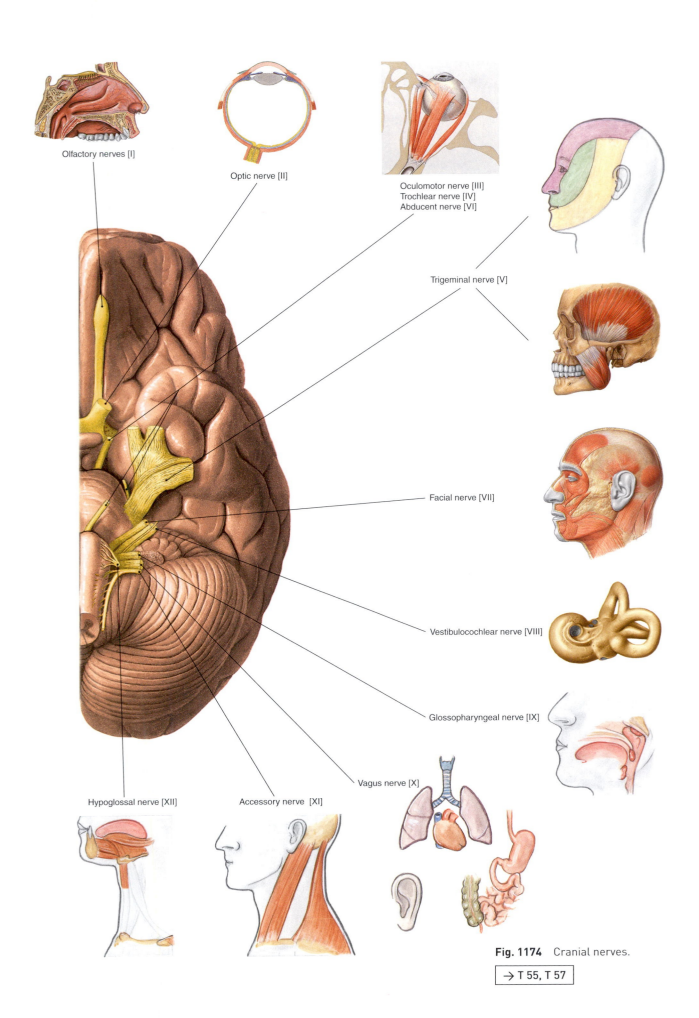

Olfactory nerves [I]

Optic nerve [II]

Oculomotor nerve [III]
Trochlear nerve [IV]
Abducent nerve [VI]

Trigeminal nerve [V]

Facial nerve [VII]

Vestibulocochlear nerve [VIII]

Glossopharyngeal nerve [IX]

Vagus nerve [X]

Hypoglossal nerve [XII]

Accessory nerve [XI]

Fig. 1174 Cranial nerves.

→ T 55, T 57

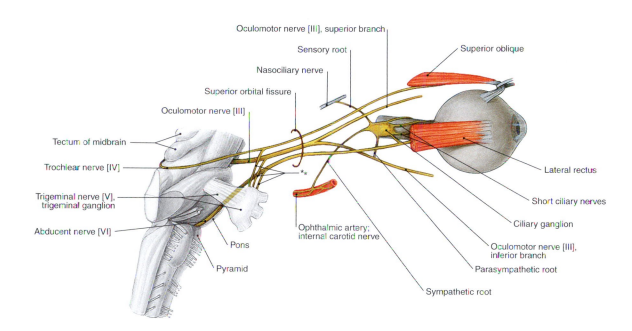

Oculomotor nerve [III], superior branch

Sensory root

Nasociliary nerve

Superior orbital fissure

Oculomotor nerve [III]

Tectum of midbrain

Trochlear nerve [IV]

Trigeminal nerve [V], trigeminal ganglion

Abducent nerve [VI]

Pons

Pyramid

Superior oblique

Lateral rectus

Short ciliary nerves

Ciliary ganglion

Oculomotor nerve [III], inferior branch

Parasympathetic root

Sympathetic root

Ophthalmic artery; internal carotid nerve

Fig. 1175 Oculomotor nerve [III], trochlear nerve [IV] and abducent nerve [VI]; viewed from the right.

$\rightarrow$ T 57 c, d, f

* Connections to the trigeminal ganglion

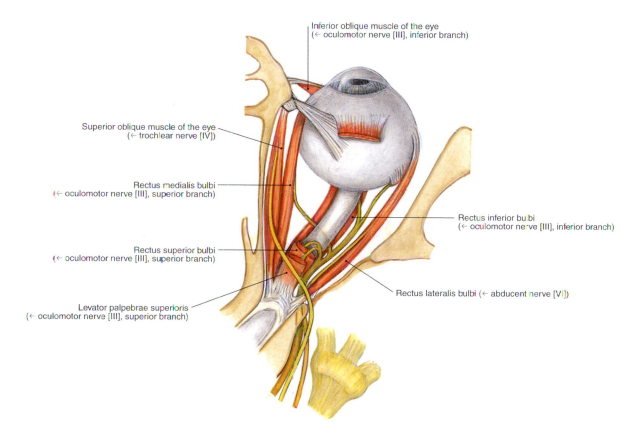

Inferior oblique muscle of the eye ($\leftarrow$ oculomotor nerve [III], inferior branch)

Superior oblique muscle of the eye ($\leftarrow$ trochlear nerve [IV])

Rectus medialis bulbi ($\leftarrow$ oculomotor nerve [III], superior branch)

Rectus superior bulbi ($\leftarrow$ oculomotor nerve [III], superior branch)

Levator palpebrae superioris ($\leftarrow$ oculomotor nerve [III], superior branch)

Rectus inferior bulbi ($\leftarrow$ oculomotor nerve [III], inferior branch)

Rectus lateralis bulbi ($\leftarrow$ abducent nerve [VI])

Fig. 1176 Innervation of the ocular muscles; superior view.

Cranial nerves

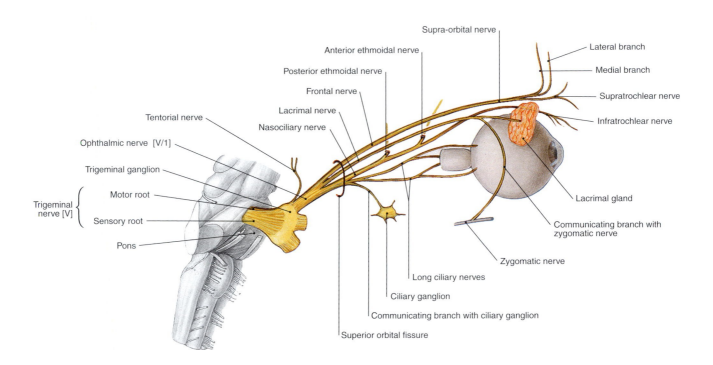

Supra-orbital nerve
Anterior ethmoidal nerve
Posterior ethmoidal nerve
Frontal nerve
Lacrimal nerve
Nasociliary nerve
Tentorial nerve
Ophthalmic nerve [V/1]
Trigeminal ganglion
Motor root
Sensory root
Pons

Trigeminal nerve [V]

Lateral branch
Medial branch
Supratrochlear nerve
Infratrochlear nerve

Lacrimal gland
Communicating branch with zygomatic nerve
Zygomatic nerve

Long ciliary nerves
Ciliary ganglion
Communicating branch with ciliary ganglion
Superior orbital fissure

→ T 57 e

Fig. 1177 Ophthalmic nerve [V/1]; viewed from the right.

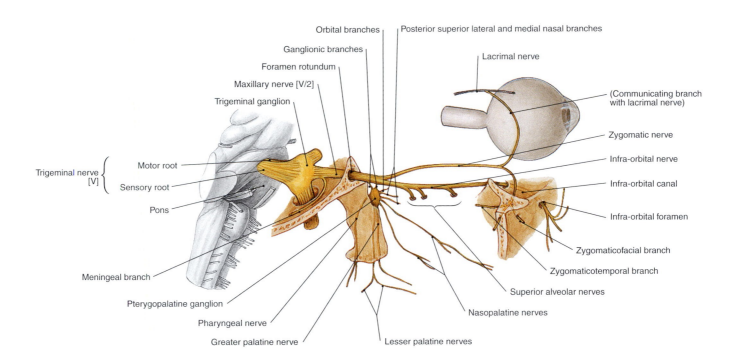

Orbital branches
Ganglionic branches
Foramen rotundum
Maxillary nerve [V/2]
Trigeminal ganglion

Posterior superior lateral and medial nasal branches
Lacrimal nerve

Trigeminal nerve [V]
Motor root
Sensory root
Pons

(Communicating branch with lacrimal nerve)
Zygomatic nerve
Infra-orbital nerve
Infra-orbital canal
Infra-orbital foramen
Zygomaticofacial branch
Zygomaticotemporal branch
Superior alveolar nerves

Meningeal branch
Pterygopalatine ganglion
Pharyngeal nerve
Greater palatine nerve
Lesser palatine nerves
Nasopalatine nerves

→ T 57 e

Fig. 1178 Maxillary nerve [V/2]; viewed from the right.

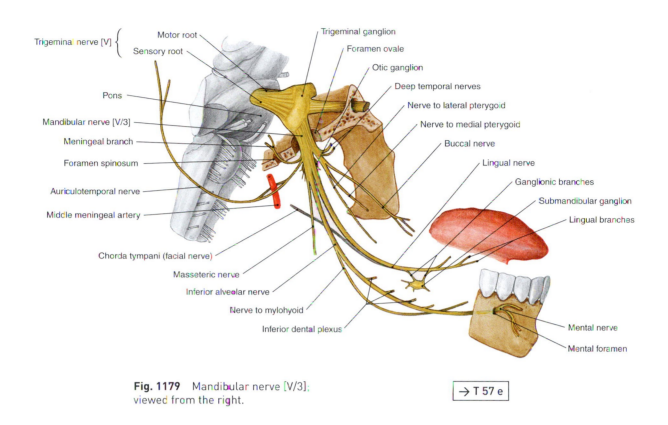

Trigeminal nerve [V] { Motor root / Sensory root

Trigeminal ganglion

Foramen ovale

Otic ganglion

Deep temporal nerves

Pons

Nerve to lateral pterygoid

Mandibular nerve [V/3]

Nerve to medial pterygoid

Meningeal branch

Buccal nerve

Foramen spinosum

Lingual nerve

Auriculotemporal nerve

Ganglionic branches

Middle meningeal artery

Submandibular ganglion

Lingual branches

Chorda tympani (facial nerve)

Masseteric nerve

Inferior alveolar nerve

Nerve to mylohyoid

Inferior dental plexus

Mental nerve

Mental foramen

Fig. 1179 Mandibular nerve [V/3]; viewed from the right.

→ T 57 e

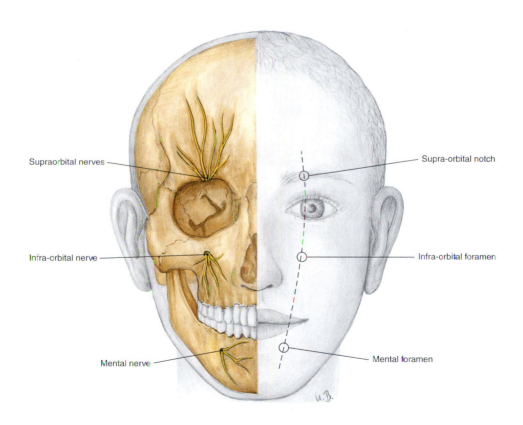

Supraorbital nerves

Supra-orbital notch

Infra-orbital nerve

Infra-orbital foramen

Mental nerve

Mental foramen

Fig. 1180 Exit points of the cutaneous branches of the trigeminal nerve [V]. Clinically, they are referred to as nerve exit points.

Cranial nerves

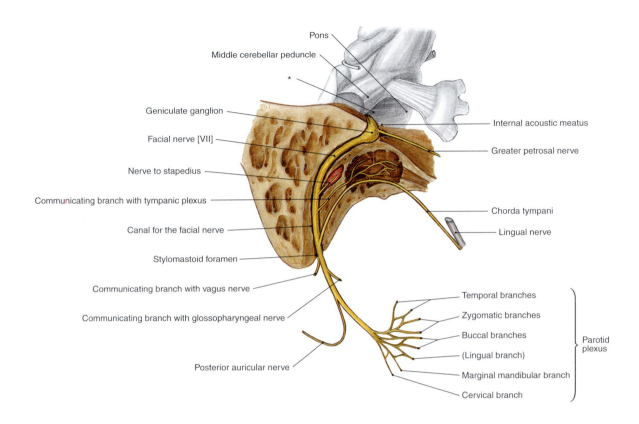

→ T 57 g

Fig. 1181 Facial nerve [VII];
the facial canal and the tympanic cavity have been opened;
viewed from the right.

* Clinical term: cerebellopontine angle

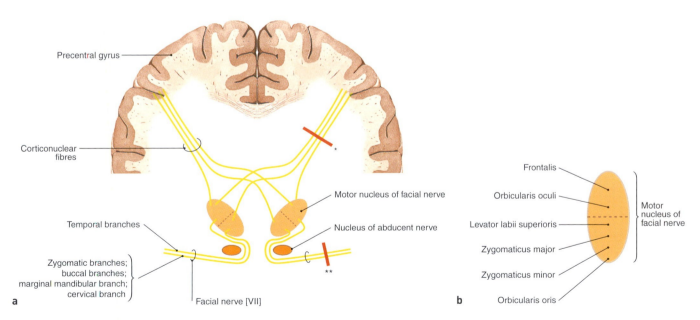

Fig. 1182 a, b Neuronal structure of the motor part
of the facial nerve [VII].
a Overview
b Representation of the facial muscles in the motor nucleus
of the facial nerve
Though the nuclei of the upper facial muscles receive innervation from both hemispheres, those of the lower facial muscles are only innervated from the contralateral side. Therefore, patients with central palsy (*) are still able to frown the brow and to close the eyelids just sufficiently. However, in patients with peripheral palsy (**) all facial muscles are paralyzed.

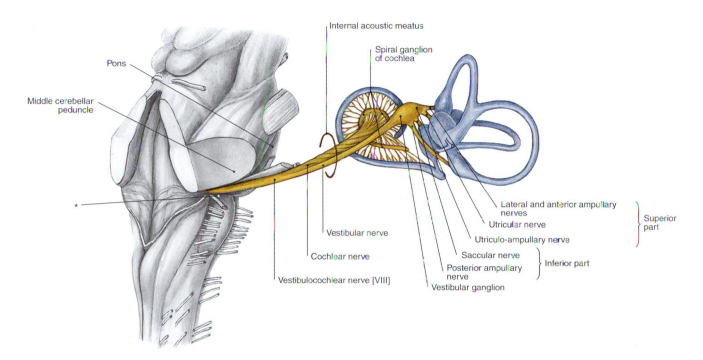

Internal acoustic meatus

Spiral ganglion of cochlea

Pons

Middle cerebellar peduncle

Lateral and anterior ampullary nerves
Utricular nerve
Utriculo-ampullary nerve
Saccular nerve
Posterior ampullary nerve
Vestibular ganglion

Superior part

Inferior part

Vestibular nerve

Cochlear nerve

Vestibulocochlear nerve [VIII]

*

Fig. 1183 Vestibulocochlear nerve [VIII]; the membranous labyrinth is greatly enlarged; posterior view from the right.

* Clinical term: cerebellopontine angle

→ T 57 h

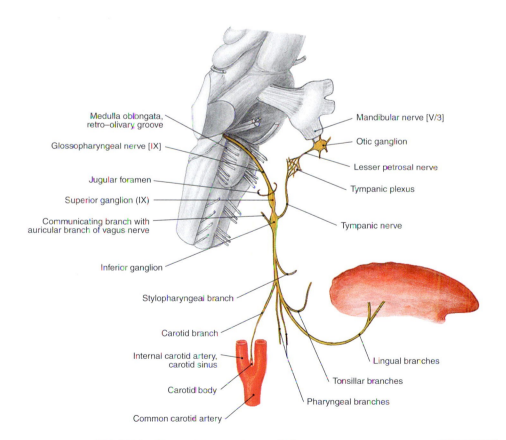

Medulla oblongata, retro–olivary groove

Glossopharyngeal nerve [IX]

Jugular foramen

Superior ganglion (IX)

Communicating branch with auricular branch of vagus nerve

Inferior ganglion

Stylopharyngeal branch

Carotid branch

Internal carotid artery, carotid sinus

Carotid body

Common carotid artery

Mandibular nerve [V/3]

Otic ganglion

Lesser petrosal nerve

Tympanic plexus

Tympanic nerve

Lingual branches

Tonsillar branches

Pharyngeal branches

Fig. 1184 Glossopharyngeal nerve [IX]; viewed from the right.

→ T 57 i

Cranial nerves

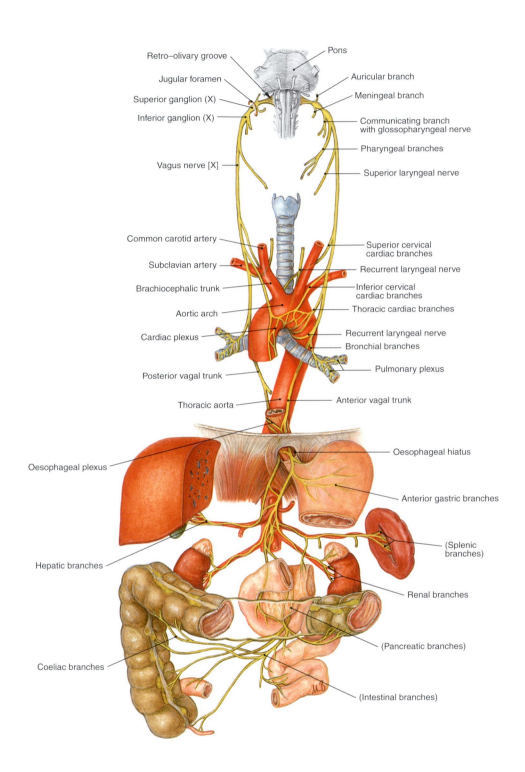

Retro–olivary groove
Jugular foramen
Superior ganglion (X)
Inferior ganglion (X)
Vagus nerve [X]
Common carotid artery
Subclavian artery
Brachiocephalic trunk
Aortic arch
Cardiac plexus
Posterior vagal trunk
Thoracic aorta
Oesophageal plexus
Hepatic branches
Coeliac branches

Pons
Auricular branch
Meningeal branch
Communicating branch with glossopharyngeal nerve
Pharyngeal branches
Superior laryngeal nerve
Superior cervical cardiac branches
Recurrent laryngeal nerve
Inferior cervical cardiac branches
Thoracic cardiac branches
Recurrent laryngeal nerve
Bronchial branches
Pulmonary plexus
Anterior vagal trunk
Oesophageal hiatus
Anterior gastric branches
(Splenic branches)
Renal branches
(Pancreatic branches)
(Intestinal branches)

→ T 57 j

Fig. 1185   Vagus nerve [X];
both nerves;
semi-schematic;
anterior view.

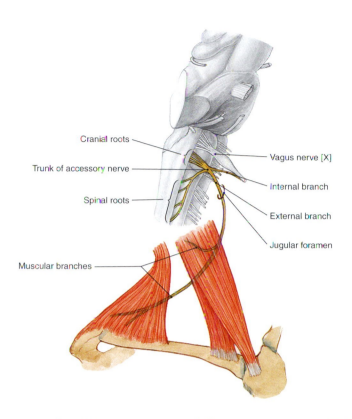

Fig. 1186 Accessory nerve [XI]; viewed from the right.

→ T 57 k

Cranial roots

Trunk of accessory nerve

Spinal roots

Muscular branches

Vagus nerve [X]

Internal branch

External branch

Jugular foramen

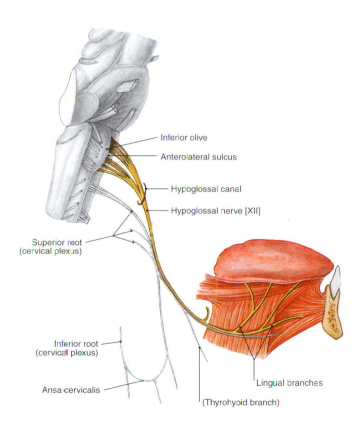

Fig. 1187 Hypoglossal nerve [XII]; viewed from the right.

→ T 57 l

Inferior olive

Anterolateral sulcus

Hypoglossal canal

Hypoglossal nerve [XII]

Superior root (cervical plexus)

Inferior root (cervical plexus)

Ansa cervicalis

(Thyrohyoid branch)

Lingual branches

Cranial nerves

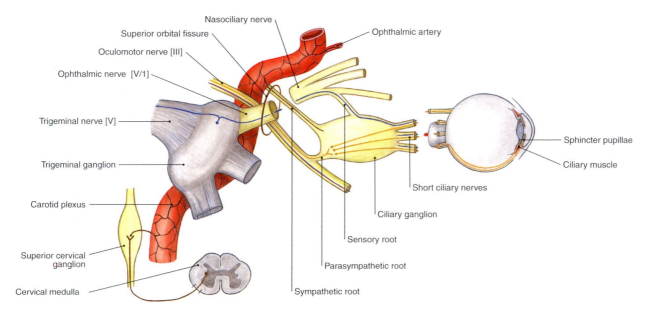

Fig. 1188 Ciliary ganglion; overview.

Nuclear region:
Accessory nucleus of the oculomotor nerve

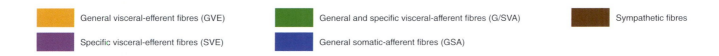

General visceral-efferent fibres (GVE)	General and specific visceral-afferent fibres (G/SVA)
Specific visceral-efferent fibres (SVE)	General somatic-afferent fibres (GSA)
	Sympathetic fibres

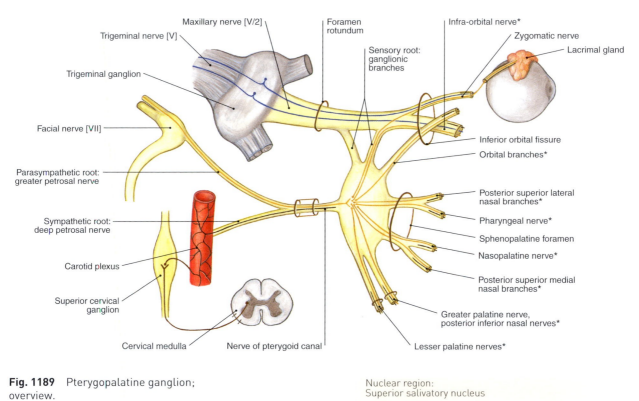

Fig. 1189 Pterygopalatine ganglion; overview.

Nuclear region:
Superior salivatory nucleus

* Innervation of the glands of the nose and the palate

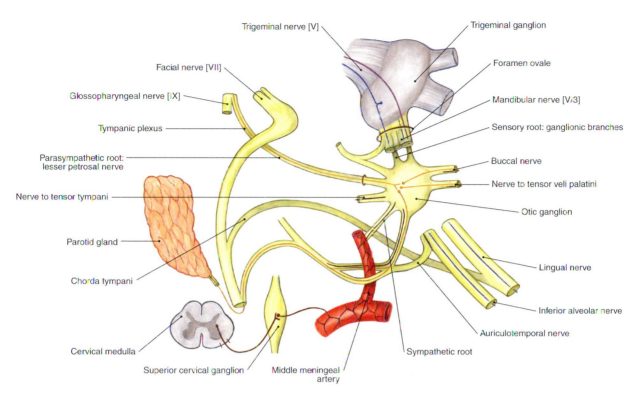

Trigeminal nerve [V]

Trigeminal ganglion

Facial nerve [VII]

Foramen ovale

Glossopharyngeal nerve [IX]

Mandibular nerve [V/3]

Tympanic plexus

Sensory root: ganglionic branches

Parasympathetic root: lesser petrosal nerve

Buccal nerve

Nerve to tensor veli palatini

Nerve to tensor tympani

Otic ganglion

Parotid gland

Lingual nerve

Chorda tympani

Inferior alveolar nerve

Auriculotemporal nerve

Cervical medulla

Sympathetic root

Superior cervical ganglion

Middle meningeal artery

Fig. 1190 Otic ganglion; overview.

Nuclear region:
Inferior salivatory nucleus

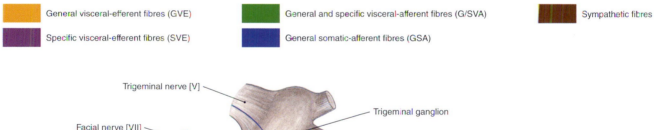

General visceral-efferent fibres (GVE)

General and specific visceral-afferent fibres (G/SVA)

Sympathetic fibres

Specific visceral-efferent fibres (SVE)

General somatic-afferent fibres (GSA)

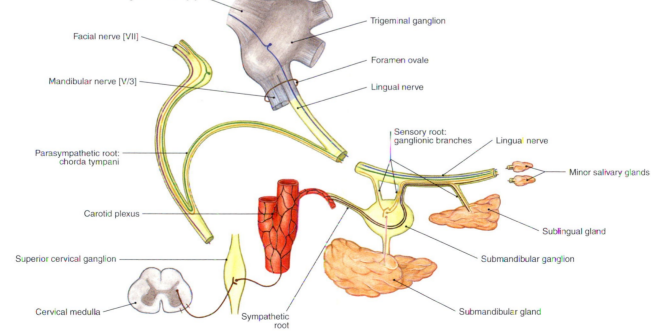

Trigeminal nerve [V]

Trigeminal ganglion

Facial nerve [VII]

Foramen ovale

Mandibular nerve [V/3]

Lingual nerve

Sensory root: ganglionic branches

Lingual nerve

Parasympathetic root: chorda tympani

Minor salivary glands

Carotid plexus

Sublingual gland

Superior cervical ganglion

Submandibular ganglion

Cervical medulla

Sympathetic root

Submandibular gland

Fig. 1191 Submandibular ganglion; overview.

Nuclear region:
Superior salivatory nucleus

Cranial nerves, topography

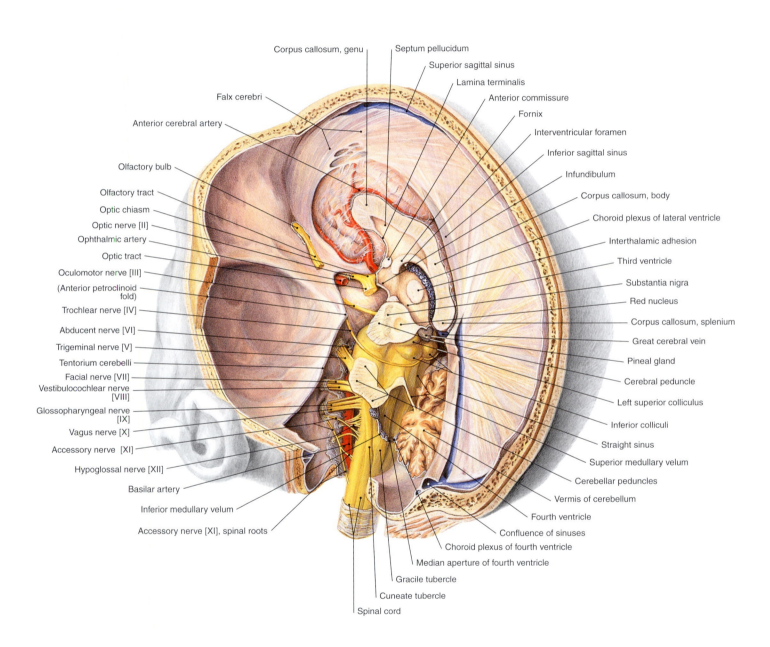

Corpus callosum, genu

Septum pellucidum

Superior sagittal sinus

Lamina terminalis

Anterior commissure

Falx cerebri

Fornix

Anterior cerebral artery

Interventricular foramen

Inferior sagittal sinus

Olfactory bulb

Infundibulum

Olfactory tract

Corpus callosum, body

Optic chiasm

Choroid plexus of lateral ventricle

Optic nerve [II]

Interthalamic adhesion

Ophthalmic artery

Optic tract

Third ventricle

Oculomotor nerve [III]

Substantia nigra

(Anterior petroclinoid fold)

Red nucleus

Trochlear nerve [IV]

Corpus callosum, splenium

Abducent nerve [VI]

Great cerebral vein

Trigeminal nerve [V]

Pineal gland

Tentorium cerebelli

Cerebral peduncle

Facial nerve [VII]

Left superior colliculus

Vestibulocochlear nerve [VIII]

Inferior colliculi

Glossopharyngeal nerve [IX]

Straight sinus

Vagus nerve [X]

Superior medullary velum

Accessory nerve [XI]

Cerebellar peduncles

Hypoglossal nerve [XII]

Vermis of cerebellum

Basilar artery

Fourth ventricle

Inferior medullary velum

Confluence of sinuses

Accessory nerve [XI], spinal roots

Choroid plexus of fourth ventricle

Median aperture of fourth ventricle

Gracile tubercle

Cuneate tubercle

Spinal cord

Fig. 1192 Course of the cranial nerves in the subarachnoid space; the left hemisphere of the cerebrum and the cerebellum as well as the tentorium cerebelli have been removed.

Cranial nerves, topography

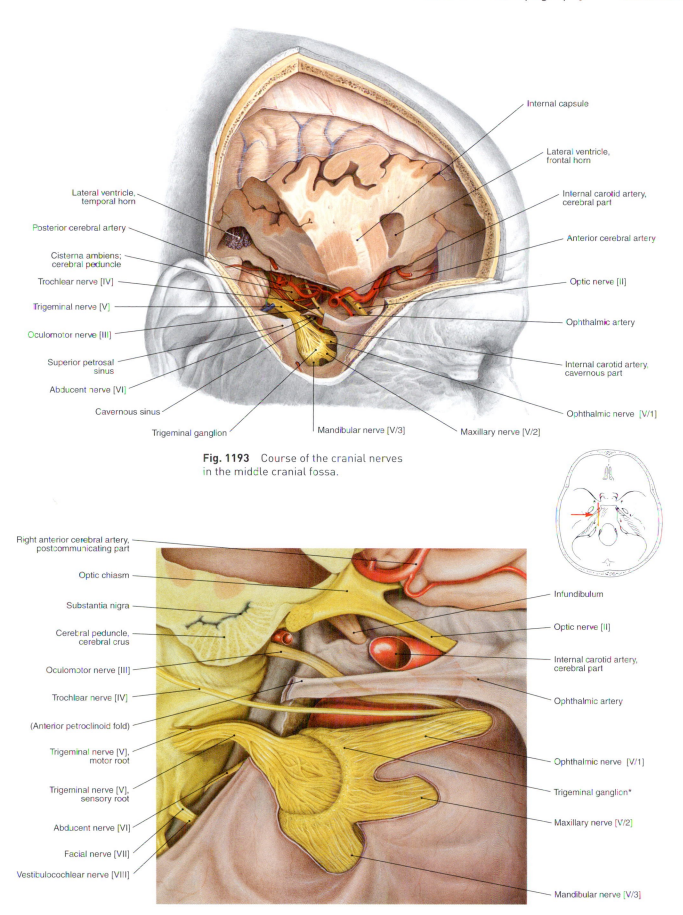

Internal capsule

Lateral ventricle, frontal horn

Internal carotid artery, cerebral part

Anterior cerebral artery

Optic nerve [II]

Ophthalmic artery

Internal carotid artery, cavernous part

Ophthalmic nerve [V/1]

Maxillary nerve [V/2]

Lateral ventricle, temporal horn

Posterior cerebral artery

Cisterna ambiens; cerebral peduncle

Trochlear nerve [IV]

Trigeminal nerve [V]

Oculomotor nerve [III]

Superior petrosal sinus

Abducent nerve [VI]

Cavernous sinus

Trigeminal ganglion

Mandibular nerve [V/3]

Fig. 1193 Course of the cranial nerves in the middle cranial fossa.

Right anterior cerebral artery, postcommunicating part

Optic chiasm

Substantia nigra

Cerebral peduncle, cerebral crus

Oculomotor nerve [III]

Trochlear nerve [IV]

(Anterior petroclinoid fold)

Trigeminal nerve [V], motor root

Trigeminal nerve [V], sensory root

Abducent nerve [VI]

Facial nerve [VII]

Vestibulocochlear nerve [VIII]

Infundibulum

Optic nerve [II]

Internal carotid artery, cerebral part

Ophthalmic artery

Ophthalmic nerve [V/1]

Trigeminal ganglion*

Maxillary nerve [V/2]

Mandibular nerve [V/3]

Fig. 1194 Arteries and nerves in the region of the sella turcica and the cavernous sinus.

* Clinical term: GASSERian ganglion

Vessels and nerves of the cranial base

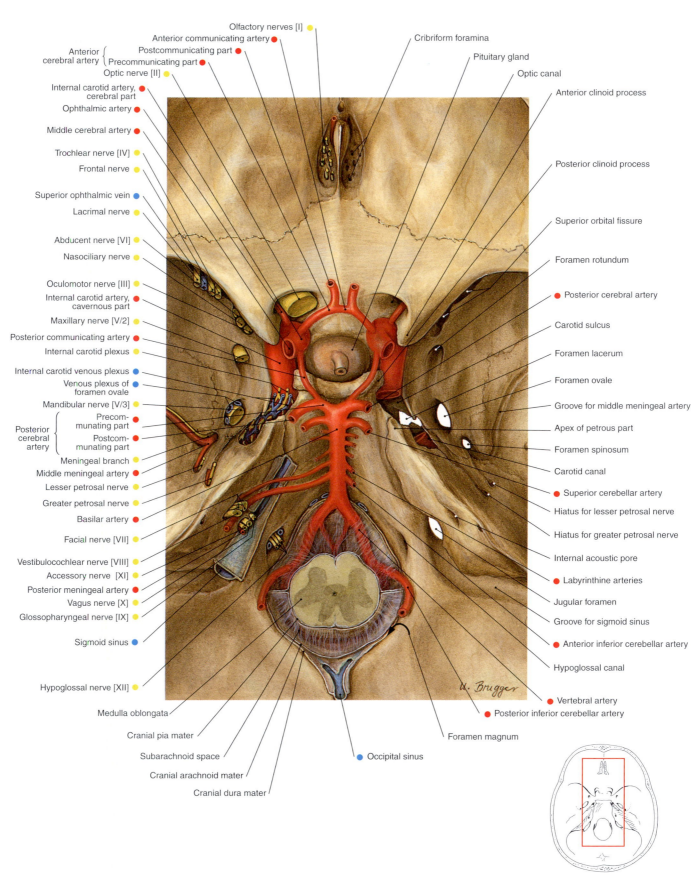

Olfactory nerves [I] ●
Anterior communicating artery ●
Anterior cerebral artery { Postcommunicating part ●
Precommunicating part ●
Optic nerve [II] ●
Internal carotid artery, ● cerebral part
Ophthalmic artery ●
Middle cerebral artery ●
Trochlear nerve [IV] ●
Frontal nerve ●
Superior ophthalmic vein ●
Lacrimal nerve ●
Abducent nerve [VI] ●
Nasociliary nerve ●
Oculomotor nerve [III] ●
Internal carotid artery, ● cavernous part
Maxillary nerve [V/2] ●
Posterior communicating artery ●
Internal carotid plexus ●
Internal carotid venous plexus ●
Venous plexus of ● foramen ovale
Mandibular nerve [V/3] ●
Posterior cerebral artery { Precom- munating part ●
Postcom- munating part ●
Meningeal branch ●
Middle meningeal artery ●
Lesser petrosal nerve ●
Greater petrosal nerve ●
Basilar artery ●
Facial nerve [VII] ●
Vestibulocochlear nerve [VIII] ●
Accessory nerve [XI] ●
Posterior meningeal artery ●
Vagus nerve [X] ●
Glossopharyngeal nerve [IX] ●
Sigmoid sinus ●
Hypoglossal nerve [XII] ●

Cribriform foramina
Pituitary gland
Optic canal
Anterior clinoid process
Posterior clinoid process
Superior orbital fissure
Foramen rotundum
● Posterior cerebral artery
Carotid sulcus
Foramen lacerum
Foramen ovale
Groove for middle meningeal artery
Apex of petrous part
Foramen spinosum
Carotid canal
● Superior cerebellar artery
Hiatus for lesser petrosal nerve
Hiatus for greater petrosal nerve
Internal acoustic pore
● Labyrinthine arteries
Jugular foramen
Groove for sigmoid sinus
● Anterior inferior cerebellar artery
Hypoglossal canal
● Vertebral artery
● Posterior inferior cerebellar artery

Medulla oblongata
Cranial pia mater
Subarachnoid space
Cranial arachnoid mater
Cranial dura mater
Foramen magnum
● Occipital sinus

→ 1172, 1173, 1268

Fig. 1195 Passage of vessels and nerves through the internal surface of cranial base and the cerebral arterial circle; superior view.

Cavernous sinus and pituitary gland

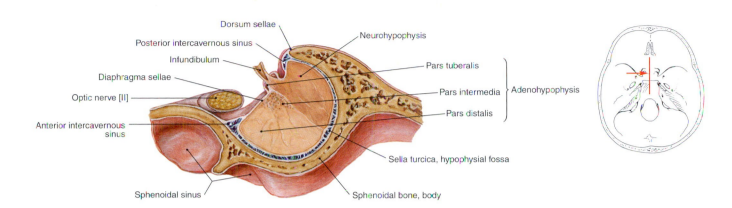

Fig. 1196 Pituitary gland.

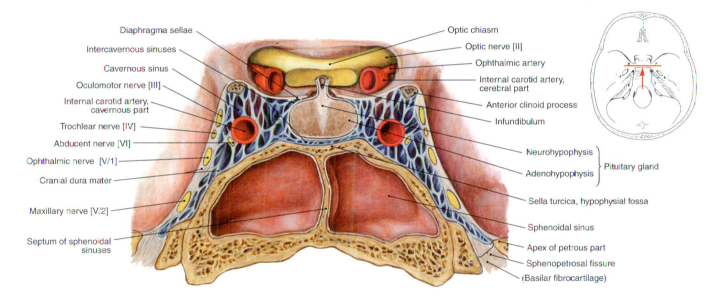

Fig. 1197 Pituitary gland and cavernous sinus.

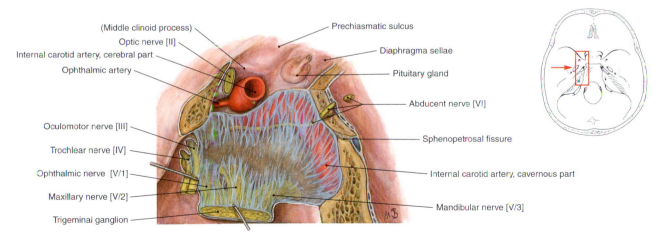

Fig. 1198 Cavernous sinus;
the part of the cranial dura mater forming the lateral wall of the
cavernous sinus has been removed;
the trigeminal ganglion has been reflected to the side.

Cranial dura mater and superior sagittal sinus

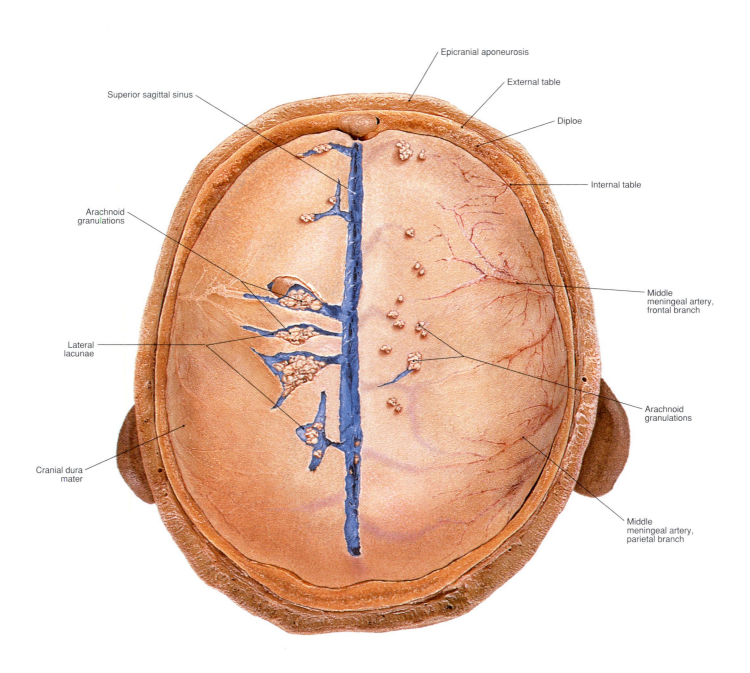

Epicranial aponeurosis

External table

Superior sagittal sinus

Diploe

Arachnoid granulations

Internal table

Lateral lacunae

Middle meningeal artery, frontal branch

Cranial dura mater

Arachnoid granulations

Middle meningeal artery, parietal branch

Fig. 1199 Cranial dura mater and superior sagittal sinus with some lateral lacunae.

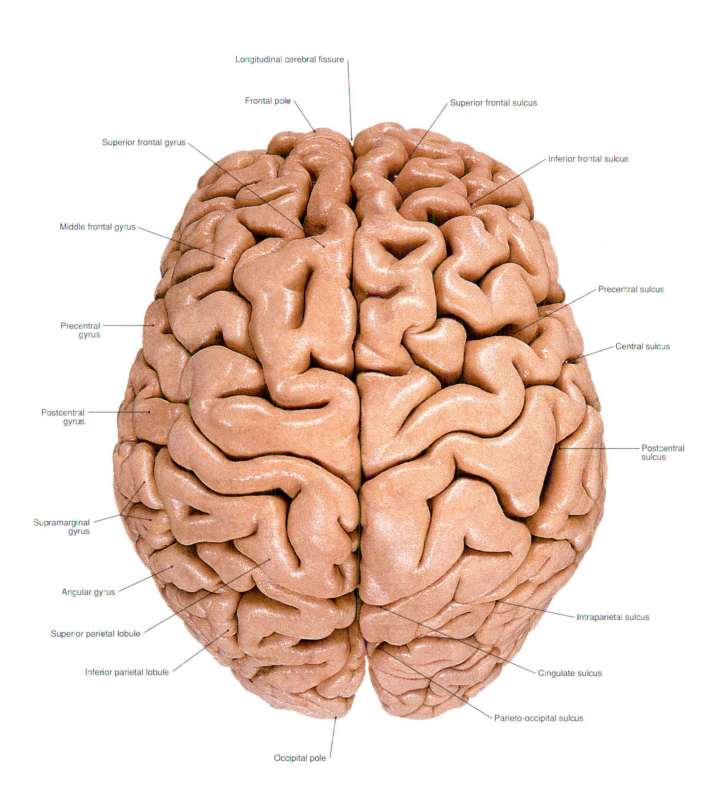

Longitudinal cerebral fissure

Frontal pole

Superior frontal gyrus

Middle frontal gyrus

Precentral gyrus

Postcentral gyrus

Supramarginal gyrus

Angular gyrus

Superior parietal lobule

Inferior parietal lobule

Occipital pole

Superior frontal sulcus

Inferior frontal sulcus

Precentral sulcus

Central sulcus

Postcentral sulcus

Intraparietal sulcus

Cingulate sulcus

Parieto-occipital sulcus

Fig. 1206   Cerebrum;
after removal of the cranial arachnoid mater;
superior view.
Formation of the gyri varies considerably.

Base of the brain

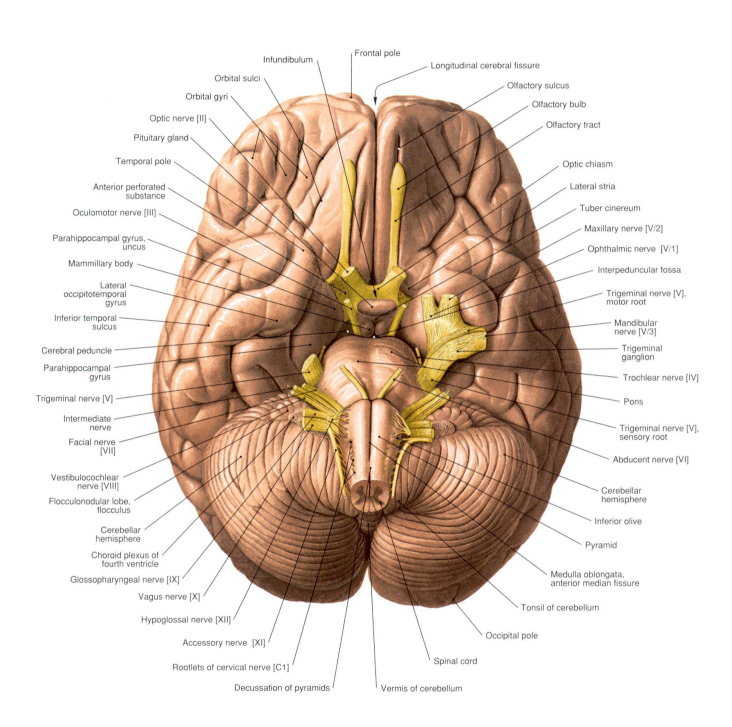

Fig. 1207 Cerebrum;
brainstem with cerebellum as well as cranial nerves;
inferior view.

Base of the brain

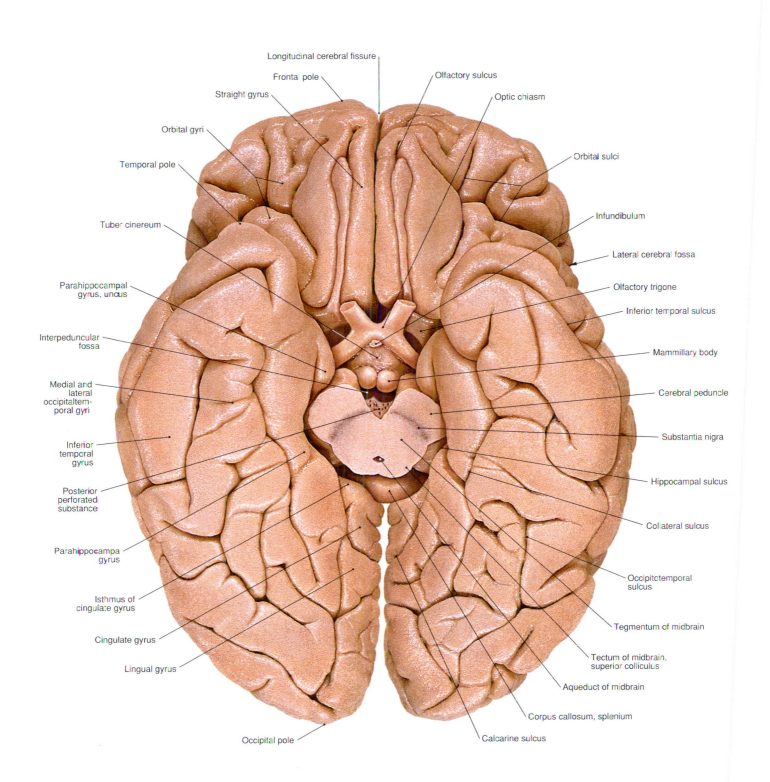

Longitudinal cerebral fissure

Frontal pole

Straight gyrus

Orbital gyri

Temporal pole

Tuber cinereum

Parahippocampal gyrus, uncus

Interpeduncular fossa

Medial and lateral occipitaltemporal gyri

Inferior temporal gyrus

Posterior perforated substance

Parahippocampal gyrus

Isthmus of cingulate gyrus

Cingulate gyrus

Lingual gyrus

Occipital pole

Olfactory sulcus

Optic chiasm

Orbital sulci

Infundibulum

Lateral cerebral fossa

Olfactory trigone

Inferior temporal sulcus

Mammillary body

Cerebral peduncle

Substantia nigra

Hippocampal sulcus

Collateral sulcus

Occipitotemporal sulcus

Tegmentum of midbrain

Tectum of midbrain, superior colliculus

Aqueduct of midbrain

Corpus callosum, splenium

Calcarine sulcus

Fig. 1208 Gyri and grooves of the cerebral hemispheres; the midbrain has been sectioned.

Lobes of the telencephalon

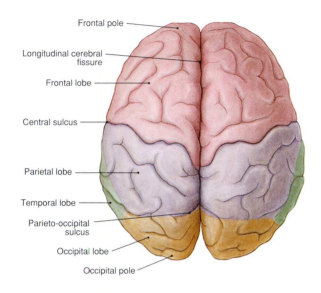

Fig. 1209 Lobes of the cerebrum; superior view.

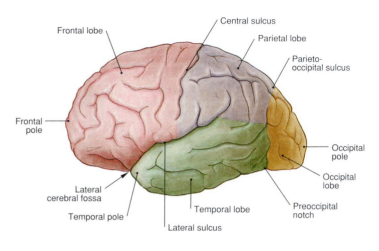

Fig. 1210 Lobes of the cerebrum; viewed from the left.

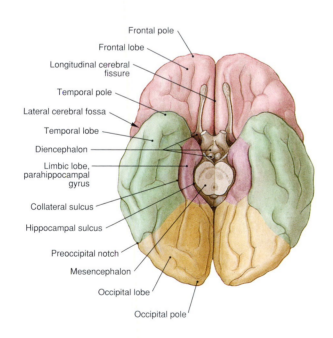

Fig. 1211 Lobes of the cerebrum; inferior view.

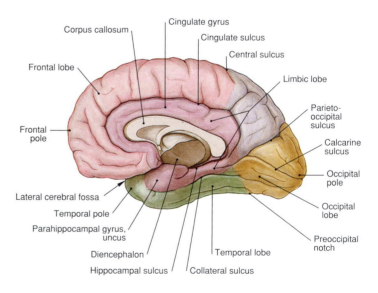

Fig. 1212 Lobes of the cerebrum; medial view.

Cerebral cortex

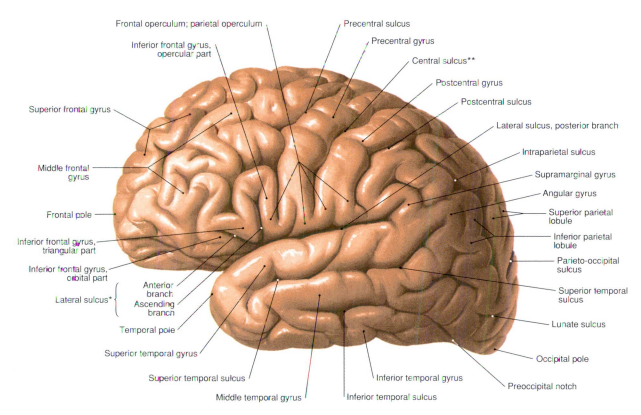

Frontal operculum; parietal operculum

Inferior frontal gyrus, opercular part

Superior frontal gyrus

Middle frontal gyrus

Frontal pole

Inferior frontal gyrus, triangular part

Inferior frontal gyrus, orbital part

Lateral sulcus*

Anterior branch
Ascending branch

Temporal pole

Superior temporal gyrus

Superior temporal sulcus

Middle temporal gyrus

Precentral sulcus

Precentral gyrus

Central sulcus**

Postcentral gyrus

Postcentral sulcus

Lateral sulcus, posterior branch

Intraparietal sulcus

Supramarginal gyrus

Angular gyrus

Superior parietal lobule

Inferior parietal lobule

Parieto-occipital sulcus

Superior temporal sulcus

Lunate sulcus

Occipital pole

Preoccipital notch

Inferior temporal gyrus

Inferior temporal sulcus

Fig. 1213   Gyri and grooves of the cerebral hemispheres; viewed from the left.

*   Sulcus of SYLVIUS
** Sulcus of ROLANDO

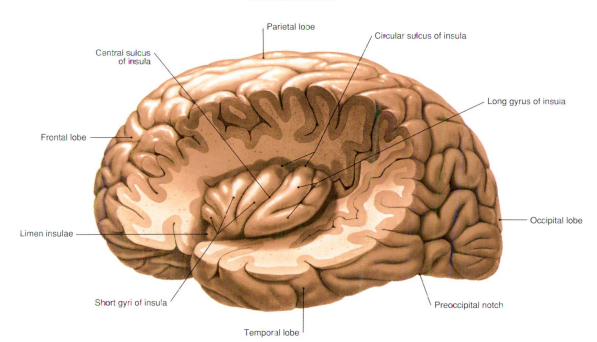

Parietal lobe

Circular sulcus of insula

Central sulcus of insula

Frontal lobe

Long gyrus of insula

Limen insulae

Occipital lobe

Short gyri of insula

Preoccipital notch

Temporal lobe

Fig. 1214   Gyri and grooves of the cerebral hemispheres; exposure of the insula after removal of the frontal, parietal and temporal opercula; viewed from the left.

Gyri of the cerebral hemispheres

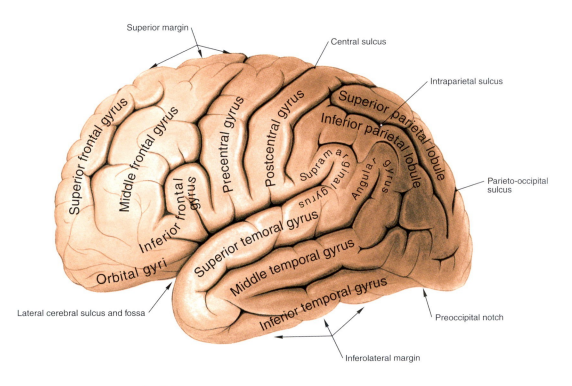

Fig. 1215 Gyri of the cerebral hemispheres; viewed from the left.

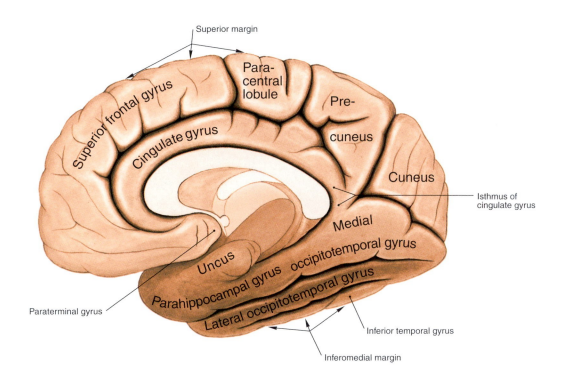

Fig. 1216 Gyri of the cerebral hemispheres; medial view.

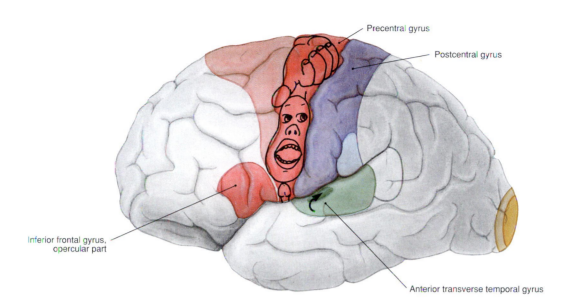

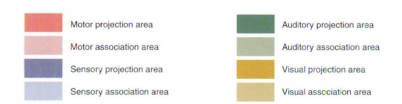

Fig. 1217 Functional cortical areas of the cerebral hemispheres according to FOERSTER; viewed from the left.

The somatotopic organisation is illustrated schematically. The primary receiving area for auditory impulses (C) extends over the upper edge of the temporal lobe onto its inner surface.

Motor projection area	Auditory projection area
Motor association area	Auditory association area
Sensory projection area	Visual projection area
Sensory association area	Visual association area

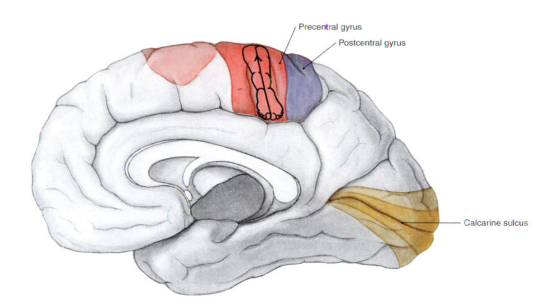

Fig. 1218 Functional cortical areas of the cerebral hemispheres according to FOERSTER; medial view.

The somatotopic organisation is illustrated schematically.

Fornix

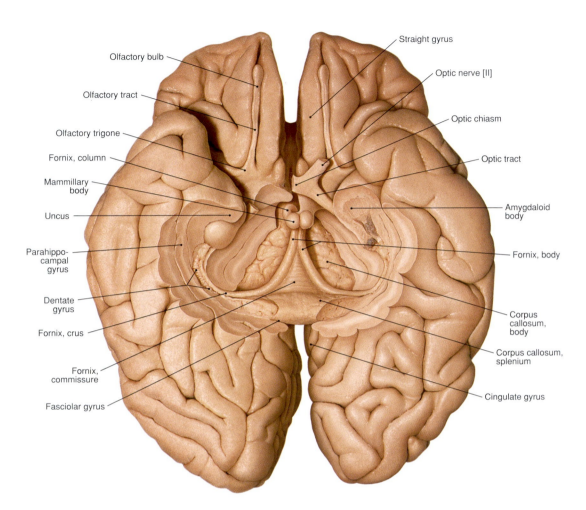

Olfactory bulb
Olfactory tract
Olfactory trigone
Fornix, column
Mammillary body
Uncus
Parahippo-campal gyrus
Dentate gyrus
Fornix, crus
Fornix, commissure
Fasciolar gyrus

Straight gyrus
Optic nerve [II]
Optic chiasm
Optic tract
Amygdaloid body
Fornix, body
Corpus callosum, body
Corpus callosum, splenium
Cingulate gyrus

Fig. 1219 Fornix;
after removal of the basal parts of the brain;
inferior view.

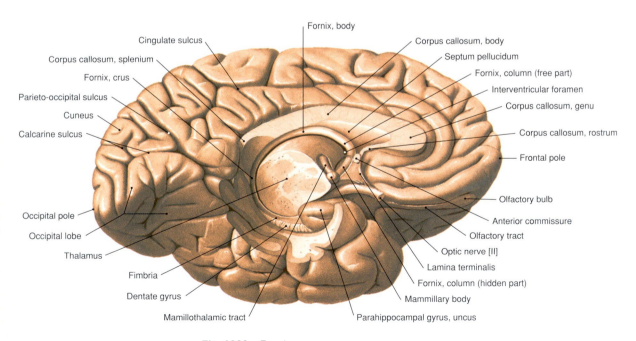

Cingulate sulcus
Corpus callosum, splenium
Fornix, crus
Parieto-occipital sulcus
Cuneus
Calcarine sulcus
Occipital pole
Occipital lobe
Thalamus
Fimbria
Dentate gyrus
Mamillothalamic tract

Fornix, body
Corpus callosum, body
Septum pellucidum
Fornix, column (free part)
Interventricular foramen
Corpus callosum, genu
Corpus callosum, rostrum
Frontal pole
Olfactory bulb
Anterior commissure
Olfactory tract
Optic nerve [II]
Lamina terminalis
Fornix, column (hidden part)
Mammillary body
Parahippocampal gyrus, uncus

Fig. 1220 Fornix;
inferomedial view.

Fornix and anterior commissure

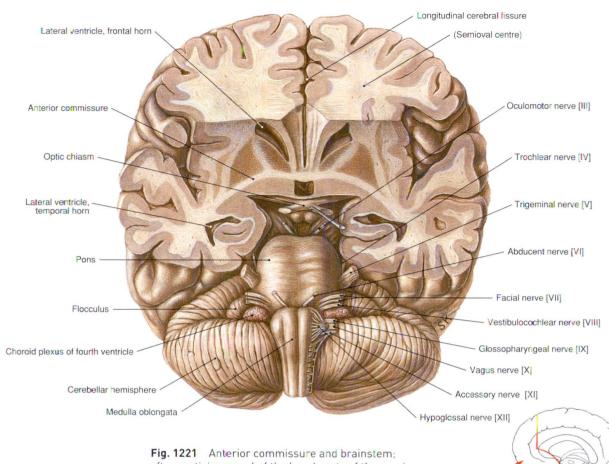

Longitudinal cerebral fissure
(Semioval centre)
Lateral ventricle, frontal horn
Anterior commissure
Optic chiasm
Lateral ventricle, temporal horn
Pons
Flocculus
Choroid plexus of fourth ventricle
Cerebellar hemisphere
Medulla oblongata
Oculomotor nerve [III]
Trochlear nerve [IV]
Trigeminal nerve [V]
Abducent nerve [VI]
Facial nerve [VII]
Vestibulocochlear nerve [VIII]
Glossopharyngeal nerve [IX]
Vagus nerve [X]
Accessory nerve [XI]
Hypoglossal nerve [XII]

Fig. 1221 Anterior commissure and brainstem;
after partial removal of the basal parts of the cerebrum;
anterior-inferior view.

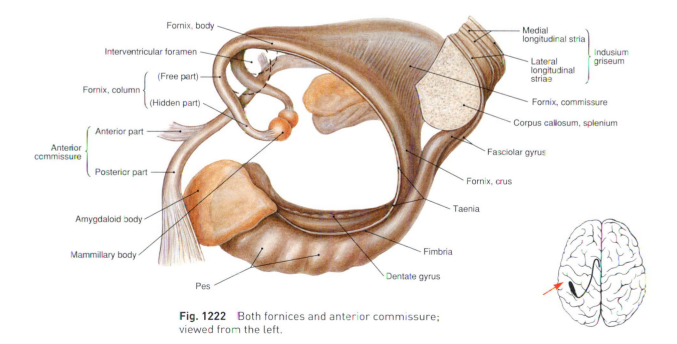

Fornix, body
Interventricular foramen
Fornix, column { (Free part) (Hidden part) }
Anterior commissure { Anterior part Posterior part }
Amygdaloid body
Mammillary body
Pes
Medial longitudinal stria
Lateral longitudinal striae } Indusium griseum
Fornix, commissure
Corpus callosum, splenium
Fasciolar gyrus
Fornix, crus
Taenia
Fimbria
Dentate gyrus

Fig. 1222 Both fornices and anterior commissure;
viewed from the left.

Basal ganglia

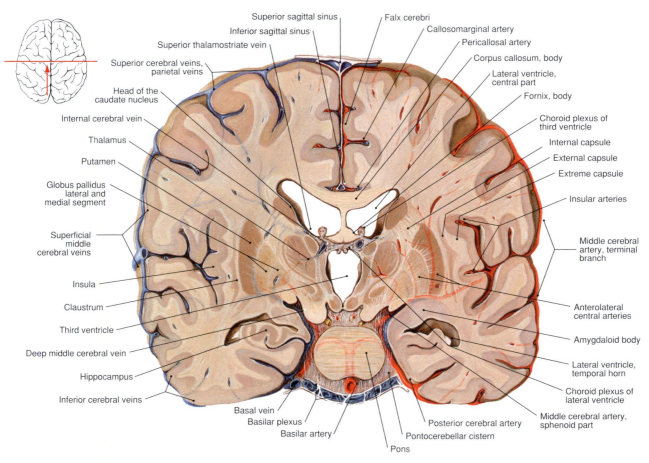

Fig. 1223 Blood supply of the basal ganglia;
frontal section;
the arteries are shown on the right and the veins on the left;
posterior view.

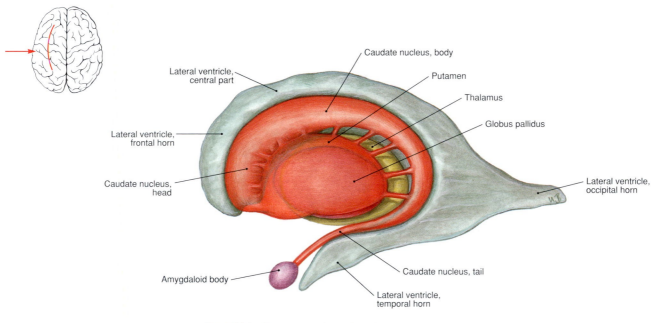

Fig. 1224 Basal ganglia and thalamus;
viewed from the left.

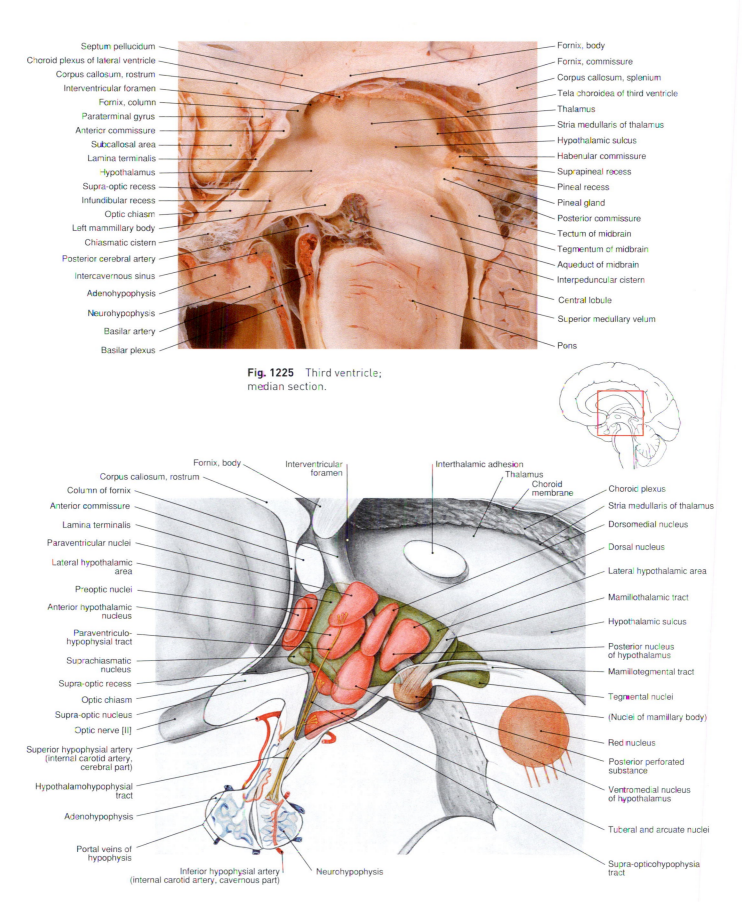

Septum pellucidum
Choroid plexus of lateral ventricle
Corpus callosum, rostrum
Interventricular foramen
Fornix, column
Paraterminal gyrus
Anterior commissure
Subcallosal area
Lamina terminalis
Hypothalamus
Supra-optic recess
Infundibular recess
Optic chiasm
Left mammillary body
Chiasmatic cistern
Posterior cerebral artery
Intercavernous sinus
Adenohypophysis
Neurohypophysis
Basilar artery
Basilar plexus

Fornix, body
Fornix, commissure
Corpus callosum, splenium
Tela choroidea of third ventricle
Thalamus
Stria medullaris of thalamus
Hypothalamic sulcus
Habenular commissure
Suprapineal recess
Pineal recess
Pineal gland
Posterior commissure
Tectum of midbrain
Tegmentum of midbrain
Aqueduct of midbrain
Interpeduncular cistern
Central lobule
Superior medullary velum
Pons

Fig. 1225 Third ventricle; median section.

Fornix, body
Corpus callosum, rostrum
Column of fornix
Anterior commissure
Lamina terminalis
Paraventricular nuclei
Lateral hypothalamic area
Preoptic nuclei
Anterior hypothalamic nucleus
Paraventriculo-hypophysial tract
Suprachiasmatic nucleus
Supra-optic recess
Optic chiasm
Supra-optic nucleus
Optic nerve [II]
Superior hypophysial artery (internal carotid artery, cerebral part)
Hypothalamohypophysial tract
Adenohypophysis
Portal veins of hypophysis
Inferior hypophysial artery (internal carotid artery, cavernous part)
Neurohypophysis

Interventricular foramen
Interthalamic adhesion
Thalamus
Choroid membrane
Choroid plexus
Stria medullaris of thalamus
Dorsomedial nucleus
Dorsal nucleus
Lateral hypothalamic area
Mamillothalamic tract
Hypothalamic sulcus
Posterior nucleus of hypothalamus
Mamillotegmental tract
Tegmental nuclei
(Nuclei of mamillary body)
Red nucleus
Posterior perforated substance
Ventromedial nucleus of hypothalamus
Tuberal and arcuate nuclei
Supra-opticohypophysial tract

Fig. 1226 Hypothalamus; overview; nuclei are illustrated translucently; medial view.

Thalamic nuclei

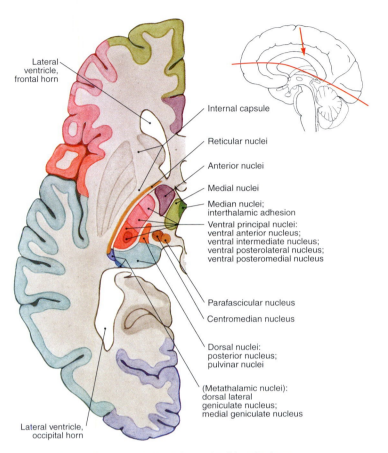

Lateral ventricle, frontal horn

Internal capsule

Reticular nuclei

Anterior nuclei

Medial nuclei

Median nuclei; interthalamic adhesion

Ventral principal nuclei: ventral anterior nucleus; ventral intermediate nucleus; ventral posterolateral nucleus; ventral posteromedial nucleus

Parafascicular nucleus

Centromedian nucleus

Dorsal nuclei: posterior nucleus; pulvinar nuclei

(Metathalamic nuclei): dorsal lateral geniculate nucleus; medial geniculate nucleus

Lateral ventricle, occipital horn

a Horizontal section through the left cerebral hemisphere

Fig. 1227 a–c Nuclei and cortical projections of the thalamus. Corresponding nuclei and cortical projections are indicated by the same colour.

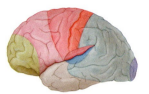

b Left cerebral hemisphere; viewed from the left

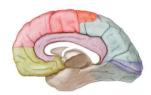

c Right cerebral hemisphere; medial view

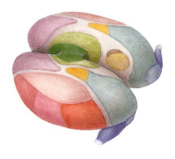

Fig. 1228 Thalamic nuclei; oblique view from posterior. For colour coding see Fig. 1227.

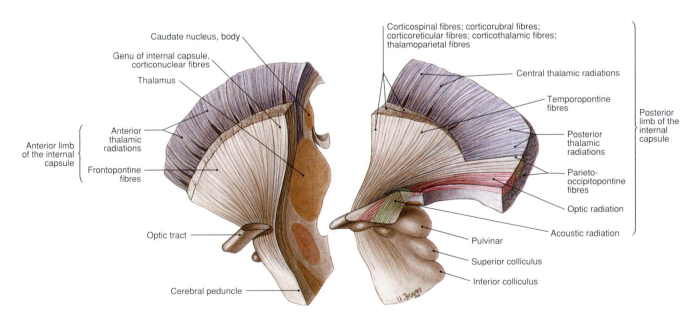

Caudate nucleus, body

Genu of internal capsule, corticonuclear fibres

Thalamus

Anterior thalamic radiations

Anterior limb of the internal capsule

Frontopontine fibres

Optic tract

Cerebral peduncle

Corticospinal fibres; corticorubral fibres; corticoreticular fibres; corticothalamic fibres; thalamoparietal fibres

Central thalamic radiations

Temporopontine fibres

Posterior limb of the internal capsule

Posterior thalamic radiations

Parieto-occipitopontine fibres

Optic radiation

Acoustic radiation

Pulvinar

Superior colliculus

Inferior colliculus

Fig. 1229 Thalamic radiation and internal capsule have been divided by a frontal section; viewed from the left.

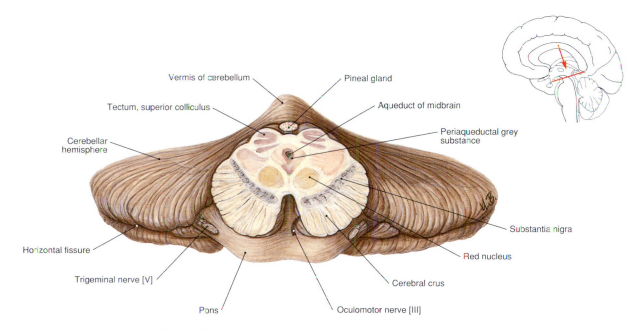

Vermis of cerebellum

Pineal gland

Tectum, superior colliculus

Aqueduct of midbrain

Cerebellar hemisphere

Periaqueductal grey substance

Substantia nigra

Horizontal fissure

Red nucleus

Trigeminal nerve [V]

Cerebral crus

Pons

Oculomotor nerve [III]

Fig. 1230 Midbrain;
cross-section at the level of the superior colliculi;
anterior view.

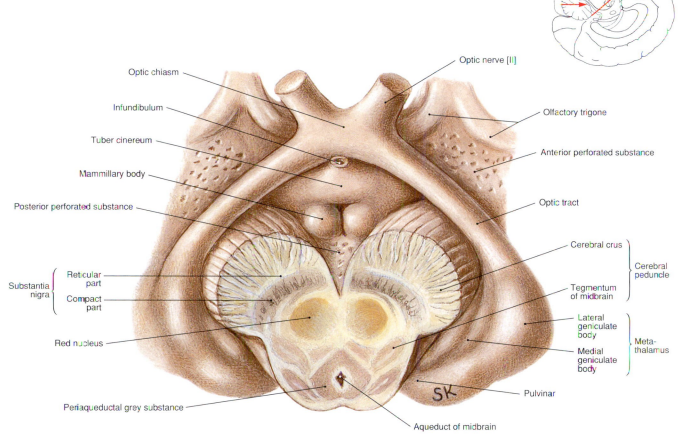

Optic chiasm

Optic nerve [II]

Infundibulum

Olfactory trigone

Tuber cinereum

Anterior perforated substance

Mammillary body

Posterior perforated substance

Optic tract

Cerebral crus

Cerebral peduncle

Substantia nigra

Reticular part

Tegmentum of midbrain

Compact part

Lateral geniculate body

Meta-thalamus

Red nucleus

Medial geniculate body

Pulvinar

Periaqueductal grey substance

Aqueduct of midbrain

SK

Fig. 1231 Midbrain and diencephalon;
after oblique section of the midbrain;
inferior view.

Midbrain and medulla oblongata

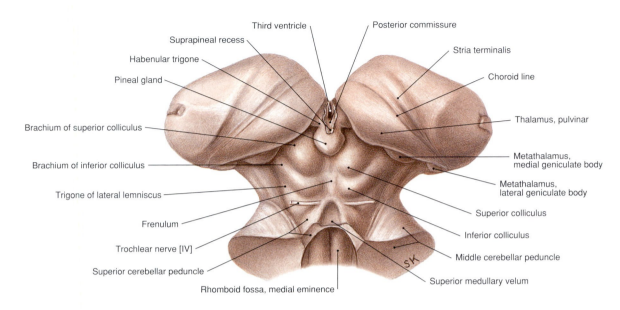

Third ventricle
Posterior commissure
Suprapineal recess
Stria terminalis
Habenular trigone
Choroid line
Pineal gland
Thalamus, pulvinar
Brachium of superior colliculus
Metathalamus, medial geniculate body
Brachium of inferior colliculus
Metathalamus, lateral geniculate body
Trigone of lateral lemniscus
Superior colliculus
Frenulum
Inferior colliculus
Trochlear nerve [IV]
Middle cerebellar peduncle
Superior cerebellar peduncle
Superior medullary velum
Rhomboid fossa, medial eminence

Fig. 1232 Midbrain and pineal gland; posterior-superior view.

527
528

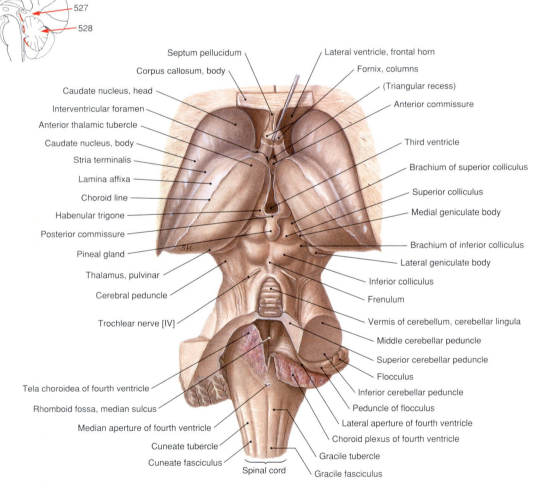

Septum pellucidum
Lateral ventricle, frontal horn
Corpus callosum, body
Fornix, columns
Caudate nucleus, head
(Triangular recess)
Interventricular foramen
Anterior commissure
Anterior thalamic tubercle
Caudate nucleus, body
Third ventricle
Stria terminalis
Brachium of superior colliculus
Lamina affixa
Superior colliculus
Choroid line
Medial geniculate body
Habenular trigone
Posterior commissure
Brachium of inferior colliculus
Pineal gland
Lateral geniculate body
Thalamus, pulvinar
Inferior colliculus
Cerebral peduncle
Frenulum
Trochlear nerve [IV]
Vermis of cerebellum, cerebellar lingula
Middle cerebellar peduncle
Superior cerebellar peduncle
Flocculus
Tela choroidea of fourth ventricle
Inferior cerebellar peduncle
Rhomboid fossa, median sulcus
Peduncle of flocculus
Median aperture of fourth ventricle
Lateral aperture of fourth ventricle
Cuneate tubercle
Choroid plexus of fourth ventricle
Cuneate fasciculus
Gracile tubercle
Spinal cord
Gracile fasciculus

Fig. 1233 Brainstem;
the pons and major parts of the cerebellum have been removed;
the tela choroidea of the fourth ventricle has been sectioned in
the median plane and reflected to the right;
posterior-superior view.

Midbrain and medulla oblongata

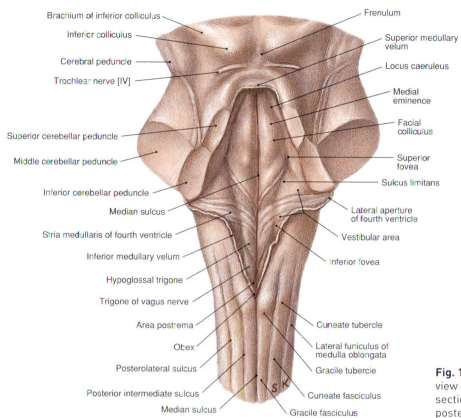

Brachium of inferior colliculus
Inferior colliculus
Cerebral peduncle
Trochlear nerve [IV]
Superior cerebellar peduncle
Middle cerebellar peduncle
Inferior cerebellar peduncle
Median sulcus
Stria medullaris of fourth ventricle
Inferior medullary velum
Hypoglossal trigone
Trigone of vagus nerve
Area postrema
Obex
Posterolateral sulcus
Posterior intermediate sulcus
Median sulcus

Frenulum
Superior medullary velum
Locus caeruleus
Medial eminence
Facial colliculus
Superior fovea
Sulcus limitans
Lateral aperture of fourth ventricle
Vestibular area
Inferior fovea
Cuneate tubercle
Lateral funiculus of medulla oblongata
Gracile tubercle
Cuneate fasciculus
Gracile fasciculus

Fig. 1234   Rhomboid fossa;
view on the floor of the fourth ventricle after
section of the cerebellar peduncles;
posterior-superior view.

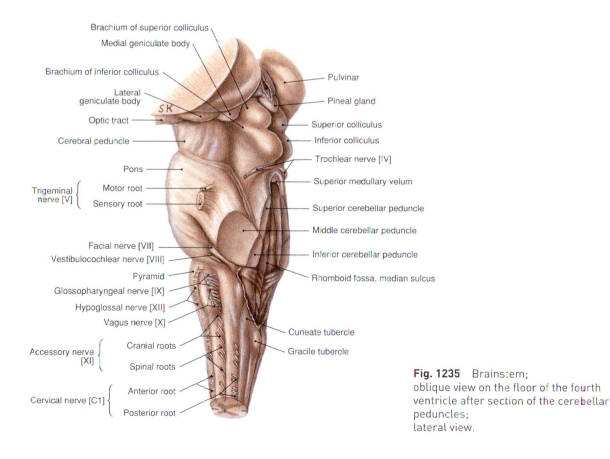

Brachium of superior colliculus
Medial geniculate body
Brachium of inferior colliculus
Lateral geniculate body
Optic tract
Cerebral peduncle
Pons
Trigeminal nerve [V] { Motor root
Sensory root }
Facial nerve [VII]
Vestibulocochlear nerve [VIII]
Pyramid
Glossopharyngeal nerve [IX]
Hypoglossal nerve [XII]
Vagus nerve [X]
Accessory nerve [XI] { Cranial roots
Spinal roots }
Cervical nerve [C1] { Anterior root
Posterior root }

Pulvinar
Pineal gland
Superior colliculus
Inferior colliculus
Trochlear nerve [IV]
Superior medullary velum
Superior cerebellar peduncle
Middle cerebellar peduncle
Inferior cerebellar peduncle
Rhomboid fossa, median sulcus
Cuneate tubercle
Gracile tubercle

Fig. 1235   Brainstem;
oblique view on the floor of the fourth
ventricle after section of the cerebellar
peduncles;
lateral view.

Nuclei of the cranial nerves

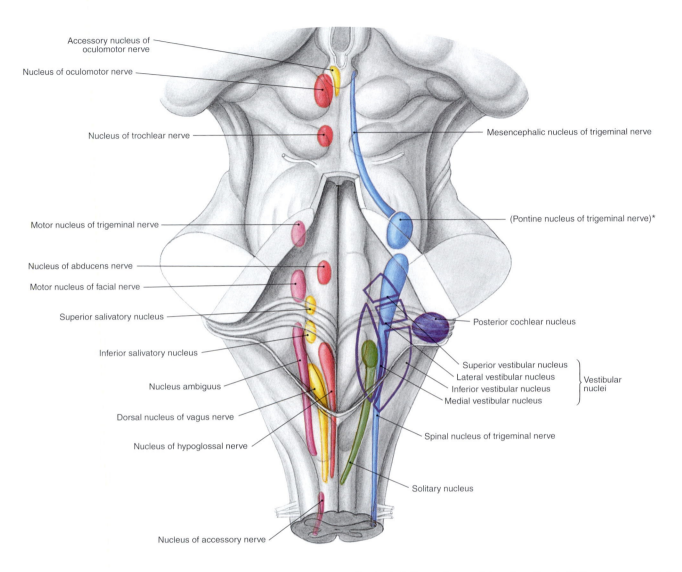

Fig. 1236 Cranial nerves; topographic overview of the nuclei; posterior view.

On the left the motor nuclei and on the right the sensory nuclei are shown.

* Clinical term: principal sensory nucleus of the trigeminal nerve

🟥 General somatic-efferent nuclei (GSE)	🟩 General and specific visceral-afferent nuclei (G/SVA)
🟨 General visceral-efferent nuclei (GVE)	🟦 General somatic-afferent nuclei (GSA)
🟪 Specific visceral-efferent nuclei (SVE)	🟪 Specific somatic-afferent nuclei (SSA)

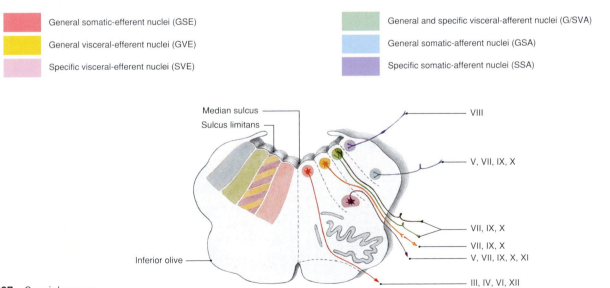

Fig. 1237 Cranial nerves; schematic cross-section through the rhomboid fossa demonstrating the nuclei.

Nuclei of the cranial nerves

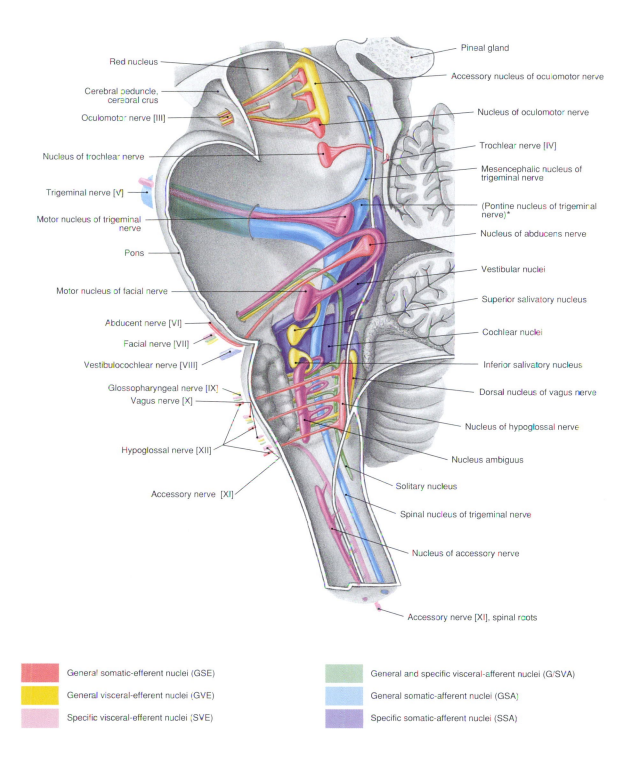

Red nucleus

Cerebral peduncle, cerebral crus

Oculomotor nerve [III]

Nucleus of trochlear nerve

Trigeminal nerve [V]

Motor nucleus of trigeminal nerve

Pons

Motor nucleus of facial nerve

Abducent nerve [VI]

Facial nerve [VII]

Vestibulocochlear nerve [VIII]

Glossopharyngeal nerve [IX]

Vagus nerve [X]

Hypoglossal nerve [XII]

Accessory nerve [XI]

Pineal gland

Accessory nucleus of oculomotor nerve

Nucleus of oculomotor nerve

Trochlear nerve [IV]

Mesencephalic nucleus of trigeminal nerve

(Pontine nucleus of trigeminal nerve)*

Nucleus of abducens nerve

Vestibular nuclei

Superior salivatory nucleus

Cochlear nuclei

Inferior salivatory nucleus

Dorsal nucleus of vagus nerve

Nucleus of hypoglossal nerve

Nucleus ambiguus

Solitary nucleus

Spinal nucleus of trigeminal nerve

Nucleus of accessory nerve

Accessory nerve [XI], spinal roots

- General somatic-efferent nuclei (GSE)
- General visceral-efferent nuclei (GVE)
- Specific visceral-efferent nuclei (SVE)
- General and specific visceral-afferent nuclei (G/SVA)
- General somatic-afferent nuclei (GSA)
- Specific somatic-afferent nuclei (SSA)

Fig. 1238 Cranial nerves;
topographic overview of the nuclei in the median plane.

* Clinical term: principal sensory nucleus of the trigeminal nerve

Cerebellum

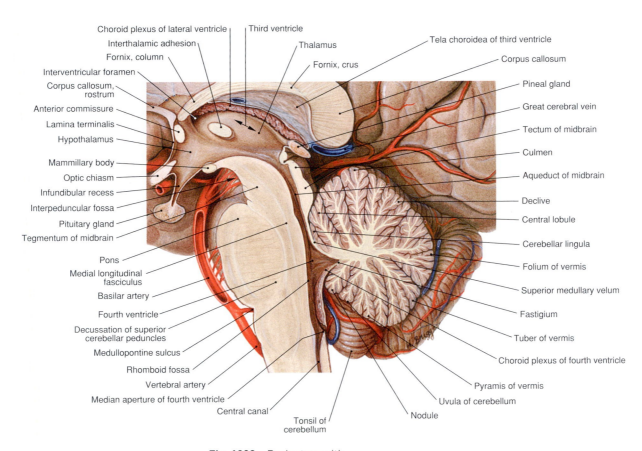

Fig. 1239　Brainstem with the cerebellum and the fourth ventricle; median section.

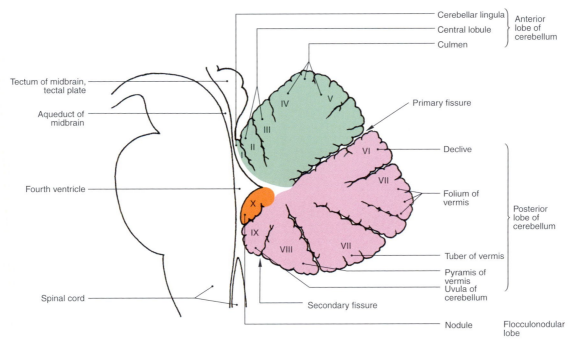

Fig. 1240　Parts of the cerebellar vermis; median section; overview.

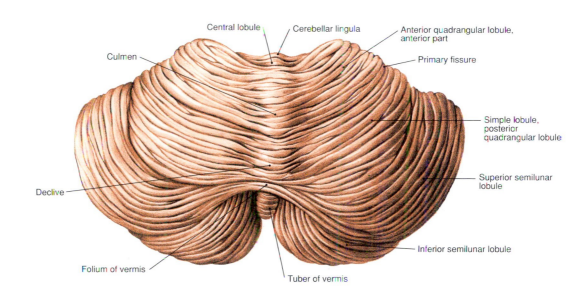

Central lobule
Cerebellar lingula
Anterior quadrangular lobule, anterior part
Culmen
Primary fissure
Simple lobule, posterior quadrangular lobule
Superior semilunar lobule
Declive
Inferior semilunar lobule
Folium of vermis
Tuber of vermis

Fig. 1241 Cerebellum; posterior-superior view.

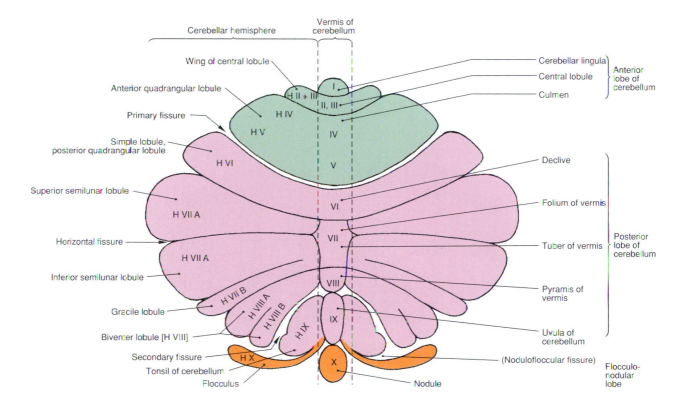

Cerebellar hemisphere
Vermis of cerebellum
Wing of central lobule
Cerebellar lingula
Central lobule
Anterior lobe of cerebellum
Anterior quadrangular lobule
H II + III
I
Culmen
Primary fissure
II, III
H IV
Simple lobule, posterior quadrangular lobule
H V
IV
H VI
V
Superior semilunar lobule
Declive
Folium of vermis
H VII A
VI
Horizontal fissure
VII
Tuber of vermis
Posterior lobe of cerebellum
H VII A
Inferior semilunar lobule
VIII
Pyramis of vermis
Gracile lobule
H VII B
H VIII A
H VIII B
IX
Biventer lobule [H VIII]
H IX
Uvula of cerebellum
Secondary fissure
H X
X
(Nodulofloccular fissure)
Flocculo-nodular lobe
Tonsil of cerebellum
Flocculus
Nodule

Fig. 1242 Cerebellum; diagram of the cerebellar cortex outstretched; overview.

Cerebellum

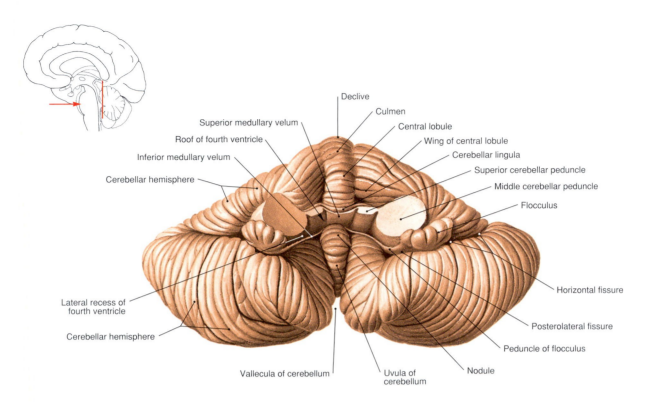

Declive
Culmen
Central lobule
Wing of central lobule
Cerebellar lingula
Superior cerebellar peduncle
Middle cerebellar peduncle
Flocculus
Superior medullary velum
Roof of fourth ventricle
Inferior medullary velum
Cerebellar hemisphere
Horizontal fissure
Posterolateral fissure
Peduncle of flocculus
Nodule
Lateral recess of fourth ventricle
Cerebellar hemisphere
Vallecula of cerebellum
Uvula of cerebellum

Fig. 1243 Cerebellum;
after section of the cerebellar peduncles;
anterior view.

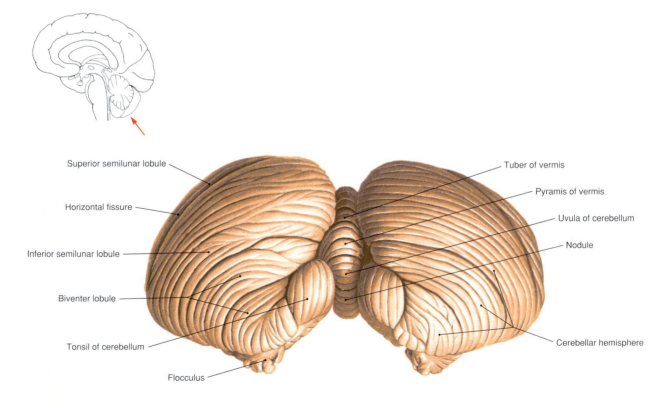

Superior semilunar lobule
Horizontal fissure
Inferior semilunar lobule
Biventer lobule
Tonsil of cerebellum
Flocculus
Tuber of vermis
Pyramis of vermis
Uvula of cerebellum
Nodule
Cerebellar hemisphere

Fig. 1244 Cerebellum;
posterior-inferior view.

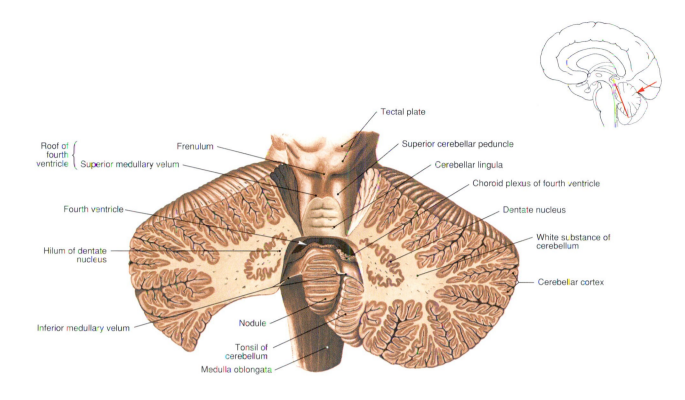

Tectal plate

Roof of fourth ventricle { Frenulum

Superior medullary velum

Superior cerebellar peduncle

Cerebellar lingula

Choroid plexus of fourth ventricle

Fourth ventricle

Dentate nucleus

White substance of cerebellum

Hilum of dentate nucleus

Cerebellar cortex

Inferior medullary velum

Nodule

Tonsil of cerebellum

Medulla oblongata

Fig. 1245 Cerebellum; oblique section; posterior view.

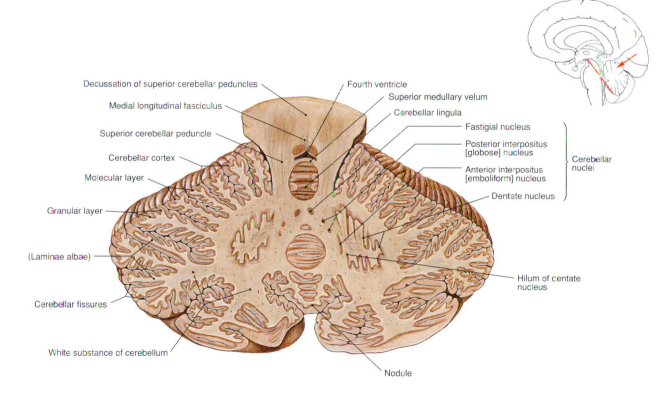

Decussation of superior cerebellar peduncles

Fourth ventricle

Medial longitudinal fasciculus

Superior medullary velum

Cerebellar lingula

Superior cerebellar peduncle

Fastigial nucleus

Cerebellar cortex

Posterior interpositus [globose] nucleus

Molecular layer

Anterior interpositus [emboliform] nucleus

} Cerebellar nuclei

Granular layer

Dentate nucleus

(Laminae albae)

Hilum of dentate nucleus

Cerebellar fissures

White substance of cerebellum

Nodule

Fig. 1246 Cerebellum; oblique section through the upper cerebellar peduncles; posterior view.

Association and commissural tracts

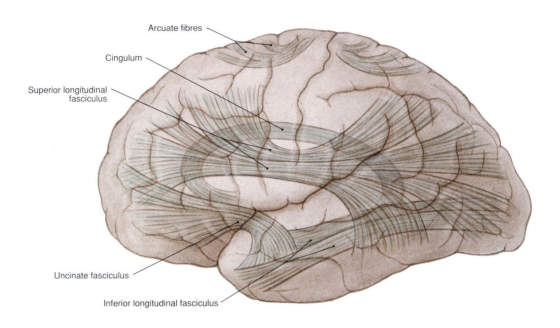

Fig. 1247 Association tracts;
projection onto the cerebral hemisphere;
overview;
viewed from the left.

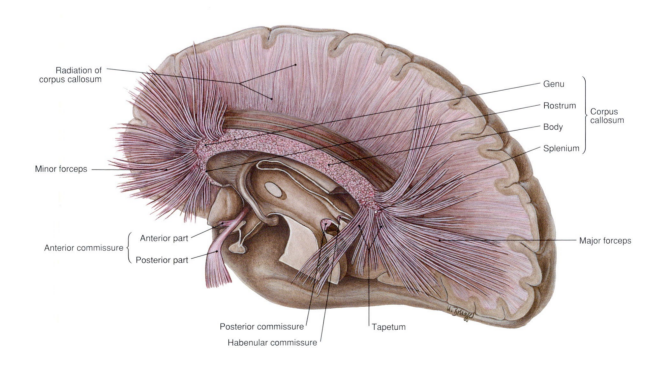

Fig. 1248 Commissural tracts;
topographic overview after extensive removal of the corpus
callosum in the paramedian plane;
single fibres of the corpus callosum are shown;
viewed from the left.

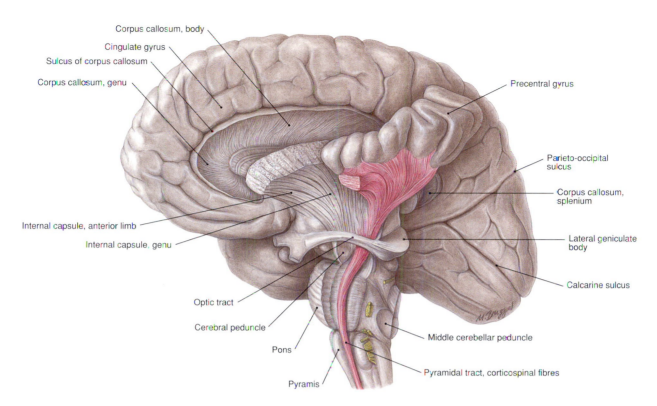

Corpus callosum, body
Cingulate gyrus
Sulcus of corpus callosum
Corpus callosum, genu

Precentral gyrus

Parieto-occipital sulcus

Corpus callosum, splenium

Internal capsule, anterior limb
Internal capsule, genu

Lateral geniculate body

Calcarine sulcus

Optic tract
Cerebral peduncle
Pons
Pyramis

Middle cerebellar peduncle

Pyramidal tract, corticospinal fibres

Fig. 1249 Projection tracts;
the internal capsule and the pyramidal tract have been exposed;
viewed from the left.

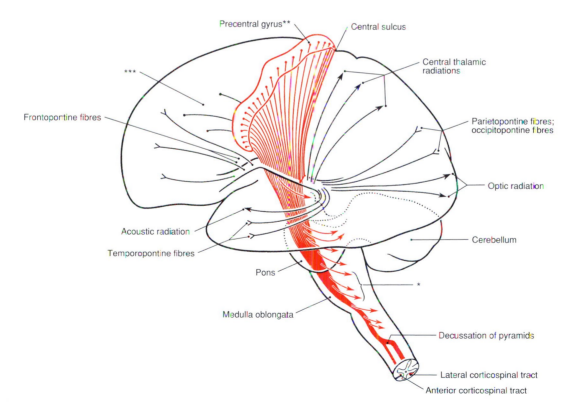

Precentral gyrus**
Central sulcus

***

Central thalamic radiations

Frontopontine fibres

Parietopontine fibres;
occipitopontine fibres

Optic radiation

Acoustic radiation

Cerebellum

Temporopontine fibres
Pons

Medulla oblongata

*

Decussation of pyramids

Lateral corticospinal tract
Anterior corticospinal tract

Fig. 1250 Internal capsule and pyramidal tract;
functional overview;
viewed from the left.

* Fibres to the tectal plate and the nuclei of the hindbrain
** Perikarya of the pyramidal tract
*** Perikarya of areas 6 and 8 (premotor cortex)

Internal capsule

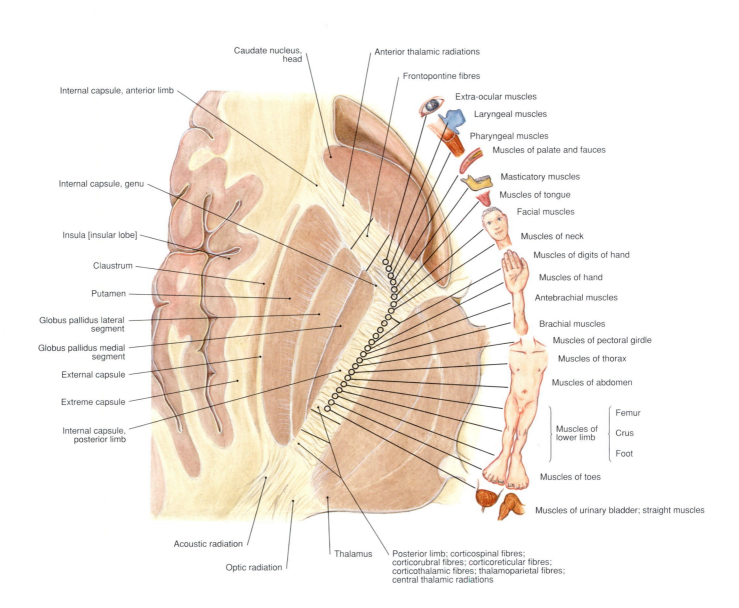

Fig. 1251 Internal capsule; functional organisation.

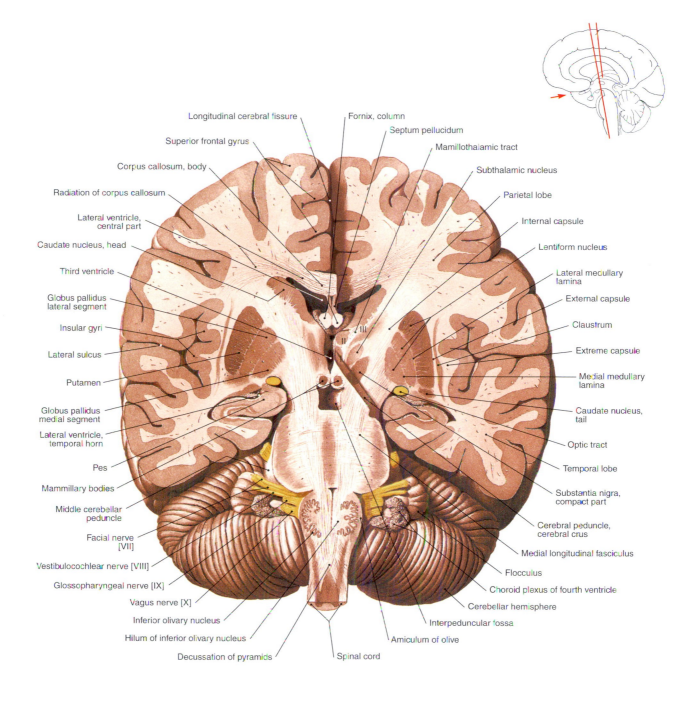

Longitudinal cerebral fissure
Superior frontal gyrus
Corpus callosum, body
Radiation of corpus callosum
Lateral ventricle, central part
Caudate nucleus, head
Third ventricle
Globus pallidus lateral segment
Insular gyri
Lateral sulcus
Putamen
Globus pallidus medial segment
Lateral ventricle, temporal horn
Pes
Mammillary bodies
Middle cerebellar peduncle
Facial nerve [VII]
Vestibulocochlear nerve [VIII]
Glossopharyngeal nerve [IX]
Vagus nerve [X]
Inferior olivary nucleus
Hilum of inferior olivary nucleus
Decussation of pyramids

Fornix, column
Septum pellucidum
Mamillothalamic tract
Subthalamic nucleus
Parietal lobe
Internal capsule
Lentiform nucleus
Lateral medullary lamina
External capsule
Claustrum
Extreme capsule
Medial medullary lamina
Caudate nucleus, tail
Optic tract
Temporal lobe
Substantia nigra, compact part
Cerebral peduncle, cerebral crus
Medial longitudinal fasciculus
Flocculus
Choroid plexus of fourth ventricle
Cerebellar hemisphere
Interpeduncular fossa
Amiculum of olive
Spinal cord

I–III = Thalamic nuclei:
I   = Median nuclei
II   = Anterior nuclei
III = Ventral principal nuclei

Fig. 1252 Pyramidal tract and basal ganglia;
obliquely staggered section through the posterior limb of the
internal capsule, the cerebral peduncles, and the medulla
oblongata.

Ventricles, projection

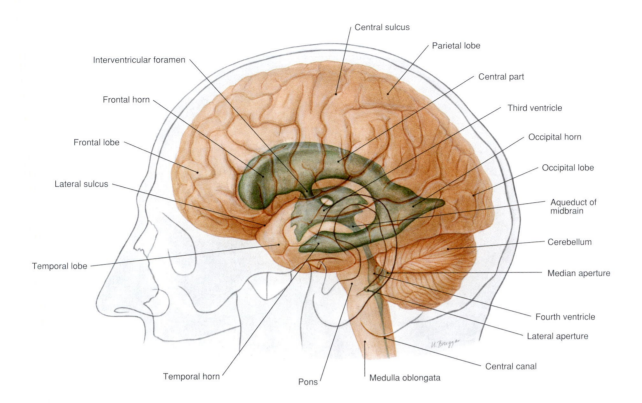

Fig. 1253 Ventricles of the brain.

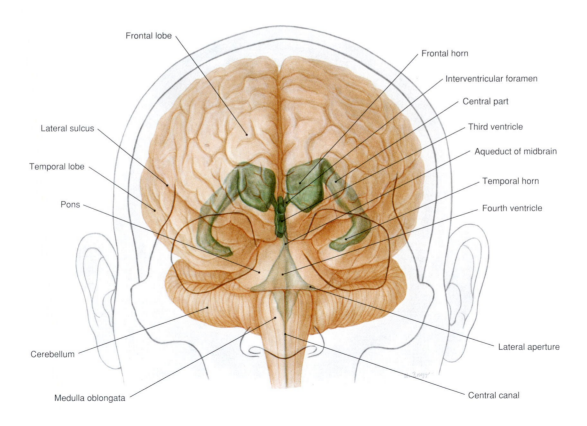

Fig. 1254 Ventricles of the brain;
anterior view.

Inner and outer liquor spaces

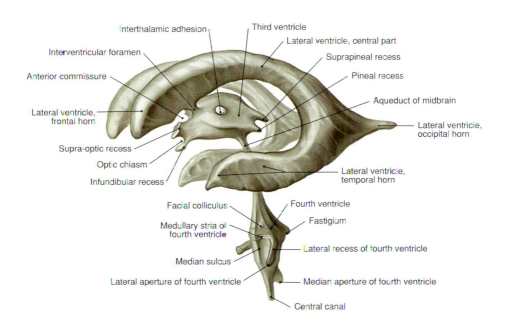

Interthalamic adhesion
Third ventricle
Interventricular foramen
Lateral ventricle, central part
Anterior commissure
Suprapineal recess
Pineal recess
Lateral ventricle, frontal horn
Aqueduct of midbrain
Lateral ventricle, occipital horn
Supra-optic recess
Optic chiasm
Infundibular recess
Lateral ventricle, temporal horn
Facial colliculus
Fourth ventricle
Medullary stria of fourth ventricle
Fastigium
Lateral recess of fourth ventricle
Median sulcus
Lateral aperture of fourth ventricle
Median aperture of fourth ventricle
Central canal

Fig. 1255 Inner liquor spaces; corrosion cast specimen; oblique view from the left.

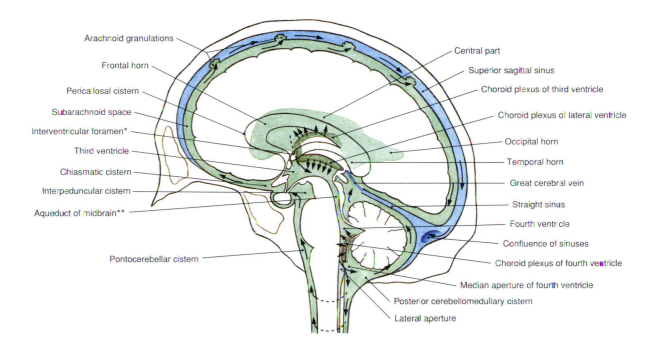

Arachnoid granulations
Central part
Frontal horn
Superior sagittal sinus
Pericallosal cistern
Choroid plexus of third ventricle
Subarachnoid space
Choroid plexus of lateral ventricle
Interventricular foramen*
Occipital horn
Third ventricle
Temporal horn
Chiasmatic cistern
Great cerebral vein
Interpeduncular cistern
Straight sinus
Aqueduct of midbrain**
Fourth ventricle
Confluence of sinuses
Pontocerebellar cistern
Choroid plexus of fourth ventricle
Median aperture of fourth ventricle
Posterior cerebellomedullary cistern
Lateral aperture

Fig. 1256 Ventricles of the brain and subarachnoid space; schema of the circulation (arrows) of the cerebrospinal fluid from the inner to the outer liquor spaces.

* Clinical term: foramen of MONRO
** Clinical term: cerebral aqueduct of SYLVIUS

Brain, topography

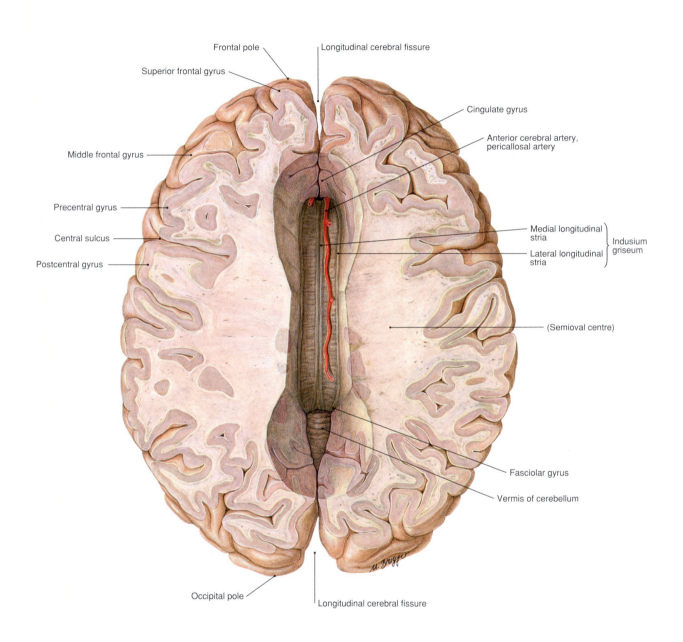

Frontal pole

Superior frontal gyrus

Longitudinal cerebral fissure

Cingulate gyrus

Anterior cerebral artery, pericallosal artery

Middle frontal gyrus

Precentral gyrus

Central sulcus

Postcentral gyrus

Medial longitudinal stria

Lateral longitudinal stria

Indusium griseum

(Semioval centre)

Fasciolar gyrus

Vermis of cerebellum

Occipital pole

Longitudinal cerebral fissure

1258

Fig. 1257 Corpus callosum;
after removal of the upper parts of the
cerebral hemispheres;
superior view.

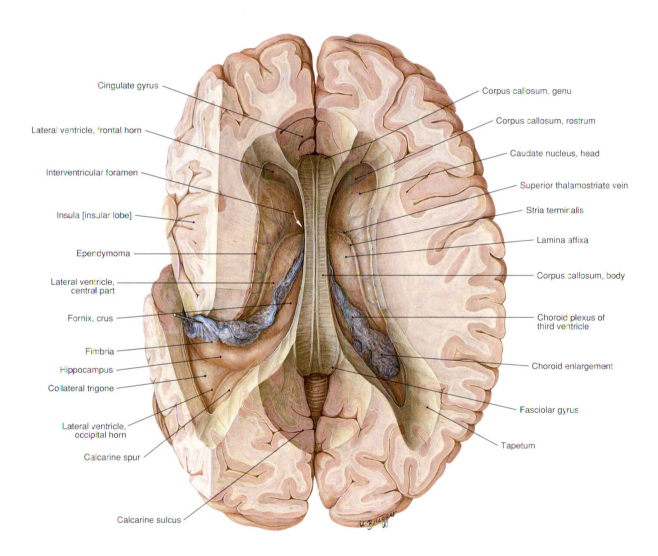

Cingulate gyrus

Lateral ventricle, frontal horn

Interventricular foramen

Insula [insular lobe]

Ependymoma

Lateral ventricle, central part

Fornix, crus

Fimbria

Hippocampus

Collateral trigone

Lateral ventricle, occipital horn

Calcarine spur

Calcarine sulcus

Corpus callosum, genu

Corpus callosum, rostrum

Caudate nucleus, head

Superior thalamostriate vein

Stria terminalis

Lamina affixa

Corpus callosum, body

Choroid plexus of third ventricle

Choroid enlargement

Fasciolar gyrus

Tapetum

Fig. 1258   Lateral ventricles;
after removal of the upper parts of the cerebral
hemispheres;
superior view.

1254

1257

Brain, topography

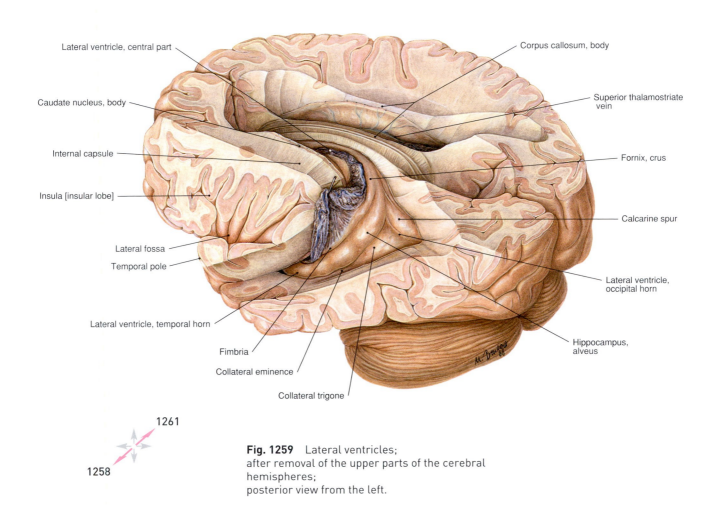

Lateral ventricle, central part

Caudate nucleus, body

Internal capsule

Insula [insular lobe]

Lateral fossa

Temporal pole

Lateral ventricle, temporal horn

Fimbria

Collateral eminence

Collateral trigone

Corpus callosum, body

Superior thalamostriate vein

Fornix, crus

Calcarine spur

Lateral ventricle, occipital horn

Hippocampus, alveus

1261

1258

Fig. 1259   Lateral ventricles;
after removal of the upper parts of the cerebral
hemispheres;
posterior view from the left.

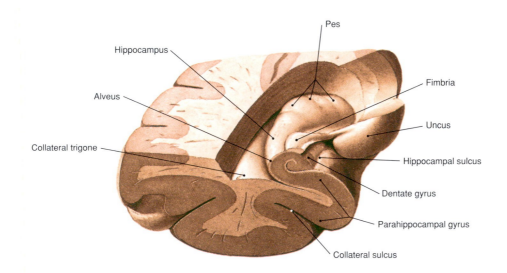

Pes

Hippocampus

Alveus

Collateral trigone

Fimbria

Uncus

Hippocampal sulcus

Dentate gyrus

Parahippocampal gyrus

Collateral sulcus

Fig. 1260   Left temporal horn of the lateral ventricle;
frontal section after removal of the temporal wall;
posterior-superior view.

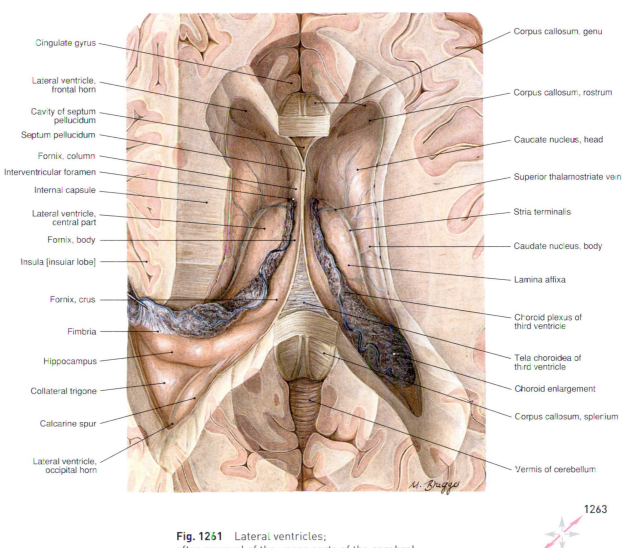

Cingulate gyrus

Lateral ventricle, frontal horn

Cavity of septum pellucidum

Septum pellucidum

Fornix, column

Interventricular foramen

Internal capsule

Lateral ventricle, central part

Fornix, body

Insula [insular lobe]

Fornix, crus

Fimbria

Hippocampus

Collateral trigone

Calcarine spur

Lateral ventricle, occipital horn

Corpus callosum, genu

Corpus callosum, rostrum

Caudate nucleus, head

Superior thalamostriate vein

Stria terminalis

Caudate nucleus, body

Lamina affixa

Choroid plexus of third ventricle

Tela choroidea of third ventricle

Choroid enlargement

Corpus callosum, splenium

Vermis of cerebellum

1263

1259

Fig. 1261 Lateral ventricles;
after removal of the upper parts of the cerebral
hemispheres and the central part of the corpus callosum;
superior view.

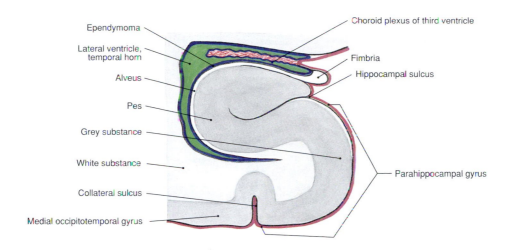

Ependymoma

Lateral ventricle, temporal horn

Alveus

Pes

Grey substance

White substance

Collateral sulcus

Medial occipitotemporal gyrus

Choroid plexus of third ventricle

Fimbria

Hippocampal sulcus

Parahippocampal gyrus

Fig. 1262 Temporal horn of the lateral ventricle;
schematic frontal section.

Brain, topography

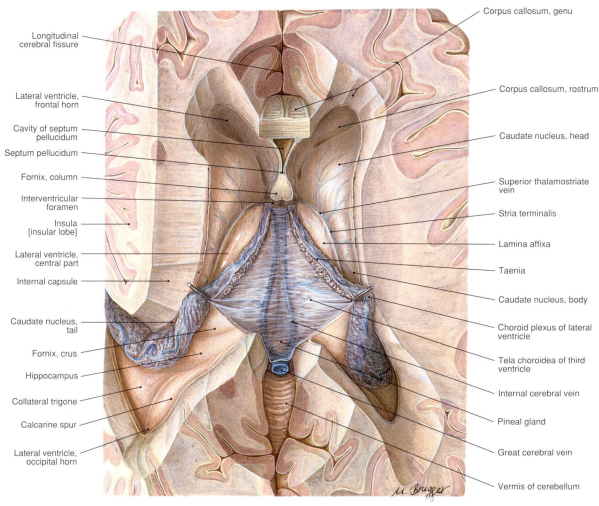

Longitudinal cerebral fissure

Lateral ventricle, frontal horn

Cavity of septum pellucidum

Septum pellucidum

Fornix, column

Interventricular foramen

Insula [insular lobe]

Lateral ventricle, central part

Internal capsule

Caudate nucleus, tail

Fornix, crus

Hippocampus

Collateral trigone

Calcarine spur

Lateral ventricle, occipital horn

Corpus callosum, genu

Corpus callosum, rostrum

Caudate nucleus, head

Superior thalamostriate vein

Stria terminalis

Lamina affixa

Taenia

Caudate nucleus, body

Choroid plexus of lateral ventricle

Tela choroidea of third ventricle

Internal cerebral vein

Pineal gland

Great cerebral vein

Vermis of cerebellum

1265
1261

Fig. 1263 Lateral ventricles; after removal of the central part of the corpus callosum and the columns of the fornix; superior view.

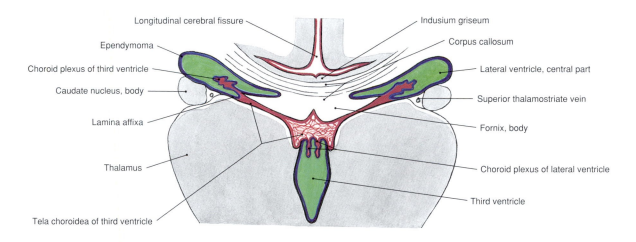

Longitudinal cerebral fissure

Ependymoma

Choroid plexus of third ventricle

Caudate nucleus, body

Lamina affixa

Thalamus

Tela choroidea of third ventricle

Indusium griseum

Corpus callosum

Lateral ventricle, central part

Superior thalamostriate vein

Fornix, body

Choroid plexus of lateral ventricle

Third ventricle

Fig. 1264 Central parts of the lateral ventricles and third ventricle; schematic frontal section.

Brain, topography

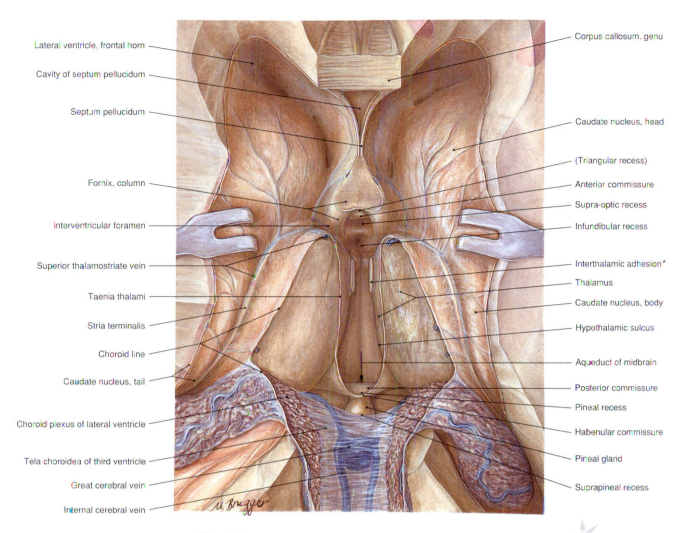

Lateral ventricle, frontal horn

Cavity of septum pellucidum

Septum pellucidum

Fornix, column

Interventricular foramen

Superior thalamostriate vein

Taenia thalami

Stria terminalis

Choroid line

Caudate nucleus, tail

Choroid plexus of lateral ventricle

Tela choroidea of third ventricle

Great cerebral vein

Internal cerebral vein

Corpus callosum, genu

Caudate nucleus, head

(Triangular recess)

Anterior commissure

Supra-optic recess

Infundibular recess

Interthalamic adhesion*

Thalamus

Caudate nucleus, body

Hypothalamic sulcus

Aqueduct of midbrain

Posterior commissure

Pineal recess

Habenular commissure

Pineal gland

Suprapineal recess

1263

Fig. 1265 Lateral ventricles and third ventricle;
parts of the cerebral hemispheres, the central part of the
corpus callosum as well as the fornix and the choroid plexus
have been removed, the tela choroidea of the third ventricle
has been reflected;
superior view.

* The interthalamic adhesion has been sectioned in the median plane.

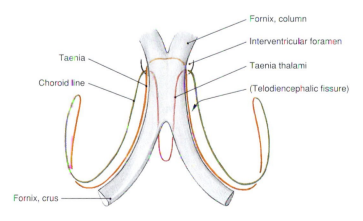

Taenia

Choroid line

Fornix, crus

Fornix, column

Interventricular foramen

Taenia thalami

(Telodiencephalic fissure)

Fig. 1266 Taeniae of the choroid plexus of the cerebrum;
superior view.

Arteries of the base of the brain

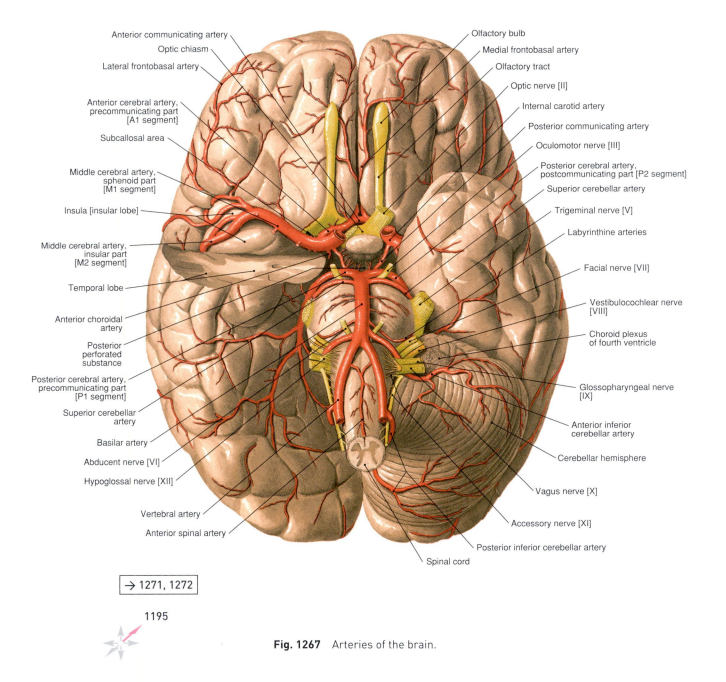

Anterior communicating artery
Optic chiasm
Lateral frontobasal artery
Anterior cerebral artery, precommunicating part [A1 segment]
Subcallosal area
Middle cerebral artery, sphenoid part [M1 segment]
Insula [insular lobe]
Middle cerebral artery, insular part [M2 segment]
Temporal lobe
Anterior choroidal artery
Posterior perforated substance
Posterior cerebral artery, precommunicating part [P1 segment]
Superior cerebellar artery
Basilar artery
Abducent nerve [VI]
Hypoglossal nerve [XII]
Vertebral artery
Anterior spinal artery

Olfactory bulb
Medial frontobasal artery
Olfactory tract
Optic nerve [II]
Internal carotid artery
Posterior communicating artery
Oculomotor nerve [III]
Posterior cerebral artery, postcommunicating part [P2 segment]
Superior cerebellar artery
Trigeminal nerve [V]
Labyrinthine arteries
Facial nerve [VII]
Vestibulocochlear nerve [VIII]
Choroid plexus of fourth ventricle
Glossopharyngeal nerve [IX]
Anterior inferior cerebellar artery
Cerebellar hemisphere
Vagus nerve [X]
Accessory nerve [XI]
Posterior inferior cerebellar artery
Spinal cord

→ 1271, 1272

1195

Fig. 1267 Arteries of the brain.

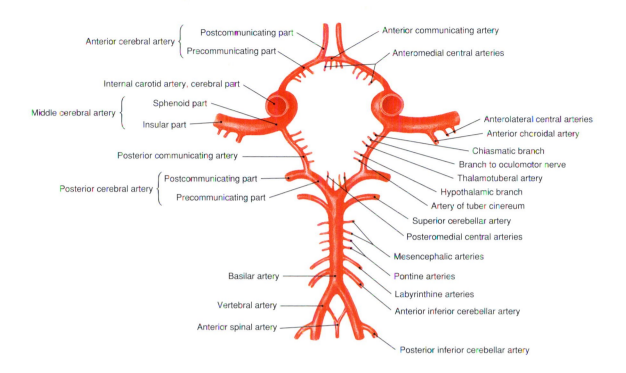

Anterior cerebral artery {
Postcommunicating part
Precommunicating part

Anterior communicating artery
Anteromedial central arteries

Internal carotid artery, cerebral part

Middle cerebral artery {
Sphenoid part
Insular part

Anterolateral central arteries
Anterior choroidal artery
Chiasmatic branch
Branch to oculomotor nerve
Thalamotuberal artery
Hypothalamic branch
Artery of tuber cinereum
Superior cerebellar artery
Posteromedial central arteries
Mesencephalic arteries
Pontine arteries
Labyrinthine arteries
Anterior inferior cerebellar artery

Posterior communicating artery

Posterior cerebral artery {
Postcommunicating part
Precommunicating part

Basilar artery

Vertebral artery

Anterior spinal artery

Posterior inferior cerebellar artery

Fig. 1268 Arterial circle of the brain [WILLIS].

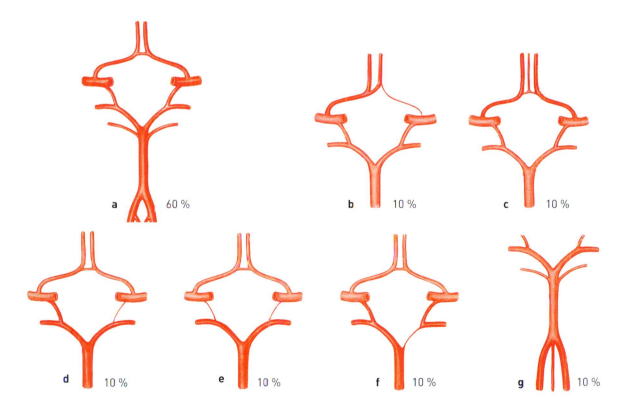

a   60 %   b   10 %   c   10 %

d   10 %   e   10 %   f   10 %   g   10 %

Fig. 1269 a–g   Arterial circle of the brain.

a–c Variations of the anterior portion
d–f Variations of the posterior portion
g   Very far inferior union of the vertebral arteries

Arteries of the brain

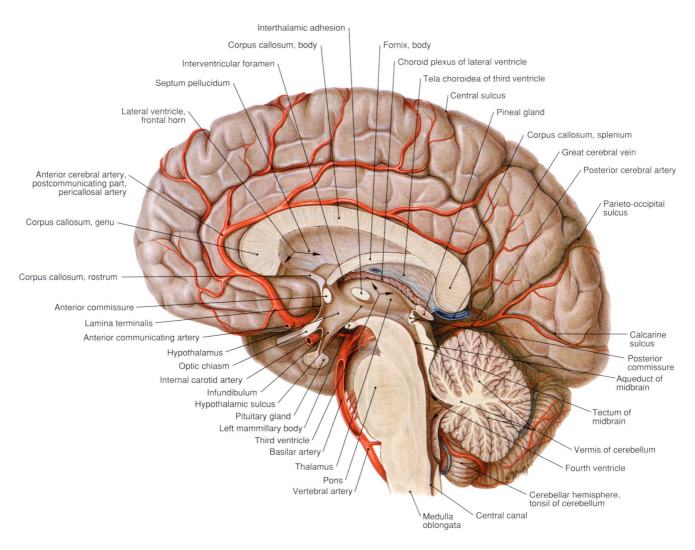

Interthalamic adhesion

Corpus callosum, body

Interventricular foramen

Septum pellucidum

Lateral ventricle, frontal horn

Anterior cerebral artery, postcommunicating part, pericallosal artery

Corpus callosum, genu

Corpus callosum, rostrum

Anterior commissure

Lamina terminalis

Anterior communicating artery

Hypothalamus

Optic chiasm

Internal carotid artery

Infundibulum

Hypothalamic sulcus

Pituitary gland

Left mammillary body

Third ventricle

Basilar artery

Thalamus

Pons

Vertebral artery

Medulla oblongata

Central canal

Fornix, body

Choroid plexus of lateral ventricle

Tela choroidea of third ventricle

Central sulcus

Pineal gland

Corpus callosum, splenium

Great cerebral vein

Posterior cerebral artery

Parieto-occipital sulcus

Calcarine sulcus

Posterior commissure

Aqueduct of midbrain

Tectum of midbrain

Vermis of cerebellum

Fourth ventricle

Cerebellar hemisphere, tonsil of cerebellum

Fig. 1270 Medial surface of the brain; diencephalon and brainstem; staggered median section; viewed from the left.

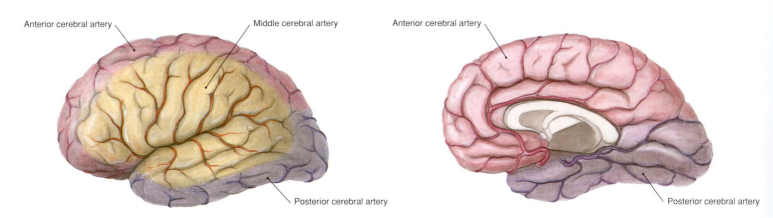

Anterior cerebral artery

Middle cerebral artery

Posterior cerebral artery

Anterior cerebral artery

Posterior cerebral artery

Fig. 1271 Arterial supply of the brain; viewed from the left.

Fig. 1272 Arterial supply of the brain; medial view.

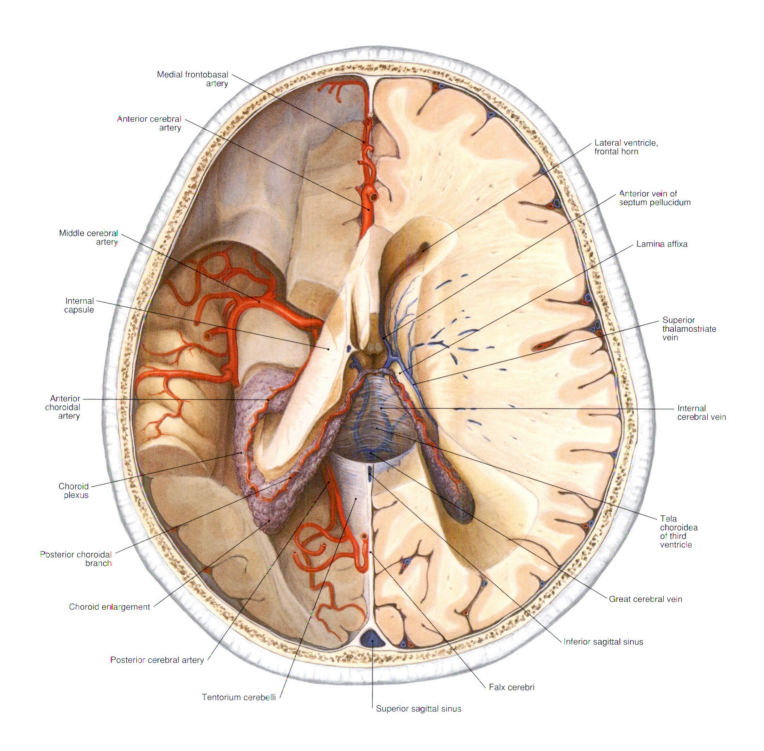

Medial frontobasal
artery

Anterior cerebral
artery

Middle cerebral
artery

Internal
capsule

Anterior
choroidal
artery

Choroid
plexus

Posterior choroidal
branch

Choroid enlargement

Posterior cerebral artery

Tentorium cerebelli

Superior sagittal sinus

Lateral ventricle,
frontal horn

Anterior vein of
septum pellucidum

Lamina affixa

Superior
thalamostriate
vein

Internal
cerebral vein

Tela
choroidea
of third
ventricle

Great cerebral vein

Inferior sagittal sinus

Falx cerebri

Fig. 1273   Arteries and veins of the brain.

Veins of the brain

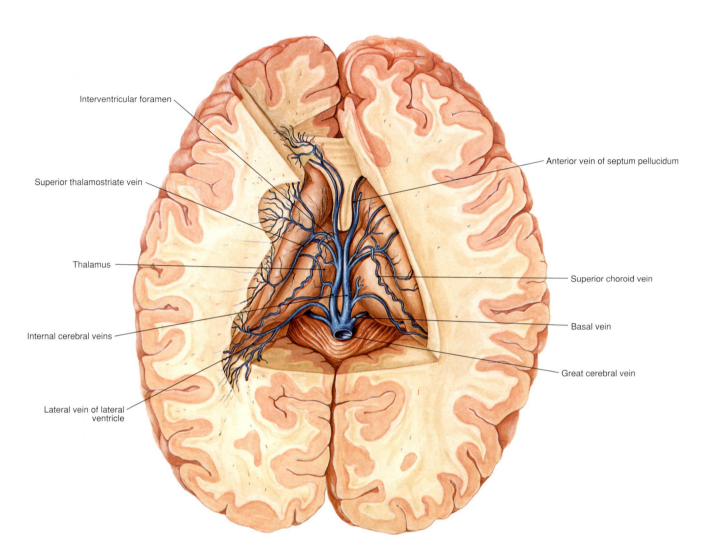

Interventricular foramen

Superior thalamostriate vein

Thalamus

Internal cerebral veins

Lateral vein of lateral ventricle

Anterior vein of septum pellucidum

Superior choroid vein

Basal vein

Great cerebral vein

Fig. 1274 Deep veins of the brain.
The internal cerebral veins run within the tela choroidea of the third ventricle.

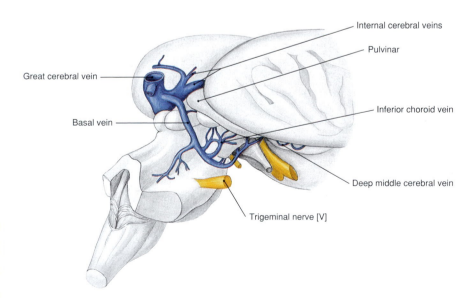

Internal cerebral veins

Pulvinar

Great cerebral vein

Inferior choroid vein

Basal vein

Deep middle cerebral vein

Trigeminal nerve [V]

Fig. 1275 Deep veins of the brain; posterior view from the right.

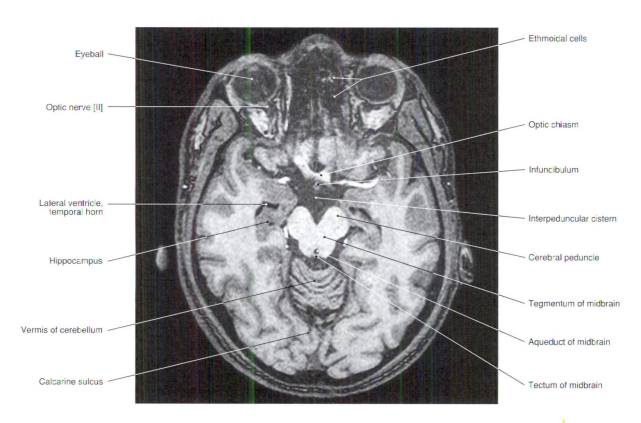

Eyeball

Optic nerve [II]

Lateral ventricle, temporal horn

Hippocampus

Vermis of cerebellum

Calcarine sulcus

Ethmoidal cells

Optic chiasm

Infuncibulum

Interpeduncular cistern

Cerebral peduncle

Tegmentum of midbrain

Aqueduct of midbrain

Tectum of midbrain

Fig. 1276 Brain;
magnetic resonance tomographic image (MRI);
horizontal section at the level of the midbrain and the
temporal horns of the lateral ventricles;
superior view.

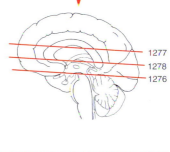

1277
1278
1276

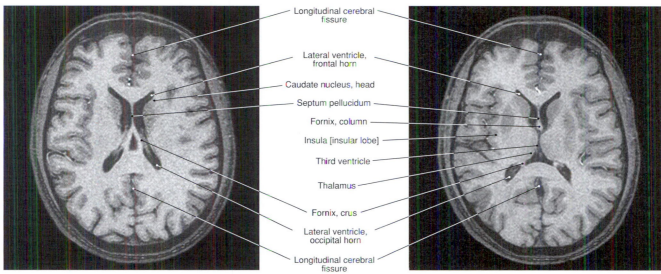

Longitudinal cerebral fissure

Lateral ventricle, frontal horn

Caudate nucleus, head

Septum pellucidum

Fornix, column

Insula [insular lobe]

Third ventricle

Thalamus

Fornix, crus

Lateral ventricle, occipital horn

Longitudinal cerebral fissure

Fig. 1277 Brain;
magnetic resonance tomographic image (MRI);
horizontal section at the level of the central parts
of the lateral ventricles;
superior view.

Fig. 1278 Brain;
magnetic resonance tomographic image (MRI);
horizontal section at the level of the third ventricle
and the opening of the temporal horns of the
lateral ventricles;
superior view.

Brain, sections

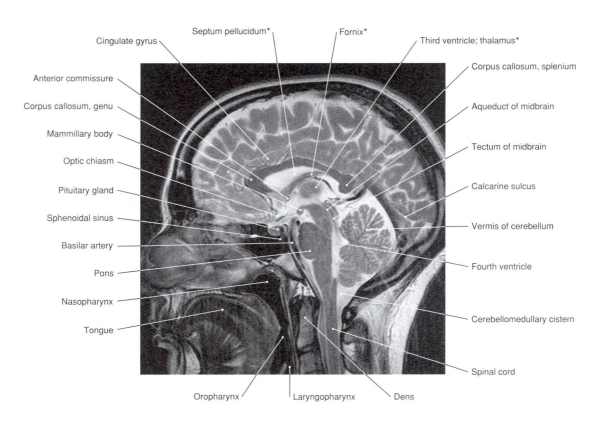

Cingulate gyrus
Septum pellucidum*
Fornix*
Third ventricle; thalamus*
Anterior commissure
Corpus callosum, splenium
Corpus callosum, genu
Aqueduct of midbrain
Mammillary body
Tectum of midbrain
Optic chiasm
Calcarine sulcus
Pituitary gland
Vermis of cerebellum
Sphenoidal sinus
Basilar artery
Fourth ventricle
Pons
Nasopharynx
Tongue
Cerebellomedullary cistern
Spinal cord
Oropharynx
Laryngopharynx
Dens

Fig. 1279 Brain;
magnetic resonance tomographic image (MRI);
median section. The structures marked with * appear
partly falsified as a consequence of the "partial-volume-effect".

1280
1279

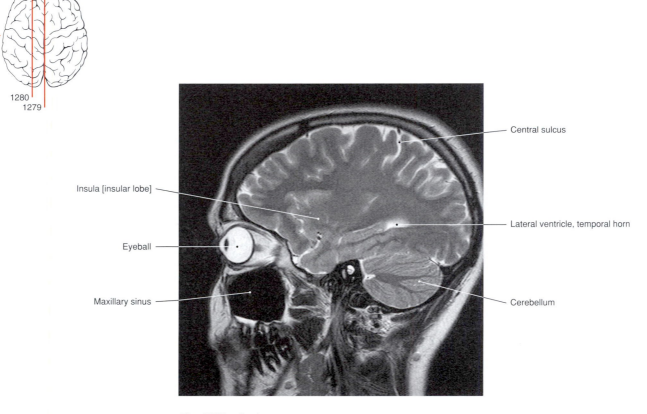

Central sulcus
Insula [insular lobe]
Lateral ventricle, temporal horn
Eyeball
Maxillary sinus
Cerebellum

Fig. 1280 Brain;
magnetic resonance tomographic image (MRI);
sagittal section.

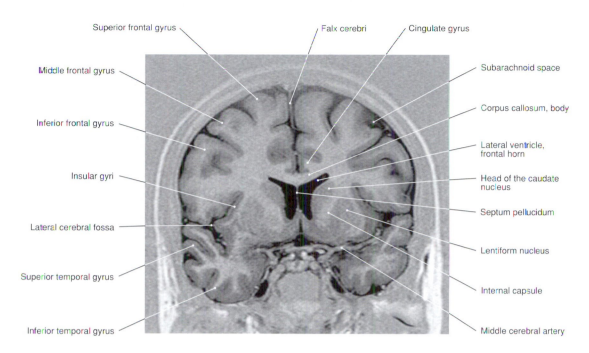

Superior frontal gyrus
Middle frontal gyrus
Inferior frontal gyrus
Insular gyri
Lateral cerebral fossa
Superior temporal gyrus
Inferior temporal gyrus

Falx cerebri
Cingulate gyrus

Subarachnoid space
Corpus callosum, body
Lateral ventricle, frontal horn
Head of the caudate nucleus
Septum pellucidum
Lentiform nucleus
Internal capsule
Middle cerebral artery

Fig. 1281   Brain;
magnetic resonance tomographic image (MRI);
frontal section.

1281   1282

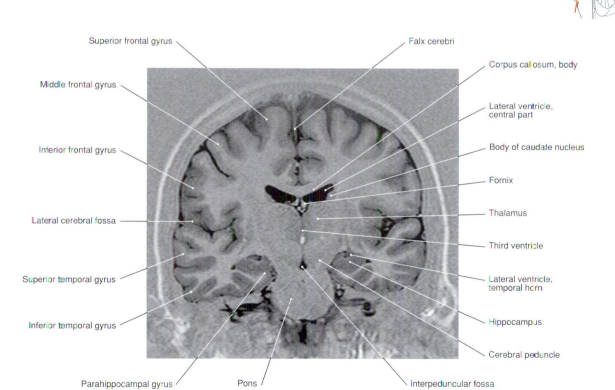

Superior frontal gyrus
Middle frontal gyrus
Interior frontal gyrus
Lateral cerebral fossa
Superior temporal gyrus
Inferior temporal gyrus

Falx cerebri

Corpus callosum, body
Lateral ventricle, central part
Body of caudate nucleus
Fornix
Thalamus
Third ventricle
Lateral ventricle, temporal horn
Hippocampus
Cerebral peduncle

Parahippocampal gyrus
Pons
Interpeduncular fossa

Fig. 1282   Brain;
magnetic resonance tomographic image (MRI);
frontal section.

Brain, frontal sections

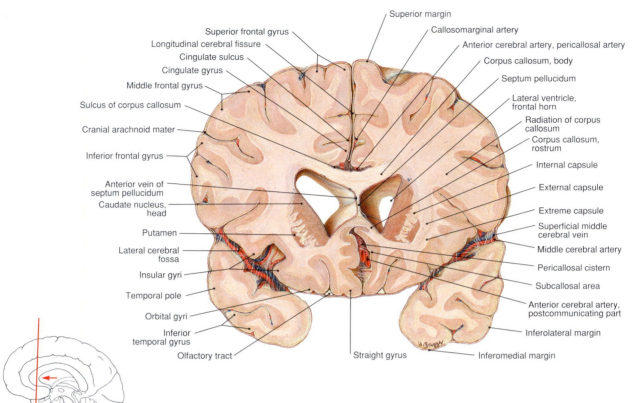

Superior frontal gyrus
Longitudinal cerebral fissure
Cingulate sulcus
Cingulate gyrus
Middle frontal gyrus
Sulcus of corpus callosum
Cranial arachnoid mater
Inferior frontal gyrus
Anterior vein of septum pellucidum
Caudate nucleus, head
Putamen
Lateral cerebral fossa
Insular gyri
Temporal pole
Orbital gyri
Inferior temporal gyrus
Olfactory tract

Superior margin
Callosomarginal artery
Anterior cerebral artery, pericallosal artery
Corpus callosum, body
Septum pellucidum
Lateral ventricle, frontal horn
Radiation of corpus callosum
Corpus callosum, rostrum
Internal capsule
External capsule
Extreme capsule
Superficial middle cerebral vein
Middle cerebral artery
Pericallosal cistern
Subcallosal area
Anterior cerebral artery, postcommunicating part
Inferolateral margin
Inferomedial margin
Straight gyrus

Fig. 1283 Brain;
frontal section at the level of the anterior parts
of the frontal horns of the lateral ventricles.

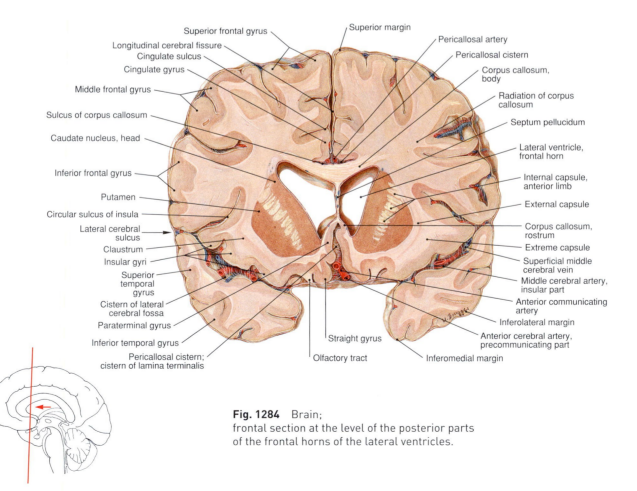

Superior frontal gyrus
Longitudinal cerebral fissure
Cingulate sulcus
Cingulate gyrus
Middle frontal gyrus
Sulcus of corpus callosum
Caudate nucleus, head
Inferior frontal gyrus
Putamen
Circular sulcus of insula
Lateral cerebral sulcus
Claustrum
Insular gyri
Superior temporal gyrus
Cistern of lateral cerebral fossa
Paraterminal gyrus
Inferior temporal gyrus
Pericallosal cistern; cistern of lamina terminalis

Superior margin
Pericallosal artery
Pericallosal cistern
Corpus callosum, body
Radiation of corpus callosum
Septum pellucidum
Lateral ventricle, frontal horn
Internal capsule, anterior limb
External capsule
Corpus callosum, rostrum
Extreme capsule
Superficial middle cerebral vein
Middle cerebral artery, insular part
Anterior communicating artery
Inferolateral margin
Anterior cerebral artery, precommunicating part
Inferomedial margin
Straight gyrus
Olfactory tract

Fig. 1284 Brain;
frontal section at the level of the posterior parts
of the frontal horns of the lateral ventricles.

Brain, frontal sections

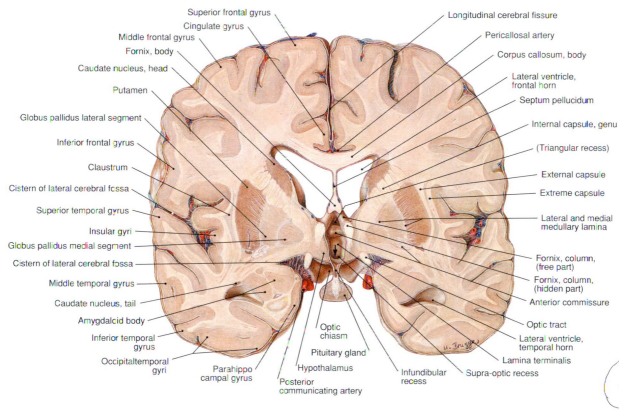

Superior frontal gyrus
Cingulate gyrus
Middle frontal gyrus
Fornix, body
Caudate nucleus, head
Putamen
Globus pallidus lateral segment
Inferior frontal gyrus
Claustrum
Cistern of lateral cerebral fossa
Superior temporal gyrus
Insular gyri
Globus pallidus medial segment
Cistern of lateral cerebral fossa
Middle temporal gyrus
Caudate nucleus, tail
Amygdalcid body
Inferior temporal gyrus
Occipitaltemporal gyri
Parahippocampal gyrus
Posterior communicating artery
Hypothalamus
Pituitary gland
Optic chiasm

Longitudinal cerebral fissure
Pericallosal artery
Corpus callosum, body
Lateral ventricle, frontal horn
Septum pellucidum
Internal capsule, genu
(Triangular recess)
External capsule
Extreme capsule
Lateral and medial medullary lamina
Fornix, column, (free part)
Fornix, column, (hidden part)
Anterior commissure
Optic tract
Lateral ventricle, temporal horn
Lamina terminalis
Supra-optic recess
Infundibular recess

Fig. 1285 Brain;
frontal section at the level of the interventricular foramina.

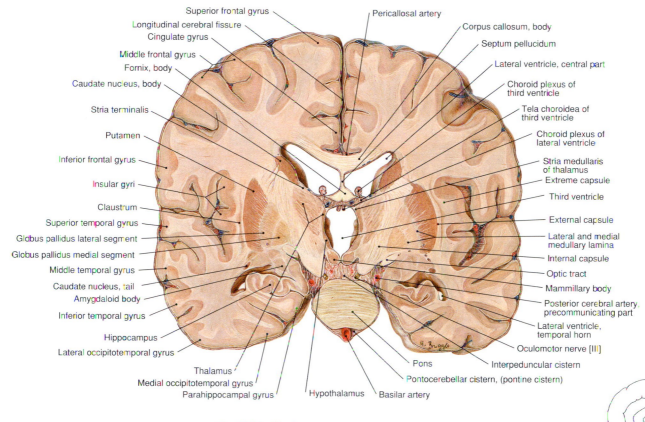

Superior frontal gyrus
Longitudinal cerebral fissure
Cingulate gyrus
Middle frontal gyrus
Fornix, body
Caudate nucleus, body
Stria terminalis
Putamen
Inferior frontal gyrus
Insular gyri
Claustrum
Superior temporal gyrus
Globus pallidus lateral segment
Globus pallidus medial segment
Middle temporal gyrus
Caudate nucleus, tail
Amygdaloid body
Inferior temporal gyrus
Hippocampus
Lateral occipitotemporal gyrus
Thalamus
Medial occipitotemporal gyrus
Parahippocampal gyrus
Hypothalamus
Basilar artery
Pontocerebellar cistern, (pontine cistern)
Pons
Interpeduncular cistern

Pericallosal artery
Corpus callosum, body
Septum pellucidum
Lateral ventricle, central part
Choroid plexus of third ventricle
Tela choroidea of third ventricle
Choroid plexus of lateral ventricle
Stria medullaris of thalamus
Extreme capsule
Third ventricle
External capsule
Lateral and medial medullary lamina
Internal capsule
Optic tract
Mammillary body
Posterior cerebral artery, precommunicating part
Lateral ventricle, temporal horn
Oculomotor nerve [III]

Fig. 1286 Brain;
frontal section at the level of the mamillary bodies.

Brain, frontal sections

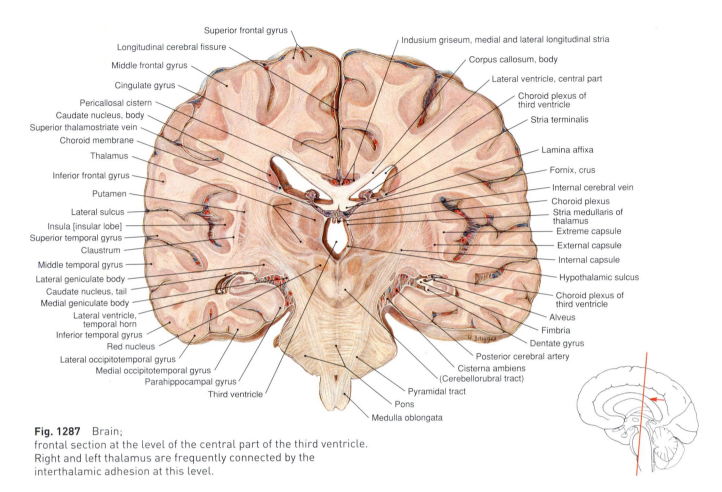

Superior frontal gyrus
Longitudinal cerebral fissure
Middle frontal gyrus
Cingulate gyrus
Pericallosal cistern
Caudate nucleus, body
Superior thalamostriate vein
Choroid membrane
Thalamus
Inferior frontal gyrus
Putamen
Lateral sulcus
Insula [insular lobe]
Superior temporal gyrus
Claustrum
Middle temporal gyrus
Lateral geniculate body
Caudate nucleus, tail
Medial geniculate body
Lateral ventricle, temporal horn
Inferior temporal gyrus
Red nucleus
Lateral occipitotemporal gyrus
Medial occipitotemporal gyrus
Parahippocampal gyrus
Third ventricle

Indusium griseum, medial and lateral longitudinal stria
Corpus callosum, body
Lateral ventricle, central part
Choroid plexus of third ventricle
Stria terminalis
Lamina affixa
Fornix, crus
Internal cerebral vein
Choroid plexus
Stria medullaris of thalamus
Extreme capsule
External capsule
Internal capsule
Hypothalamic sulcus
Choroid plexus of third ventricle
Alveus
Fimbria
Dentate gyrus
Posterior cerebral artery
Cisterna ambiens (Cerebellorubral tract)
Pyramidal tract
Pons
Medulla oblongata

Fig. 1287 Brain;
frontal section at the level of the central part of the third ventricle.
Right and left thalamus are frequently connected by the
interthalamic adhesion at this level.

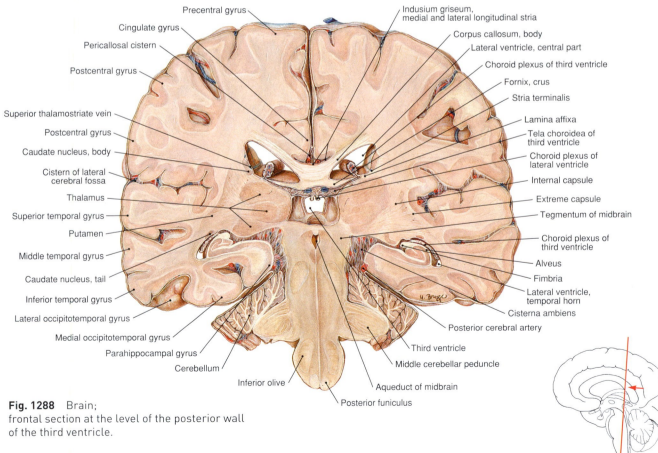

Precentral gyrus
Cingulate gyrus
Pericallosal cistern
Postcentral gyrus
Superior thalamostriate vein
Postcentral gyrus
Caudate nucleus, body
Cistern of lateral cerebral fossa
Thalamus
Superior temporal gyrus
Putamen
Middle temporal gyrus
Caudate nucleus, tail
Inferior temporal gyrus
Lateral occipitotemporal gyrus
Medial occipitotemporal gyrus
Parahippocampal gyrus
Cerebellum
Inferior olive

Indusium griseum, medial and lateral longitudinal stria
Corpus callosum, body
Lateral ventricle, central part
Choroid plexus of third ventricle
Fornix, crus
Stria terminalis
Lamina affixa
Tela choroidea of third ventricle
Choroid plexus of lateral ventricle
Internal capsule
Extreme capsule
Tegmentum of midbrain
Choroid plexus of third ventricle
Alveus
Fimbria
Lateral ventricle, temporal horn
Cisterna ambiens
Posterior cerebral artery
Third ventricle
Middle cerebellar peduncle
Aqueduct of midbrain
Posterior funiculus

Fig. 1288 Brain;
frontal section at the level of the posterior wall
of the third ventricle.

Brain, frontal sections

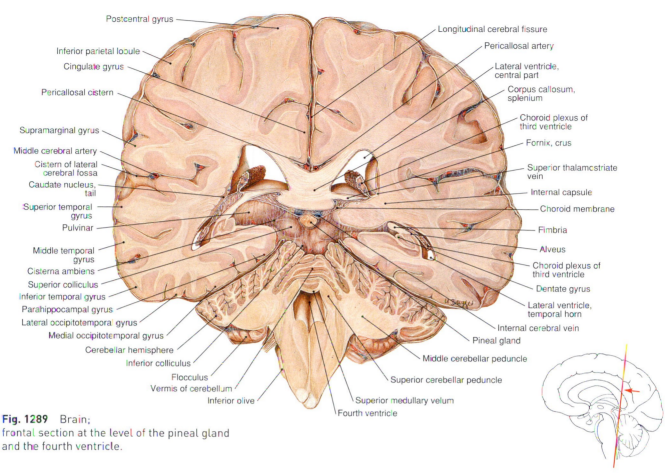

Postcentral gyrus

Inferior parietal lobule

Cingulate gyrus

Pericallosal cistern

Supramarginal gyrus

Middle cerebral artery

Cistern of lateral cerebral fossa

Caudate nucleus, tail

Superior temporal gyrus

Pulvinar

Middle temporal gyrus

Cisterna ambiens

Superior colliculus

Inferior temporal gyrus

Parahippocampal gyrus

Lateral occipitotemporal gyrus

Medial occipitotemporal gyrus

Cerebellar hemisphere

Inferior colliculus

Flocculus

Vermis of cerebellum

Inferior olive

Longitudinal cerebral fissure

Pericallosal artery

Lateral ventricle, central part

Corpus callosum, splenium

Choroid plexus of third ventricle

Fornix, crus

Superior thalamostriate vein

Internal capsule

Choroid membrane

Fimbria

Alveus

Choroid plexus of third ventricle

Dentate gyrus

Lateral ventricle, temporal horn

Internal cerebral vein

Pineal gland

Middle cerebellar peduncle

Superior cerebellar peduncle

Superior medullary velum

Fourth ventricle

Fig. 1289 Brain;
frontal section at the level of the pineal gland and the fourth ventricle.

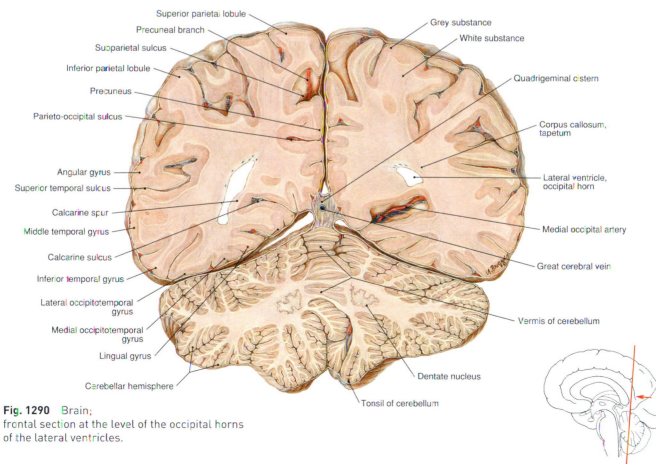

Superior parietal lobule

Precuneal branch

Subparietal sulcus

Inferior parietal lobule

Precuneus

Parieto-occipital sulcus

Angular gyrus

Superior temporal sulcus

Calcarine spur

Middle temporal gyrus

Calcarine sulcus

Inferior temporal gyrus

Lateral occipitotemporal gyrus

Medial occipitotemporal gyrus

Lingual gyrus

Cerebellar hemisphere

Tonsil of cerebellum

Grey substance

White substance

Quadrigeminal cistern

Corpus callosum, tapetum

Lateral ventricle, occipital horn

Medial occipital artery

Great cerebral vein

Vermis of cerebellum

Dentate nucleus

Fig. 1290 Brain;
frontal section at the level of the occipital horns of the lateral ventricles.

Brain, horizontal section

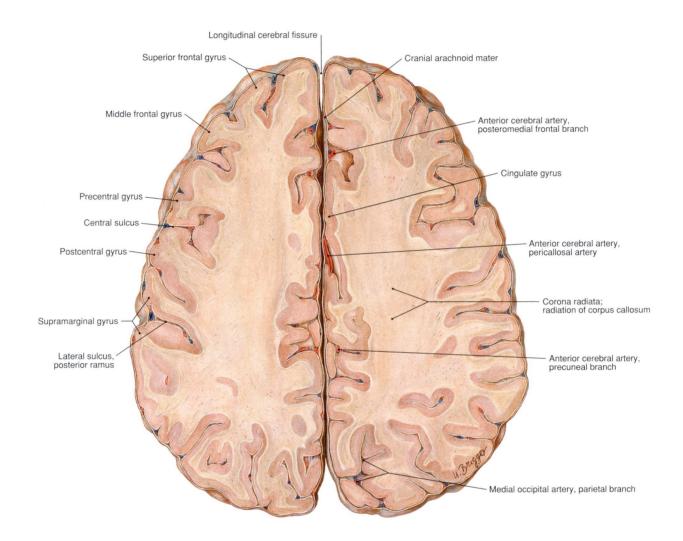

Longitudinal cerebral fissure

Superior frontal gyrus

Middle frontal gyrus

Precentral gyrus

Central sulcus

Postcentral gyrus

Supramarginal gyrus

Lateral sulcus, posterior ramus

Cranial arachnoid mater

Anterior cerebral artery, posteromedial frontal branch

Cingulate gyrus

Anterior cerebral artery, pericallosal artery

Corona radiata; radiation of corpus callosum

Anterior cerebral artery, precuneal branch

Medial occipital artery, parietal branch

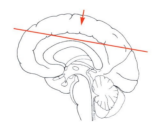

Fig. 1291 Brain; horizontal section just above the corpus callosum. In Fig. 1283–1303, the subarachnoid space appears somewhat enlarged, particularly in the region of the hemispheric sulci, due to the fact that these specimens were taken from elderly individuals.

Brain, horizontal section

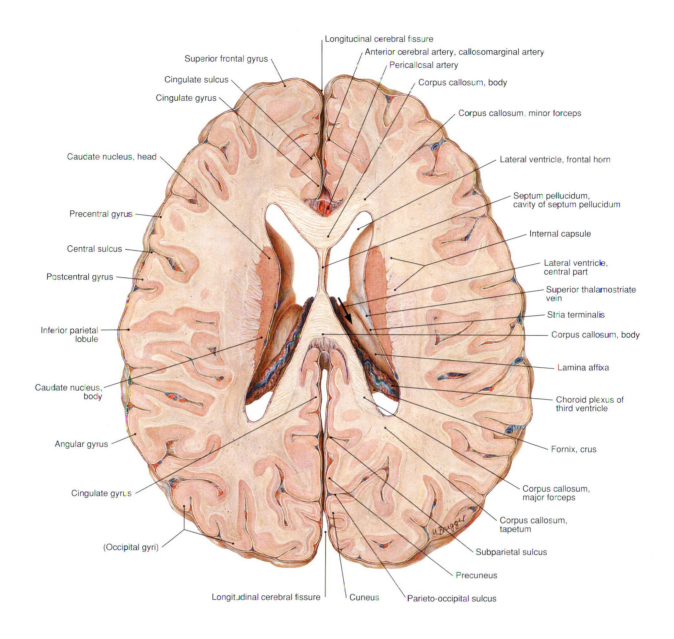

Longitudinal cerebral fissure

Superior frontal gyrus

Anterior cerebral artery, callosomarginal artery

Pericallosal artery

Cingulate sulcus

Corpus callosum, body

Cingulate gyrus

Corpus callosum, minor forceps

Caudate nucleus, head

Lateral ventricle, frontal horn

Septum pellucidum,
cavity of septum pellucidum

Precentral gyrus

Internal capsule

Central sulcus

Lateral ventricle,
central part

Postcentral gyrus

Superior thalamostriate
vein

Stria terminalis

Corpus callosum, body

Inferior parietal
lobule

Lamina affixa

Caudate nucleus,
body

Choroid plexus of
third ventricle

Angular gyrus

Fornix, crus

Cingulate gyrus

Corpus callosum,
major forceps

Corpus callosum,
tapetum

(Occipital gyri)

Subparietal sulcus

Precuneus

Longitudinal cerebral fissure

Cuneus

Parieto-occipital sulcus

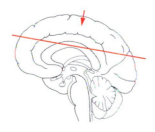

Fig. 1292 Brain;
horizontal section at the level of
the central part of the lateral ventricles.

Brain, horizontal section

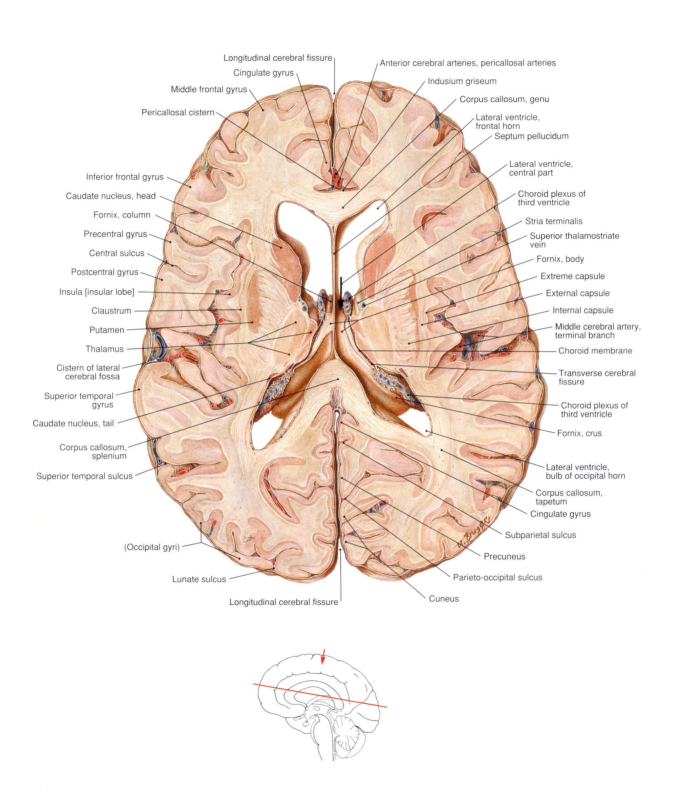

Longitudinal cerebral fissure
Cingulate gyrus
Middle frontal gyrus
Pericallosal cistern
Inferior frontal gyrus
Caudate nucleus, head
Fornix, column
Precentral gyrus
Central sulcus
Postcentral gyrus
Insula [insular lobe]
Claustrum
Putamen
Thalamus
Cistern of lateral cerebral fossa
Superior temporal gyrus
Caudate nucleus, tail
Corpus callosum, splenium
Superior temporal sulcus
(Occipital gyri)
Lunate sulcus
Longitudinal cerebral fissure

Anterior cerebral arteries, pericallosal arteries
Indusium griseum
Corpus callosum, genu
Lateral ventricle, frontal horn
Septum pellucidum
Lateral ventricle, central part
Choroid plexus of third ventricle
Stria terminalis
Superior thalamostriate vein
Fornix, body
Extreme capsule
External capsule
Internal capsule
Middle cerebral artery, terminal branch
Choroid membrane
Transverse cerebral fissure
Choroid plexus of third ventricle
Fornix, crus
Lateral ventricle, bulb of occipital horn
Corpus callosum, tapetum
Cingulate gyrus
Subparietal sulcus
Precuneus
Parieto-occipital sulcus
Cuneus

Fig. 1293 Brain;
horizontal section at the level of the floor of
the central part of the lateral ventricles.

Brain, horizontal section

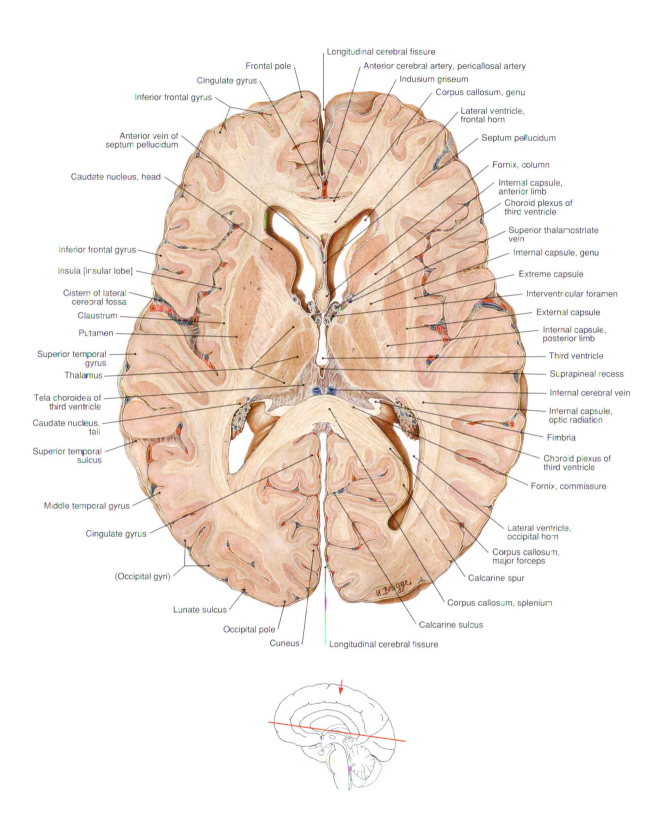

Longitudinal cerebral fissure
Frontal pole
Anterior cerebral artery, pericallosal artery
Cingulate gyrus
Indusium griseum
Inferior frontal gyrus
Corpus callosum, genu
Lateral ventricle, frontal horn
Anterior vein of septum pellucidum
Septum pellucidum
Caudate nucleus, head
Fornix, column
Internal capsule, anterior limb
Choroid plexus of third ventricle
Inferior frontal gyrus
Superior thalamostriate vein
Insula [insular lobe]
Internal capsule, genu
Cistern of lateral cerebral fossa
Extreme capsule
Claustrum
Interventricular foramen
Putamen
External capsule
Superior temporal gyrus
Internal capsule, posterior limb
Thalamus
Third ventricle
Tela choroidea of third ventricle
Suprapineal recess
Internal cerebral vein
Caudate nucleus, tail
Internal capsule, optic radiation
Superior temporal sulcus
Fimbria
Choroid plexus of third ventricle
Middle temporal gyrus
Fornix, commissure
Cingulate gyrus
Lateral ventricle, occipital horn
(Occipital gyri)
Corpus callosum, major forceps
Calcarine spur
Lunate sulcus
Corpus callosum, splenium
Occipital pole
Calcarine sulcus
Cuneus
Longitudinal cerebral fissure

Fig. 1294 Brain;
horizontal section at the level of the upper part
of the third ventricle.

Brain, horizontal section

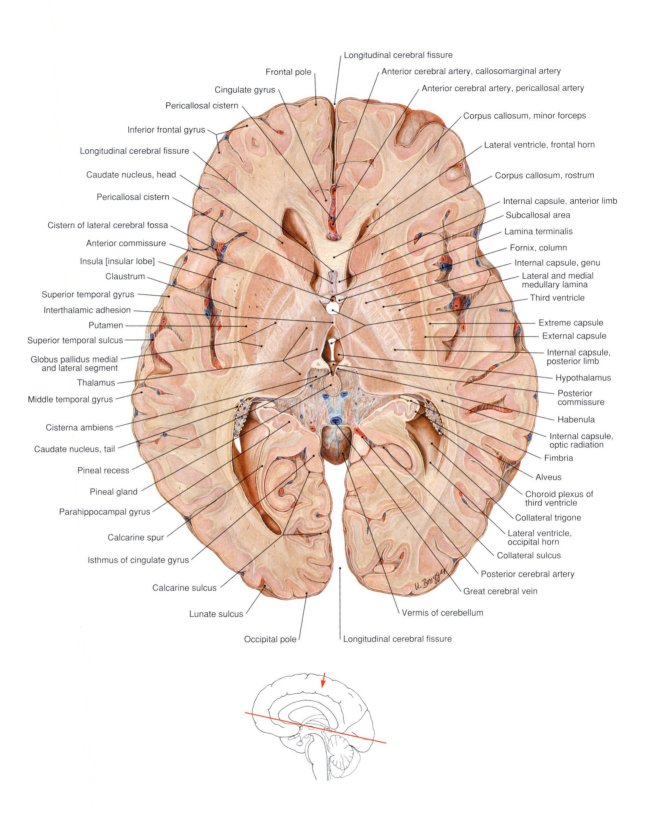

Longitudinal cerebral fissure
Frontal pole
Anterior cerebral artery, callosomarginal artery
Cingulate gyrus
Anterior cerebral artery, pericallosal artery
Pericallosal cistern
Corpus callosum, minor forceps
Inferior frontal gyrus
Lateral ventricle, frontal horn
Longitudinal cerebral fissure
Corpus callosum, rostrum
Caudate nucleus, head
Internal capsule, anterior limb
Pericallosal cistern
Subcallosal area
Cistern of lateral cerebral fossa
Lamina terminalis
Anterior commissure
Fornix, column
Insula [insular lobe]
Internal capsule, genu
Claustrum
Lateral and medial medullary lamina
Superior temporal gyrus
Third ventricle
Interthalamic adhesion
Extreme capsule
Putamen
External capsule
Superior temporal sulcus
Internal capsule, posterior limb
Globus pallidus medial and lateral segment
Hypothalamus
Thalamus
Posterior commissure
Middle temporal gyrus
Habenula
Cisterna ambiens
Internal capsule, optic radiation
Caudate nucleus, tail
Fimbria
Pineal recess
Alveus
Pineal gland
Choroid plexus of third ventricle
Parahippocampal gyrus
Collateral trigone
Calcarine spur
Lateral ventricle, occipital horn
Isthmus of cingulate gyrus
Collateral sulcus
Calcarine sulcus
Posterior cerebral artery
Lunate sulcus
Great cerebral vein
Occipital pole
Vermis of cerebellum
Longitudinal cerebral fissure

Fig. 1295   Brain;
horizontal section through the centre of the third
ventricle at the level of the interthalamic adhesion.

Brain, horizontal section

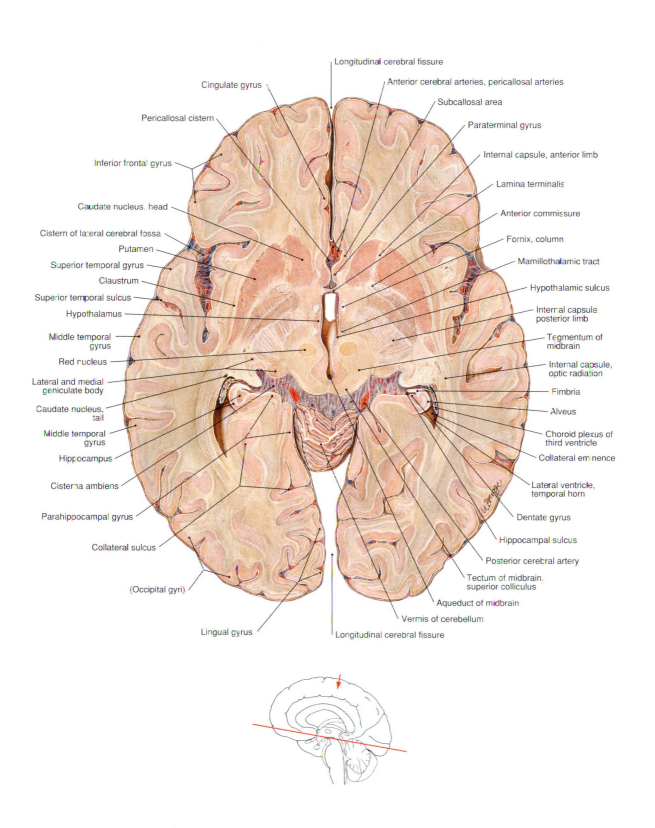

Cingulate gyrus

Pericallosal cistern

Inferior frontal gyrus

Caudate nucleus, head

Cistern of lateral cerebral fossa

Putamen

Superior temporal gyrus

Claustrum

Superior temporal sulcus

Hypothalamus

Middle temporal gyrus

Red nucleus

Lateral and medial geniculate body

Caudate nucleus, tail

Middle temporal gyrus

Hippocampus

Cisterna ambiens

Parahippocampal gyrus

Collateral sulcus

(Occipital gyri)

Lingual gyrus

Longitudinal cerebral fissure

Anterior cerebral arteries, pericallosal arteries

Subcallosal area

Paraterminal gyrus

Internal capsule, anterior limb

Lamina terminalis

Anterior commissure

Fornix, column

Mamillothalamic tract

Hypothalamic sulcus

Internal capsule, posterior limb

Tegmentum of midbrain

Internal capsule, optic radiation

Fimbria

Alveus

Choroid plexus of third ventricle

Collateral eminence

Lateral ventricle, temporal horn

Dentate gyrus

Hippocampal sulcus

Posterior cerebral artery

Tectum of midbrain, superior colliculus

Aqueduct of midbrain

Vermis of cerebellum

Longitudinal cerebral fissure

Fig. 1296 Brain;
horizontal section through the third ventricle at the level
of the opening of the cerebral aqueduct.

Brain, horizontal section

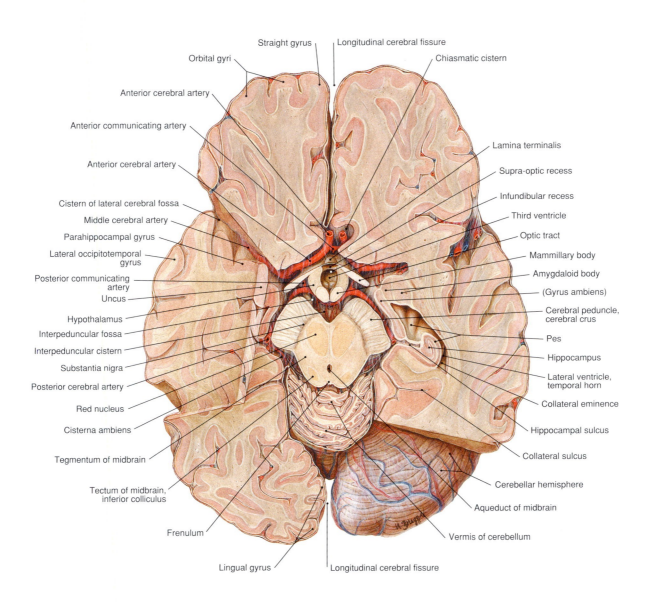

Straight gyrus
Longitudinal cerebral fissure
Orbital gyri
Chiasmatic cistern
Anterior cerebral artery
Lamina terminalis
Anterior communicating artery
Supra-optic recess
Anterior cerebral artery
Infundibular recess
Third ventricle
Cistern of lateral cerebral fossa
Optic tract
Middle cerebral artery
Parahippocampal gyrus
Mammillary body
Lateral occipitotemporal gyrus
Amygdaloid body
Posterior communicating artery
(Gyrus ambiens)
Uncus
Cerebral peduncle, cerebral crus
Hypothalamus
Pes
Interpeduncular fossa
Hippocampus
Interpeduncular cistern
Lateral ventricle, temporal horn
Substantia nigra
Posterior cerebral artery
Collateral eminence
Red nucleus
Hippocampal sulcus
Cisterna ambiens
Collateral sulcus
Tegmentum of midbrain
Cerebellar hemisphere
Tectum of midbrain, inferior colliculus
Aqueduct of midbrain
Frenulum
Vermis of cerebellum
Lingual gyrus
Longitudinal cerebral fissure

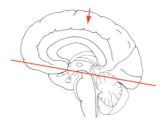

Fig. 1297 Brain;
staggered horizontal section through the floor of the third
ventricle at the level of the mamillary bodies.

Brain, sagittal section

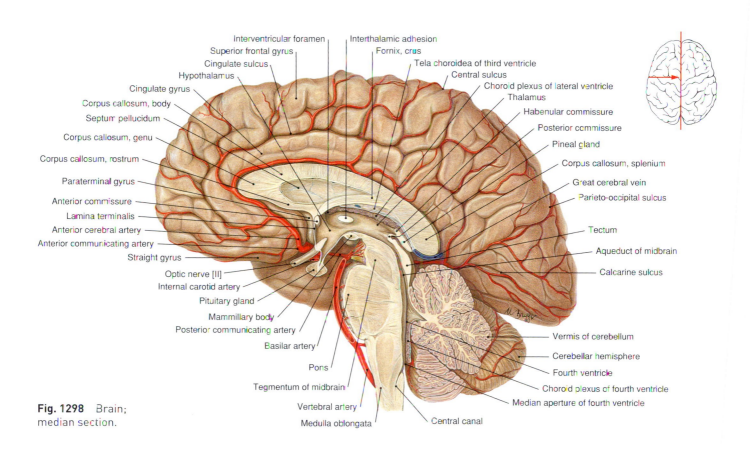

Interventricular foramen
Superior frontal gyrus
Cingulate sulcus
Hypothalamus
Cingulate gyrus
Corpus callosum, body
Septum pellucidum
Corpus callosum, genu
Corpus callosum, rostrum
Paraterminal gyrus
Anterior commissure
Lamina terminalis
Anterior cerebral artery
Anterior communicating artery
Straight gyrus
Optic nerve [II]
Internal carotid artery
Pituitary gland
Mammillary body
Posterior communicating artery
Basilar artery
Pons
Tegmentum of midbrain
Vertebral artery
Medulla oblongata

Interthalamic adhesion
Fornix, crus
Tela choroidea of third ventricle
Central sulcus
Choroid plexus of lateral ventricle
Thalamus
Habenular commissure
Posterior commissure
Pineal gland
Corpus callosum, splenium
Great cerebral vein
Parieto-occipital sulcus
Tectum
Aqueduct of midbrain
Calcarine sulcus

Vermis of cerebellum
Cerebellar hemisphere
Fourth ventricle
Choroid plexus of fourth ventricle
Median aperture of fourth ventricle
Central canal

Fig. 1298 Brain;
median section.

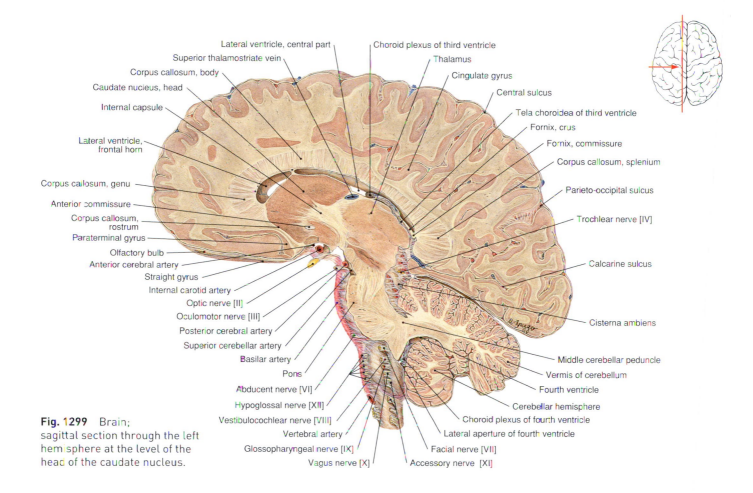

Lateral ventricle, central part
Superior thalamostriate vein
Corpus callosum, body
Caudate nucleus, head
Internal capsule
Lateral ventricle, frontal horn
Corpus callosum, genu
Anterior commissure
Corpus callosum, rostrum
Paraterminal gyrus
Olfactory bulb
Anterior cerebral artery
Straight gyrus
Internal carotid artery
Optic nerve [II]
Oculomotor nerve [III]
Posterior cerebral artery
Superior cerebellar artery
Basilar artery
Pons
Abducent nerve [VI]
Hypoglossal nerve [XII]
Vestibulocochlear nerve [VIII]
Vertebral artery
Glossopharyngeal nerve [IX]
Vagus nerve [X]

Choroid plexus of third ventricle
Thalamus
Cingulate gyrus
Central sulcus
Tela choroidea of third ventricle
Fornix, crus
Fornix, commissure
Corpus callosum, splenium
Parieto-occipital sulcus
Trochlear nerve [IV]
Calcarine sulcus
Cisterna ambiens
Middle cerebellar peduncle
Vermis of cerebellum
Fourth ventricle
Cerebellar hemisphere
Choroid plexus of fourth ventricle
Lateral aperture of fourth ventricle
Facial nerve [VII]
Accessory nerve [XI]

Fig. 1299 Brain;
sagittal section through the left
hemisphere at the level of the
head of the caudate nucleus.

Brain, sagittal sections

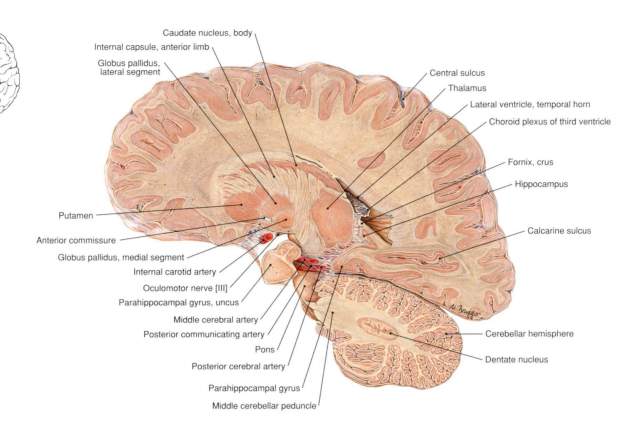

Caudate nucleus, body
Internal capsule, anterior limb
Globus pallidus, lateral segment
Central sulcus
Thalamus
Lateral ventricle, temporal horn
Choroid plexus of third ventricle
Fornix, crus
Hippocampus
Putamen
Anterior commissure
Calcarine sulcus
Globus pallidus, medial segment
Internal carotid artery
Oculomotor nerve [III]
Parahippocampal gyrus, uncus
Middle cerebral artery
Posterior communicating artery
Pons
Cerebellar hemisphere
Dentate nucleus
Posterior cerebral artery
Parahippocampal gyrus
Middle cerebellar peduncle

Fig. 1300 Brain;
sagittal section through the left hemisphere
at the level of the body of the caudate nucleus.

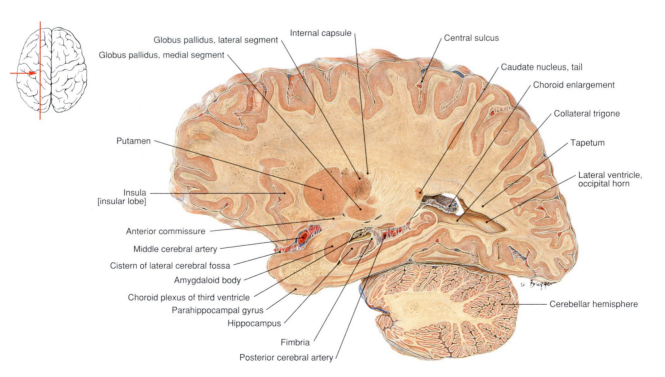

Globus pallidus, lateral segment
Internal capsule
Central sulcus
Globus pallidus, medial segment
Caudate nucleus, tail
Choroid enlargement
Collateral trigone
Putamen
Tapetum
Insula [insular lobe]
Lateral ventricle, occipital horn
Anterior commissure
Middle cerebral artery
Cistern of lateral cerebral fossa
Amygdaloid body
Choroid plexus of third ventricle
Parahippocampal gyrus
Cerebellar hemisphere
Hippocampus
Fimbria
Posterior cerebral artery

Fig. 1301 Brain;
sagittal section through the left hemisphere
at the level of the amygdaloid body.

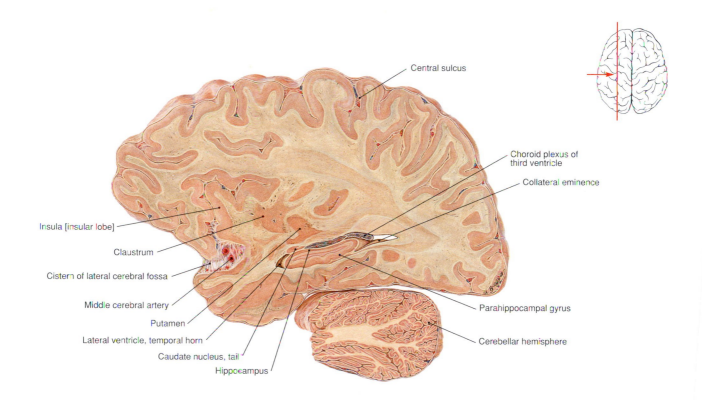

Central sulcus

Choroid plexus of
third ventricle

Collateral eminence

Insula [insular lobe]

Claustrum

Cistern of lateral cerebral fossa

Middle cerebral artery

Putamen

Lateral ventricle, temporal horn

Caudate nucleus, tail

Hippocampus

Parahippocampal gyrus

Cerebellar hemisphere

Fig. 1302 Brain;
sagittal section through the left hemisphere
at the level of the apex of the temporal horn.

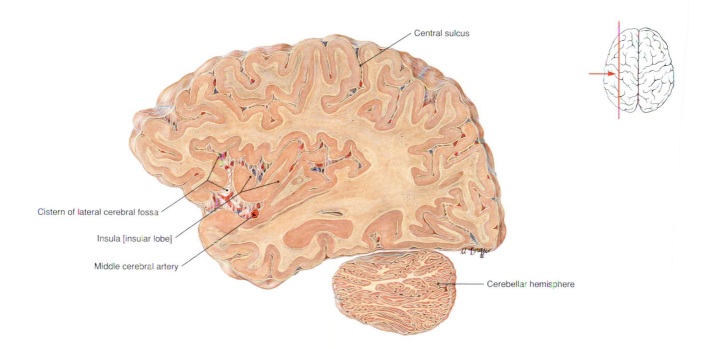

Central sulcus

Cistern of lateral cerebral fossa

Insula [insular lobe]

Middle cerebral artery

Cerebellar hemisphere

Fig. 1303 Brain;
sagittal section through the left hemisphere
at the level of the insula.

Situs of the spinal cord

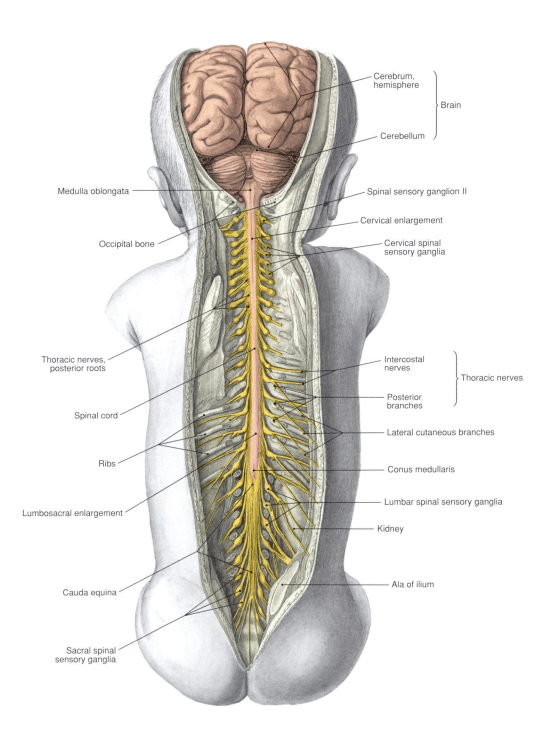

Cerebrum, hemisphere

Brain

Cerebellum

Medulla oblongata

Spinal sensory ganglion II

Cervical enlargement

Occipital bone

Cervical spinal sensory ganglia

Thoracic nerves, posterior roots

Intercostal nerves

Thoracic nerves

Posterior branches

Spinal cord

Lateral cutaneous branches

Ribs

Conus medullaris

Lumbar spinal sensory ganglia

Lumbosacral enlargement

Kidney

Cauda equina

Ala of ilium

Sacral spinal sensory ganglia

Fig. 1304 Brain; spinal cord and spinal nerves; brain and spinal nerves in a neonate.
In the neonate, the spinal cord extends two vertebral segments further caudally compared to the adult.

Segmental structure of the spinal cord

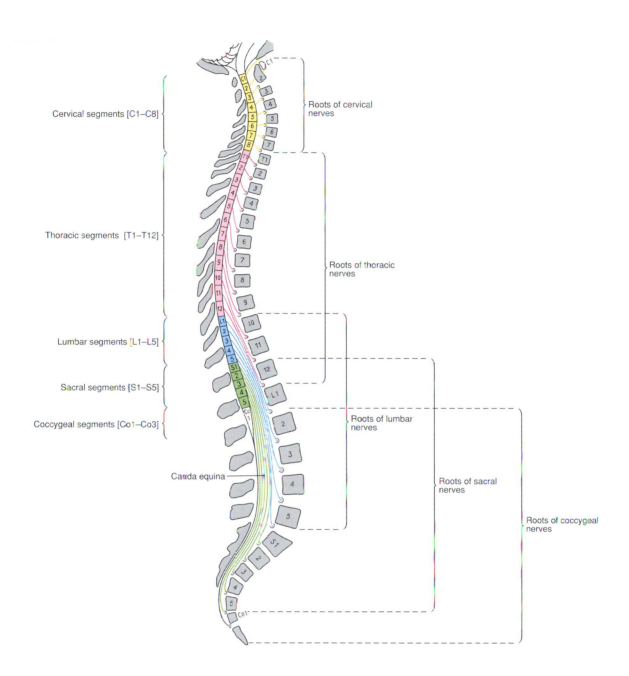

Cervical segments [C1–C8]

Roots of cervical nerves

Thoracic segments [T1–T12]

Roots of thoracic nerves

Lumbar segments [L1–L5]

Sacral segments [S1–S5]

Coccygeal segments [Co1–Co3]

Roots of lumbar nerves

Cauda equina

Roots of sacral nerves

Roots of coccygeal nerves

Fig. 1305 Spinal cord segments and spinal nerve roots; schematic median section.

As the spinal cord does not follow the growth of the vertebral column, the course of the spinal roots towards their corresponding segmental intervertebral foramina becomes steeper from cranial to caudal. In the neonate, the spinal cord ends at the level of the spinous process of the fourth lumbar vertebra, whereas in the adult, it extends normally only to the second lumbar vertebra.

Spinal cord

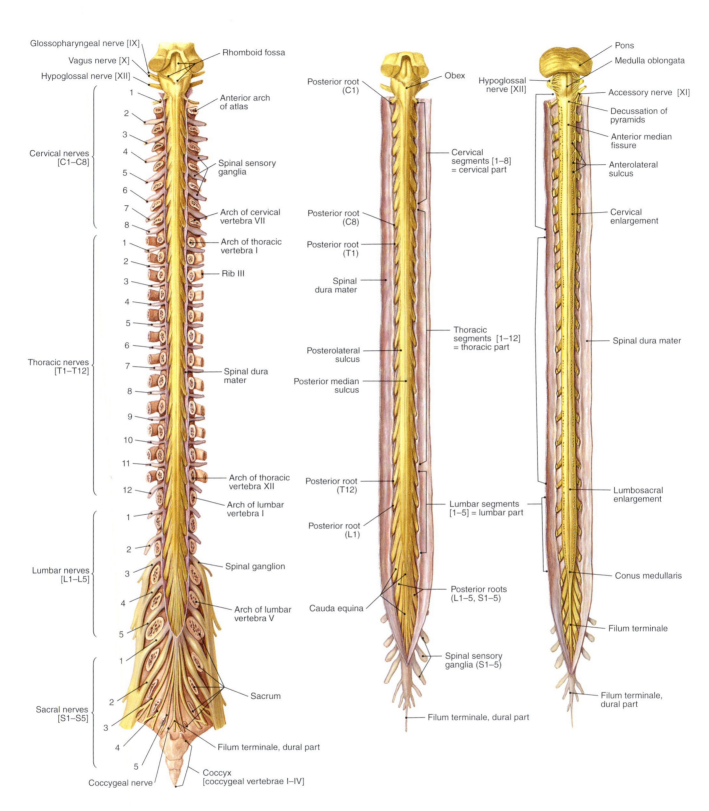

Glossopharyngeal nerve [IX]
Vagus nerve [X]
Hypoglossal nerve [XII]
Rhomboid fossa
Anterior arch of atlas
Cervical nerves [C1–C8]
1
2
3
4
5
6
7
8
Spinal sensory ganglia
Arch of cervical vertebra VII
Arch of thoracic vertebra I
Rib III
Thoracic nerves [T1–T12]
1
2
3
4
5
6
7
8
9
10
11
12
Spinal dura mater
Arch of thoracic vertebra XII
Arch of lumbar vertebra I
Lumbar nerves [L1–L5]
1
2
3
4
5
Spinal ganglion
Arch of lumbar vertebra V
Sacral nerves [S1–S5]
1
2
3
4
5
Sacrum
Filum terminale, dural part
Coccyx [coccygeal vertebrae I–IV]
Coccygeal nerve

Posterior root (C1)
Obex
Cervical segments [1–8] = cervical part
Posterior root (C8)
Posterior root (T1)
Spinal dura mater
Thoracic segments [1–12] = thoracic part
Posterolateral sulcus
Posterior median sulcus
Posterior root (T12)
Lumbar segments [1–5] = lumbar part
Posterior root (L1)
Posterior roots (L1–5, S1–5)
Cauda equina
Spinal sensory ganglia (S1–5)
Filum terminale, dural part

Pons
Medulla oblongata
Hypoglossal nerve [XII]
Accessory nerve [XI]
Decussation of pyramids
Anterior median fissure
Anterolateral sulcus
Cervical enlargement
Spinal dura mater
Lumbosacral enlargement
Conus medullaris
Filum terminale
Filum terminale, dural part

Fig. 1306 Spinal cord and spinal nerves; situs of the spinal cord; dorsal view.
As spinal cord segments are numbered according to the spinal nerves, and the uppermost spinal nerve is counted as the first cervical nerve, there are actually eight cervical segments.

Fig. 1307 Spinal cord and spinal nerves; the spinal dura mater has been opened; dorsal view.

Fig. 1308 Spinal cord and spinal nerves; the spinal dura mater has been opened; ventral view.

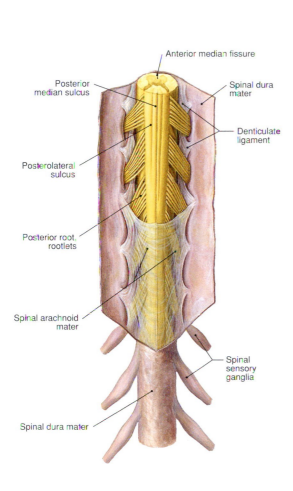

Anterior median fissure

Posterior median sulcus

Spinal dura mater

Denticulate ligament

Posterolateral sulcus

Posterior root, rootlets

Spinal arachnoid mater

Spinal sensory ganglia

Spinal dura mater

Fig. 1309 Spinal cord and spinal meninges; dorsal view.

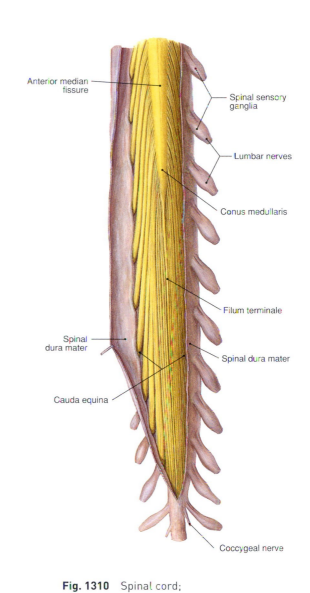

Anterior median fissure

Spinal sensory ganglia

Lumbar nerves

Conus medullaris

Filum terminale

Spinal dura mater

Spinal dura mater

Cauda equina

Coccygeal nerve

Fig. 1310 Spinal cord; caudal part with the cauda equina; ventral view.

→ 550

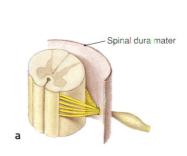

Spinal dura mater

a

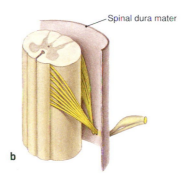

Spinal dura mater

b

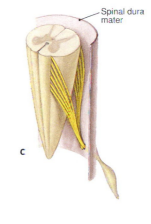

Spinal dura mater

c

Fig. 1311 a–c Spinal nerve roots; typical course within the subarachnoid space.
a Cervical segment
b Thoracic segment
c Lumbar segment

Arteries of the spinal cord

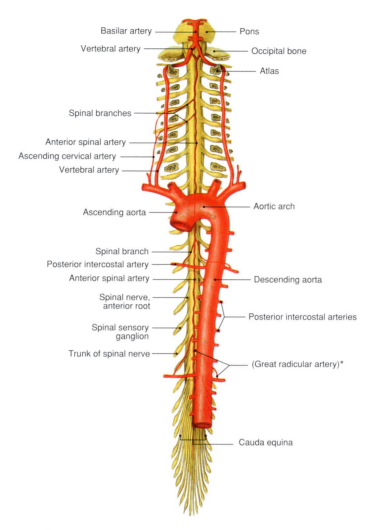

Basilar artery — Pons

Vertebral artery — Occipital bone

— Atlas

Spinal branches

Anterior spinal artery

Ascending cervical artery

Vertebral artery

Ascending aorta — Aortic arch

Spinal branch

Posterior intercostal artery

Anterior spinal artery — Descending aorta

Spinal nerve, anterior root

Spinal sensory ganglion — Posterior intercostal arteries

Trunk of spinal nerve

(Great radicular artery)*

— Cauda equina

Fig. 1312   Arteries of the spinal cord.

* Clinical term: artery of ADAMKIEWICZ

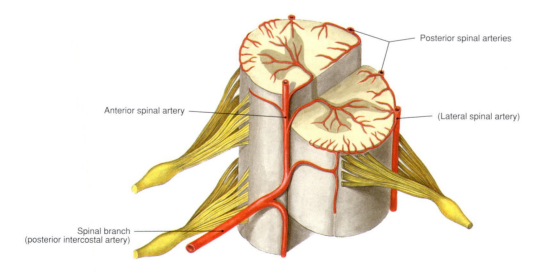

Posterior spinal arteries

Anterior spinal artery

(Lateral spinal artery)

Spinal branch
(posterior intercostal artery)

Fig. 1313   Arteries of the spinal cord.

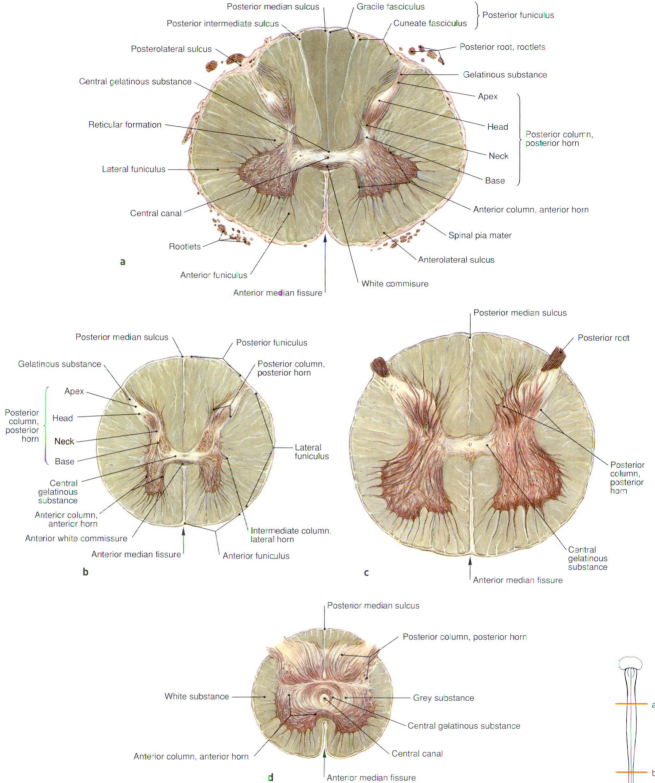

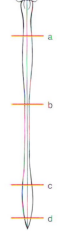

Fig. 1314 a–d Spinal cord;
cross-sections; myelin stain; approx. 500%.
a Cervical part
b Thoracic part
c Lumbar part
d Sacral part

Functional organisation of the spinal cord

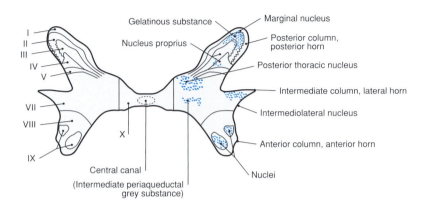

Fig. 1315 Spinal cord;
laminar organisation of the grey matter according to its
cytoarchitecture (according to REXED, 1952), exemplified
by the tenth thoracic segment (T10).
Formation and number of the laminae vary in different
spinal cord segments.

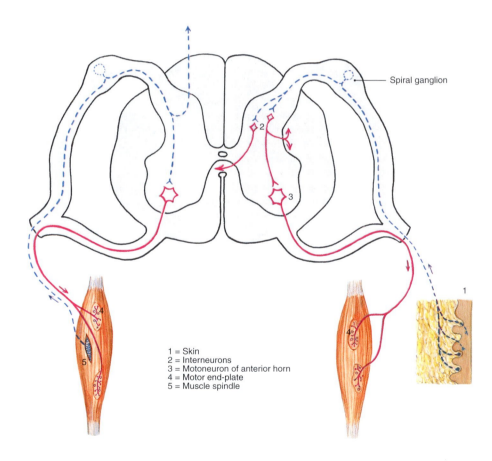

1 = Skin
2 = Interneurons
3 = Motoneuron of anterior horn
4 = Motor end-plate
5 = Muscle spindle

Fig. 1316 Reflexes at the spinal cord;
left: monosynaptic reflex (bineuronal, proprioceptive, myostatic, e.g.,
patellar tendon reflex, Achilles tendon reflex, etc.);
right: polysynaptic reflex (polyneuronal, e.g., abdominal reflex,
cremasteric reflex, plantar reflex, etc.).

Functional organisation of the spinal cord

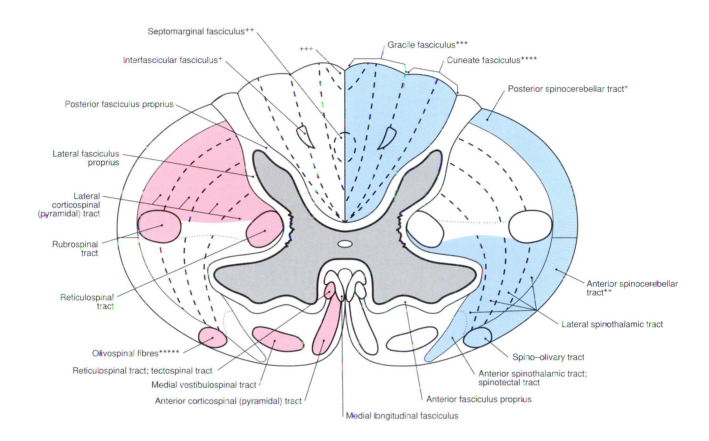

Septomarginal fasciculus++

+++

Interfascicular fasciculus+

Gracile fasciculus***

Cuneate fasciculus****

Posterior fasciculus proprius

Posterior spinocerebellar tract*

Lateral fasciculus proprius

Lateral corticospinal (pyramidal) tract

Rubrospinal tract

Reticulospinal tract

Anterior spinocerebellar tract**

Lateral spinothalamic tract

Olivospinal fibres*****

Spino–olivary tract

Reticulospinal tract; tectospinal tract

Anterior spinothalamic tract; spinotectal tract

Medial vestibulospinal tract

Anterior fasciculus proprius

Anterior corticospinal (pyramidal) tract

Medial longitudinal fasciculus

Fig. 1317 Spinal cord;
schematic organisation of the white matter exemplified
by a lower cervical segment.
Afferent (= ascending) pathways in blue;
efferent (= descending) pathways in red.

*	Clinical term: FLECHSIG's tract
**	Clinical term: GOWER's tract
***	Clinical term: GOLL's tract
****	Clinical term: BURDACH's tract
*****	The actual existence of these fibres has not definitely been documented.

The regions indicated by +, ++, and +++ designate descending
collateral tracts of the posterior fasciculi.

+	SCHULTZE's comma tract (cervical part)
++	FLECHSIG's oval bundle (thoracic part)
+++	Triangle of PHILIPPE-GOMBAULT (lumbar and sacral parts)

Pathways of the spinal cord

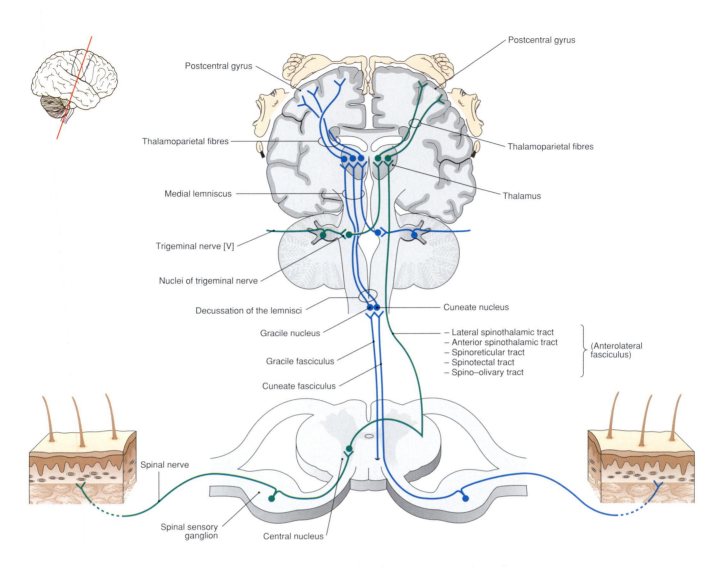

Fig. 1318   Pathways for epicritic (blue) and protopathic (green) sensibility.

Ascending pathways

Pathway for epicritic sensibility (tactile pathway)
(Precise differentiation of pressure and touch)

1. neuron (uncrossed)
   From receptors (exteroceptors) in the skin and the mucosa, as well as the periosteum, the joints and the muscle spindles etc., to the cuneate and gracile nucleus in the medulla oblongata: gracile and cuneate fasciculus (perikarya in the spinal ganglia): descending collaterals (see Fig. 1317).
2. neuron (crossed)
   From the medulla oblongata (cuneate and gracile nucleus) to the thalamus (medial lemniscus, perikarya in the cuneate and gracile nucleus).
3. neuron (uncrossed)
   From the thalamus to the cerebral cortex, particularly to the postcentral gyrus (thalamocortical fibres, perikarya in the thalamus).

Pathway for protopathic sensibility (pain pathway)
(Pain, temperature, general pressure sensation)

1. neuron (uncrossed)
   From receptors (exteroceptors) of the skin and the mucosa etc., to the posterior horn, laminae I–V (perikarya in the spinal ganglia).
2. neuron (crossed, some fibres possibly uncrossed)
   From the posterior horn to the thalamus, in the reticular formation and to the midbrain tectum (anterior and lateral spinothalamic tracts, spinoreticular tract, spinotectal tract; perikarya in the posterior column).
3. neuron (uncrossed)
   From the thalamus among others to the cerebral cortex, particularly to the postcentral gyrus (thalamocortical fibres, perikarya in the thalamus).

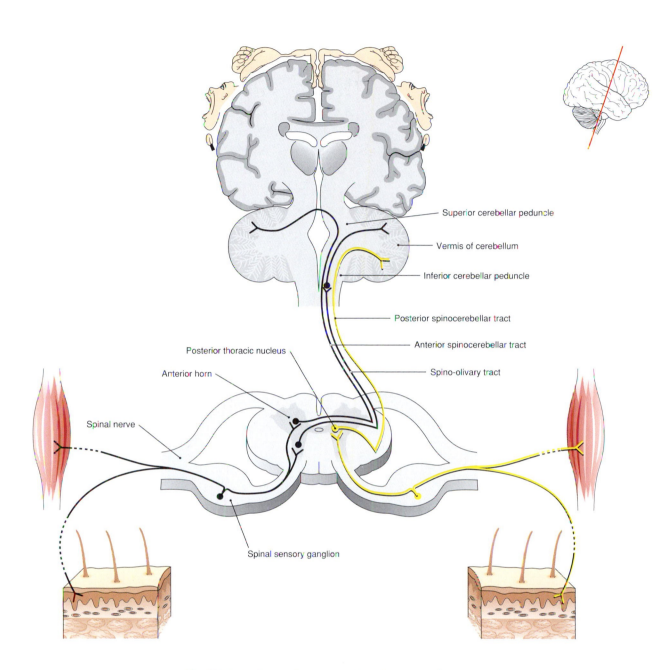

Superior cerebellar peduncle

Vermis of cerebellum

Inferior cerebellar peduncle

Posterior spinocerebellar tract

Anterior spinocerebellar tract

Spino-olivary tract

Posterior thoracic nucleus

Anterior horn

Spinal nerve

Spinal sensory ganglion

Fig. 1319 Pathways for unconscious deep sensibility.

Ascending pathways

Pathway for unconscious deep sensibility
(Unconscious, but precise spatial differentiation as a prerequisite for movement coordination by the cerebellum)

Via the anterior cerebellar tract

1. neuron (uncrossed)
   From receptors (proprioceptors) in muscles, tendons, and the connective tissue to the nuclei of the intermediate zone and the anterior column (perikarya in the spinal ganglia).
2. neuron (crossed)
   From the anterior horn within the anterior spinocerebellar tract of the anterolateral tract to the cerebellum via the superior cerebellar peduncle (perikarya in the intermediate zone and the anterior horn).

Via the posterior cerebellar tract

1. neuron (uncrossed)
   From end organs (proprioceptors) in muscles, tendons, and the connective tissue to the nuclei of the posterior column and the thoracic nucleus (perikarya in the spinal ganglia).
2. neuron (uncrossed)
   From the posterior horn and the thoracic nucleus within the posterior spinocerebellar tract of the lateral tract to the cerebellum via the inferior cerebellar peduncle (perikarya in the thoracic nucleus and at the base of the posterior column).

Pathways of the spinal cord

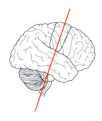

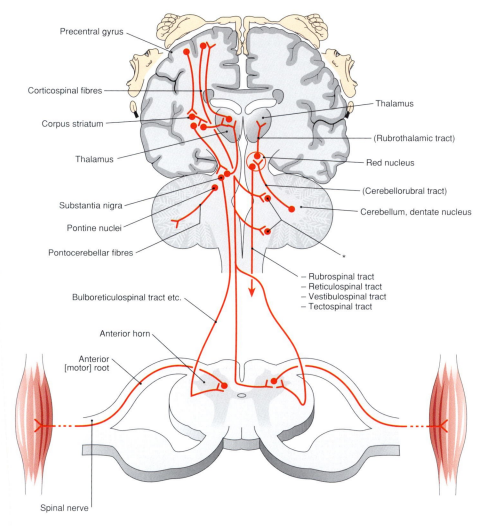

Precentral gyrus

Corticospinal fibres

Corpus striatum

Thalamus

Substantia nigra

Pontine nuclei

Pontocerebellar fibres

Bulboreticulospinal tract etc.

Anterior horn

Anterior [motor] root

Spinal nerve

Thalamus

(Rubrothalamic tract)

Red nucleus

(Cerebellorubral tract)

Cerebellum, dentate nucleus

*

− Rubrospinal tract
− Reticulospinal tract
− Vestibulospinal tract
− Tectospinal tract

Fig. 1320   Pathways of the motor system.

*   Motor nuclei of cranial nerves

Descending pathways

The motor system comprises a large number of nuclear regions and tracts. The "motor final path" are the motoneurons. Despite the extraordinary complexity of these circuits, the traditional organisation will be maintained for didactic reasons.

(So-called) Pyramidal tract

1. (central) neuron (crossed)
   From the cerebral cortex through the internal capsule and the cerebral peduncles to interneurons within the anterior and posterior column (lateral corticospinal tract, anterior corticospinal tract, perikarya in the precentral gyrus). Branching off of fibres to the nuclei of the cranial nerves (corticonuclear fibres and bulbar corticonuclear fibres).
2. (peripheral) neuron (motor end pathway, α-motoneurons)
   From the anterior horn to the motor end plates of the skeletal musculature (motoneurons, perikarya in the anterior horn).

(So-called) Extrapyramidal motor system

1. central neurons (crossed and uncrossed)
   From the cerebral cortex, particularly the precentral gyrus and the adjacent cortical areas including synapses to the basal ganglia, thalamus, subthalamic nucleus, red nucleus, substantia nigra, cerebellum, etc. and feedback loops to the interneurons of the anterior column (rubrospinal tract, medial and lateral vestibulospinal tract, reticulospinal tract, tectospinal tract).
2. peripheral neuron (motor end pathway, α-motoneurons)
   From the anterior horn to the motor end-plates of the skeletal muscles (motoneurons; perikarya in the anterior horn).

Lesions of the spinal cord

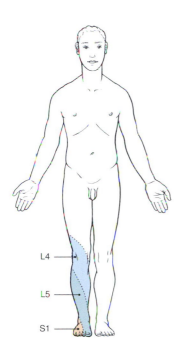

Fig. 1321 Dysfunctional cutaneous innervation due to palsy of certain, frequently affected spinal nerves.

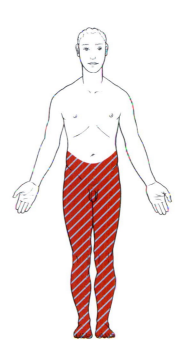

Fig. 1322 Complete paraplegia at the level of the eleventh thoracic segment.
Paralysis of the complete motor and sensory system.

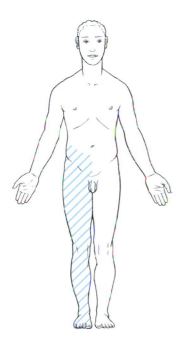

Fig. 1323 Paralysis of the tracts of the right posterior funiculus at the level of the eleventh thoracic segment.
Loss of fine tactile sensation as well as loss of sense of position and vibration (rough touch sensation remains functional).

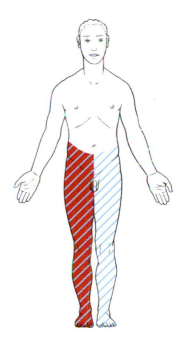

Fig. 1324 Hemiplegia (BROWN-SÉQUARD) due to disruption of the half of the spinal cord on the right side at the level of the eleventh thoracic segment.
On the right side (ipsilaterally): loss of motor function (initially flaccid, later spastic); loss of fine tactile sensation as well as loss of sense of position and vibration (rough touch sensation remains functional).
On the left side (contralaterally): loss of pain and temperature sensation.

Eyelids

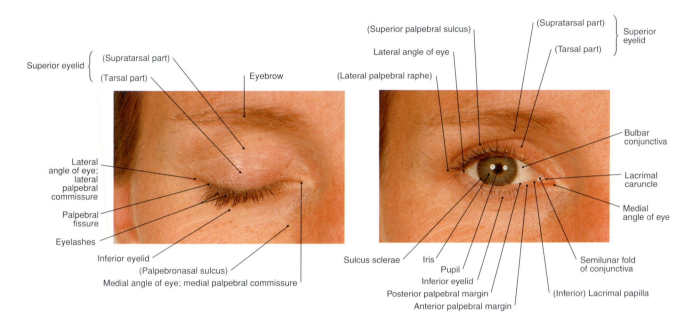

Superior eyelid { (Supratarsal part) (Tarsal part)

Eyebrow

Lateral angle of eye; lateral palpebral commissure

Palpebral fissure

Eyelashes

Inferior eyelid

(Palpebronasal sulcus)

Medial angle of eye; medial palpebral commissure

(Superior palpebral sulcus)

Lateral angle of eye

(Lateral palpebral raphe)

(Supratarsal part) } Superior eyelid

(Tarsal part)

Bulbar conjunctiva

Lacrimal caruncle

Medial angle of eye

Sulcus sclerae   Iris   Semilunar fold of conjunctiva

Pupil

Inferior eyelid

Posterior palpebral margin   (Inferior) Lacrimal papilla

Anterior palpebral margin

Fig. 1325   Eyelids.

Fig. 1326   Eye and eyelids.

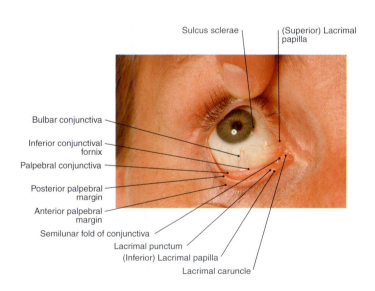

Sulcus sclerae   (Superior) Lacrimal papilla

Bulbar conjunctiva

Inferior conjunctival fornix

Palpebral conjunctiva

Posterior palpebral margin

Anterior palpebral margin

Semilunar fold of conjunctiva

Lacrimal punctum

(Inferior) Lacrimal papilla

Lacrimal caruncle

Fig. 1327   Eye and eyelids.

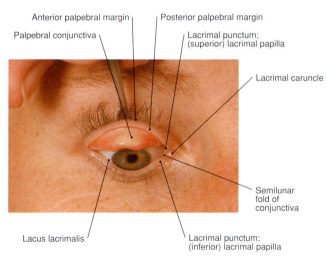

Anterior palpebral margin   Posterior palpebral margin

Palpebral conjunctiva

Lacrimal punctum; (superior) lacrimal papilla

Lacrimal caruncle

Semilunar fold of conjunctiva

Lacus lacrimalis   Lacrimal punctum; (inferior) lacrimal papilla

Fig. 1328   Eye and eyelids.
Eversion of the upper eyelid (extropionisation) is hindered by the stiffness of the tarsus, but can be facilitated with the aid of a small hook.

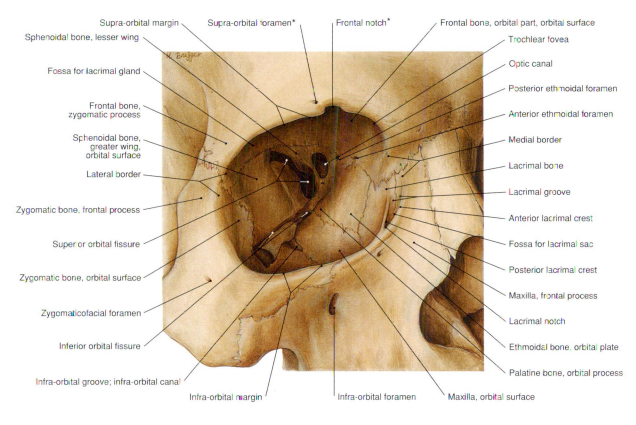

Supra-orbital margin
Supra-orbital foramen*
Frontal notch*
Frontal bone, orbital part, orbital surface
Sphenoidal bone, lesser wing
Trochlear fovea
Fossa for lacrimal gland
Optic canal
Posterior ethmoidal foramen
Frontal bone, zygomatic process
Anterior ethmoidal foramen
Sphenoidal bone, greater wing, orbital surface
Medial border
Lacrimal bone
Lateral border
Lacrimal groove
Zygomatic bone, frontal process
Anterior lacrimal crest
Superior orbital fissure
Fossa for lacrimal sac
Zygomatic bone, orbital surface
Posterior lacrimal crest
Maxilla, frontal process
Zygomaticofacial foramen
Lacrimal notch
Inferior orbital fissure
Ethmoidal bone, orbital plate
Palatine bone, orbital process
Infra-orbital groove; infra-orbital canal
Infra-orbital margin
Infra-orbital foramen
Maxilla, orbital surface

Fig. 1329 Orbit; oblique view from lateral.

* These structures can be present as foramina or notches.

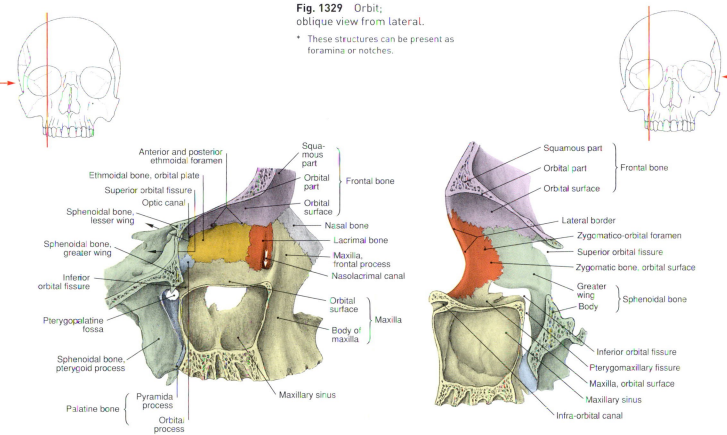

Anterior and posterior ethmoidal foramen
Squamous part
Ethmoidal bone, orbital plate
Orbital part } Frontal bone
Superior orbital fissure
Orbital surface
Optic canal
Nasal bone
Sphenoidal bone, lesser wing
Lacrimal bone
Sphenoidal bone, greater wing
Maxilla, frontal process
Inferior orbital fissure
Nasolacrimal canal
Pterygopalatine fossa
Orbital surface } Maxilla
Body of maxilla
Sphenoidal bone, pterygoid process
Pyramidal process
Palatine bone {
Orbital process
Maxillary sinus

Fig. 1330 Medial wall of the orbit; lateral view.

Squamous part
Orbital part } Frontal bone
Orbital surface
Lateral border
Zygomatico-orbital foramen
Superior orbital fissure
Zygomatic bone, orbital surface
Greater wing
Body } Sphenoidal bone
Inferior orbital fissure
Pterygomaxillary fissure
Maxilla, orbital surface
Maxillary sinus
Infra-orbital canal

Fig. 1331 Lateral wall of the orbit; medial view.

Eyelids

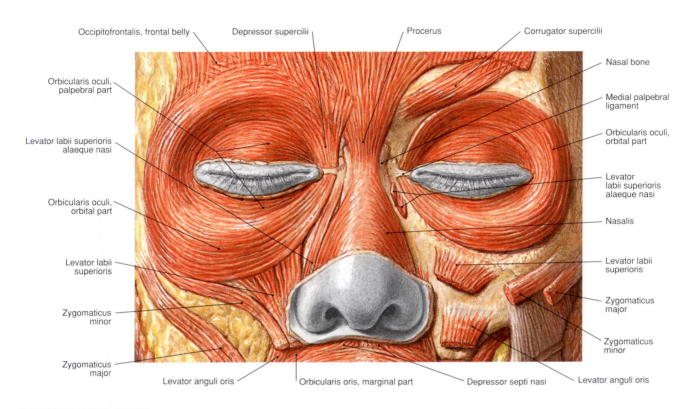

Occipitofrontalis, frontal belly — Depressor supercilii — Procerus — Corrugator supercilii

Orbicularis oculi, palpebral part

Levator labii superioris alaeque nasi

Orbicularis oculi, orbital part

Levator labii superioris

Zygomaticus minor

Zygomaticus major

Nasal bone

Medial palpebral ligament

Orbicularis oculi, orbital part

Levator labii superioris alaeque nasi

Nasalis

Levator labii superioris

Zygomaticus major

Zygomaticus minor

Levator anguli oris — Orbicularis oris, marginal part — Depressor septi nasi — Levator anguli oris

→ 119, 120, T 1 a, c, d, e

Fig. 1332 Facial muscles.

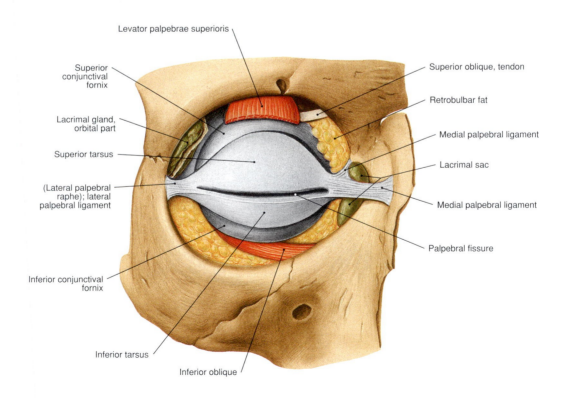

Levator palpebrae superioris

Superior conjunctival fornix

Lacrimal gland, orbital part

Superior tarsus

(Lateral palpebral raphe); lateral palpebral ligament

Inferior conjunctival fornix

Inferior tarsus

Inferior oblique

Superior oblique, tendon

Retrobulbar fat

Medial palpebral ligament

Lacrimal sac

Medial palpebral ligament

Palpebral fissure

Fig. 1333 Orbital opening with eyelids.

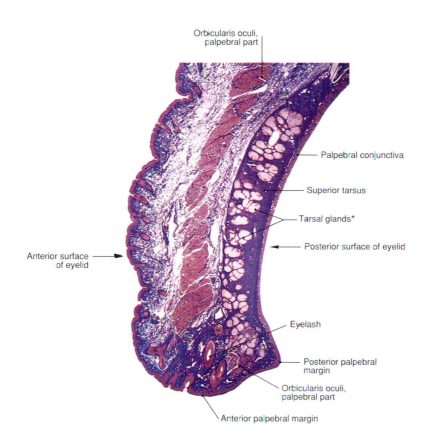

Orbicularis oculi, palpebral part

Palpebral conjunctiva

Superior tarsus

Tarsal glands*

Posterior surface of eyelid

Anterior surface of eyelid

Eyelash

Posterior palpebral margin

Orbicularis oculi, palpebral part

Anterior palpebral margin

Fig. 1334 Upper eyelid;
photograph of a microscopic specimen;
azan stain;
sagittal section, magnified.

* Clinical term: MEIBOMian glands

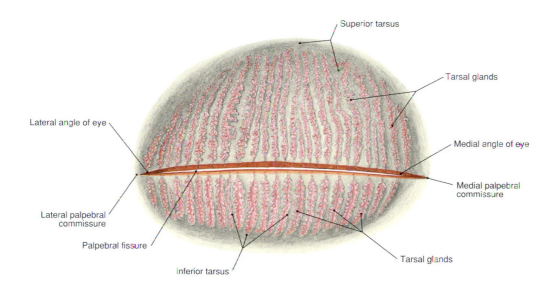

Superior tarsus

Tarsal glands

Lateral angle of eye

Medial angle of eye

Medial palpebral commissure

Lateral palpebral commissure

Palpebral fissure

Tarsal glands

Inferior tarsus

Fig. 1335 Eyelids;
translucent specimen illustrating the excretory
ductules of the tarsal glands;
posterior view.

Lacrimal apparatus

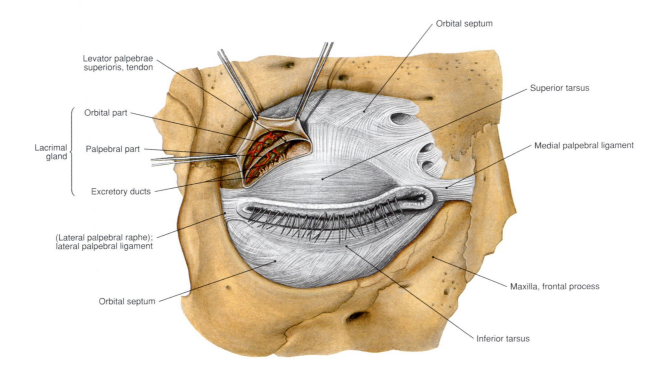

Levator palpebrae superioris, tendon

Orbital septum

Superior tarsus

Lacrimal gland
- Orbital part
- Palpebral part
- Excretory ducts

Medial palpebral ligament

(Lateral palpebral raphe); lateral palpebral ligament

Orbital septum

Maxilla, frontal process

Inferior tarsus

Fig. 1336 Orbital opening with eyelids and lacrimal gland.

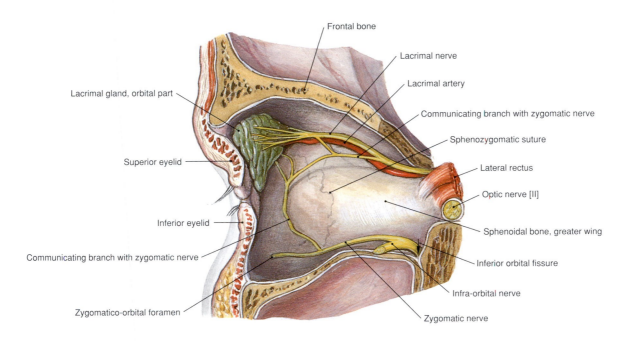

Frontal bone

Lacrimal nerve

Lacrimal artery

Lacrimal gland, orbital part

Communicating branch with zygomatic nerve

Sphenozygomatic suture

Superior eyelid

Lateral rectus

Optic nerve [II]

Inferior eyelid

Sphenoidal bone, greater wing

Communicating branch with zygomatic nerve

Inferior orbital fissure

Infra-orbital nerve

Zygomatico-orbital foramen

Zygomatic nerve

Fig. 1337 Innervation of the lacrimal gland; medial view.

Lacrimal apparatus

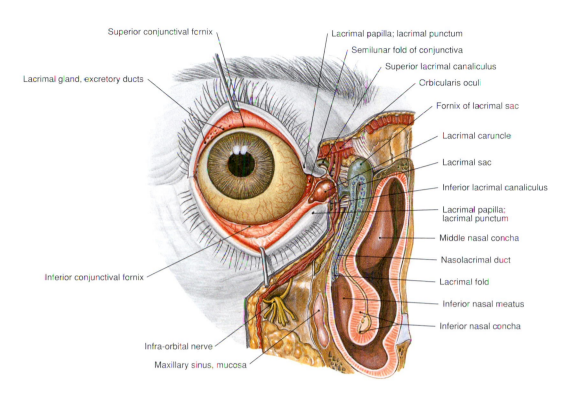

Superior conjunctival fornix
Lacrimal gland, excretory ducts
Inferior conjunctival fornix
Infra-orbital nerve
Maxillary sinus, mucosa

Lacrimal papilla; lacrimal punctum
Semilunar fold of conjunctiva
Superior lacrimal canaliculus
Orbicularis oculi
Fornix of lacrimal sac
Lacrimal caruncle
Lacrimal sac
Inferior lacrimal canaliculus
Lacrimal papilla; lacrimal punctum
Middle nasal concha
Nasolacrimal duct
Lacrimal fold
Inferior nasal meatus
Inferior nasal concha

Fig. 1338 Lacrimal apparatus;
the eyelids have been pulled away from the eyeball;
the nasolacrimal duct has been opened up to the inferior nasal meatus.

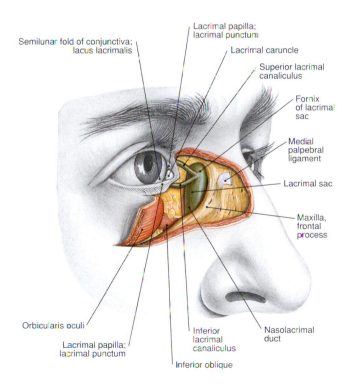

Semilunar fold of conjunctiva; lacus lacrimalis
Lacrimal papilla; lacrimal punctum
Lacrimal caruncle
Superior lacrimal canaliculus
Fornix of lacrimal sac
Medial palpebral ligament
Lacrimal sac
Maxilla, frontal process
Orbicularis oculi
Lacrimal papilla; lacrimal punctum
Inferior lacrimal canaliculus
Inferior oblique
Nasolacrimal duct

Fig. 1339 Lacrimal apparatus.

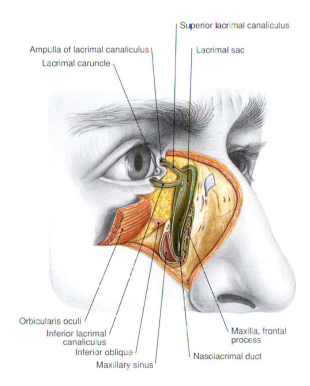

Ampulla of lacrimal canaliculus
Lacrimal caruncle
Superior lacrimal canaliculus
Lacrimal sac
Orbicularis oculi
Inferior lacrimal canaliculus
Inferior oblique
Maxillary sinus
Maxilla, frontal process
Nasolacrimal duct

Fig. 1340 Lacrimal apparatus;
the nasolacrimal duct and the nasolacrimal canal
have been opened.

Extra-ocular muscles

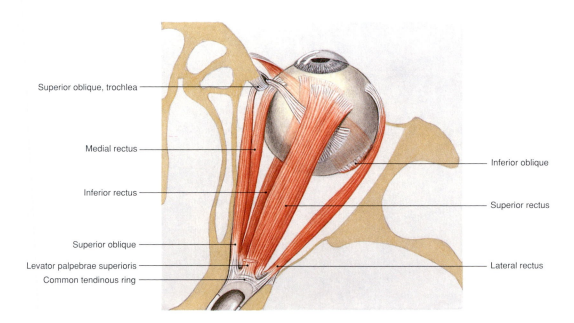

Superior oblique, trochlea

Medial rectus

Inferior rectus

Superior oblique

Levator palpebrae superioris

Common tendinous ring

Inferior oblique

Superior rectus

Lateral rectus

Fig. 1341 Extra-ocular muscles;
schema;
superior view.

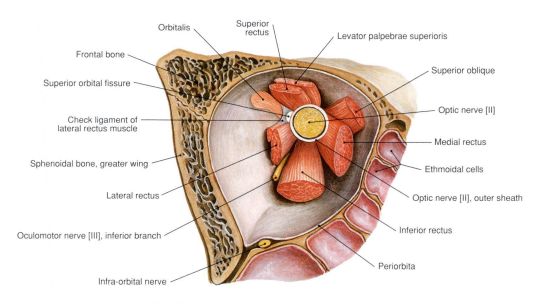

Orbitalis

Superior rectus

Levator palpebrae superioris

Frontal bone

Superior orbital fissure

Superior oblique

Check ligament of
lateral rectus muscle

Optic nerve [II]

Sphenoidal bone, greater wing

Medial rectus

Lateral rectus

Ethmoidal cells

Oculomotor nerve [III], inferior branch

Optic nerve [II], outer sheath

Inferior rectus

Infra-orbital nerve

Periorbita

Fig. 1342 Extra-ocular muscles;
anterior view.

Extra-ocular muscles

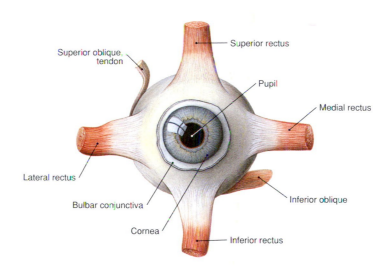

Fig. 1343 Extra-ocular muscles.

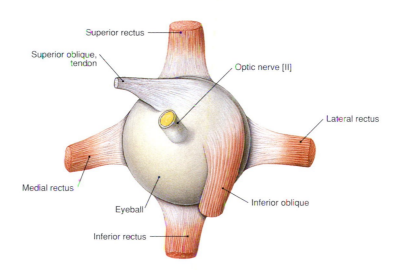

Fig. 1344 Extra-ocular muscles; posterior view.

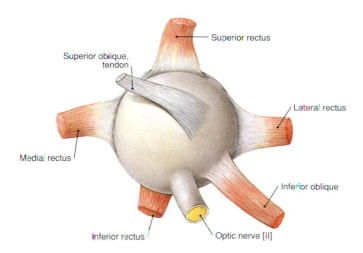

Fig. 1345 Extra-ocular muscles; posterior-superior view.

Extra-ocular muscles

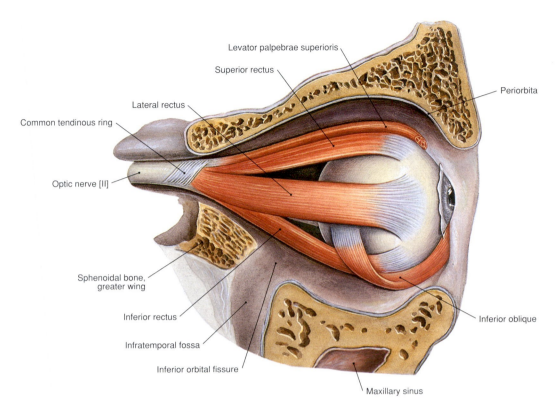

Fig. 1346 Extra-ocular muscles; lateral view.

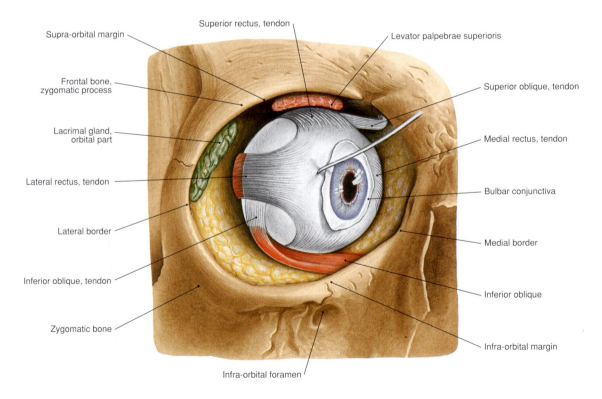

Fig. 1347 Extra-ocular muscles; oblique view from anterior.

Extra-ocular muscles

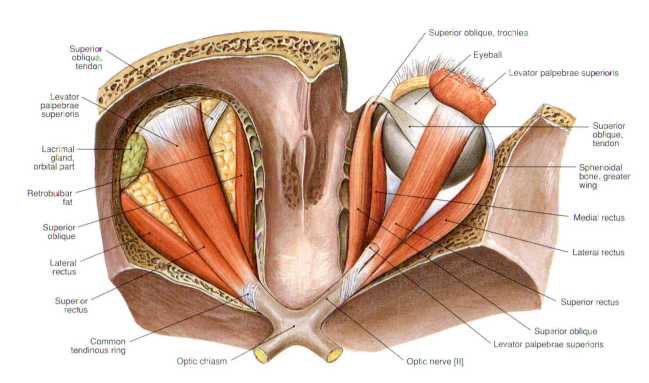

Superior oblique, trochlea
Eyeball
Levator palpebrae superioris
Superior oblique, tendon
Sphenoidal bone, greater wing
Medial rectus
Lateral rectus
Superior rectus
Superior oblique
Levator palpebrae superioris
Optic nerve [II]

Superior oblique, tendon
Levator palpebrae superioris
Lacrimal gland, orbital part
Retrobulbar fat
Superior oblique
Lateral rectus
Superior rectus
Common tendinous ring
Optic chiasm

Fig. 1348 Extra-ocular muscles; superior view.

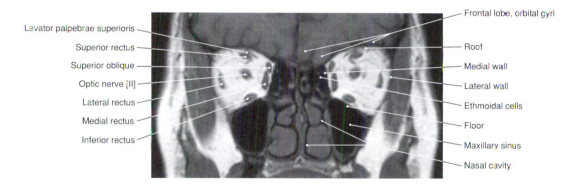

Levator palpebrae superioris
Superior rectus
Superior oblique
Optic nerve [II]
Lateral rectus
Medial rectus
Inferior rectus

Frontal lobe, orbital gyri
Roof
Medial wall
Lateral wall
Ethmoidal cells
Floor
Maxillary sinus
Nasal cavity

Fig. 1349 Extra-ocular muscles; magnetic resonance tomographic image (MRI); frontal section through the middle of the orbit; anterior view.

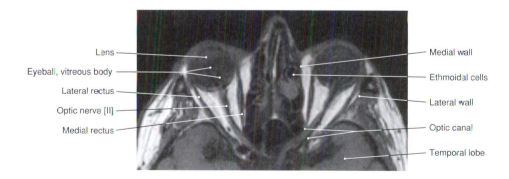

Lens
Eyeball, vitreous body
Lateral rectus
Optic nerve [II]
Medial rectus

Medial wall
Ethmoidal cells
Lateral wall
Optic canal
Temporal lobe

Fig. 1350 Eyeball and extra-ocular muscles; magnetic resonance tomographic image (MRI); horizontal section at the level of the optic nerve; superior view.

Eyeball, structure

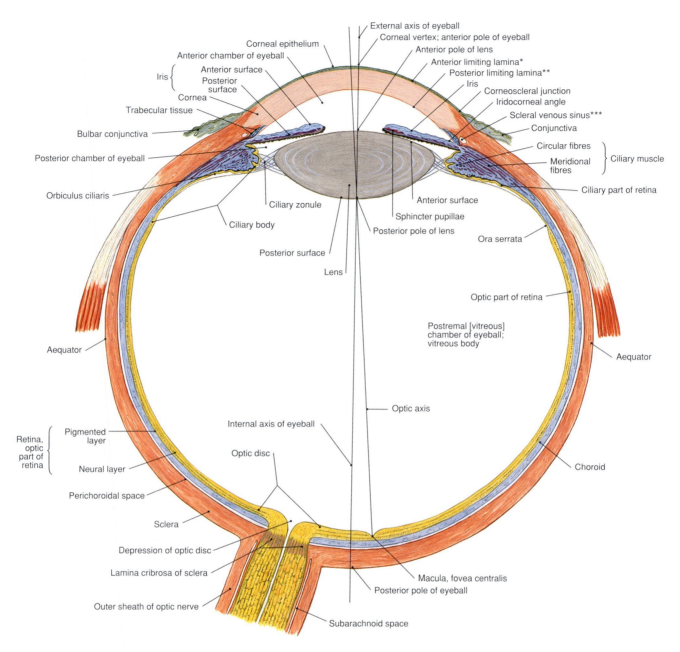

Fig. 1351 Eyeball;
schematic horizontal section at the level of the
exit of the optic nerve.

*   Clinical term: BOWMAN's membrane
**   Clinical term: DESCEMET's membrane
*** Clinical term: canal of SCHLEMM

Dimensions of the eyeball

(Average values according to the anatomic and ophthalmologic literature)

External bulbar axis	24.0 mm	Radius of curvature of the sclera	13.0 mm
		Radius of curvature of the cornea	7.8 mm
Internal bulbar axis	22.5 mm		
		Power of the entire eye (distance vision)	59 dioptres
Thickness of the cornea	0.5 mm		
Depth of the anterior chamber	3.6 mm	Power of the cornea	43 dioptres
		Power of the lens (distance vision)	19 dioptres
Thickness of the lens	3.6 mm		
Distance between lens and retina	15.6 mm	Interpupillary distance	6 1–69 mm
Thickness of the retina	0.3 mm		

Blood vessels of the eyeball!

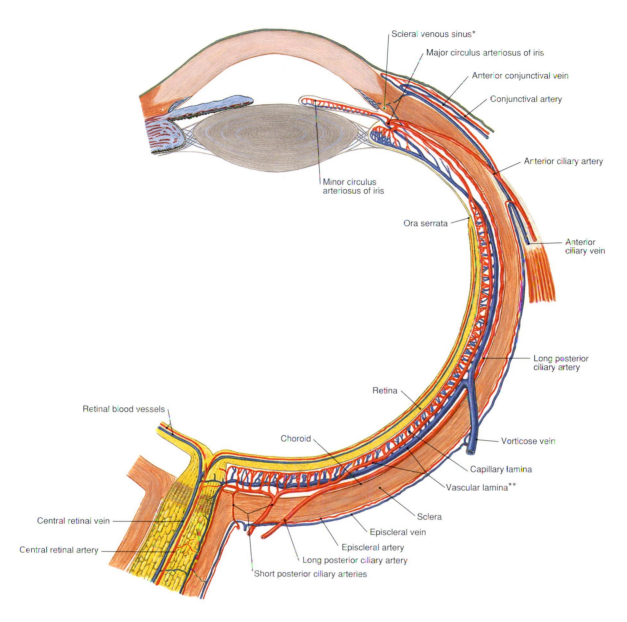

Fig. 1352 Blood vessels of the eyeball.

*   Clinical term: canal of SCHLEMM

** Clinical term: uvea

Layers of the eyeball

Fibrous layer of the eyeball
– Cornea (pronounced curvature, translucent)
– Sclera (lesser curvature, opaque; bluish-white in
  infancy, yellowish-white in senescence)

Vascular layer of the eyeball
– Iris with the central circular opening, the pupil
– Ciliary body with the ciliary muscle, the ciliary process,
  the ciliary zonule with the zonular fibres and the
  zonular spaces
– Choroid

Inner layer of the eyeball (retina)
– Nonvisual retina (from the pupillary-iridial margin, to the ora
  serrata)
    Iridial part of the retina (single-layered, heavily pigmented),
    ciliary part of the retina (single-layered, unpigmented)
– Optic part of the retina (stratified)
  1. neuron: vision cells (rod cells – brightness;
     cone cells – colour)
  2. neuron: bipolar ganglion cells within the retina
     (ganglion of the retina)
  3. neuron: multi-polar ganglion cells (optic ganglion),
     whose long axons form the optic nerve and continue in
     the optic tract

Ciliary body and iris

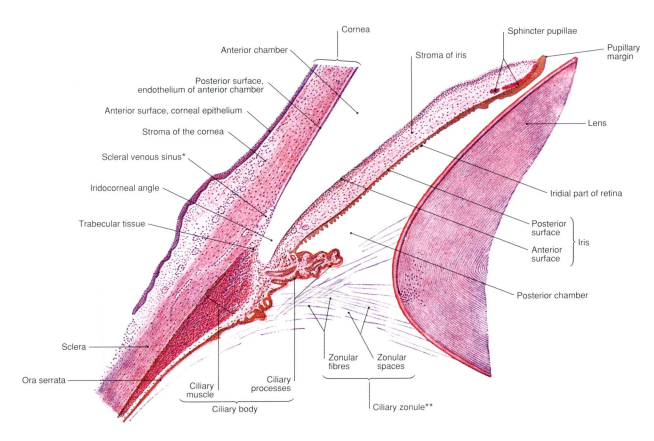

Fig. 1353   Eyeball;
schematic horizontal section at the level of
the pupil.

*   Clinical term: canal of SCHLEMM
** Clinical term: zonule of ZINN

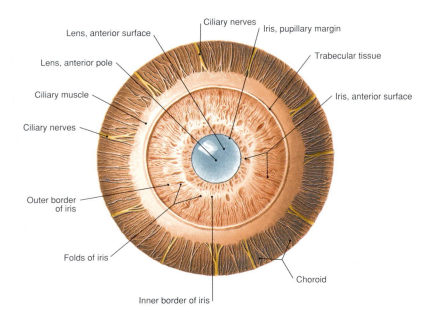

Fig. 1354   Iris and pupil;
after removal of the sclera and cornea;
anterior view.

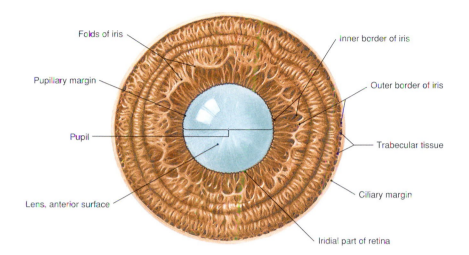

Folds of iris

Pupillary margin

Pupil

Lens, anterior surface

Inner border of iris

Outer border of iris

Trabecular tissue

Ciliary margin

Iridial part of retina

Fig. 1355   Iris;
after removal of the cornea;
anterior view.

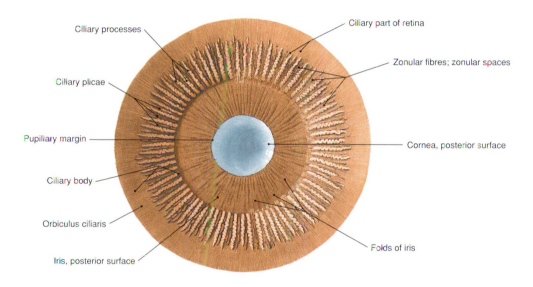

Ciliary processes

Ciliary plicae

Pupillary margin

Ciliary body

Orbiculus ciliaris

Iris, posterior surface

Ciliary part of retina

Zonular fibres; zonular spaces

Cornea, posterior surface

Folds of iris

Fig. 1356   Iris;
posterior view.

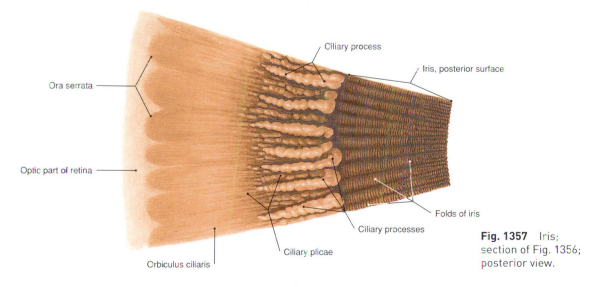

Ora serrata

Optic part of retina

Orbiculus ciliaris

Ciliary plicae

Ciliary process

Iris, posterior surface

Folds of iris

Ciliary processes

Fig. 1357   Iris;
section of Fig. 1356;
posterior view.

Lens

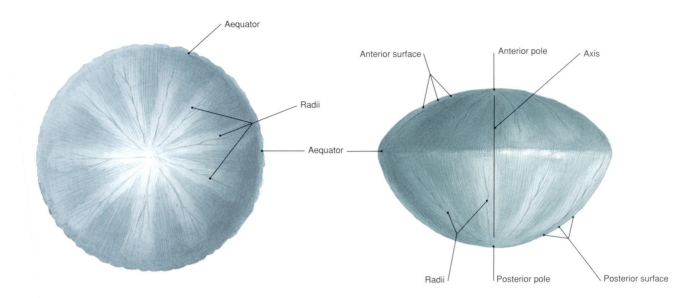

Fig. 1358 Lens;
anterior view.

Fig. 1359 Lens;
viewed from the equator.

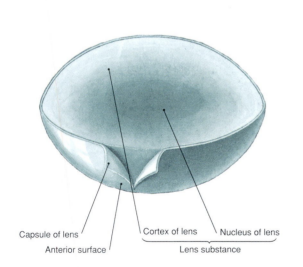

Fig. 1360 Lens;
oblique view from anterior.

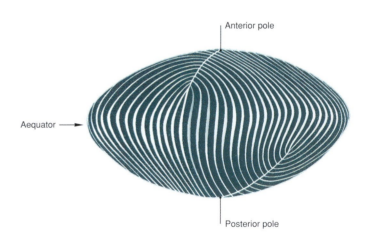

Fig. 1361 Lens;
schema of the lens fibres in a neonate;
viewed from the equator.

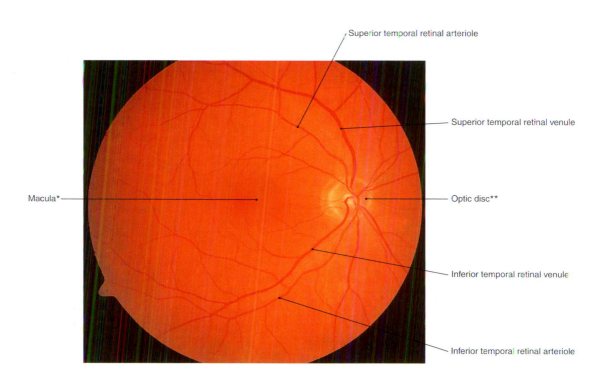

Superior temporal retinal arteriole

Superior temporal retinal venule

Optic disc**

Inferior temporal retinal venule

Inferior temporal retinal arteriole

Macula*

Fig. 1362 Ocular fundus;
ophthalmoscopic picture of the central region;
anterior view.

* Clinical term: yellow spot
** Clinical term: papilla or blind spot

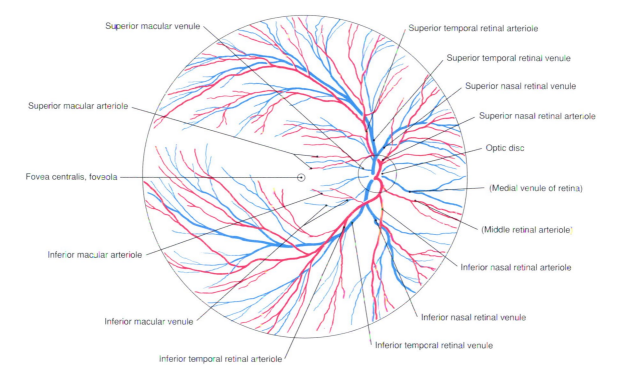

Superior macular venule

Superior temporal retinal arteriole

Superior temporal retinal venule

Superior nasal retinal venule

Superior macular arteriole

Superior nasal retinal arteriole

Optic disc

Fovea centralis, foveola

(Medial venule of retina)

(Middle retinal arteriole)

Inferior macular arteriole

Inferior nasal retinal arteriole

Inferior nasal retinal venule

Inferior macular venule

Inferior temporal retinal venule

Inferior temporal retinal arteriole

Fig. 1363 Blood vessels of the retina;
schema of the course of the vessels;
anterior view.

Optic nerve

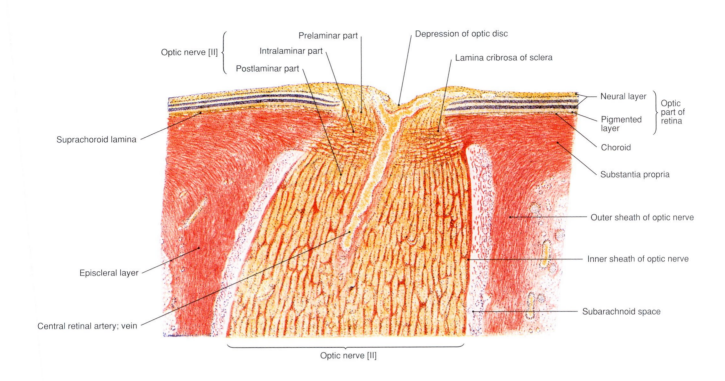

Optic nerve [II]
- Prelaminar part
- Intralaminar part
- Postlaminar part

Depression of optic disc

Lamina cribrosa of sclera

Neural layer
Pigmented layer
} Optic part of retina

Choroid

Substantia propria

Outer sheath of optic nerve

Inner sheath of optic nerve

Subarachnoid space

Suprachoroid lamina

Episcleral layer

Central retinal artery; vein

Optic nerve [II]

Fig. 1364 Optic nerve [II];
horizontal section at its exit from the eyeball.

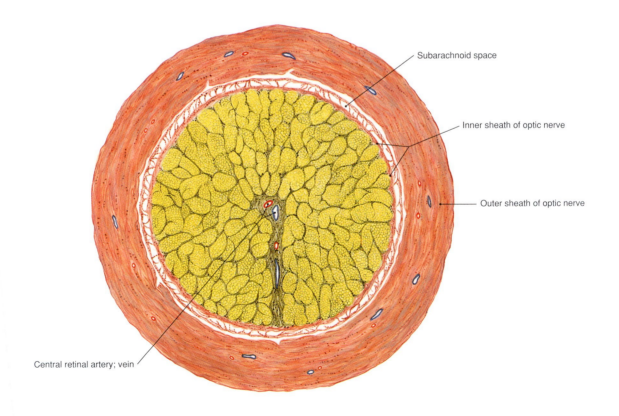

Subarachnoid space

Inner sheath of optic nerve

Outer sheath of optic nerve

Central retinal artery; vein

Fig. 1365 Optic nerve [II];
cross-section near the eyeball.

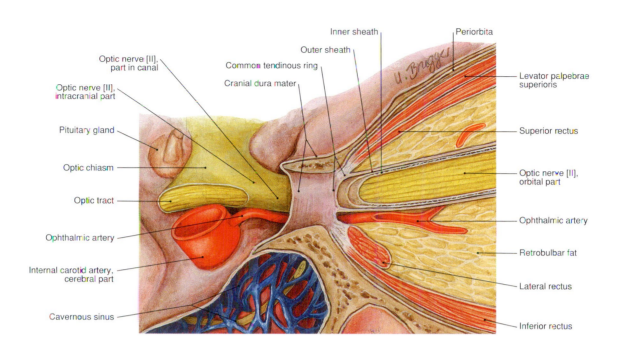

Optic nerve [II], part in canal
Optic nerve [II], intracranial part
Pituitary gland
Optic chiasm
Optic tract
Ophthalmic artery
Internal carotid artery, cerebral part
Cavernous sinus

Inner sheath
Outer sheath
Common tendinous ring
Cranial dura mater

Periorbita
Levator palpebrae superioris
Superior rectus
Optic nerve [II], orbital part
Ophthalmic artery
Retrobulbar fat
Lateral rectus
Inferior rectus

Fig. 1366 Optic nerve [II];
the optic canal has been opened;
viewed from the right.

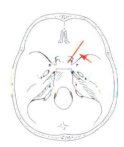

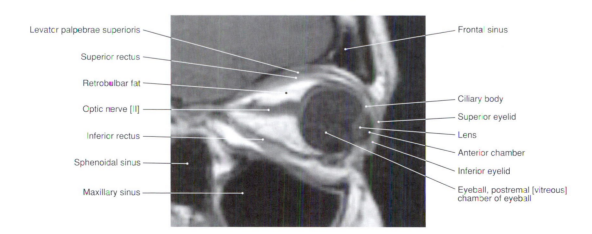

Levator palpebrae superioris
Superior rectus
Retrobulbar fat
Optic nerve [II]
Inferior rectus
Sphenoidal sinus
Maxillary sinus

Frontal sinus
Ciliary body
Superior eyelid
Lens
Anterior chamber
Inferior eyelid
Eyeball, postremal [vitreous] chamber of eyeball

Fig. 1367 Orbit;
magnetic resonance tomographic image (MRI);
vertical section along the optic nerve;
viewed from the right.

→ 1379

Optic pathway and blood vessels

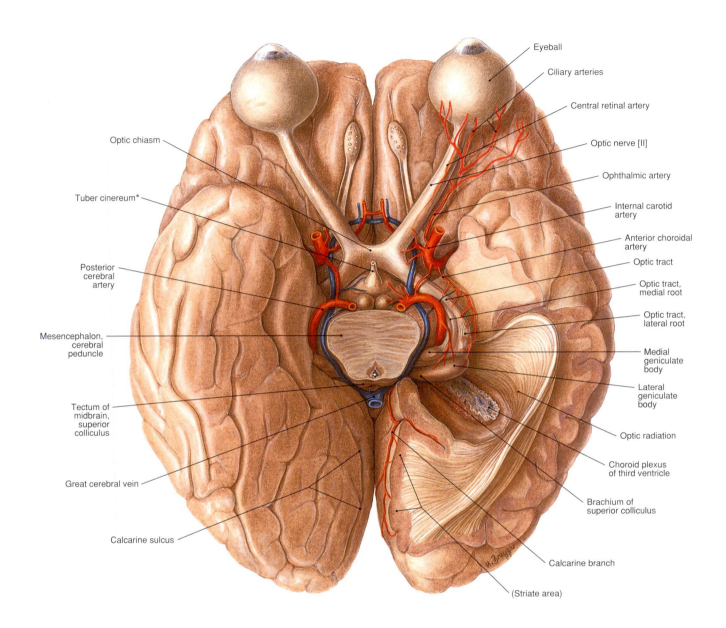

Eyeball

Ciliary arteries

Central retinal artery

Optic nerve [II]

Ophthalmic artery

Internal carotid artery

Anterior choroidal artery

Optic tract

Optic tract, medial root

Optic tract, lateral root

Medial geniculate body

Lateral geniculate body

Optic radiation

Choroid plexus of third ventricle

Brachium of superior colliculus

Calcarine branch

(Striate area)

Optic chiasm

Tuber cinereum*

Posterior cerebral artery

Mesencephalon, cerebral peduncle

Tectum of midbrain, superior colliculus

Great cerebral vein

Calcarine sulcus

Fig. 1368 Brain and blood supply of the parts of the optic pathway; inferior view.
The pituitary gland has been removed at its infundibulum (*). Due to the close proximity of the pituitary gland and the optic chiasm, pituitary tumours can cause visual disturbances.

Optic pathway

1. neuron: rod cells and cone cells of the retina
2. neuron: bipolar ganglion cells of the retina (perikarya in the retinal ganglion)
3. neuron: multi-polar ganglion cells of the retina (perikarya in the optic ganglion)
   The axons of the optic ganglion cells extend primarily to the lateral geniculate body (lateral root), although several fibres also extend to the pretectal area and the superior colliculus (medial root), as well as to the hypothalamus.

They run within the optic nerve to the optic chiasm, where the fibres from the nasal part of the ocular fundus cross to the opposite side. Each optic tract contains fibres, which transmit information from the contralateral half of the visual field.

4. neuron: Its axons travel primarily from the lateral geniculate body to areas 17 and 18 of the cerebral cortex (striate area) in the region surrounding the calcarine sulcus.

Optic pathway

1 Common visual field
1a Visual field of the left eye
1b Visual field of the right eye
2a Projection on the left retina
2b Projection on the right retina

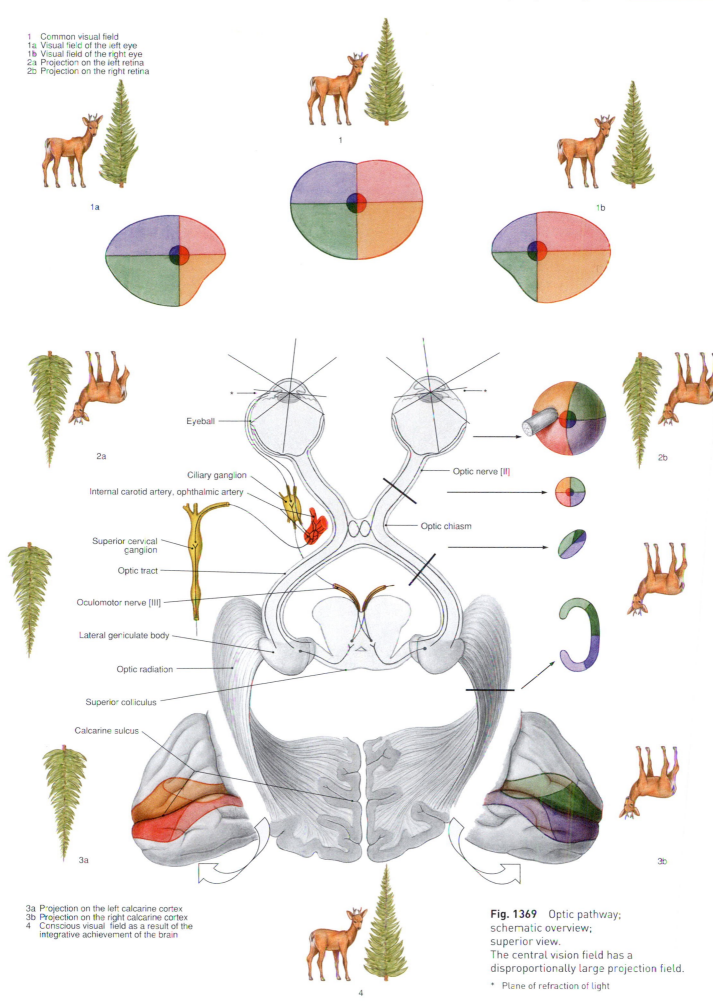

Eyeball

Ciliary ganglion

Internal carotid artery, ophthalmic artery

Superior cervical ganglion

Optic tract

Oculomotor nerve [III]

Lateral geniculate body

Optic radiation

Superior colliculus

Calcarine sulcus

Optic nerve [II]

Optic chiasm

3a Projection on the left calcarine cortex
3b Projection on the right calcarine cortex
4 Conscious visual field as a result of the
   integrative achievement of the brain

Fig. 1369 Optic pathway;
schematic overview;
superior view.
The central vision field has a
disproportionally large projection field.

* Plane of refraction of light

Orbit, topography

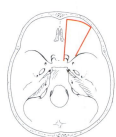

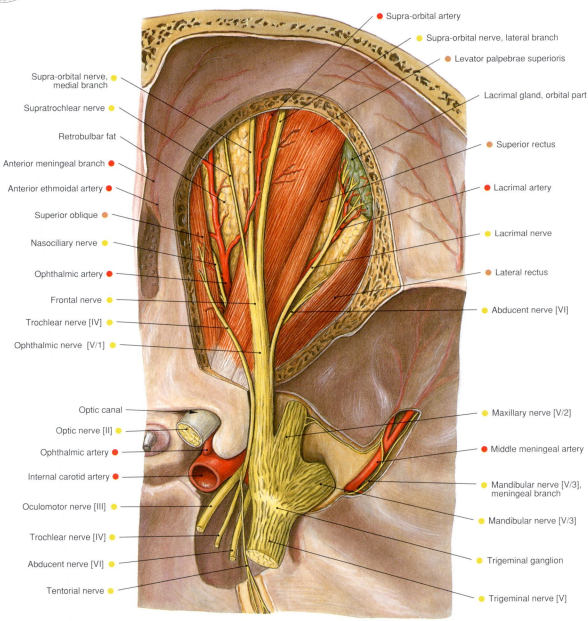

Supra-orbital artery ●

Supra-orbital nerve, lateral branch ●

Levator palpebrae superioris ●

Supra-orbital nerve, medial branch ●

Supratrochlear nerve ●

Retrobulbar fat

Anterior meningeal branch ●

Anterior ethmoidal artery ●

Superior oblique ●

Nasociliary nerve ●

Ophthalmic artery ●

Frontal nerve ●

Trochlear nerve [IV] ●

Ophthalmic nerve [V/1] ●

Lacrimal gland, orbital part

Superior rectus ●

Lacrimal artery ●

Lacrimal nerve ●

Lateral rectus ●

Abducent nerve [VI] ●

Optic canal

Optic nerve [II] ●

Ophthalmic artery ●

Internal carotid artery ●

Oculomotor nerve [III] ●

Trochlear nerve [IV] ●

Abducent nerve [VI] ●

Tentorial nerve ●

Maxillary nerve [V/2] ●

Middle meningeal artery ●

Mandibular nerve [V/3], meningeal branch ●

Mandibular nerve [V/3] ●

Trigeminal ganglion ●

Trigeminal nerve [V] ●

1371

Fig. 1370 Arteries and nerves of the orbit; superior view.

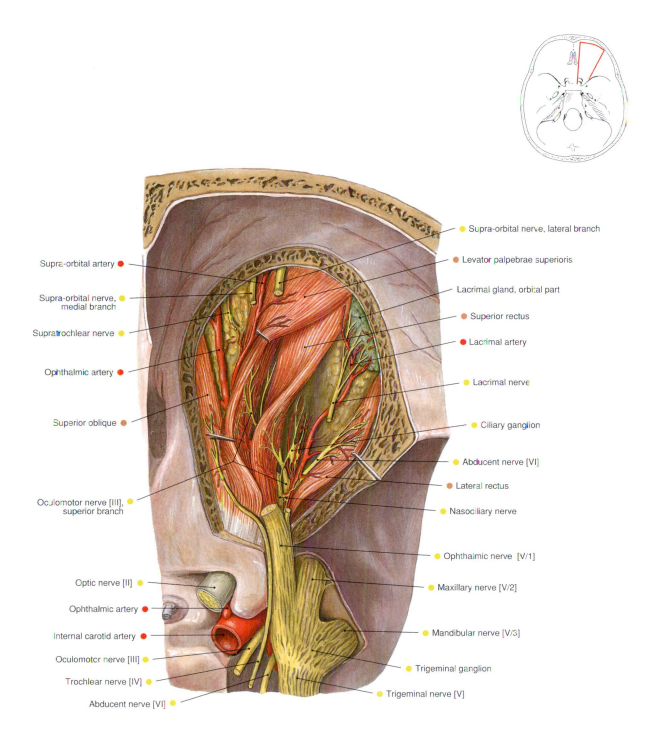

Supra-orbital artery ●

Supra-orbital nerve, medial branch ●

Supratrochlear nerve ●

Ophthalmic artery ●

Superior oblique ●

Oculomotor nerve [III], superior branch ●

Optic nerve [II] ●

Ophthalmic artery ●

Internal carotid artery ●

Oculomotor nerve [III] ●

Trochlear nerve [IV] ●

Abducent nerve [VI] ●

● Supra-orbital nerve, lateral branch

● Levator palpebrae superioris

Lacrimal gland, orbital part

● Superior rectus

● Lacrimal artery

● Lacrimal nerve

● Ciliary ganglion

● Abducent nerve [VI]

● Lateral rectus

● Nasociliary nerve

● Ophthalmic nerve [V/1]

● Maxillary nerve [V/2]

● Mandibular nerve [V/3]

● Trigeminal ganglion

● Trigeminal nerve [V]

Fig. 1371   Arteries and nerves of the orbit; after removal of the roof of the orbit; superior view.

1372

1370

Orbit, topography

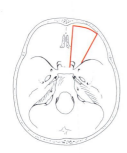

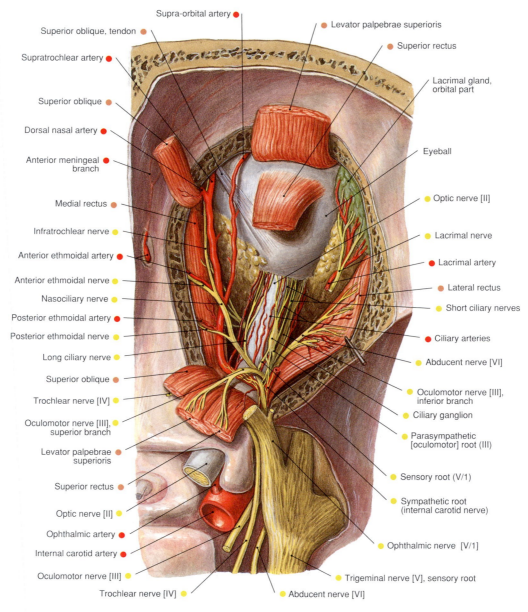

Supra-orbital artery

Superior oblique, tendon

Supratrochlear artery

Superior oblique

Dorsal nasal artery

Anterior meningeal branch

Medial rectus

Infratrochlear nerve

Anterior ethmoidal artery

Anterior ethmoidal nerve

Nasociliary nerve

Posterior ethmoidal artery

Posterior ethmoidal nerve

Long ciliary nerve

Superior oblique

Trochlear nerve [IV]

Oculomotor nerve [III], superior branch

Levator palpebrae superioris

Superior rectus

Optic nerve [II]

Ophthalmic artery

Internal carotid artery

Oculomotor nerve [III]

Trochlear nerve [IV]

Levator palpebrae superioris

Superior rectus

Lacrimal gland, orbital part

Eyeball

Optic nerve [II]

Lacrimal nerve

Lacrimal artery

Lateral rectus

Short ciliary nerves

Ciliary arteries

Abducent nerve [VI]

Oculomotor nerve [III], inferior branch

Ciliary ganglion

Parasympathetic [oculomotor] root (III)

Sensory root (V/1)

Sympathetic root (internal carotid nerve)

Ophthalmic nerve [V/1]

Trigeminal nerve [V], sensory root

Abducent nerve [VI]

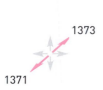

1373

1371

Fig. 1372 Arteries and nerves of the orbit; after partial removal of the levator palpebrae superioris, the rectus superior and the obliquus superior muscle; superior view.

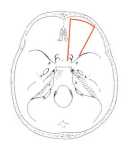

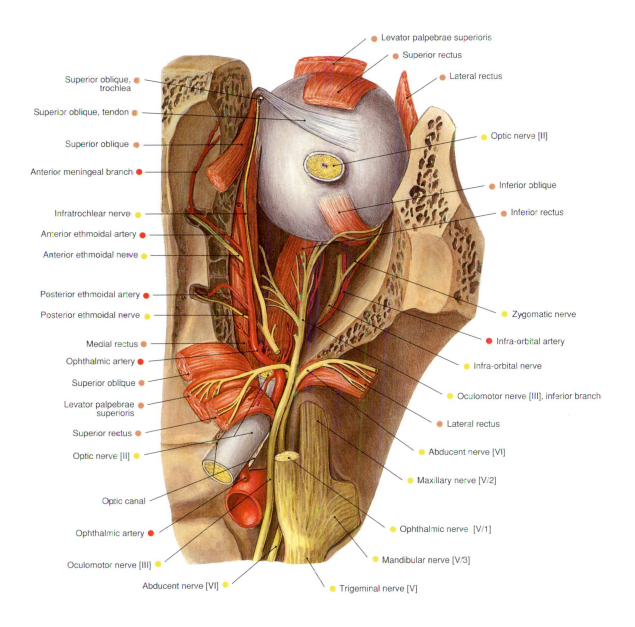

Levator palpebrae superioris
Superior rectus
Lateral rectus

Superior oblique, trochlea

Superior oblique, tendon

Superior oblique

Anterior meningeal branch

Optic nerve [II]

Inferior oblique

Inferior rectus

Infratrochlear nerve

Anterior ethmoidal artery

Anterior ethmoidal nerve

Posterior ethmoidal artery

Posterior ethmoidal nerve

Zygomatic nerve

Infra-orbital artery

Medial rectus

Ophthalmic artery

Superior oblique

Levator palpebrae superioris

Superior rectus

Optic nerve [II]

Infra-orbital nerve

Oculomotor nerve [III], inferior branch

Lateral rectus

Abducent nerve [VI]

Maxillary nerve [V/2]

Optic canal

Ophthalmic artery

Ophthalmic nerve [V/1]

Mandibular nerve [V/3]

Oculomotor nerve [III]

Abducent nerve [VI]

Trigeminal nerve [V]

Fig. 1373 Arteries and nerves of the orbit; after removal of the roof of the orbit; superior view.

1372

Blood vessels of the orbit

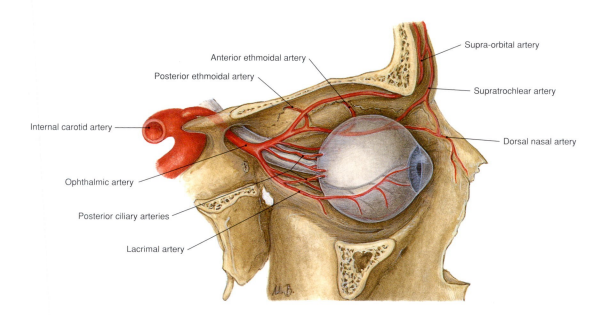

Anterior ethmoidal artery

Posterior ethmoidal artery

Internal carotid artery

Ophthalmic artery

Posterior ciliary arteries

Lacrimal artery

Supra-orbital artery

Supratrochlear artery

Dorsal nasal artery

Fig. 1374 Arteries of the orbit;
lateral view.

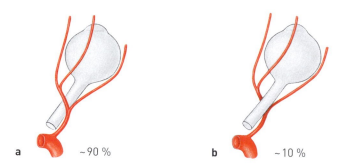

a ~90 %

b ~10 %

Fig. 1375 a, b Variations of the ophthalmic artery;
superior view.

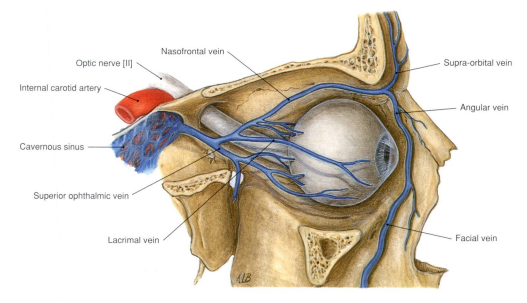

Optic nerve [II]

Internal carotid artery

Nasofrontal vein

Cavernous sinus

Superior ophthalmic vein

Lacrimal vein

Supra-orbital vein

Angular vein

Facial vein

Fig. 1376 Veins of the orbit;
lateral view.

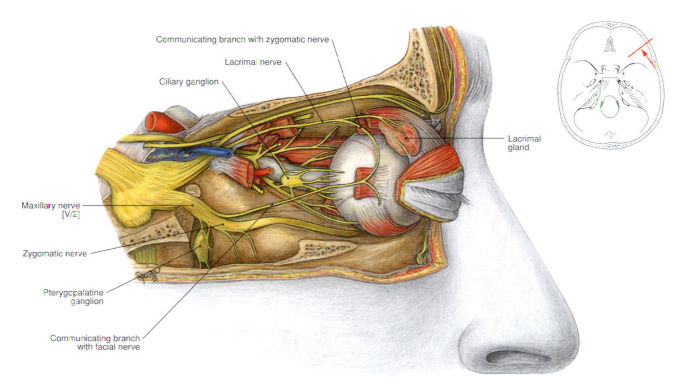

Communicating branch with zygomatic nerve

Lacrimal nerve

Ciliary ganglion

Lacrimal gland

Maxillary nerve [V/2]

Zygomatic nerve

Pterygopalatine ganglion

Communicating branch with facial nerve

Fig. 1377 Orbit;
viewed from the right.

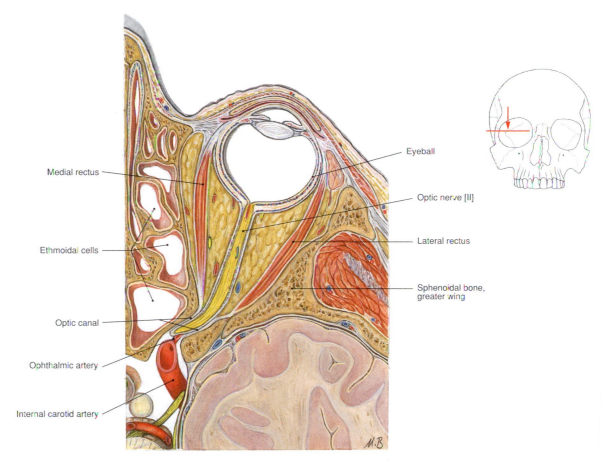

Medial rectus

Eyeball

Optic nerve [II]

Lateral rectus

Ethmoidal cells

Sphenoidal bone, greater wing

Optic canal

Ophthalmic artery

Internal carotid artery

Fig. 1378 Orbit;
horizontal section;
superior view.

Orbit, sections

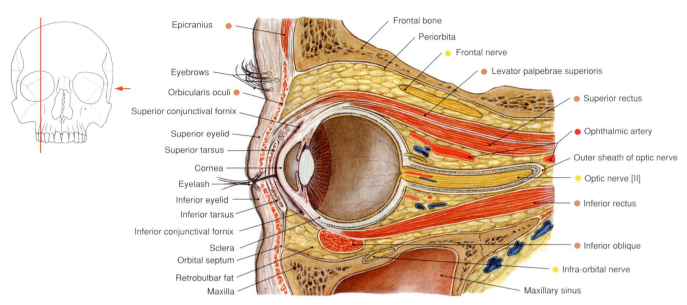

Epicranius
Eyebrows
Orbicularis oculi
Superior conjunctival fornix
Superior eyelid
Superior tarsus
Cornea
Eyelash
Inferior eyelid
Inferior tarsus
Inferior conjunctival fornix
Sclera
Orbital septum
Retrobulbar fat
Maxilla

Frontal bone
Periorbita
Frontal nerve
Levator palpebrae superioris
Superior rectus
Ophthalmic artery
Outer sheath of optic nerve
Optic nerve [II]
Inferior rectus
Inferior oblique
Infra-orbital nerve
Maxillary sinus

Fig. 1379 Orbit;
vertical section through the eyeball and the optic nerve;
medial view.

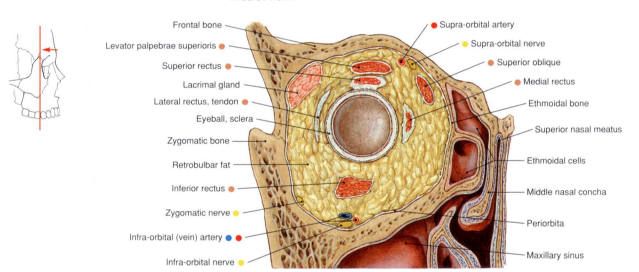

Frontal bone
Levator palpebrae superioris
Superior rectus
Lacrimal gland
Lateral rectus, tendon
Eyeball, sclera
Zygomatic bone
Retrobulbar fat
Inferior rectus
Zygomatic nerve
Infra-orbital (vein) artery
Infra-orbital nerve

Supra-orbital artery
Supra-orbital nerve
Superior oblique
Medial rectus
Ethmoidal bone
Superior nasal meatus
Ethmoidal cells
Middle nasal concha
Periorbita
Maxillary sinus

Fig. 1380 Orbit;
frontal section at the level of the posterior part of the eyeball;
anterior view.

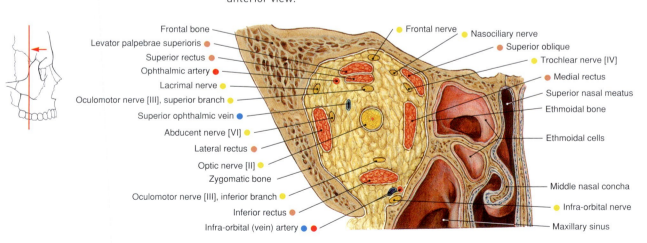

Frontal bone
Levator palpebrae superioris
Superior rectus
Ophthalmic artery
Lacrimal nerve
Oculomotor nerve [III], superior branch
Superior ophthalmic vein
Abducent nerve [VI]
Lateral rectus
Optic nerve [II]
Zygomatic bone
Oculomotor nerve [III], inferior branch
Inferior rectus
Infra-orbital (vein) artery

Frontal nerve
Nasociliary nerve
Superior oblique
Trochlear nerve [IV]
Medial rectus
Superior nasal meatus
Ethmoidal bone
Ethmoidal cells
Middle nasal concha
Infra-orbital nerve
Maxillary sinus

Fig. 1381 Orbit;
frontal section at the level of the middle of the extracranial
course of the optic nerve;
anterior view.

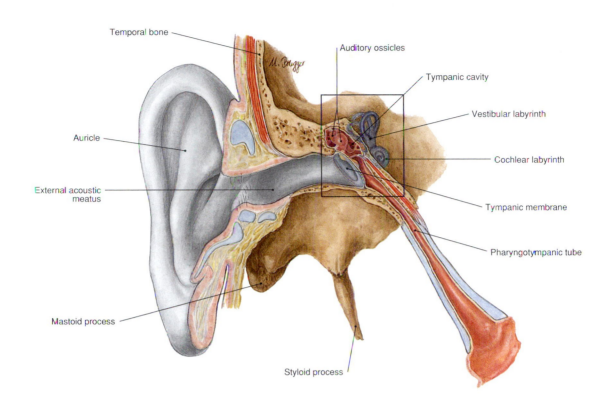

Fig. 1382   Ear.

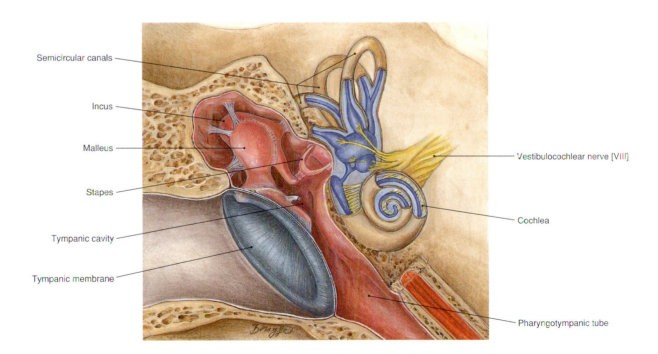

Fig. 1383   Middle and inner ear;
section from Fig. 1382;
anterior view.

Auricle

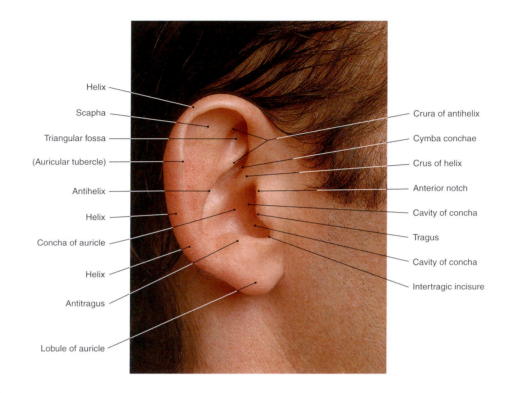

Helix
Scapha
Triangular fossa
(Auricular tubercle)
Antihelix
Helix
Concha of auricle
Helix
Antitragus
Lobule of auricle

Crura of antihelix
Cymba conchae
Crus of helix
Anterior notch
Cavity of concha
Tragus
Cavity of concha
Intertragic incisure

Fig. 1384 Auricle.

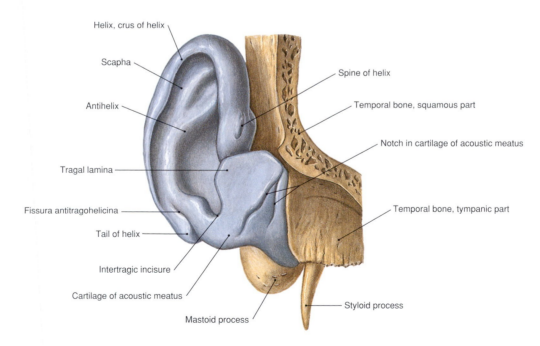

Helix, crus of helix
Scapha
Antihelix
Tragal lamina
Fissura antitragohelicina
Tail of helix
Intertragic incisure
Cartilage of acoustic meatus
Mastoid process

Spine of helix
Temporal bone, squamous part
Notch in cartilage of acoustic meatus
Temporal bone, tympanic part
Styloid process

Fig. 1385 Auricular cartilage.

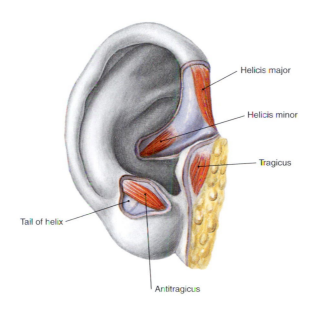

Fig. 1386 Auricular muscles.

Helicis major

Helicis minor

Tragicus

Tail of helix

Antitragicus

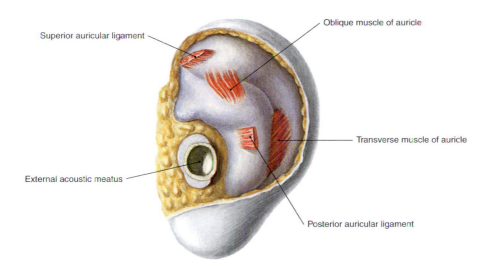

Fig. 1387 Auricular muscles.

Superior auricular ligament

Oblique muscle of auricle

Transverse muscle of auricle

External acoustic meatus

Posterior auricular ligament

External acoustic meatus and tympanic membrane

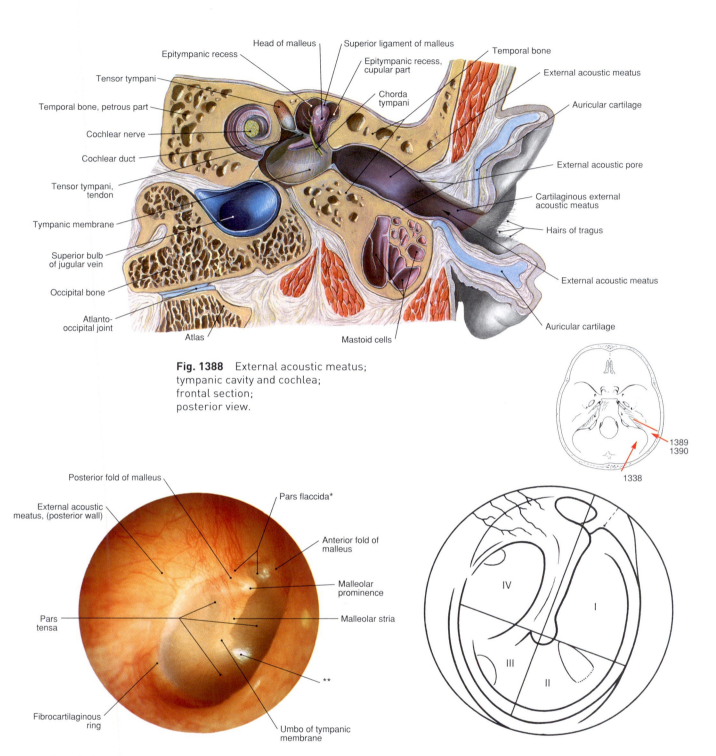

Head of malleus

Superior ligament of malleus

Epitympanic recess

Tensor tympani

Epitympanic recess, cupular part

Temporal bone

Temporal bone, petrous part

Chorda tympani

External acoustic meatus

Cochlear nerve

Auricular cartilage

Cochlear duct

External acoustic pore

Tensor tympani, tendon

Cartilaginous external acoustic meatus

Tympanic membrane

Hairs of tragus

Superior bulb of jugular vein

External acoustic meatus

Occipital bone

Atlanto-occipital joint

Auricular cartilage

Atlas

Mastoid cells

Fig. 1388 External acoustic meatus; tympanic cavity and cochlea; frontal section; posterior view.

1389
1390

1338

Posterior fold of malleus

Pars flaccida*

External acoustic meatus, (posterior wall)

Anterior fold of malleus

Malleolar prominence

Pars tensa

Malleolar stria

**

Fibrocartilaginous ring

Umbo of tympanic membrane

Fig. 1389 Tympanic membrane; otoscopic image; lateral view.

* Clinical term: SHRAPNELL's membrane
** Typically occurring reflection of light

IV

I

III

II

Fig. 1390 Tympanic membrane; quadrant schema; lateral view.

In order to obtain a complete otoscopic overview of the cutaneous surface of the tympanic membrane, the external acoustic meatus must be stretched by pulling the auricle upwards and posteriorly.
To facilitate orientation, the tympanic membrane is usually divided into four quadrants (I–IV).

The longer diameter of the tympanic membrane in the adult is 10–11 mm, the shorter diameter is approx. 9 mm. The light source characteristically produces a triangular reflection of light at the umbo in the region of quadrant II.

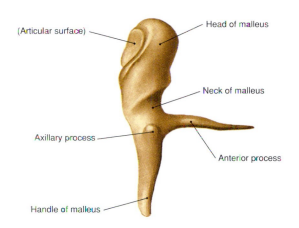

(Articular surface)

Head of malleus

Neck of malleus

Axillary process

Anterior process

Handle of malleus

Fig. 1391 Malleus; lateral view.

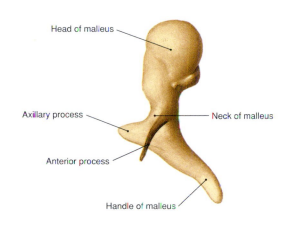

Head of malleus

Axillary process

Neck of malleus

Anterior process

Handle of malleus

Fig. 1392 Malleus; anterior view.

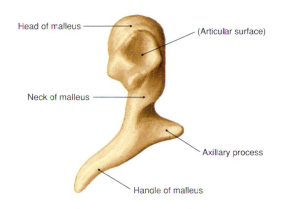

Head of malleus

(Articular surface)

Neck of malleus

Axillary process

Handle of malleus

Fig. 1393 Malleus; posterior view.

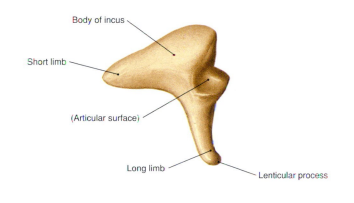

Body of incus

Short limb

(Articular surface)

Long limb

Lenticular process

Fig. 1394 Incus; lateral view.

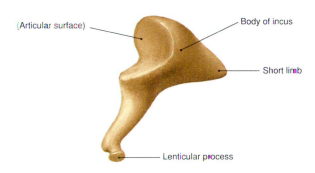

(Articular surface)

Body of incus

Short limb

Lenticular process

Fig. 1395 Incus; medial view.

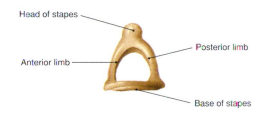

Head of stapes

Anterior limb

Posterior limb

Base of stapes

Fig. 1396 Stapes; superior view.

Auditory ossicles

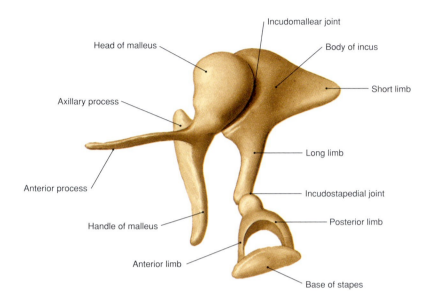

Incudomallear joint

Head of malleus

Body of incus

Short limb

Axillary process

Long limb

Anterior process

Incudostapedial joint

Handle of malleus

Posterior limb

Anterior limb

Base of stapes

Fig. 1397 Auditory ossicles;
superomedial view.

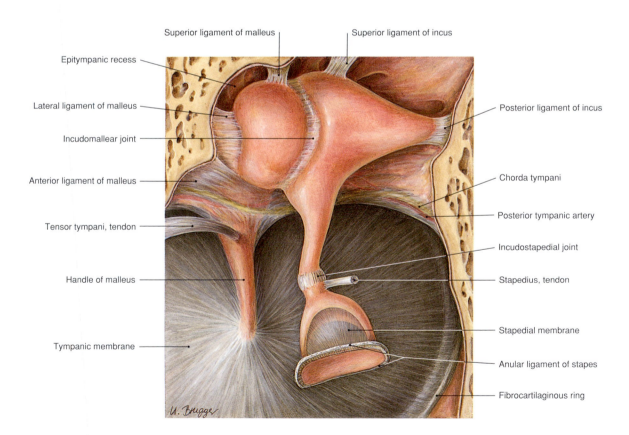

Superior ligament of malleus

Superior ligament of incus

Epitympanic recess

Lateral ligament of malleus

Posterior ligament of incus

Incudomallear joint

Anterior ligament of malleus

Chorda tympani

Posterior tympanic artery

Tensor tympani, tendon

Incudostapedial joint

Handle of malleus

Stapedius, tendon

Stapedial membrane

Tympanic membrane

Anular ligament of stapes

Fibrocartilaginous ring

Fig. 1398 Joints and ligaments of the auditory ossicles;
covered with mucosa;
superomedial view.

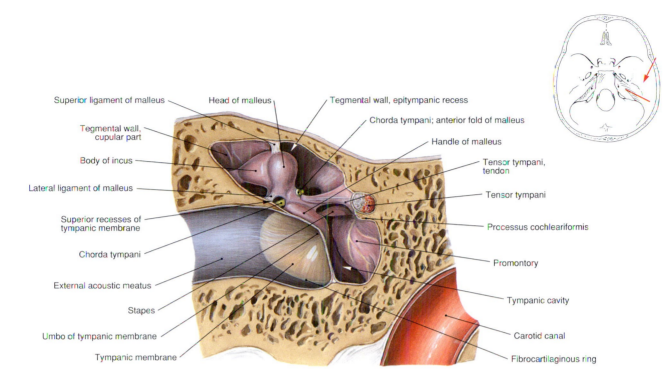

Superior ligament of malleus
Tegmental wall, cupular part
Body of incus
Lateral ligament of malleus
Superior recesses of tympanic membrane
Chorda tympani
External acoustic meatus
Stapes
Umbo of tympanic membrane
Tympanic membrane

Head of malleus
Tegmental wall, epitympanic recess
Chorda tympani; anterior fold of malleus
Handle of malleus
Tensor tympani, tendon
Tensor tympani
Processus cochleariformis
Promontory
Tympanic cavity
Carotid canal
Fibrocartilaginous ring

Fig. 1399 Tympanic cavity; frontal section; anterior view.

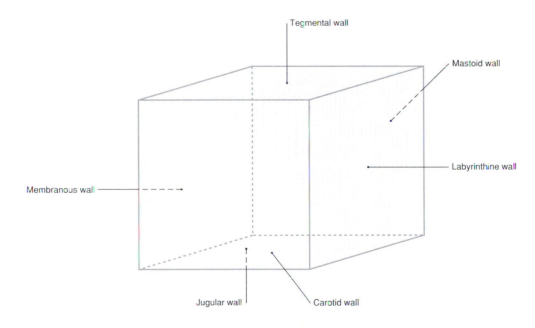

Tegmental wall
Mastoid wall
Labyrinthine wall
Membranous wall
Jugular wall
Carotid wall

Fig. 1400 Walls of the tympanic cavity; schema for orientation.

Tympanic cavity

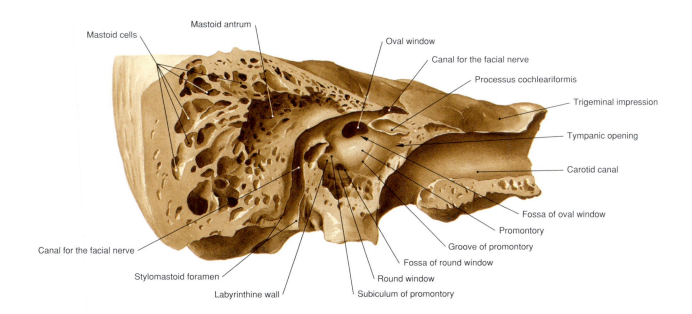

Mastoid cells

Mastoid antrum

Oval window

Canal for the facial nerve

Processus cochleariformis

Trigeminal impression

Tympanic opening

Carotid canal

Fossa of oval window

Promontory

Groove of promontory

Fossa of round window

Round window

Subiculum of promontory

Labyrinthine wall

Stylomastoid foramen

Canal for the facial nerve

Fig. 1401 Medial wall of the tympanic cavity;
after removal of the lateral wall and the adjacent parts of the
anterior and superior wall;
the facial canal and the carotid canal have been opened;
anterolateral view.

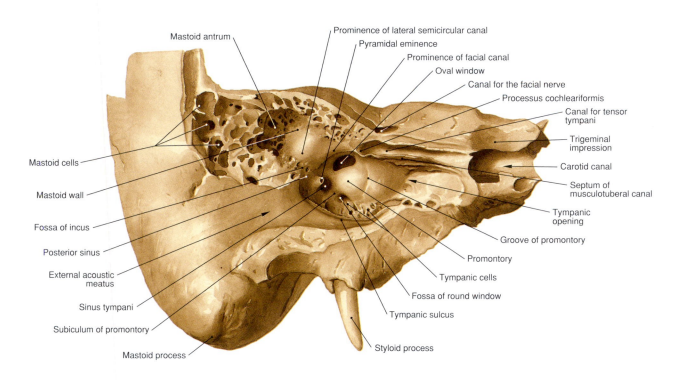

Mastoid antrum

Prominence of lateral semicircular canal

Pyramidal eminence

Prominence of facial canal

Oval window

Canal for the facial nerve

Processus cochleariformis

Canal for tensor tympani

Trigeminal impression

Carotid canal

Septum of musculotuberal canal

Tympanic opening

Groove of promontory

Promontory

Tympanic cells

Fossa of round window

Tympanic sulcus

Styloid process

Mastoid cells

Mastoid wall

Fossa of incus

Posterior sinus

External acoustic meatus

Sinus tympani

Subiculum of promontory

Mastoid process

Fig. 1402 Medial wall of the tympanic cavity;
vertical section along the longitudinal axis of the petrous part of
the temporal bone;
anterolateral view.

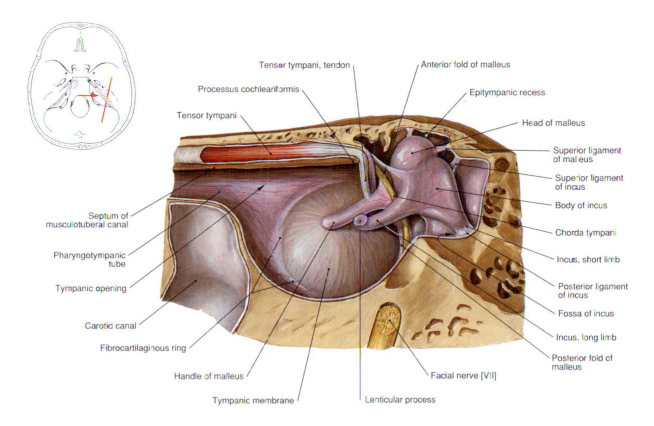

Tensor tympani, tendon
Anterior fold of malleus
Processus cochleariformis
Epitympanic recess
Tensor tympani
Head of malleus
Superior ligament of malleus
Superior ligament of incus
Body of incus
Septum of musculotuberal canal
Chorda tympani
Pharyngotympanic tube
Incus, short limb
Tympanic opening
Posterior ligament of incus
Carotid canal
Fossa of incus
Fibrocartilaginous ring
Incus, long limb
Posterior fold of malleus
Handle of malleus
Facial nerve [VII]
Tympanic membrane
Lenticular process

Fig. 1403 Lateral wall of the tympanic cavity; medial view.

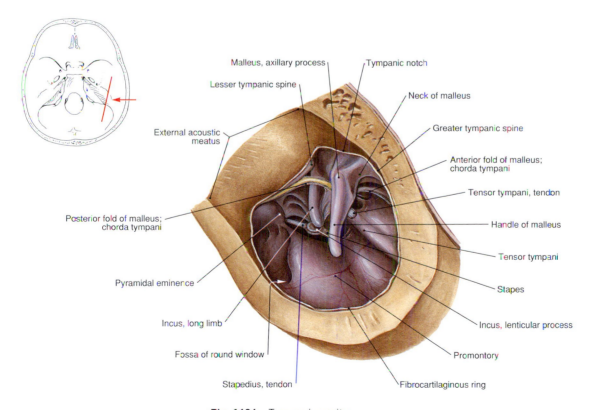

Malleus, axillary process
Tympanic notch
Lesser tympanic spine
Neck of malleus
Greater tympanic spine
External acoustic meatus
Anterior fold of malleus; chorda tympani
Tensor tympani, tendon
Posterior fold of malleus; chorda tympani
Handle of malleus
Tensor tympani
Pyramidal eminence
Stapes
Incus, long limb
Incus, lenticular process
Fossa of round window
Promontory
Stapedius, tendon
Fibrocartilaginous ring

Fig. 1404 Tympanic cavity; after removal of the tympanic membrane; lateral view.

Auditory tube

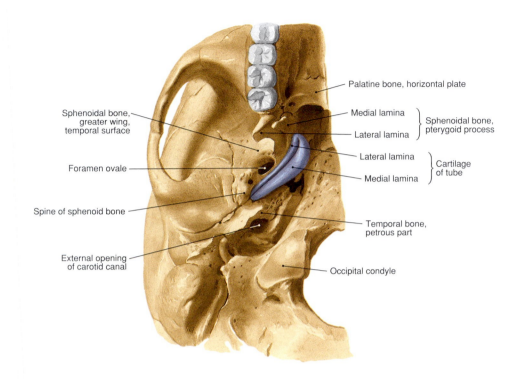

Fig. 1405 Cartilage of the auditory tube;
exposed at the base of the skull;
inferior view.

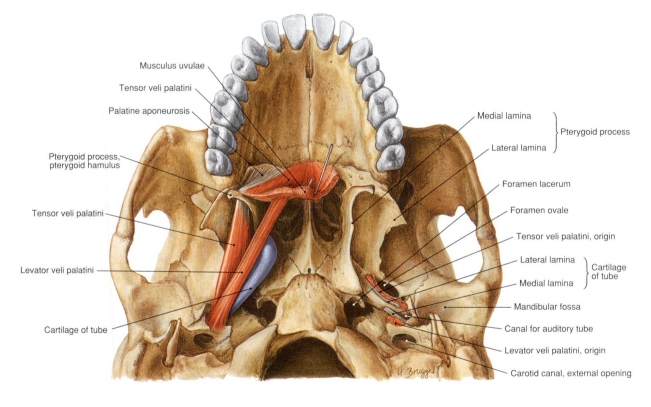

→ 246, 249, T 3
Fig. 1406 Levator and tensor veli palatini muscles
and the cartilage of the auditory tube.

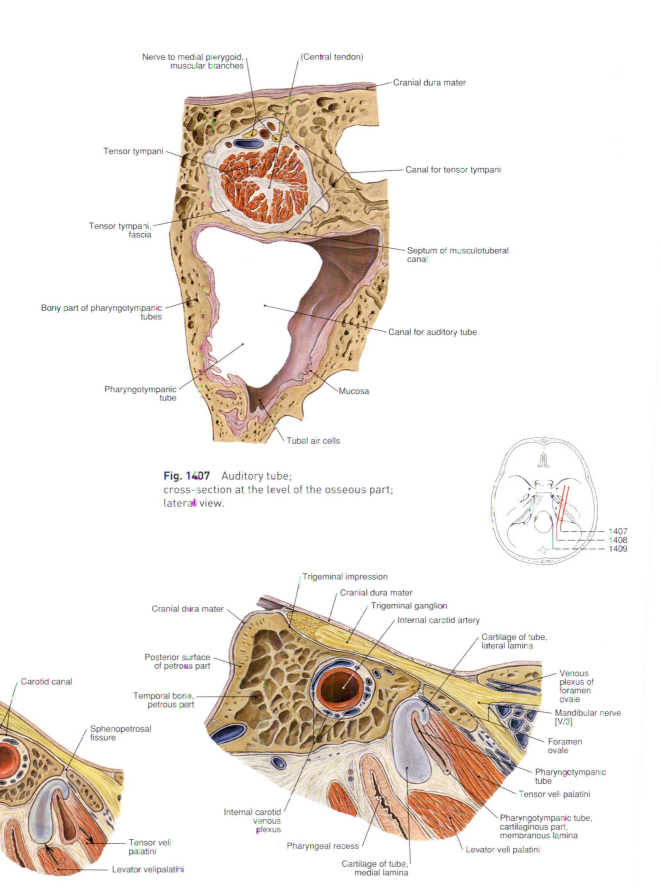

Nerve to medial pterygoid, muscular branches

(Central tendon)

Cranial dura mater

Tensor tympani

Canal for tensor tympani

Tensor tympani, fascia

Septum of musculotuberal canal

Bony part of pharyngotympanic tubes

Canal for auditory tube

Pharyngotympanic tube

Mucosa

Tubal air cells

Fig. 1407 Auditory tube; cross-section at the level of the osseous part; lateral view.

1407
1408
1409

Trigeminal impression

Cranial dura mater

Cranial dura mater

Trigeminal ganglion

Internal carotid artery

Posterior surface of petrous part

Cartilage of tube, lateral lamina

Carotid canal

Temporal bone, petrous part

Venous plexus of foramen ovale

Sphenopetrosal fissure

Mandibular nerve [V/3]

Foramen ovale

Pharyngotympanic tube

Tensor veli palatini

Internal carotid venous plexus

Pharyngotympanic tube, cartilaginous part, membranous lamina

Tensor veli palatini

Pharyngeal recess

Levator veli palatini

Levator velipalatini

Cartilage of tube, medial lamina

Fig. 1408 Auditory tube; cross-section at the level of the lateral aspect of the cartilaginous part; lateral view.

Fig. 1409 Auditory tube; cross-section at the level of the medial aspect of the cartilaginous part; lateral view.

Bony labyrinth

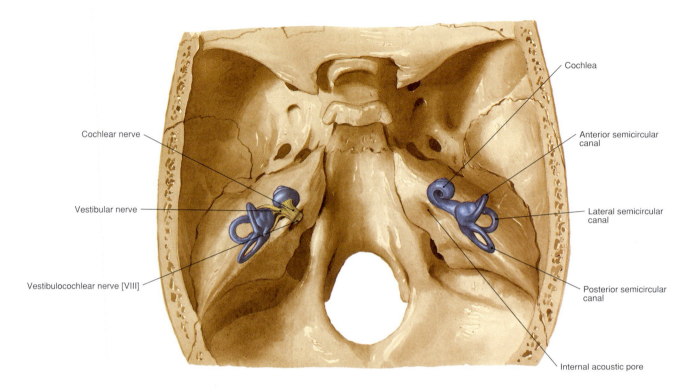

Cochlear nerve

Vestibular nerve

Vestibulocochlear nerve [VIII]

Cochlea

Anterior semicircular canal

Lateral semicircular canal

Posterior semicircular canal

Internal acoustic pore

Fig. 1410 Inner ear and vestibulocochlear nerve [VIII]; cast specimen projected onto the petrous part of the temporal bone illustrating its natural position; superior view.

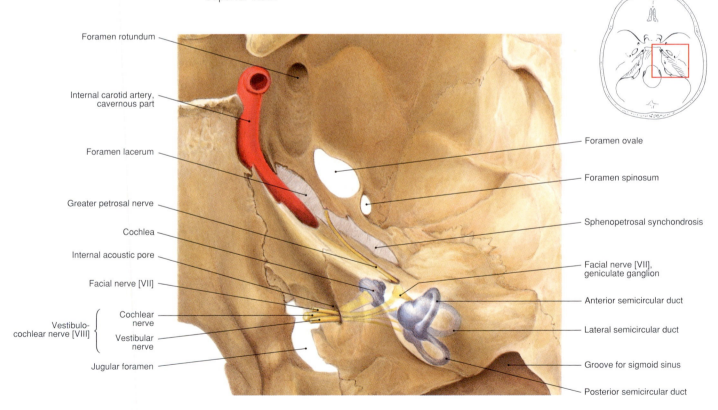

Foramen rotundum

Internal carotid artery, cavernous part

Foramen lacerum

Greater petrosal nerve

Cochlea

Internal acoustic pore

Facial nerve [VII]

Vestibulo-cochlear nerve [VIII] { Cochlear nerve

Vestibular nerve

Jugular foramen

Foramen ovale

Foramen spinosum

Sphenopetrosal synchondrosis

Facial nerve [VII], geniculate ganglion

Anterior semicircular duct

Lateral semicircular duct

Groove for sigmoid sinus

Posterior semicircular duct

→ 1173

Fig. 1411 Inner ear with the facial nerve and the vestibulocochlear nerve; projected onto the petrous part of the temporal bone; superior view.

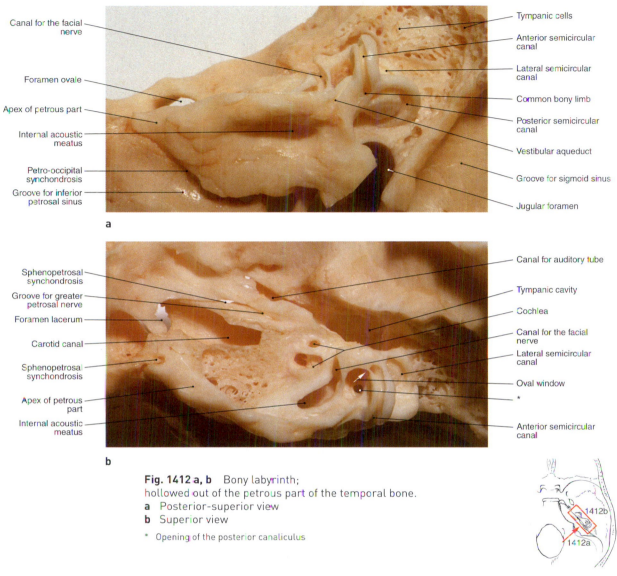

Canal for the facial nerve

Foramen ovale

Apex of petrous part

Internal acoustic meatus

Petro-occipital synchondrosis

Groove for inferior petrosal sinus

Tympanic cells

Anterior semicircular canal

Lateral semicircular canal

Common bony limb

Posterior semicircular canal

Vestibular aqueduct

Groove for sigmoid sinus

Jugular foramen

a

Sphenopetrosal synchondrosis

Groove for greater petrosal nerve

Foramen lacerum

Carotid canal

Sphenopetrosal synchondrosis

Apex of petrous part

Internal acoustic meatus

Canal for auditory tube

Tympanic cavity

Cochlea

Canal for the facial nerve

Lateral semicircular canal

Oval window

*

Anterior semicircular canal

b

Fig. 1412 a, b Bony labyrinth;
hollowed out of the petrous part of the temporal bone.
a Posterior-superior view
b Superior view

* Opening of the posterior canaliculus

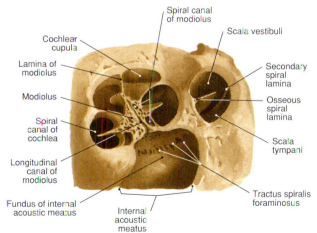

Spiral canal of modiolus

Cochlear cupula

Lamina of modiolus

Modiolus

Spiral canal of cochlea

Longitudinal canal of modiolus

Fundus of internal acoustic meatus

Internal acoustic meatus

Scala vestibuli

Secondary spiral lamina

Osseous spiral lamina

Scala tympani

Tractus spiralis foraminosus

Fig. 1413 Spiral canal of the cochlea;
opened along the axis of the modiolus;
superior view.

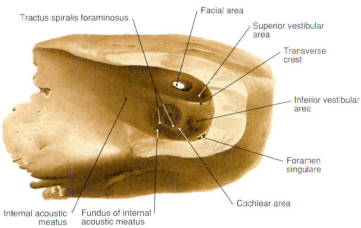

Tractus spiralis foraminosus

Facial area

Superior vestibular area

Transverse crest

Inferior vestibular area

Foramen singulare

Cochlear area

Internal acoustic meatus

Fundus of internal acoustic meatus

Fig. 1414 Internal acoustic meatus
and fundus of the internal acoustic meatus;
after partial removal of the posterior wall;
medial view.

→ 1173

Bony labyrinth

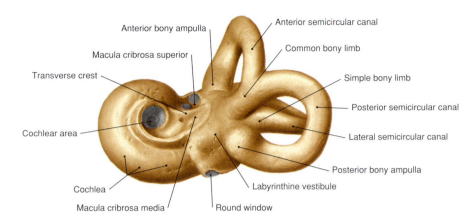

Fig. 1415 Bony labyrinth;
the osseous lining of the membranous labyrinth has been
hollowed out of the petrous part of the temporal bone;
oblique view from posterior.

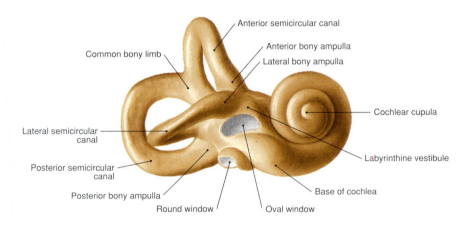

Fig. 1416 Bony labyrinth;
the osseous lining of the membranous labyrinth has been
hollowed out of the petrous part of the temporal bone;
lateral view.

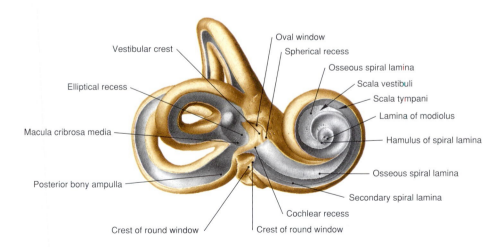

Fig. 1417 Bony labyrinth;
cavities have been hollowed out;
anterolateral view.

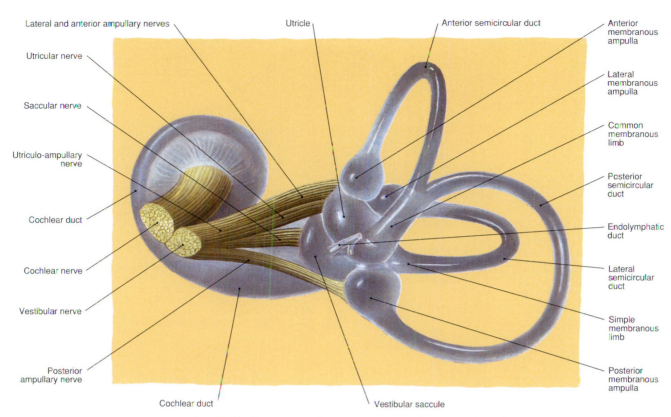

Lateral and anterior ampullary nerves

Utricular nerve

Saccular nerve

Utriculo-ampullary nerve

Cochlear duct

Cochlear nerve

Vestibular nerve

Posterior ampullary nerve

Cochlear duct

Utricle

Vestibular saccule

Anterior semicircular duct

Anterior membranous ampulla

Lateral membranous ampulla

Common membranous limb

Posterior semicircular duct

Endolymphatic duct

Lateral semicircular duct

Simple membranous limb

Posterior membranous ampulla

Fig. 1418 Vestibulocochlear nerve and membranous labyrinth; semi-schematic overview; posterior view.

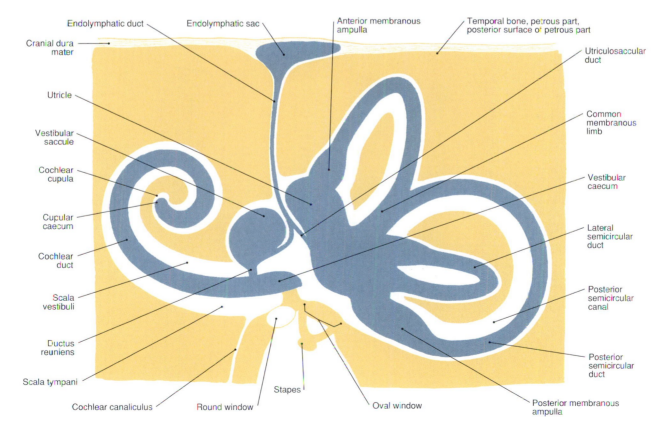

Endolymphatic duct

Cranial dura mater

Utricle

Vestibular saccule

Cochlear cupula

Cupular caecum

Cochlear duct

Scala vestibuli

Ductus reuniens

Scala tympani

Cochlear canaliculus

Endolymphatic sac

Round window

Stapes

Anterior membranous ampulla

Temporal bone, petrous part, posterior surface of petrous part

Utriculosaccular duct

Common membranous limb

Vestibular caecum

Lateral semicircular duct

Posterior semicircular canal

Posterior semicircular duct

Oval window

Posterior membranous ampulla

Fig. 1419 Membranous labyrinth; overview.

Cochlea

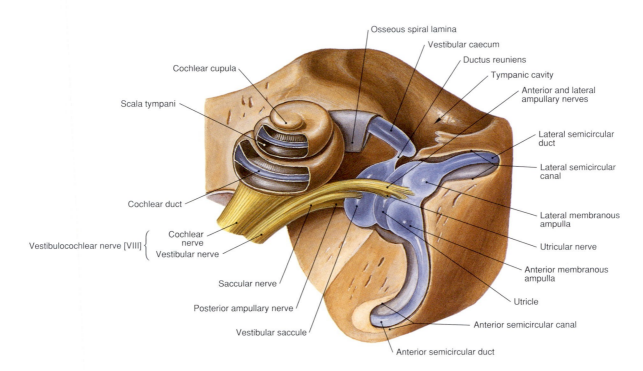

Fig. 1420 Vestibulocochlear nerve and membranous labyrinth; superior view.

Osseous spiral lamina
Vestibular caecum
Ductus reuniens
Tympanic cavity
Anterior and lateral ampullary nerves
Lateral semicircular duct
Lateral semicircular canal
Lateral membranous ampulla
Utricular nerve
Anterior membranous ampulla
Utricle
Anterior semicircular canal

Cochlear cupula
Scala tympani
Cochlear duct
Vestibulocochlear nerve [VIII] { Cochlear nerve / Vestibular nerve
Saccular nerve
Posterior ampullary nerve
Vestibular saccule
Anterior semicircular duct

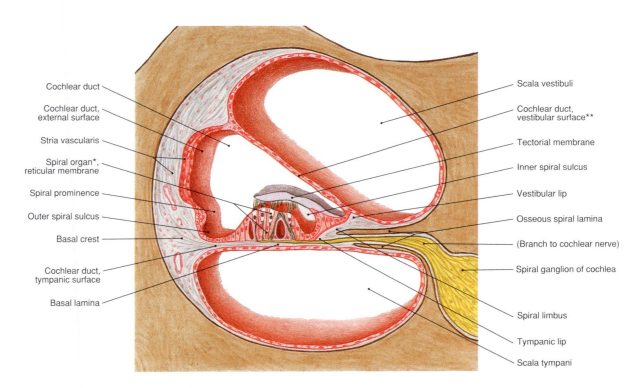

Fig. 1421 Cochlea with the spiral organ.

* Clinical term: organ of CORTI
** Clinical term: REISSNER's membrane

Cochlear duct
Cochlear duct, external surface
Stria vascularis
Spiral organ*, reticular membrane
Spiral prominence
Outer spiral sulcus
Basal crest
Cochlear duct, tympanic surface
Basal lamina

Scala vestibuli
Cochlear duct, vestibular surface**
Tectorial membrane
Inner spiral sulcus
Vestibular lip
Osseous spiral lamina
(Branch to cochlear nerve)
Spiral ganglion of cochlea
Spiral limbus
Tympanic lip
Scala tympani

Equilibrium organ, structure

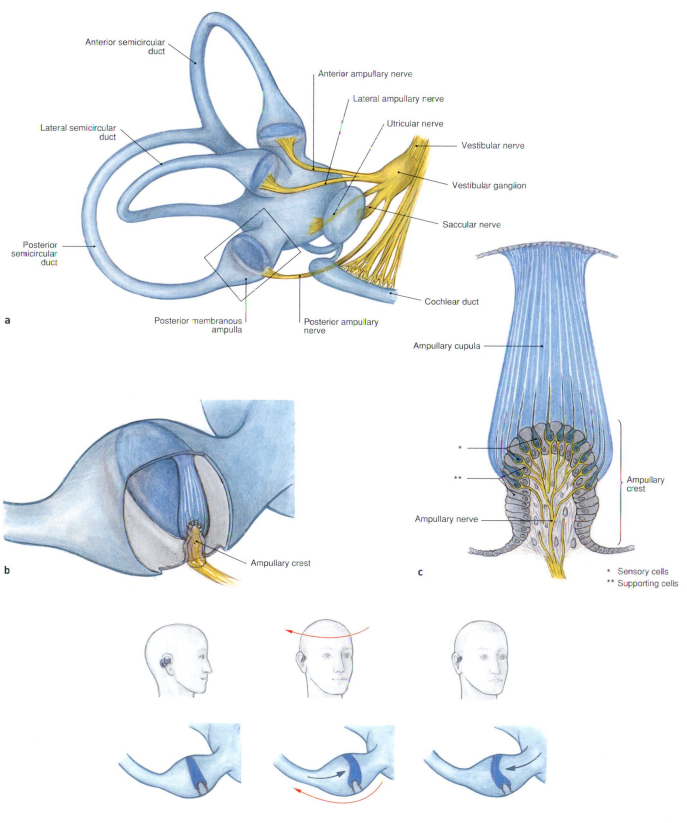

Anterior semicircular duct

Anterior ampullary nerve

Lateral ampullary nerve

Utricular nerve

Vestibular nerve

Lateral semicircular duct

Vestibular ganglion

Saccular nerve

Posterior semicircular duct

Cochlear duct

a

Posterior membranous ampulla

Posterior ampullary nerve

Ampullary cupula

* Sensory cells

** Supporting cells

Ampullary crest

Ampullary nerve

Ampullary crest

b

c

Resting state | Rotation of the head to the right side | Stop of rotation

d

Fig. 1422 a–d Equilibrium organ.
a Anterior view
b Higher magnification of the area indicated in a: the anterior part of the posterior membranous ampulla has been opened.

c Cross-section through the ampullary crest
d Function of the cupula of the lateral semicircular duct, during rotation of the head

Hearing and equilibrium

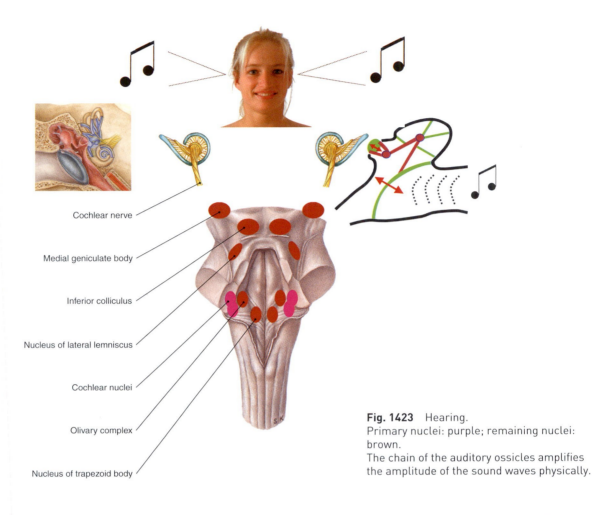

Cochlear nerve

Medial geniculate body

Inferior colliculus

Nucleus of lateral lemniscus

Cochlear nuclei

Olivary complex

Nucleus of trapezoid body

Fig. 1423 Hearing.
Primary nuclei: purple; remaining nuclei: brown.
The chain of the auditory ossicles amplifies the amplitude of the sound waves physically.

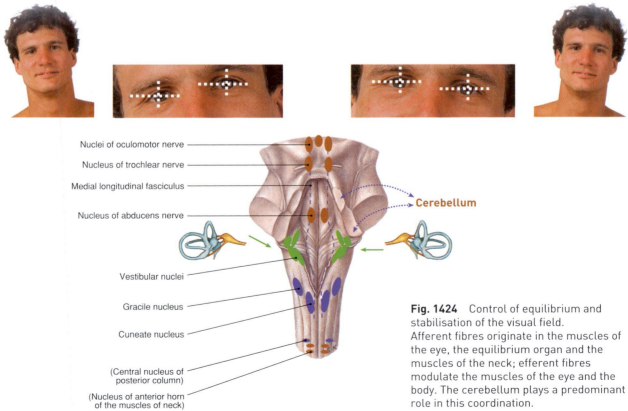

Nuclei of oculomotor nerve

Nucleus of trochlear nerve

Medial longitudinal fasciculus

Nucleus of abducens nerve

Cerebellum

Vestibular nuclei

Gracile nucleus

Cuneate nucleus

(Central nucleus of posterior column)

(Nucleus of anterior horn of the muscles of neck)

Fig. 1424 Control of equilibrium and stabilisation of the visual field.
Afferent fibres originate in the muscles of the eye, the equilibrium organ and the muscles of the neck; efferent fibres modulate the muscles of the eye and the body. The cerebellum plays a predominant role in this coordination.

Auditory and equilibrium pathway

Auditory pathway

1. neuron: Bipolar cells in the spiral cochlear ganglion. After exiting the small apertures of the foraminous spiral tract within the internal acoustic meatus, the fibres form the cochlear nerve and unite with the vestibular nerve at the floor of the internal acoustic meatus to form the vestibulocochlear nerve [VIII]. Fibres from the basal cochlear parts traverse to the posterior cochlear nucleus and those from the apical parts terminate in the anterior cochlear nucleus.

2. neuron: Multi-polar ganglion cells of the cochlear nuclei. The fibres from the anterior cochlear nucleus pass mainly within the trapezoid body to the opposite side and form the lateral lemnicus, which provides a connection to the inferior colliculus. A few fibres join the lateral lemniscus of the same side. The axons of the posterior cochlear nucleus cross superficially to the rhomboid fossa and enter the lateral lemniscus of the opposite side.

3. or 4. neuron: From the inferior colliculus connections are made with the medial geniculate body.

4. or 5. neuron: The acoustic radiation connects the medial geniculate body to HESCHL's transverse gyrus and with WERNICKE's centre in the temporal lobe.

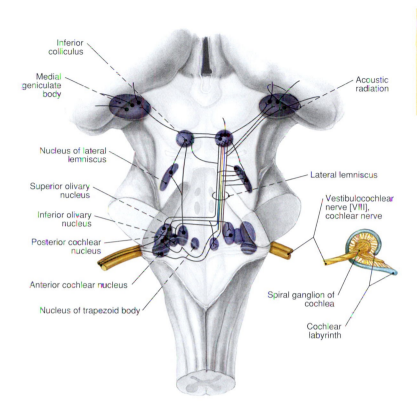

Fig. 1425 Auditory pathway; overview.

Equilibrium pathway

1. neuron: Bipolar cells in the vestibular ganglion. Their neurites pass the inferior and superior vestibular areas to form the vestibular nerve at the floor of the internal acoustic meatus, which together with the cochlear nerve then forms the vestibulocochlear nerve [VIII]. These fibres terminate at the vestibular nuclei in the lateral angle of the floor of the rhomboid fossa.

2. and subsequent neurons: Fibres originating in the lateral vestibular nucleus (DEITERS' nucleus) traverse within the lateral vestibulospinal tract to the anterior column of the spinal cord.
   Fibres originating in the superior vestibular nucleus (nucleus of BECHTEREW), the medial vestibular nucleus (SCHWALBE's nucleus) as well as the inferior vestibular nucleus (ROLLER's nucleus) traverse to the cerebellum and connect to the motor nuclei of the cranial nerves III, IV and VI, mostly via the medial longitudinal fasciculus.
   The medial vestibular nucleus and the inferior vestibular nucleus send fibres along the medial vestibulospinal tract to the anterior column of the spinal cord.

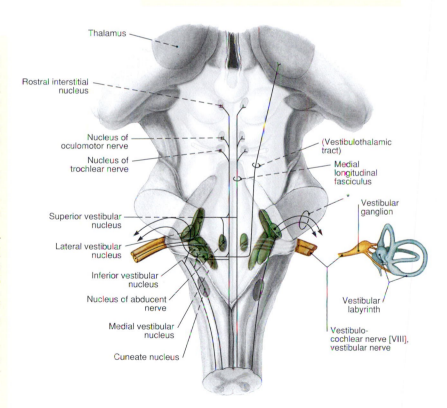

Fig. 1426 Equilibrium pathway; overview.

* Connections to the cerebellum

Nerves in the petrous part of the temporal bone

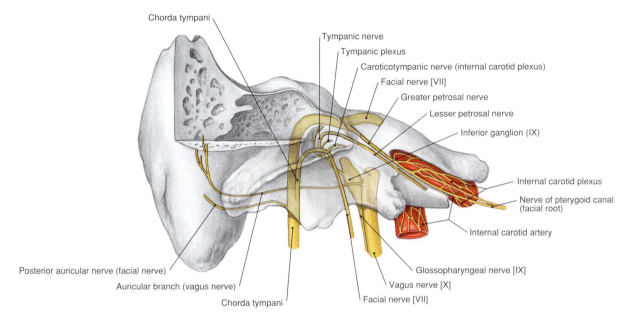

Chorda tympani

Tympanic nerve

Tympanic plexus

Caroticotympanic nerve (internal carotid plexus)

Facial nerve [VII]

Greater petrosal nerve

Lesser petrosal nerve

Inferior ganglion (IX)

Internal carotid plexus

Nerve of pterygoid canal (facial root)

Internal carotid artery

Glossopharyngeal nerve [IX]

Vagus nerve [X]

Facial nerve [VII]

Chorda tympani

Auricular branch (vagus nerve)

Posterior auricular nerve (facial nerve)

→ 1181

Fig. 1427 Facial nerve;
glossopharyngeal nerve;
and vagus nerve [X];
the petrous part of the temporal bone has been partly sectioned;
the nerves are illustrated translucently;
anterior view.

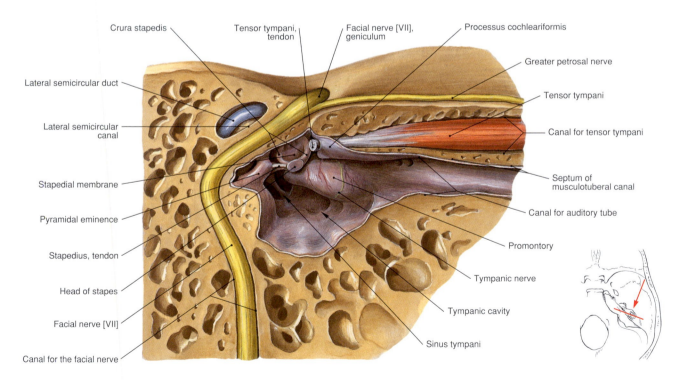

Crura stapedis

Tensor tympani, tendon

Facial nerve [VII], geniculum

Processus cochleariformis

Greater petrosal nerve

Tensor tympani

Lateral semicircular duct

Lateral semicircular canal

Canal for tensor tympani

Septum of musculotuberal canal

Stapedial membrane

Pyramidal eminence

Canal for auditory tube

Promontory

Stapedius, tendon

Tympanic nerve

Head of stapes

Tympanic cavity

Facial nerve [VII]

Sinus tympani

Canal for the facial nerve

Fig. 1428 Facial nerve and tympanic cavity;
vertical section along the longitudinal axis of the
petrous part of the temporal bone;
the facial canal has been opened;
anterior view.

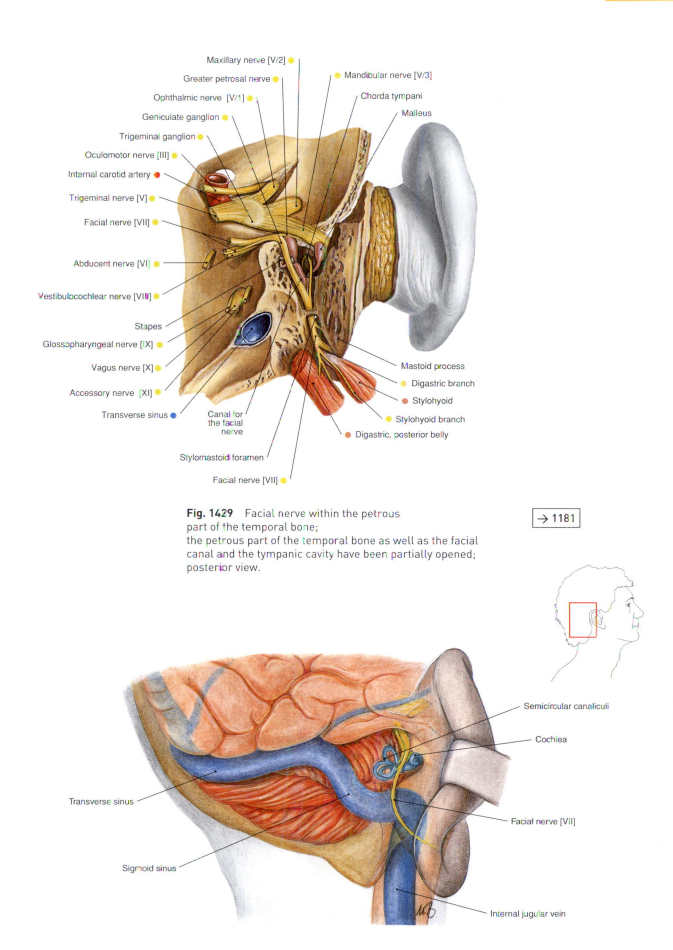

Maxillary nerve [V/2] ●
Greater petrosal nerve ●
Ophthalmic nerve [V/1] ●
Geniculate ganglion ●
Trigeminal ganglion ●
Oculomotor nerve [III] ●
Internal carotid artery ●
Trigeminal nerve [V] ●
Facial nerve [VII] ●
Abducent nerve [VI] ●
Vestibulocochlear nerve [VIII] ●
Stapes
Glossopharyngeal nerve [IX] ●
Vagus nerve [X] ●
Accessory nerve [XI] ●
Transverse sinus ●
Canal for the facial nerve
Stylomastoid foramen
Facial nerve [VII] ●

Mandibular nerve [V/3] ●
Chorda tympani
Malleus

Mastoid process
Digastric branch ●
Stylohyoid ●
Stylohyoid branch ●
Digastric, posterior belly ●

Fig. 1429 Facial nerve within the petrous part of the temporal bone;
the petrous part of the temporal bone as well as the facial canal and the tympanic cavity have been partially opened; posterior view.

→ 1181

Semicircular canaliculi
Cochlea
Transverse sinus
Facial nerve [VII]
Sigmoid sinus
Internal jugular vein

Fig. 1430 Lateral projection of the inner ear.

Petrous part of the temporal bone, imaging

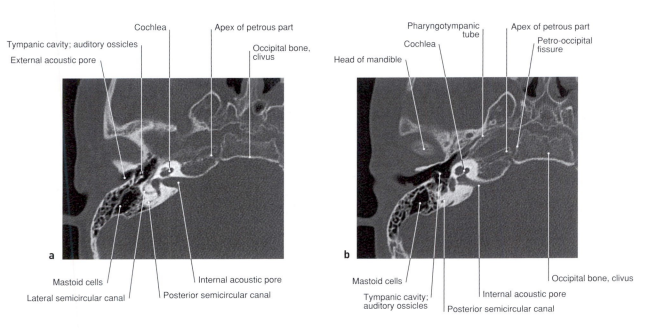

Cochlea
Apex of petrous part
Tympanic cavity; auditory ossicles
Occipital bone, clivus
External acoustic pore

Pharyngotympanic tube
Apex of petrous part
Cochlea
Petro-occipital fissure
Head of mandible

Mastoid cells
Internal acoustic pore
Lateral semicircular canal
Posterior semicircular canal

Mastoid cells
Occipital bone, clivus
Tympanic cavity; auditory ossicles
Internal acoustic pore
Posterior semicircular canal

Fig. 1431 a, b   Petrous part of the temporal bone,;
high-resolution computed tomographic horizontal sections (HRCT);
inferior view.
a   Through the lateral semicircular canal
b   Inferior to the lateral semicircular canal

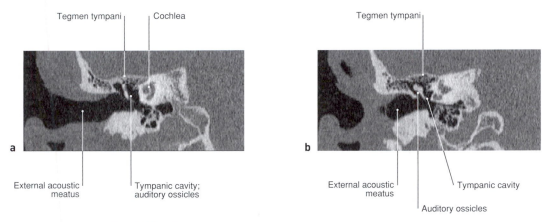

Tegmen tympani
Cochlea

Tegmen tympani

External acoustic meatus
Tympanic cavity; auditory ossicles

External acoustic meatus
Tympanic cavity
Auditory ossicles

Fig. 1432 a, b   Ear;
high-resolution computed tomographic frontal sections (HRCT);
anterior view.
a   Through the base of the cochlea
b   Through the external acoustic meatus

Index

The numbers refer to the page numbers.
The numbers with "T" refer to the numbers of the tables in the separate booklet.